Food Labeling: Analysis, Understanding, and Perception

Food Labeling: Analysis, Understanding, and Perception

Editors

Daniela Martini
Davide Menozzi

MDPI • Basel • Beijing • Wuhan • Barcelona • Belgrade • Manchester • Tokyo • Cluj • Tianjin

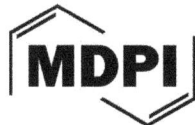

Editors
Daniela Martini
Dept. Food, Environmental
and Nutritional Sciences
(DeFENS)
University of Milan
Milan
Italy

Davide Menozzi
Dept. Food and Drug
University of Parma
Parma
Italy

Editorial Office
MDPI
St. Alban-Anlage 66
4052 Basel, Switzerland

This is a reprint of articles from the Special Issue published online in the open access journal *Nutrients* (ISSN 2072-6643) (available at: www.mdpi.com/journal/nutrients/special_issues/Food_Labeling).

For citation purposes, cite each article independently as indicated on the article page online and as indicated below:

LastName, A.A.; LastName, B.B.; LastName, C.C. Article Title. *Journal Name* **Year**, *Volume Number*, Page Range.

ISBN 978-3-0365-1255-6 (Hbk)
ISBN 978-3-0365-1254-9 (PDF)

© 2022 by the authors. Articles in this book are Open Access and distributed under the Creative Commons Attribution (CC BY) license, which allows users to download, copy and build upon published articles, as long as the author and publisher are properly credited, which ensures maximum dissemination and a wider impact of our publications.

The book as a whole is distributed by MDPI under the terms and conditions of the Creative Commons license CC BY-NC-ND.

Contents

About the Editors . . . . **vii**

Daniela Martini and Davide Menozzi
Food Labeling: Analysis, Understanding, and Perception
Reprinted from: *Nutrients* **2021**, *13*, 268, doi:10.3390/nu13010268 . . . . **1**

Marika Dello Russo, Carmela Spagnuolo, Stefania Moccia, Donato Angelino, Nicoletta Pellegrini and Daniela Martini et al.
Nutritional Quality of Pasta Sold on the Italian Market: The Food Labelling of Italian Products (FLIP) Study
Reprinted from: *Nutrients* **2021**, *13*, 171, doi:10.3390/nu13010171 . . . . **7**

Alyne Michelle Botelho, Anice Milbratz de Camargo, Kharla Janinny Medeiros, Gabriella Beatriz Irmão, Moira Dean and Giovanna Medeiros Rataichesck Fiates
Supermarket Circulars Promoting the Sales of 'Healthy' Foods: Analysis Based on Degree of Processing
Reprinted from: *Nutrients* **2020**, *12*, 2877, doi:10.3390/nu12092877 . . . . **19**

Noé Ontiveros, Jesús Aristeo-López Gallardo, Jesús Gilberto Arámburo-Gálvez, Carlos Eduardo Beltrán-Cárdenas, Oscar Gerardo Figueroa-Salcido and José Antonio Mora-Melgem et al.
Characteristics of Allergen Labelling and Precautionary Allergen Labelling in Packaged Food Products Available in Latin America
Reprinted from: *Nutrients* **2020**, *12*, 2698, doi:10.3390/nu12092698 . . . . **33**

Davide Menozzi, Thong Tien Nguyen, Giovanni Sogari, Dimitar Taskov, Sterenn Lucas and José Luis Santiago Castro-Rial et al.
Consumers' Preferences and Willingness to Pay for Fish Products with Health and Environmental Labels: Evidence from Five European Countries
Reprinted from: *Nutrients* **2020**, *12*, 2650, doi:10.3390/nu12092650 . . . . **45**

Paweł Bryła
Who Reads Food Labels? Selected Predictors of Consumer Interest in Front-of-Package and Back-of-Package Labels during and after the Purchase
Reprinted from: *Nutrients* **2020**, *12*, 2605, doi:10.3390/nu12092605 . . . . **65**

Livia S. A. Augustin, Anne-Marie Aas, Arnie Astrup, Fiona S. Atkinson, Sara Baer-Sinnott and Alan W. Barclay et al.
Dietary Fibre Consensus from the International Carbohydrate Quality Consortium (ICQC)
Reprinted from: *Nutrients* **2020**, *12*, 2553, doi:10.3390/nu12092553 . . . . **85**

Klaudia Modlinska, Dominika Adamczyk, Katarzyna Goncikowska, Dominika Maison and Wojciech Pisula
The Effect of Labelling and Visual Properties on the Acceptance of Foods Containing Insects
Reprinted from: *Nutrients* **2020**, *12*, 2498, doi:10.3390/nu12092498 . . . . **97**

Danielle J. Azzopardi, Kathleen E. Lacy and Julie L. Woods
Energy Density of New Food Products Targeted to Children
Reprinted from: *Nutrients* **2020**, *12*, 2242, doi:10.3390/nu12082242 . . . . **117**

Francesco Bimbo, Luigi Roselli, Domenico Carlucci and Bernardo Corrado de Gennaro
Consumer Misuse of Country-of-Origin Label: Insights from the Italian Extra-Virgin Olive Oil Market
Reprinted from: *Nutrients* **2020**, *12*, 2150, doi:10.3390/nu12072150 135

Brigitta Plasek, Zoltán Lakner and Ágoston Temesi
Factors that Influence the Perceived Healthiness of Food—Review
Reprinted from: *Nutrients* **2020**, *12*, 1881, doi:10.3390/nu12061881 147

Yi-Chun Chen, Ya-Li Huang, Yi-Wen Chien and Mei Chun Chen
The Effect of an Online Sugar Fact Intervention: Change of Mothers with Young Children
Reprinted from: *Nutrients* **2020**, *12*, 1859, doi:10.3390/nu12061859 167

Péter Czine, Áron Török, Károly Pető, Péter Horváth and Péter Balogh
The Impact of the Food Labeling and Other Factors on Consumer Preferences Using Discrete Choice Modeling—The Example of Traditional Pork Sausage
Reprinted from: *Nutrients* **2020**, *12*, 1768, doi:10.3390/nu12061768 183

Christopher P.F. Marinangeli, Scott V. Harding, Andrea J. Glenn, Laura Chiavaroli, Andreea Zurbau and David J.A. Jenkins et al.
Destigmatizing Carbohydrate with Food Labeling: The Use of Non-Mandatory Labelling to Highlight Quality Carbohydrate Foods
Reprinted from: *Nutrients* **2020**, *12*, 1725, doi:10.3390/nu12061725 201

Sofía Rincón-Gallardo Patiño, Mi Zhou, Fabio Da Silva Gomes, Robin Lemaire, Valisa Hedrick and Elena Serrano et al.
Effects of Menu Labeling Policies on Transnational Restaurant Chains to Promote a Healthy Diet: A Scoping Review to Inform Policy and Research
Reprinted from: *Nutrients* **2020**, *12*, 1544, doi:10.3390/nu12061544 231

Maddison Breen, Hollie James, Anna Rangan and Luke Gemming
Prevalence of Product Claims and Marketing Buzzwords Found on Health Food Snack Products Does Not Relate to Nutrient Profile
Reprinted from: *Nutrients* **2020**, *12*, 1513, doi:10.3390/nu12051513 259

Margherita Dall'Asta, Donato Angelino, Nicoletta Pellegrini and Daniela Martini
The Nutritional Quality of Organic and Conventional Food Products Sold in Italy: Results from the Food Labelling of Italian Products (FLIP) Study
Reprinted from: *Nutrients* **2020**, *12*, 1273, doi:10.3390/nu12051273 273

María José Yusta-Boyo, Laura M. Bermejo, Marta García-Solano, Ana M. López-Sobaler, Rosa M. Ortega and Marta García-Pérez et al.
Sugar Content in Processed Foods in Spain and a Comparison of Mandatory Nutrition Labelling and Laboratory Values
Reprinted from: *Nutrients* **2020**, *12*, 1078, doi:10.3390/nu12041078 287

Fiona E. Pelly, Libby Swanepoel, Joseph Rinella and Sheri Cooper
Consumers' Perceptions of the Australian Health Star Rating Labelling Scheme
Reprinted from: *Nutrients* **2020**, *12*, 704, doi:10.3390/nu12030704 307

Bethany D. Merillat and Claudia González-Vallejo
How Much Sugar is in My Drink? The Power of Visual Cues
Reprinted from: *Nutrients* **2020**, *12*, 394, doi:10.3390/nu12020394 317

Jonas Potthoff, Annalisa La Face and Anne Schienle
The Color Nutrition Information Paradox: Effects of Suggested Sugar Content on Food Cue Reactivity in Healthy Young Women
Reprinted from: *Nutrients* **2020**, *12*, 312, doi:10.3390/nu12020312 . . . . **331**

Paweł Bryła
Selected Predictors of the Importance Attached to Salt Content Information on the Food Packaging (a Study among Polish Consumers)
Reprinted from: *Nutrients* **2020**, *12*, 293, doi:10.3390/nu12020293 . . . . **343**

Donato Angelino, Alice Rosi, Margherita Dall'Asta, Nicoletta Pellegrini and Daniela Martini
Evaluation of the Nutritional Quality of Breakfast Cereals Sold on the Italian Market: The Food Labelling of Italian Products (FLIP) Study
Reprinted from: *Nutrients* **2019**, *11*, 2827, doi:10.3390/nu11112827 . . . . **359**

Klazine Van der Horst, Tamara Bucher, Kerith Duncanson, Beatrice Murawski and David Labbe
Consumer Understanding, Perception and Interpretation of Serving Size Information on Food Labels: A Scoping Review
Reprinted from: *Nutrients* **2019**, *11*, 2189, doi:10.3390/nu11092189 . . . . **371**

Zenobia Talati, Manon Egnell, Serge Hercberg, Chantal Julia and Simone Pettigrew
Consumers' Perceptions of Five Front-of-Package Nutrition Labels: An Experimental Study Across 12 Countries
Reprinted from: *Nutrients* **2019**, *11*, 1934, doi:10.3390/nu11081934 . . . . **391**

Manon Egnell, Zenobia Talati, Marion Gombaud, Pilar Galan, Serge Hercberg and Simone Pettigrew et al.
Consumers' Responses to Front-of-Pack Nutrition Labelling: Results from a Sample from The Netherlands
Reprinted from: *Nutrients* **2019**, *11*, 1817, doi:10.3390/nu11081817 . . . . **407**

About the Editors

Daniela Martini

Daniela Martini is an assistant professor of human nutrition at the University of Milan, Italy. She is also member of the Board of Directors for the Italian Society of Human Nutrition (SINU) and coordinates the SINU Young Working Group. Her expertise includes food regulation (i.e., food labelling, nutrition, and health claims), the analysis of antioxidant compounds in foods, and the evaluation of the role of foods and dietary patterns in the modulation of markers of health.

Davide Menozzi

Davide Menozzi is an associate professor of agricultural economics and rural appraisal at the University of Parma, Italy. His main research interests include analyses of consumer behavior and preferences, the economics of food quality schemes, and the evaluation of the socioeconomic sustainability of dietary behaviors. He teaches graduate and undergraduate agricultural economics courses at the University of Parma. He is an active member of the Italian Association of Agricultural and Applied Economists (AIEAA) and the European Association of Agricultural Economists (EAAE).

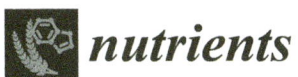

Editorial

Food Labeling: Analysis, Understanding, and Perception

Daniela Martini [1,*] and Davide Menozzi [2,*]

1. Department of Food, Environmental and Nutritional Sciences (DeFENS), Università degli Studi di Milano, 20133 Milan, Italy
2. Department of Food and Drug, University of Parma, 43124 Parma, Italy
* Correspondence: daniela.martini@unimi.it (D.M.); davide.menozzi@unipr.it (D.M.)

Citation: Martini, D.; Menozzi, D. Food Labeling: Analysis, Understanding, and Perception. *Nutrients* 2021, 13, 268. https://doi.org/10.3390/nu13010268

Received: 13 January 2021
Accepted: 15 January 2021
Published: 19 January 2021

Publisher's Note: MDPI stays neutral with regard to jurisdictional claims in published maps and institutional affiliations.

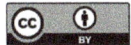

Copyright: © 2021 by the authors. Licensee MDPI, Basel, Switzerland. This article is an open access article distributed under the terms and conditions of the Creative Commons Attribution (CC BY) license (https://creativecommons.org/licenses/by/4.0/).

Food labels are the first informative tool found by the customers during shopping, and are informative in terms of ingredients, nutrient content, and the presence of allergens of the selected product. However, food labeling also represents a marketing tool and may influence perception of the food quality and, in turn, the dietary choice of consumers. For this reason, there is growing research in the food labeling field and in the evaluation of its effects on consumers, food operators, and the whole market [1,2]. This is supported by a wide range of manuscripts published in recent years, for instance, with the specific purpose to better investigate how specific information on the food packaging may influence food purchases and consumption and, in general, dietary behavior [3–8]

The Special Issue "*Food Labeling: Analysis, Understanding, and Perception*" was conceived with the intention to further explore current efforts in food labeling research and welcomed original studies, as well as reviews of the literature, focusing on: (i) the analysis of the nutrient profile of products with different characteristics reported on the food labels, i.e., nutrition and health claims (NHCs), organic, gluten-free (GF); (ii) the nutrient profile underlying front-of-pack (FOP) nutrition labels and their graphical design in different countries; (iii) the consumers' perception, knowledge, and understanding of the information provided on food labeling; (iv) the impact of information on food labeling (e.g., FOP information, serving size) on consumers' willingness to pay and food choice; (v) the attitudes, beliefs, and perceptions and behavioral and socioeconomic determinants regarding the use of food labels.

This Special Issue provides a series of 25 contributions, with 20 original papers, four narrative reviews, and one commentary. This last article is a consensus by eminent exponents of the International Carbohydrate Quality Consortium (ICQC) [9], which underlines the importance of dietary fiber, which is not always mandatory on food labeling (e.g., Reg. (EU) No 1169/2011) [10]. The authors supported the need for including fiber values in food labeling by distinguishing between intrinsic and added fiber, which may also help to achieve the recommended intake by consumers. The need to consider other information on food labels has also been discussed by Marinangeli and colleagues [11], who reviewed the regulatory frameworks and examples of associated non-mandatory food labeling claims currently employed to highlight healthy carbohydrate foods to consumers. Among the information, the authors considered NHCs related to dietary fiber, glycemic index, and glycemic response, and the presence of whole carbohydrate foods and ingredients that are intact or reconstituted (e.g., whole grains).

Some studies focused on the analysis of the nutritional quality of specific food groups and/or specific nutrients. Three studies were performed within the Food Labeling of Italian Products (FLIP) [12–14], a project aiming to evaluate the nutritional quality of packaged products currently sold in the online shops of several retailers in Italy [15–17]. Specifically, two studies focused on the analysis of the food labeling of breakfast cereals [12] and pasta [14]. The first study reported an elevated inter-product variability among breakfast cereals currently sold in Italy, with only limited differences when products with NHCs and GF declarations were compared with products not carrying this information [12].

Similarly, the study performed on pasta revealed that pasta types currently on the Italian market largely vary in terms of nutrition profile, with stuffed pasta characterized by a high salt content [14]. This last aspect supports the importance of providing nutrition facts of product to consumers to help them in making informed food choices. The last study performed within the FLIP project compared the nutritional quality of organic and conventional food products, highlighting that, with just a few exceptions, prepacked organic products are not of a superior nutritional quality than conventional ones, based on the mandatory information present on their packaging [13].

Yusta-Bojo et al. [18] focused on the sugar content in the most-consumed processed foods in Spain and compared the sugar values declared on the label (LVs) with laboratory analysis values (AVs). The study findings evidenced a high adequacy of LVs with the EU labeling tolerance requirements, with only cured ham presenting significant differences between the median AVs and LVs. Lastly, Azzopardi et al. investigated the energy density (ED) of food products targeted at children sold in Australia, finding a high proportion of products with a high ED (i.e., >950 kJ/100 g) among the 548 food items considered [19]. The same study observed that the health star rating (HSR) system, one of the FOP systems introduced in Australia in 2014, did not consistently discriminate between ED levels, particularly for high-ED foods.

The HSR was also studied in another study focused on consumers' perception [20] and performed with fifteen Australian grocery shoppers. Intriguingly, the findings from this study showed that the HSR was perceived as a simple, easy-to-understand, and useful tool, despite a certain grade of skepticism concerning its conception. The consumers' perception and responses to FOP labels was also considered in another two papers published by Egnell et al. [21] and Talati et al. [22], showing results from the Netherlands and across another 12 countries, respectively, supporting that this represents a widely explored field of research. In detail, the first study [21] compared the perception and understanding of five FOP labels (HSR, Nutri-Score, multiple traffic lights (MTLs), reference intake, and warning symbols) among 1032 Dutch participants, finding a favorable perception, with Nutri-Score showing the highest performance in helping consumers to rank the products according to their nutritional quality. Conversely, in a similar study performed with over 12,000 participants across 12 countries, MTLs obtained the most favorable ratings, with mixed or neutral perceptions of the other FOP labels [22]. A third study by Breen et al. [23] compared NHCs, the HSR, and the price of snack foods sold in health food (HF) stores and aisles with the ones sold in regular areas (RAs) of supermarkets. The results showed that snack foods of HF stores displayed a significantly higher number of product claims compared to RA foods, together with a higher HSR and cost.

Botelho et al. [24] analyzed the FOP of food items shown in specific sections of the circulars of two Brazilian supermarket chains during a 10-week period, classifying them by their "unprocessed/minimally processed" versus "ultraprocessed" (UP) items and the presence and type of claims on the FOP. The NOVA systems represent another way of classifying foods that has receiving growing interest and which is based on the degree of food processing [25]. In this Special Issue, authors found that more than 50% of the items sold in the health and wellness section were UP and reported a high presence of reduced and increased nutrient content claims, suggesting that supermarkets' circulars often promote the sale of UP foods.

Besides the study of consumers' perception of FOP, it is worth investigating the predictors of consumer interest in FOP and back-of-pack labels. This was the object of a Polish study [26] which found that self-rated knowledge about nutrition healthiness is the only significant predictor in over 1000 Polish consumers, while neither demographic nor socioeconomic variables were significant predictors of interest towards food labels. Plasek and coworkers [27] focused on six categories of actors that seem to influence the perceived healthiness of foods: (i) the communication information (such as FOPs and NHCs), (ii) the product category, (iii) the shape and color of the product packaging, (iv) the ingredients of the product, (v) the organic origin of the product, and (vi) the sensory characteristics of food. Bryla [28] also found that FOP label reading is one of the predictors of the importance linked to salt content in over 1000 Polish consumers, in addition to other predictors such as the importance and attention to NHCs and the respondent's age.

Two studies applied hypothetical discrete choice experiments to analyzing consumers' choices and willingness to pay (WTP) for, respectively, fish products [29] and pork sausages [30]. Menozzi and colleagues interviewed 2500 fish consumers in five European countries to assess the relative importance and WTP for different fish species and labeled attributes (i.e., sustainability label, NHCs, product presentation, production system, and price). The findings showed positive premiums for sustainability label, NHCs, and wild-caught alternatives, with high heterogeneity across countries and species [29]. Czine et al. [30] investigated whether product characteristics indicated on food labels of sausage made from traditional Hungarian mangalica pork might influence consumers' choices. The authors found respondents' preference for the label of origin indicating meat from registered animals, and purchasing from the farmers' market is preferred over the butcher and hyper-/supermarket.

Country-of-origin (COO) labeling effects were analyzed by Bimbo et al. [31]. The authors tested the price differential associated with the COO information for extra-virgin olive oil (EVOO) in Italy, employing a hedonic price model on the purchase of EVOO products collected from 982 consumers at the supermarket checkouts. Although the mandatory COO labeling regulation for EVOO can be an effective tool for consumers to identify the origin of the product and for producers to differentiate products, the results evidenced a significant share of consumers unable to correctly identify the origin of the EVOO purchased, mostly among consumers who reported having purchased Italian EVOO.

Two experiments were conducted to analyze the effects of visual aids and color nutrition information (CNI) on sugar-sweetened beverages [32] and sweet food consumption [33]. Merillat et al. [32] assessed the effects of visual aids on judgments of sugar quantity in popular drinks and the choices of 261 individuals recruited in the USA. In the experimental condition, participants viewed beverages along with test tubes filled with the total amount of sugar in each drink and this led to a lower intention to consume any of the beverages, suggesting that this simple visual aid intervention affected judgments and choices towards curtailing sugar intake. Using an eye-tracking technique, Potthoff et al. [33] evaluated the effect of CNI based on a traffic light system adopted in Austria; participants in this study viewed images depicting sweets preceded by a colored circle informing about the sugar content of the food, with and without nutrition information. The results showed that the intervention had the opposite of the intended effect and the authors questioned whether CNI is helpful to influence initial cue reactivity toward sweet foods.

A quasi-experimental online trial on the choice of sugar foods was performed by Chen et al. [34] in Taiwan. The authors analyzed how mothers' choices of low-sugar food were affected by theory-driven nutrition interventions, finding that, after the intervention, they exhibited enhanced sugar and nutrition label knowledge, perceived behavioral control, behavioral intentions, and behavior.

Another experiment was conducted by Modlinska et al. [35] with 99 Polish individuals to assess the influence of food labeling (insect content) and appearance (traces of insect-like ingredients) on the participants' perception. The results showed that products labeled as containing insects are consumed with reluctance and in lower quantities despite their appearance, regardless of the form in which the insects are served. The authors provided recommendations for labeling strategies to help to reduce the effect of disgust.

As already mentioned, food labeling does not include only nutritional information, and this is why a series of papers focused on other aspects is included. For instance, Ontiveros and colleagues [36] focused on allergens, by evaluating the characteristics of food allergen labeling and precautionary allergen labeling (PAL) in over 10,000 products sold in six Latin American countries. The authors found a high (>87.4%) compliance with local regulations, but countries without specific regulations for allergen labeling had two-fold more products containing allergens in their ingredients lists but no food allergen labeling, compared to countries with regulations. These results suggest that the lack of regulations for the characteristics of allergen labeling increases the risk of accidental exposure to allergens of interest.

Another interesting topic was reviewed by Van der Horst and coworkers [37], who investigated how healthy adults perceive and interpret serving size information on food packages and its influence on product perception and consumption. In their systematic review, the authors observed an overall poor conception of serving size, while the few included studies showed that labeled serving size affects portion size selection and consumption.

Finally, Rincón-Gallardo Patiño et al. [38] investigated restaurant menu labeling policies and their effects on menu reformulation. The authors found three voluntary and eight mandatory menu labeling policies primarily for energy disclosures, developed in upper-middle- and high-income countries, whereas none was found in low- or middle-income countries. The subsequent analysis conducted by the authors showed reductions in energy for newly introduced menu items only in the US. Implications for policy, practice, and research are also provided.

Overall, the studies included in the Special Issue provide new insights in this field of research, with relevant recommendations for policy makers, business operators, and researchers for developing more effective labeling strategies, allowing consumers to make informed dietary choices. At the same time, many authors reported the need for performing further investigations to confirm and expand current findings.

Funding: This research received no external funding.

Institutional Review Board Statement: Not applicable.

Informed Consent Statement: Not applicable.

Data Availability Statement: Not applicable.

Conflicts of Interest: The authors declare no conflict of interest.

References

1. Shangguan, S.; Afshin, A.; Shulkin, M.; Ma, W.; Marsden, D.; Smith, J.; Saheb-Kashaf, M.; Shi, P.; Micha, R.; Imamura, F.; et al. A Meta-Analysis of Food Labeling Effects on Consumer Diet Behaviors and Industry Practices. *Am. J. Prev. Med.* **2019**, *56*, 300–314. [CrossRef] [PubMed]
2. Cecchini, M.; Warin, L. Impact of food labelling systems on food choices and eating behaviours: A systematic review and meta-analysis of randomized studies. *Obes. Rev.* **2016**, *17*, 201–210. [CrossRef] [PubMed]
3. Mora-García, C.; Tobar, L.; Young, J. The Effect of Randomly Providing Nutri-Score Information on Actual Purchases in Colombia. *Nutrients* **2019**, *11*, 491. [CrossRef] [PubMed]
4. de Morais Sato, P.; Mais, L.A.; Khandpur, N.; Ulian, M.D.; Bortoletto Martins, A.P.; Garcia, M.T.; Spinillo, C.G.; Urquizar Rojas, C.F.; Jaime, P.C.; Scagliusi, F.B. Consumers' opinions on warning labels on food packages: A qualitative study in Brazil. *PLoS ONE* **2019**, *14*, e0218813. [CrossRef]
5. Miller, L.; Cassady, D.; Applegate, E.; Beckett, L.; Wilson, M.; Gibson, T.; Ellwood, K. Relationships among Food Label Use, Motivation, and Dietary Quality. *Nutrients* **2015**, *7*, 1068–1080. [CrossRef]
6. Sogari, G.; Li, J.; Lefebvre, M.; Menozzi, D.; Pellegrini, N.; Cirelli, M.; Gómez, M.I.; Mora, C. The Influence of Health Messages in Nudging Consumption of Whole Grain Pasta. *Nutrients* **2019**, *11*, 2993. [CrossRef]
7. Oostenbach, L.H.; Slits, E.; Robinson, E.; Sacks, G. Systematic review of the impact of nutrition claims related to fat, sugar and energy content on food choices and energy intake. *BMC Public Health* **2019**, *19*, 1296. [CrossRef]
8. Benson, T.; Lavelle, F.; McCloat, A.; Mooney, T.; Bucher, T.; Egan, B.; Dean, M. Are the Claims to Blame? A Qualitative Study to Understand the Effects of Nutrition and Health Claims on Perceptions and Consumption of Food. *Nutrients* **2019**, *11*, 2058. [CrossRef]
9. Augustin, L.S.A.; Aas, A.-M.; Astrup, A.; Atkinson, F.S.; Baer-Sinnott, S.; Barclay, A.W.; Brand-Miller, J.C.; Brighenti, F.; Bullo, M.; Buyken, A.E.; et al. Dietary Fibre Consensus from the International Carbohydrate Quality Consortium (ICQC). *Nutrients* **2020**, *12*, 2553. [CrossRef]
10. European Commission. European Union Council Regulation No 1169/2011 on the provision of food information to consumers. *Off. J. Eur. Union* **2011**, *L304*, 18–63.
11. Marinangeli, C.P.F.; Harding, S.V.; Glenn, A.J.; Chiavaroli, L.; Zurbau, A.; Jenkins, D.J.A.; Kendall, C.W.C.; Miller, K.B.; Sievenpiper, J.L. Destigmatizing Carbohydrate with Food Labeling: The Use of Non-Mandatory Labelling to Highlight Quality Carbohydrate Foods. *Nutrients* **2020**, *12*, 1725. [CrossRef] [PubMed]

12. Angelino, D.; Rosi, A.; Dall'Asta, M.; Pellegrini, N.; Martini, D. Evaluation of the nutritional quality of breakfast cereals sold on the italian market: The food labelling of italian products (FLIP) study. *Nutrients* 2019, *11*, 2827. [CrossRef]
13. Dall'Asta, M.; Angelino, D.; Pellegrini, N.; Martini, D. The Nutritional Quality of Organic and Conventional Food Products Sold in Italy: Results from the Food Labelling of Italian Products (FLIP) Study. *Nutrients* 2020, *12*, 1273. [CrossRef] [PubMed]
14. Dello Russo, M.; Spagnuolo, C.; Moccia, S.; Angelino, D.; Martini, D. Nutritional Quality of Pasta Sold on the Italian Market: The Food Labelling of Italian Products (FLIP) Study. *Nutrients* 2021, *13*, 171. [CrossRef] [PubMed]
15. Angelino, D.; Rosi, A.; Vici, G.; Dello Russo, M.; Pellegrini, N.; Martini, D. Nutritional Quality of Plant-Based Drinks Sold in Italy: The Food Labelling of Italian Products (FLIP) Study. *Foods* 2020, *9*, 682. [CrossRef] [PubMed]
16. Dall'Asta, M.; Rosi, A.; Angelino, D.; Pellegrini, N.; Martini, D. Evaluation of nutritional quality of biscuits and sweet snacks sold on the Italian market: The Food Labelling of Italian Products (FLIP) study. *Public Health Nutr.* 2020, *23*, 2811–2818. [CrossRef]
17. Angelino, D.; Rosi, A.; Ruggiero, E.; Nucci, D.; Paolella, G.; Pignone, V.; Pellegrini, N.; Martini, D. Analysis of Food Labels to Evaluate the Nutritional Quality of Bread Products and Substitutes Sold in Italy: Results from the Food Labelling of Italian Products (FLIP) Study. *Foods* 2020, *9*, 1905. [CrossRef]
18. Yusta-Boyo, M.J.; Bermejo, L.M.; García-Solano, M.; López-Sobaler, A.M.; Ortega, R.M.; García-Pérez, M.; Dal-Re Saavedra, M.Á. Sugar Content in Processed Foods in Spain and a Comparison of Mandatory Nutrition Labelling and Laboratory Values. *Nutrients* 2020, *12*, 1078. [CrossRef]
19. Azzopardi, D.J.; Lacy, K.E.; Woods, J.L. Energy Density of New Food Products Targeted to Children. *Nutrients* 2020, *12*, 2242. [CrossRef]
20. Pelly, F.E.; Swanepoel, L.; Rinella, J.; Cooper, S. Consumers' Perceptions of the Australian Health Star Rating Labelling Scheme. *Nutrients* 2020, *12*, 704. [CrossRef]
21. Egnell, M.; Talati, Z.; Gombaud, M.; Galan, P.; Hercberg, S.; Pettigrew, S.; Julia, C. Consumers' Responses to Front-of-Pack Nutrition Labelling: Results from a Sample from The Netherlands. *Nutrients* 2019, *11*, 1817. [CrossRef] [PubMed]
22. Talati, Z.; Egnell, M.; Hercberg, S.; Julia, C.; Pettigrew, S. Consumers' Perceptions of Five Front-of-Package Nutrition Labels: An Experimental Study Across 12 Countries. *Nutrients* 2019, *11*, 1934. [CrossRef] [PubMed]
23. Breen, M.; James, H.; Rangan, A.; Gemming, L. Prevalence of Product Claims and Marketing Buzzwords Found on Health Food Snack Products Does Not Relate to Nutrient Profile. *Nutrients* 2020, *12*, 1513. [CrossRef] [PubMed]
24. Botelho, A.M.; de Camargo, A.M.; Medeiros, K.J.; Irmão, G.B.; Dean, M.; Fiates, G.M.R. Supermarket Circulars Promoting the Sales of 'Healthy' Foods: Analysis Based on Degree of Processing. *Nutrients* 2020, *12*, 2877. [CrossRef]
25. Monteiro, C.A.; Cannon, G.; Moubarac, J.-C.; Levy, R.B.; Louzada, M.L.C.; Jaime, P.C. The UN Decade of Nutrition, the NOVA food classification and the trouble with ultra-processing. *Public Health Nutr.* 2018, *21*, 5–17. [CrossRef]
26. Bryła, P. Who Reads Food Labels? Selected Predictors of Consumer Interest in Front-of-Package and Back-of-Package Labels during and after the Purchase. *Nutrients* 2020, *12*, 2605. [CrossRef]
27. Plasek, B.; Lakner, Z.; Temesi, Á. Factors that Influence the Perceived Healthiness of Food—Review. *Nutrients* 2020, *12*, 1881. [CrossRef]
28. Bryła, P. Selected Predictors of the Importance Attached to Salt Content Information on the Food Packaging (a Study among Polish Consumers). *Nutrients* 2020, *12*, 293. [CrossRef]
29. Menozzi, D.; Nguyen, T.T.; Sogari, G.; Taskov, D.; Lucas, S.; Castro-Rial, J.L.S.; Mora, C. Consumers' Preferences and Willingness to Pay for Fish Products with Health and Environmental Labels: Evidence from Five European Countries. *Nutrients* 2020, *12*, 2650. [CrossRef]
30. Czine, P.; Török, Á.; Pető, K.; Horváth, P.; Balogh, P. The Impact of the Food Labeling and Other Factors on Consumer Preferences Using Discrete Choice Modeling—The Example of Traditional Pork Sausage. *Nutrients* 2020, *12*, 1768. [CrossRef]
31. Bimbo, F.; Roselli, L.; Carlucci, D.; de Gennaro, B.C. Consumer Misuse of Country-of-Origin Label: Insights from the Italian Extra-Virgin Olive Oil Market. *Nutrients* 2020, *12*, 2150. [CrossRef] [PubMed]
32. Merillat, B.D.; González-Vallejo, C. How Much Sugar is in My Drink? The Power of Visual Cues. *Nutrients* 2020, *12*, 394. [CrossRef] [PubMed]
33. Potthoff, J.; La Face, A.; Schienle, A. The Color Nutrition Information Paradox: Effects of Suggested Sugar Content on Food Cue Reactivity in Healthy Young Women. *Nutrients* 2020, *12*, 312. [CrossRef] [PubMed]
34. Chen, Y.-C.; Huang, Y.-L.; Chien, Y.-W.; Chen, M.C. The Effect of an Online Sugar Fact Intervention: Change of Mothers with Young Children. *Nutrients* 2020, *12*, 1859. [CrossRef] [PubMed]
35. Modlinska, K.; Adamczyk, D.; Goncikowska, K.; Maison, D.; Pisula, W. The Effect of Labelling and Visual Properties on the Acceptance of Foods Containing Insects. *Nutrients* 2020, *12*, 2498. [CrossRef]
36. Ontiveros, N.; Gallardo, J.A.-L.; Arámburo-Gálvez, J.G.; Beltrán-Cárdenas, C.E.; Figueroa-Salcido, O.G.; Mora-Melgem, J.A.; Granda-Restrepo, D.M.; Rodríguez-Bellegarrigue, C.I.; de Vergara-Jiménez, M.J.; Cárdenas-Torres, F.I.; et al. Characteristics of Allergen Labelling and Precautionary Allergen Labelling in Packaged Food Products Available in Latin America. *Nutrients* 2020, *12*, 2698. [CrossRef]
37. Van der Horst, K.; Bucher, T.; Duncanson, K.; Murawski, B.; Labbe, D. Consumer Understanding, Perception and Interpretation of Serving Size Information on Food Labels: A Scoping Review. *Nutrients* 2019, *11*, 2189. [CrossRef]
38. Rincón-Gallardo Patiño, S.; Zhou, M.; Da Silva Gomes, F.; Lemaire, R.; Hedrick, V.; Serrano, E.; Kraak, V.I. Effects of Menu Labeling Policies on Transnational Restaurant Chains to Promote a Healthy Diet: A Scoping Review to Inform Policy and Research. *Nutrients* 2020, *12*, 1544. [CrossRef]

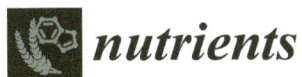

Article

Nutritional Quality of Pasta Sold on the Italian Market: The Food Labelling of Italian Products (FLIP) Study

Marika Dello Russo [1,†], Carmela Spagnuolo [1,†], Stefania Moccia [1,†], Donato Angelino [2], Nicoletta Pellegrini [3,*], Daniela Martini [4] and on behalf of the Italian Society of Human Nutrition (SINU) Young Working Group [‡]

1. Institute of Food Sciences, National Research Council, 83100 Avellino, Italy; marika.dellorusso@isa.cnr.it (M.D.R.); carmela.spagnuolo@isa.cnr.it (C.S.); stefania.moccia@isa.cnr.it (S.M.)
2. Faculty of Bioscience and Technology for Food, Agriculture and Environment, University of Teramo, 64100 Teramo, Italy; dangelino@unite.it
3. Department of Agricultural, Food, Environmental and Animal Sciences, University of Udine, 33100 Udine, Italy
4. Department of Food, Environmental and Nutritional Sciences (DeFENS), Università degli Studi di Milano, 20133 Milan, Italy; daniela.martini@unimi.it
* Correspondence: nicoletta.pellegrini@uniud.it; Tel.: +39-043-255-8183
† These authors contributed equally to this work.
‡ Membership of the SINU Young Working Group is provided in the Acknowledgments.

Abstract: Pasta represents a staple food in many populations and, in recent years, an increasing number of pasta items has been placed on the market to satisfy needs and trends. The aims of this work were: (i) to investigate the nutritional composition of the different types of pasta currently sold in Italy by collecting the nutrition facts on their packaging; (ii) to compare energy, nutrient and salt content per 100 g and serving in fresh and dried pasta; (iii) to compare the nutrition declaration in pairs of products with and without different declarations (i.e., gluten free (GF), organic, and nutrition claims (NC)). A total of 756 items, made available by 13 retailers present on the Italian market, were included in the analysis. Data showed a wide difference between dried and fresh pasta, with high inter-type variability. A negligible amount of salt was observed in all types of pasta, except for stuffed products, which had a median high quantity of salt (>1 g/100 g and ~1.5 g/serving). Organic pasta had higher fibre and lower protein contents compared to conventional pasta. GF products were higher in carbohydrate and fat but lower in fibre and protein than not-GF products, while only a higher fibre content was found in pasta with NC compared to products not boasting claims. Overall, the results show high variability in terms of nutrition composition among the pasta items currently on the market, supporting the importance of reading and understanding food labels for making informed food choices.

Keywords: pasta; food labelling; nutrition declaration; nutritional composition; gluten free; nutrition claims

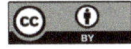

1. Introduction

Pasta is one of the most widespread staple foods, known at least since the time of the Etruscans, who learned how to work the wheat by grinding it, mixing it with water, levelling it in thin doughs, and cooking it on a red-hot stone. According to Italian law [1], "dried pasta" must be made with water and durum wheat semolina, while "fresh pasta" can be made with soft wheat and has a higher moisture content than "dried pasta". There are also laws regarding the preparation of "special pasta", which contains other ingredients than wheat and water: "egg pasta", manufactured with durum wheat and hen's eggs, and "stuffed pasta", which includes "fresh pasta" filled with different ingredients, as in the case of ravioli or lasagne. In this scenario, the manufacturing process of pasta is continuously updated over the years to face food needs and trends. For example, a wide range of pasta containing different ingredients, such as vegetable extracts, i.e., spinach and tomato, is currently available on the market.

A survey carried out by the International Pasta Organisation in 2014 reported that about 14.3 million tons of pasta are annually produced worldwide, mainly in Italy, the United States, Brazil, Turkey and Russia. Italians are the main pasta consumers, with 25.3 kg per capita per year, followed by Tunisians (16 kg), Venezuelans (12.2 kg) and Greeks (11.5 kg) [2]. Pasta consumption has faced a decrease in the last years, probably because of, among other reasons, the myth about dodging carbohydrate-rich foods as a "strategy" for losing weight [3]. However, it is worth noting that pasta is a key component of many healthy eating patterns, above all the Mediterranean Diet, and its consumption has been positively associated with a low body mass index and prevention of overweight and obesity risk conditions [4–8]. Among the possible reasons explaining the positive effects it has on health, pasta generally has a good nutritional quality, due to low amounts of fat and available carbohydrates. Moreover, pasta can be also a suitable vehicle for the incorporation of beneficial components, such as fibre or probiotics [9,10], considering its low cost, long shelf life, and wide range of acceptability in many consumers groups [11]. However, pasta is a very heterogeneous category, including several types of products which often differ not only in shape but most importantly in ingredients, and thus, in nutrition composition. Nevertheless, dietary recommendations do not take into account this variability for suggestions in portion sizes and frequency of consumption. Moreover, it should be carefully considered that pasta is often consumed in association with other ingredients, i.e., oil and/or grated cheese, or elaborated sauces, which can largely contribute to the energy value of the entire serving. Regardless of this aspect, the knowledge of the nutritional quality of pasta itself can be useful for evaluating the nutritional characteristics of the dish and helping consumers in their purchase. However, an overview of the nutritional quality of all the products named as "pasta" on the label is still missing in the literature.

In Europe, the nutrition information of pasta, and generally of pre-packed foods, is available to the consumer on the food label in accordance with Council Regulation No 1169/2011 [12], together with other mandatory information (i.e., list of ingredients, net amount, and name of producer). Moreover, other voluntary information can be reported on the pack, including nutrition claims (NC) and health claims (HC), the reduced presence or absence of gluten, or organic certification [12–14]. Research has shown that reading and understanding the nutrition facts and the claims reported on the label can help consumers in making healthy food choices [15]. However, it has been evidenced that the presence of NC or HC or the absence of gluten on the label can be misperceived as a guarantee of a better nutritional quality of the product [16–19]. Thus, consumers should be guided towards more informed and conscious food choices, which may lead to better dietary behaviours. In this context, the Food Labelling of Italian Products (FLIP) Study was conceived to systematically investigate the overall quality of the pre-packed foods of the most important food groups sold on the Italian market by collecting the nutrition declaration on their packaging [20,21]. The present study specifically focuses on pasta: there is, indeed, a wide variety of different pasta products sold on the shelves, and many of them boast nutrition claims and other information. A comparison of energy, nutrient, and salt content in pairs of products with and without the different declarations considered in the study (i.e., gluten free (GF), organic and their counterparts, as well as NC) was performed. Moreover, even if pasta is commonly consumed accompanied by other ingredients and sauces, the nutritional characteristics of pasta itself might be different among the various types, which may influence the nutritional quality of the entire meal. Based on these premises, it is important to investigate the nutritional composition of pasta sold in the market, also considering that the serving size can be widely different among the different types of pasta. To the best of our knowledge, no study has been carried out yet to comprehensively and systematically investigate the nutritional composition of the different varieties of pasta sold in Italy.

2. Materials and Methods

2.1. Food Product Selection

In the present study, information about pasta products was taken from the online shopping website of the main retailers present on the Italian market, as reported in a previous paper [21]. The online research was performed from July 2018 until March 2019.

All the prepacked pasta items with mandatory food information on the package, as requested by the Council Regulation (EC) no. 1169/2011 [12], were included. Conversely, the following products were excluded: not pre-packed, not available online during the collection data phase, with partial package images and/or unclear nutrition declaration, and/or an incomplete list of the ingredients. Pasta items were divided in two categories (fresh and dry), and for both, four types of pasta were selected and analysed: semolina, egg, stuffed, and special pasta.

2.2. Data Extraction and Analysis

For all the selected products, data from the complete images of the package were collected. The quali-quantitative data reported on the label of all products were recorded, including: company name, brand name, descriptive name, energy (kcal/100 g), total fat (g/100 g), saturated fatty acids (SFA, g/100 g), total carbohydrates (g/100 g), sugars (g/100 g), protein (g/100 g), and salt (g/100 g). In addition to the mandatory nutrition information indicated in the Council Regulation (EC) 1169/2011 [12], fibre content (g/100 g) was also collected. Descriptive name was used to classify the retrieved items in the two categories (fresh and dried pasta), each one including four types (semolina, egg, special, and stuffed pasta).

Once these values were retrieved, data of the energy and nutrient contents were also presented per standard serving by using the Italian suggested serving sizes for pasta [22]. The considered standard serving was 80 g for all types of dried pasta, 100 g for fresh semolina and egg pasta, and 125 g for fresh stuffed pasta.

Finally, information on the presence or absence of organic certification, GF declaration, and NC, was collected. Taking into account the disparity in the number of products with and without organic, GF, and NC declarations, the comparison of energy, nutrient, and salt content per 100 g in products with and without declarations was performed on only pairs of products, with three independent selections for each declaration. For each of the three declarations (organic, GF, NC), a similar item without declaration from the same brand was selected for each product by considering the category of pasta (i.e., fresh or dried) and type (i.e., semolina, egg, special, stuffed). For instance, for each fresh egg pasta GF, a corresponding fresh egg pasta item not GF from the same brand was chosen. When no items from the same brand but without the declaration were available, a similar item from the same category and type but another brand was randomly selected. Regarding GF products, the selection and the choice of pairs were limited to cereal-based products, thus excluding legume-based pasta, due to the high heterogeneity in terms of nutrition contents between these two types of products.

The precision of the extracted data was independently double-checked by two researchers (M.D.R. and S.M.), and inaccuracies were solved through secondary extractions by a third researcher (C.S.). After data collection, a dataset was created, grouping products into the four categories of interest: semolina pasta, egg pasta, stuffed pasta, and special pasta.

For the analysis of salt content, products were classified as "very low salt content" if they had <0.12 g of salt/100 g and "low salt content" if products had <0.3 g of salt/100 g, following the indications by Regulation (EC) No 1924/2006 [13]. The remaining products were instead classified as "medium salt content" (>0.3 but < 1 g of salt/100 g) and "high salt content" ($\geq$ 1 g of salt/100 g) as reported by the Italian Society of Human Nutrition (www.sinu.it) in the dissemination materials produced for the "World salt awareness week" performed in the framework of the World Action on Salt and Health (http://www.worldactiononsalt.com/).

2.3. Statistical Analysis

The Statistical Package for Social Sciences software (IBM SPSS Statistics, Version 24.0, IBM corp., Chicago, IL) was used to perform the statistical analysis, with a significance level set at $p < 0.05$. The normality of data distribution was firstly verified through the Kolmogorov-Smirnov test and rejected. Therefore, variables were expressed as median and interquartile range. Differences in terms of energy, macronutrients, and salt content among different types of pasta were explored using the Kruskal-Wallis test for independent samples with multiple pairwise comparisons. Analysis per 100 g was performed separately within and not between the two pasta categories (fresh and dried pasta), due to the difference in their moisture content. The analysis per serving was instead performed among all different types of pasta. The Mann-Whitney non-parametric test for two independent samples was applied for the comparisons of organic, GF, or NC pasta with their relative counterparts.

3. Results

3.1. Number and Types of Products

A total of 756 different items were analysed, categorised in fresh pasta ($n = 269$) and dried pasta ($n = 487$) based on their legal name.

Moreover, according to the nutritional characteristics of the different types of pasta, products within each category were further grouped into four pasta types (i.e., semolina, egg, stuffed, and special pasta that include other ingredients, such as rice, quinoa, amaranth, and legumes). Among fresh pasta, stuffed pasta had the largest number of items ($n = 208$), followed by egg pasta ($n = 45$) and semolina pasta ($n = 16$), and only one special pasta item, which was, thus, not considered in the following analysis. Conversely, egg pasta prevailed among dried pasta ($n = 206$), followed by semolina ($n = 157$) and special pasta ($n = 119$), while only five stuffed pasta items were found.

To compare the nutritional composition between products with and without specific declarations, the analysis was carried out on 49 pairs of organic/conventional items, 90 GF/gluten-containing products. Finally, 45 products with at least one NC declaration and 45 without NC were considered.

3.2. Nutritional Composition of Pasta per 100 g

As reported in Table 1, there was a high variability of energy and nutrient contents among fresh and dried pasta ($p < 0.05$) when different pasta types, within each category, were analysed. Considering fresh pasta, egg pasta had total median energy of 293 (288–308) kcal/100 g, which was slightly but significantly higher than stuffed pasta, which had total median energy of 274 (248–293) kcal/100 g, and semolina pasta, which had total median energy of 272 (261–273) kcal/100 g. Different results were found for energy median values of dried pasta types, where no differences were observed between egg and stuffed pasta (369 (365–374) kcal/100 g and 394 (393–403) kcal/100 g, respectively), even though they had significantly higher energy values than special and semolina pasta (351 (347–358) kcal/100 g and 354 (351–357) kcal/100 g, respectively). Overall, carbohydrates were the most abundant macronutrients, ranging from 54% of energy in stuffed fresh pasta to 71% of energy in semolina dried pasta.

In the fresh pasta category, stuffed pasta showed a significantly higher content of total fat, SFA, sugar, and salt, but a significantly lower amount of carbohydrate, compared to the other pasta types. Among the dried pasta, semolina and special pasta had a significantly lower total fat, SFA, and protein content and a greater amount of carbohydrates compared to egg- and stuffed-pasta (Table 1).

Regarding salt content, only stuffed pasta, both fresh and dried, had a median high quantity of salt (>1 g/100 g). Considering all the items (i.e., fresh and dried), low content of salt (<0.3 g/100 g) was reported by 68.1% of the products, while a medium (>0.3 g/100 g but <1 g/100 g) and high (≥1 g/100 g) category of salt content was reported for 10.9% and 21.1%, respectively. As shown in Figure 1, the type of pasta with the highest salt content was stuffed pasta. Indeed, 98.6% of stuffed products had a medium or high salt content. Conversely, no special pasta items and only 0.6% of semolina products had a high salt content.

Table 1. Energy and nutritional composition across categories of pasta.

	Fresh Pasta				Dried Pasta				
	All (n = 269)	Semolina (n = 16)	Egg (n = 45)	Stuffed (n = 208)	All (n = 487)	Semolina (n = 157)	Egg (n = 206)	Stuffed (n = 5)	Special (n = 119)
Energy (kcal/100 g)	280 (253–295)	272 (261–273) [b]	293 (288–308) [a]	274 (248–293) [b]	359 (352–368)	354 (351–357) [b]	369 (365–374) [a]	394 (393–403) [a]	351 (347–358) [b]
Total Fat (g/100 g)	7.3 (4.7–9.2)	1.3 (1.2–1.6)	3.0 (2.6–3.4) [b]	8.1 (6.5–10.0) [a]	2.5 (1.5–4.0)	1.5 (1.3–1.9) [c]	4.0 (3.8–4.7) [b]	12.5 (12.2–13.0) [a]	1.8 (1.4–2.4) [c]
SFA (g/100 g)	2.7 (1.6–3.8)	0.3 (0.3–0.3) [b]	1.0 (0.7–1.3) [b]	3.1 (2.4–4.1) [a]	0.7 (0.3–1.2)	0.4 (0.3–0.5) [b]	1.3 (1.2–1.5) [a]	3.0 (2.7–3.8) [a]	0.4 (0.3–0.5) [b]
Total Carb (g/100 g)	39.9 (33.6–47.0)	54.9 (46.4–55.0) [a]	54.0 (52.0–57.8) [a]	37.2 (32.0–41.0) [b]	68.0 (66.0–71.5)	71.0 (69.5–72.0) [a]	67.0 (66.0–68.0) [b]	51.7 (51.0–52.9) [b]	69.6 (64.0–76.0) [a]
Sugars (g/100 g)	2.4 (1.4–4.0)	1.5 (1.5–1.6) [b]	1.3 (1.1–1.5) [b]	3.1 (1.7–4.6) [a]	2.8 (2.2–3.2)	3.2 (2.9–3.5) [a]	2.8 (2.4–3.0) [b]	3.2 (2.0–3.3) [ab]	1.4 (0.6–2.6) [c]
Fibre (g/100 g) [#]	2.4 (2.0–3.1)	2.5 (2.5–6.0) [a]	2.3 (2.1–2.4) [b]	2.5 (2.0–3.1) [b]	3.0 (2.8–3.8)	3.0 (2.7–3.6)	3.0 (2.8–3.5)	5.0 (3.3–7.5)	3.5 (2.2–6.5)
Protein (g/100 g)	10.0 (9.0–12.0)	9.0 (9.0–9.2) [b]	11.0 (10.2–11.2) [a]	10.0 (8.9–13.0) [a]	14.0 (12.0–15.0)	13.0 (12.0–14.0) [b]	14.5 (14.0–15.0) [a]	15.3 (15.0–15.5) [a]	12.0 (6.8–14.0) [b]
Salt (g/100 g)	1.1 (0.6–1.4)	0.0 (0.0–0.0) [b]	0.1 (0.1–0.2) [b]	1.2 (0.9–1.4) [a]	0.0 (0.0–0.1)	0.0 (0.0–0.0) [b]	0.1 (0.1–0.1) [a]	1.0 (1.0–1.0) [a]	0.0 (0.0–0.0) [b]

Values are expressed as median (25th–75th percentile). SFA: saturated fatty acid; Carb: carbohydrate. For each category, different superscript lowercase letters in the same row indicate significant differences among types (Kruskal–Wallis test for independent samples with multiple pairwise comparisons). [#] Number of items reporting fibre: Fresh pasta (All n = 198; Semolina n = 15; Egg n = 34; Stuffed n = 149), Dried pasta (All n = 449; Semolina n = 135; Egg n = 193; Stuffed n = 5; Special n = 116).

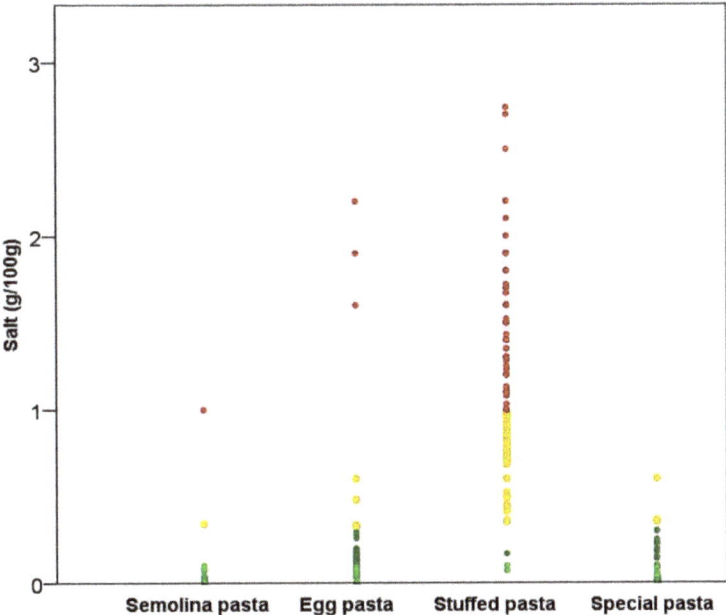

Figure 1. Salt content of the pasta products. Coloured dots refer to the classification for salt content by Council Regulation (EC) No 1924/2006 [13]: light green = very low salt content (<0.12 g/100 g); green = low salt content (<0.3 g/100 g); yellow = medium salt content (<1 g/100 g); red = high salt content (≥1 g/100 g).

Table 2 shows the nutritional content of organic, GF, and NC pasta and their respective counterparts. No differences were observed when considering organic declaration, except for a lower protein content (12.0 (11.0–14.0) vs. 13.7 (13.0–14.6) g/100 g) and higher fibre content (3.0 (2.8–3.4) vs. 2.8 (2.7–3.0) g/100 g) in organic pasta compared to conventional pasta. GF products showed a significantly higher content of total carbohydrate and fat and a lower content of sugar, fibre and protein compared to the non-containing gluten counterpart (Table 2). No differences were identified when products with NC were compared to their counterpart, except for fibre content, which was significantly higher in pasta with NC.

Table 2. Energy and nutrition facts in products with and without specific declarations, on selected pairs of products (as reported in Materials and Methods section).

	Organic		GF		NC	
	Yes (n = 49)	No (n = 49)	Yes (n = 90)	No (n = 90)	Yes (n = 45)	No (n = 45)
Energy (kcal/100 g)	357 (351–365)	359 (354–366)	349 (283–358)	353 (291–356)	350 (346–361)	349 (346–359)
Fat (g/100 g)	2.0 (1.4–3.8)	2.0 (1.4–3.9)	2.3 (1.5–7.1)	1.6 (1.4–6.0) *	2.1 (1.5–3.3)	2.4 (1.7–3.3)
SFA (g/100 g)	0.6 (0.3–1.0)	0.5 (0.4–1.3)	0.7 (0.3–2.6)	0.4 (0.3–2.4)	0.4 (0.3–1.0)	0.4 (0.3–0.9)
Carbohydrates (g/100 g)	70.6 (67.5–72.0)	69.0 (67.0–70.8)	73.7 (42.0–77.2)	70.1 (42.0–71.5) *	66.5 (64.6–68.0)	66.0 (63.0–69.4)
Sugars (g/100 g)	2.6 (2.4–3.5)	2.9 (2.6–3.5)	0.7 (0.4–1.3)	3.2 (2.9–3.7) *	2.7 (2.3–3.2)	2.5 (1.5–3.0)
Fibre (g/100 g) [#]	3.0 (2.8–3.4)	2.8 (2.7–3.0) *	2.3 (2.0–3.1)	2.7 (2.5–3.0) *	6.1 (3.4–7.0)	4.0 (2.8–6.5) *
Protein (g/100 g)	12.0 (11.0–14.0)	13.7 (13.0–14.6) *	7.2 (6.5–8.5)	12.6 (11.2–13.5) *	13.0 (11.1–14.2)	13.0 (10.5–14.0)
Salt (g/100 g)	0.0 (0.0–0.1)	0.0 (0.0–0.1)	0.0 (0.0–0.8)	0.0 (0.0–1.0)	0.0 (0.0–0.1)	0.0 (0.0–0.1)

Values are expressed as median (25th–75th percentile). SFA: saturated fatty acid; GF: gluten free; NC: nutrition claim. For each category, asterisks indicate significant differences between groups (Mann-Whitney non-parametric test for two independent samples), $p < 0.05$.
[#] Number of items reporting fibre: organic = 45/43; GF = 82/74; NC = 45/43 (yes/no).

3.3. Nutritional Composition per Serving Size

In order to better investigate the nutrition content of all pasta types, a further evaluation of nutrition facts (energy, nutrients, and salt) per standard serving was performed (Figure 2). This analysis was performed because the different types of pasta can be considered as alternatives as indicated in the Reference Intakes of nutrients and energy for the Italian population [22]. The analysis was carried out without dried stuffed pasta, because only five items were present. Regarding the energy content per standard serving, for fresh stuffed pasta (342 (310–366) kcal/serving) it was significantly higher than for the other pasta types, while no statistical differences were observed among fresh semolina (272 (258–273) kcal/serving), dried semolina (283 (281–286) kcal/serving), and dried special pasta (281 (278–286) kcal/serving), and between fresh egg (293 (288–308) kcal/serving) and dried egg pasta (295 (292–299) kcal/serving). The same trend was observed for total fats. Regarding the carbohydrate content per standard serving, fresh stuffed pasta and dried special pasta showed the greatest variability. In fact, the median carbohydrate content per standard serving of fresh stuffed pasta was significantly lower than other pasta types, except for fresh semolina pasta; moreover, dried semolina pasta had a median content similar to dried special pasta but significantly higher compared to all the other pasta types. Fibre content of dried special pasta had great variability and its median content did not show significant differences from fresh and dried semolina pasta. The median quantity of protein per serving was significantly higher in stuffed pasta compared to the others, except for dried egg pasta. Considering the salt content per standard serving, only fresh stuffed pasta had a median high quantity of salt (1.5 g/serving).

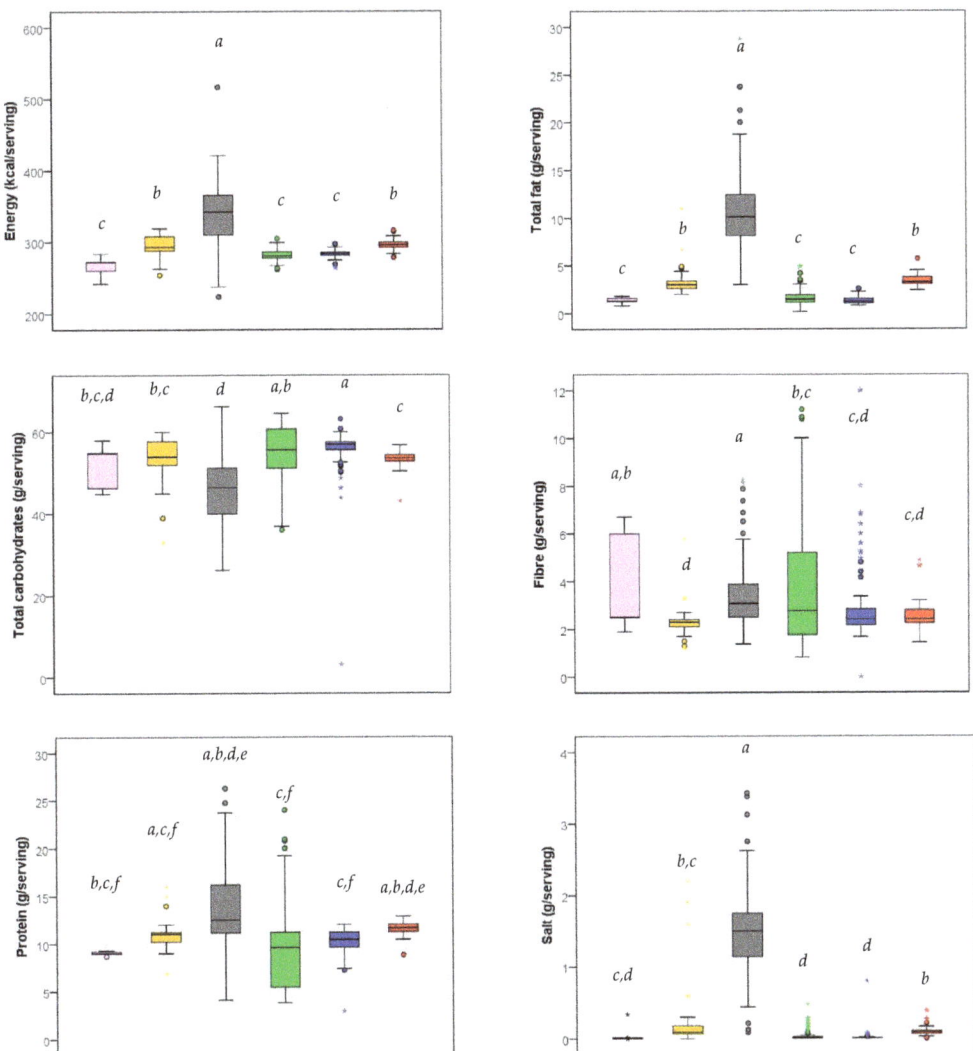

Figure 2. Box plot for energy and nutrition facts per standard serving across categories of pasta. Standard serving was 80 g for all types of dried pasta, 100 g for fresh semolina and egg pasta, and 125 g for fresh stuffed pasta. For each category, different letters indicate significant differences among pasta types (Kruskal–Wallis test for independent samples with multiple pairwise comparisons). ▢ fresh semolina (n = 16), ▢ fresh egg (n = 45), ▢ fresh stuffed (n = 208), ▢ dried special (n = 119), ▢ dried semolina (n = 157), ▢ dried egg (n = 206).

4. Discussion

To the best of our knowledge, the present study evaluated, for the first time, the nutritional quality of the different pasta products sold on the Italian market, taking into account the mandatory and some voluntary nutrition information printed on the packaging.

The first intriguing finding is related to the high number of items retrieved on the market. On the one hand, this number confirms Italians as the number one producers and consumers of pasta. It is worth remembering that pasta is indeed a widely common staple food and it is a key product in the Mediterranean dietary pattern [23]—to such an extent that the Italian Food Dietary Guidelines suggests the consumption of one serving of pasta per day (or rice or other cereals) [24]. On the other hand, the several different types of pasta found on the market confirm the great interest of food companies in satisfying the emerging needs and trends of the customers, not only in terms of format but mostly for the many ingredients that can be used for pasta-making.

Data of the nutrition facts evidenced wide differences in terms of energy and nutrients across the two different pasta categories under study, i.e., fresh and dried pasta. Differences were also found among the types of pasta, particularly for stuffed pasta, showing a lower carbohydrate and a higher fat, sugar, and energy content with respect to the other pasta types. Such a difference observed for stuffed pasta is probably mainly due to the filling, of which the weight usually represents half of the total weight. For the same reason, this type of pasta was characterised by the highest median content of salt, with almost all stuffed products (98.6%) having a medium or high salt content. Conversely, the results indicated a negligible amount of salt, the least amount of all pasta types. This is why semolina pasta and other types of pasta are generally prepared at home as well as in the restaurant, canteens, etc. by adding salt in the boiling water; however, the final salt content is likely lower than those reported on the food label of stuffed pasta [25,26].

These results are even more evident by analysing the nutrition declaration per serving size instead of 100 g, mainly because the reference serving for stuffed pasta is generally higher than the ones for dried and fresh semolina and egg pasta [22]. This led to an increased differentiation between the nutritional quality of the different types of pasta, for instance with fresh stuffed pasta providing the highest energy per portion despite no differences were found for 100 g.

Regarding salt, values per serving confirmed the ones obtained per 100 g, highlighting that a portion of stuffed pasta contributes to a high extent to the daily intake of salt, on average equivalent to about 33% of the 5 g/day indicated as the goal by the World Health Organisation (WHO) [27] and over 2 g/serving size for 10% of the stuffed items. It is worth remembering that an excessive consumption of salt in a diet increases blood pressure and consequently the risk of adverse effects on cardiovascular health [28,29]. These results highlight, on the one hand, the importance of nutritional education and increasing knowledge in the population in taking into consideration the serving size, which can deeply influence the nutrient intake; on the other hand, the results suggest that not only food per se, but also the preparation of foods (e.g., adding salt to boiling water), has a key role in the daily intake of nutrients. For example, the high salt content in stuffed pasta suggests that the addition of salt to boiling water should be avoided, even though this is not usually reported on the pack; in some cases, it is even suggested to add salt.

To investigate the nutrition quality of the different categories and types of pasta, we also compared the nutrition facts of products with and without three different declarations, i.e., GF, organic, and NC. This aspect was taken into consideration because consumers' perception may be influenced by several types of declarations, with the so-called "halo effect" [30]. It has, indeed, been evidenced that consumers perceive foods with claims (e.g., NC) or specific front-of-pack labelling [31], as well as GF products [32] and organic foods [33], healthier than their counterparts. Thus, this misperception may influence food habits, which, in turn, may in some cases lead to an overconsumption [34]. To investigate whether the presence of declaration may affect the nutrition quality of the pasta, we selected and compared the nutrition declaration in an equal number of products with and without each of these declarations on the pack, similarly to what already done in a previous study aimed at comparing the nutritional quality of organic vs. conventional products [20]. This choice was due to the gap of product numbers with and without these declarations currently on the market. The first comparison was made between GF and gluten-containing pasta. Our results suggest that GF products had higher carbohydrates and fat contents and lower fibre, sugar, and protein contents compared to the gluten-containing products. It is worth noting that the use of legume flours/ingredients is increasing in order to enhance the nutritional profile of GF products, resulting in significantly higher fibre and protein contents and a lower amount of carbohydrates compared to conventional semolina pasta [35,36]. However, these types of pasta have not been taken into consideration, as there were no gluten-containing counterparts for the comparison. Our results confirm the findings of an Italian survey considering GF pasta sold on the Italian market, although the authors also found a higher energy, SFA, and salt amount in GF pasta compared to the regular ones [37]. Moreover, our results are partially in agreement with the ones found by a Spanish research considering a total of 53 pasta items, 15 of which were GF [38]. The authors confirmed higher total fats and lower sugars for GF pasta, but they also found higher protein and SFA than gluten-containing pasta. Contrasting results in terms of lipid contents have been found in a UK study focusing on both GF and regular whole grain and white pasta [39]. In fact, UK white GF pasta (111 items) showed a lower content of total fat and SFA than the counterparts (96 items), whereas these data were not confirmed for the whole grain items [39].

Regarding the nutritional profile of products boasting NC, only fibre content was significantly higher than in products without claims. This is plausibly due to the fact the almost all NCs found in these products were related to fibre (i.e., 38 items "source or rich in fibre"), while only 7 items boasted a NC claim related to protein. Intriguingly, a survey conducted on 87 pasta and rice items sold on the Irish market found that 31% of the products considered boasted a NC or a HC and that most of the NC referred to fat (including saturated fats) and carbohydrates, followed by sugars and protein [40]. Overall, data from the present study support the hypothesis that NC should not be considered as marker of the overall quality of food products, as already indicated in previous studies on different types of products [21]. This suggests that more effort should be made in nutrition education to avoid misperceptions, which lead to inappropriate food choices and possibly overconsumption [41].

Finally, we also compared the nutritional quality of organic and conventional pasta. In agreement with studies comparing conventional and organic durum wheat products [42–44], our data only showed a significantly lower protein content and a higher fibre amount in organic pasta with respect to the conventional counterpart. Even though no other significant difference between organic and conventional products was found, these variations were not due to the co-existence of other characteristics, such as a different number of wholemeal in the organic vs. the conventional counterparts, as none of the 49 paired items were wholemeal. These results are in line with a previous publication, where it was highlighted that the organic certification cannot be intended as a marker of the general nutritional quality of the products [20].

Our work showed strengths and limitations, mainly attributable to the methodology used for product selection. On the one hand, we analysed for the first time the nutritional composition of a high number of different pasta products retrieved from the major retailers present on the Italian market that have a home-shopping website, thus including the majority of pasta sold in Italy. On the other hand, the exclusion of products sold by local groceries and discounts as well as shops dedicated to special foods, i.e., GF items, might have limited the product analysis. Another limitation of the study concerns the different origin of the nutritional data on the label, which could be based on laboratory analysis or calculation from the ingredients used or generally established and accepted data, creating a putative bias in data origin. Moreover, the high variability of filling characteristics found among stuffed pasta items made tricky the intra- and inter-type comparisons of the nutritional quality. Finally, the comparison of the nutritional quality between the pairs of products with and without declarations could be considered a limitation. However, including all the 756 items in the analysis would have affected the findings because of the large difference in the number of products of the same type, with and without declarations such as GF, organic, or NC. Conversely, the comparison of items of the same brand was a way to avoid that the brand name can act as a possible cause of bias.

5. Conclusions

To the best of our knowledge, this is the first study which comprehensively analysed the nutritional composition of a wide range of fresh and dried pasta products sold in the Italian market. Data showed that pasta types currently on the market are very different in terms of nutrition profile, and not really comparable. Particularly stuffed pasta was characterised by a high salt content, representing a large proportion of the maximum of 5 g/day indicated by the WHO. This last aspect particularly highlights the need to clarify as much as possible the nutrition facts of product to the consumer, as pasta is usually eaten by adding sauces and/or toppings which might further increase the energy, macronutrient, and salt intake. Linked to this, we also advised that salt, mainly the discretionary one, should be carefully reduced or avoided in cooking this type of pasta. It is, indeed, particularly crucial to increase consumer awareness about the choice of both adequate pasta type and dressing and their contribution to the nutritional quality of the entire dishes.

Overall, findings from the present study are particularly of interest and should be taken into account in dietary recommendations, which currently provide only information regarding the serving size of the different type of pasta, but not about their frequency of consumption. Stuffed pasta probably should not be regularly consumed as an alternative to semolina pasta. Thus, the awareness of the consumers about the nutrition profile of the different types of pasta could be the topic of targeted nutrition education interventions aimed to improve their knowledge and, in turn, their food habits. Finally, with this study focusing on pasta products, we confirm that organic or other declarations, i.e., NC, cannot be an overall marker of the nutritional quality of the product and, thus, this topic should also be the object of future nutrition education targeted to consumers.

Author Contributions: M.D.R., C.S., and S.M. were involved in the protocol design, data analyses, interpretation of results, and drafting of the manuscript; D.A. participated in the protocol design, data analysis, and drafting of the manuscript; N.P. participated in the protocol design and critically reviewed the manuscript; D.M. conceived the study, supervised the data collection, and had primary responsibility for the final content. Other members of the Italian Society of Human Nutrition (SINU) Young Working Group were involved in the protocol design. All authors have read and agreed to the published version of the manuscript.

Funding: This research received no external funding.

Institutional Review Board Statement: Not applicable.

Informed Consent Statement: Not applicable.

Data Availability Statement: Not applicable.

Acknowledgments: The authors wish to thank all students who participated to the development of the dataset.

SINU Young Working Group
- Margherita Dall'Asta; Department of Animal Science, Food and Nutrition, Università Cattolica del Sacro Cuore, Piacenza, Italy.
- Daniele Nucci; Veneto Institute of Oncology IOV-IRCCS, Padova, Italy.
- Gaetana Paolella; Department of Chemistry and Biology A. Zambelli, University of Salerno, Fisciano, Italy.
- Veronica Pignone; Department of Epidemiology and Prevention, IRCCS Neuromed, Pozzilli, Italy.
- Alice Rosi; Department of Food and Drug, University of Parma, Parma, Italy.
- Emilia Ruggiero; Department of Epidemiology and Prevention, IRCCS Neuromed, Pozzilli, Italy.
- Giorgia Vici; University of Camerino, Camerino, Italy.

Conflicts of Interest: The present publication has been conceived within the Italian Society of Human Nutrition (SINU) Young Group, and it has been made without any funding from food industries or other entities. The authors declare no conflict of interest.

References

1. Decreto del Presidente della Repubblica n.146. Regolamento per la revisione della normativa sulla produzione e commercializzazione di sfarinati e paste alimentari, a norma dell'articolo 50 della legge 22 febbraio 1994. *Gazz. Uff.* **2001**, *117*, 6–12.
2. IPO. The World Pasta Industry Status report-International Pasta Organization. 2014. Available online: http://www.internationalpasta.org (accessed on 13 January 2020).
3. Mintel.com. 2017. Available online: https://www.mintel.com/press-centre/food-and-drink/italys-love-of-pasta-goes-off-the-boil (accessed on 20 October 2020).
4. Pounis, G.; Castelnuovo, A.D.; Costanzo, S.; Persichillo, M.; Bonaccio, M.; Bonanni, A.; Cerletti, C.; Donati, M.B.; de Gaetano, G.; Iacoviello, L. Association of pasta consumption with body mass index and waist-to-hip ratio: Results from Moli-sani and INHES studies. *Nutr. Diabetes* **2016**, *6*, e218. [CrossRef] [PubMed]
5. Chiavaroli, L.; Kendall, C.W.C.; Braunstein, C.R.; Blanco Mejia, S.; Leiter, L.A.; Jenkins, D.J.A.; Sievenpiper, J.L. Effect of pasta in the context of low-glycaemic index dietary patterns on body weight and markers of adiposity: A systematic review and meta-analysis of randomised controlled trials in adults. *BMJ Open* **2018**, *8*, e019438. [CrossRef] [PubMed]
6. Vitale, M.; Masulli, M.; Rivellese, A.A.; Bonora, E.; Babini, A.C.; Sartore, G.; Corsi, L.; Buzzetti, R.; Citro, G.; Baldassarre, M.P.A.; et al. Pasta Consumption and connected dietary habits: Associations with glucose control, adiposity measures, and cardiovascular risk factors in people with type 2 diabetes-TOSCA.IT Study. *Nutrients* **2019**, *12*, 101. [CrossRef]
7. Huang, M.; Li, J.; Ha, M.A.; Riccardi, G.; Liu, S. A systematic review on the relations between pasta consumption and cardio-metabolic risk factors. *Nutr. Metab. Cardiovasc. Dis.* **2017**, *27*, 939–948. [CrossRef]
8. Augustin, L.S.A.; Taborelli, M.; Montella, M.; Libra, M.; La Vecchia, C.; Tavani, A.; Crispo, A.; Grimaldi, M.; Facchini, G.; Jenkins, D.J.A.; et al. Associations of dietary carbohydrates, glycaemic index and glycaemic load with risk of bladder cancer: A case-control study. *Br. J. Nutr.* **2017**, *118*, 722–729. [CrossRef]
9. Angelino, D.; Martina, A.; Rosi, A.; Veronesi, L.; Antonini, M.; Mennella, I.; Vitaglione, P.; Grioni, S.; Brighenti, F.; Zavaroni, I.; et al. Glucose- and lipid-related biomarkers are affected in healthy obese or hyperglycemic adults consuming a whole-grain pasta enriched in prebiotics and probiotics: A 12-week randomized controlled trial. *J. Nutr.* **2019**, *149*, 1714–1723. [CrossRef] [PubMed]
10. Ciccoritti, R.; Taddei, F.; Nicoletti, I.; Gazza, L.; Corradini, D.; D'Egidio, M.G.; Martini, D. Use of bran fractions and debranned kernels for the development of pasta with high nutritional and healthy potential. *Food Chem.* **2017**, *225*, 77–86. [CrossRef] [PubMed]
11. Oliviero, T.; Fogliano, V. Food design strategies to increase vegetable intake: The case of vegetable enriched pasta. *Trends Food Sci. Technol.* **2016**, *51*, 58–64. [CrossRef]
12. European Union. Regulation No. 1169/2011 on the provision of food information to consumers. *Off. J. Eur. Union* **2011**, *L304*, 18–63.
13. European Union. Regulation No. 1924/2006 on nutrition and health claims made on foods. *Off. J. Eur. Union* **2006**, *L404*, 9–25.
14. European Union. Regulation No. 828/2014 on the requirements for the provision of information to consumers on the absence or reduced presence of gluten in food. *Off. J. Eur. Union* **2014**, *L228*, 5–8.
15. Talati, Z.; Pettigrew, S.; Neal, B.; Dixon, H.; Hughes, C.; Kelly, B.; Miller, C. Consumers' responses to health claims in the context of other on-pack nutrition information: A systematic review. *Nutr. Rev.* **2017**, *75*, 260–273. [CrossRef]
16. Bialkova, S.; Sasse, L.; Fenko, A. The role of nutrition labels and advertising claims in altering consumers' evaluation and choice. *Appetite* **2016**, *96*, 38–46. [CrossRef]
17. Asioli, D.; Aschemann-Witzel, J.; Caputo, V.; Vecchio, R.; Annunziata, A.; Naes, T.; Varela, P. Making sense of the "clean label" trends: A review of consumer food choice behavior and discussion of industry implications. *Food Res. Int.* **2017**, *99*, 58–71. [CrossRef]
18. Van Buul, V.J.; Brouns, F.J. Nutrition and health claims as marketing tools. *Crit. Rev. Food Sci. Nutr.* **2015**, *55*, 1552–1560. [CrossRef]
19. Kaur, A.; Scarborough, P.; Rayner, M. A systematic review, and meta-analyses, of the impact of health-related claims on dietary choices. *Int. J. Behav. Nutr. Phys. Act.* **2017**, *14*, 93. [CrossRef]
20. Dall'Asta, M.; Angelino, D.; Pellegrini, N.; Martini, D. The nutritional quality of organic and conventional food products sold in Italy: Results from the Food Labelling of Italian Products (FLIP) study. *Nutrients* **2020**, *12*, 1273. [CrossRef]
21. Angelino, D.; Rosi, A.; Dall'Asta, M.; Pellegrini, N.; Martini, D. Evaluation of the nutritional quality of breakfast cereals sold on the Italian market: The Food Labelling of Italian Products (FLIP) study. *Nutrients* **2019**, *11*, 2827. [CrossRef]
22. SINU. *LARN-Livelli di Assunzione di Riferimento di Nutrienti ed Energia per la Popolazione Italiana*; IV Revisione; Coordinamento editoriale SINU-INRAN; SICS: Milan, Italy, 2014.
23. Giacco, R.; Vitale, M.; Riccardi, G. Pasta: Role in Diet. In *The Encyclopedia of Food and Health*; Academic Press: Oxford, UK, 2016; Volume 4, pp. 242–245.
24. CREA. *Linee Guida per una Sana Alimentazione 2018*; CREA: Rome, Italy, 2018; pp. 1–229.
25. Albrecht, J.A.; Asp, E.H.; Buzzard, I.M. Contents and retentions of sodium and other minerals in pasta cooked in unsalted or salted water. *AGRIS* **1987**, *64*, 106–109.
26. Bianchi, L.M.; Phillips, K.M.; McGinty, R.C.; Ahuja, J.K.; Pehrsson, P.R. Cooking parameters affect the sodium content of prepared pasta. *Food Chem.* **2019**, *271*, 479–487. [CrossRef]
27. WHO. *Guideline: Sodium Intake for Adults and Children*; WHO: Geneva, Switzerland, 2012; pp. 2011–2046.
28. D'Elia, L.; Manfredi, M.; Strazzullo, P.; Galletti, F.; Group, M.-S.S. Validation of an easy questionnaire on the assessment of salt habit: The MINISAL-SIIA Study Program. *Eur. J. Clin. Nutr.* **2019**, *73*, 793–800. [CrossRef] [PubMed]

29. He, F.J.; MacGregor, G.A. Reducing population salt intake worldwide: From evidence to implementation. *Prog. Cardiovasc. Dis.* **2010**, *52*, 363–382. [CrossRef]
30. Sundar, A.; Kardes, F.R. The Role of perceived variability and the health halo effect in nutritional inference and consumption. *Psychol. Mark.* **2015**, *32*, 512–521. [CrossRef]
31. Talati, Z.; Pettigrew, S.; Dixon, H.; Neal, B.; Ball, K.; Hughes, C. Do health claims and front-of-pack labels lead to a positivity bias in unhealthy foods? *Nutrients* **2016**, *8*, 787. [CrossRef] [PubMed]
32. Dunn, C.; House, L.; Shelnutt, K.P. Consumer perceptions of gluten-free products and the healthfulness of gluten-free diets. *J. Nutr. Educ. Behav.* **2014**, *46*, S184–S185. [CrossRef]
33. Küst, P. The Impact of the organic label halo effect on consumers' quality perceptions, value-in-use and well-being. *JUMS* **2019**, *4*, 241–264.
34. Oostenbach, L.H.; Slits, E.; Robinson, E.; Sacks, G. Systematic review of the impact of nutrition claims related to fat, sugar and energy content on food choices and energy intake. *BMC Public Health* **2019**, *19*, 1296. [CrossRef]
35. Laleg, K.; Cassan, D.; Barron, C.; Prabhasankar, P.; Micard, V. Structural, culinary, nutritional and anti-nutritional properties of high protein, gluten free, 100% legume pasta. *PLoS ONE* **2016**, *11*, e0160721. [CrossRef]
36. Trevisan, S.; Pasini, G.; Simonato, B. An overview of expected glycaemic response of one ingredient commercial gluten free pasta. *LWT* **2019**, *109*, 13–16. [CrossRef]
37. Cornicelli, M.; Saba, M.; Machello, N.; Silano, M.; Neuhold, S. Nutritional composition of gluten-free food versus regular food sold in the Italian market. *Dig. Liver Dis.* **2018**, *50*, 1305–1308. [CrossRef]
38. Miranda, J.; Lasa, A.; Bustamante, M.A.; Churruca, I.; Simon, E. Nutritional differences between a gluten-free diet and a diet containing equivalent products with gluten. *Plant Foods Hum. Nutr.* **2014**, *69*, 182–187. [CrossRef]
39. Fry, L.; Madden, A.M.; Fallaize, R. An investigation into the nutritional composition and cost of gluten-free versus regular food products in the UK. *J. Hum. Nutr. Diet* **2018**, *31*, 108–120. [CrossRef]
40. Lalor, F.; Kennedy, J.; Flynn, M.A.; Wall, P.G. A study of nutrition and health claims–a snapshot of what's on the Irish market. *Public Health Nutr.* **2010**, *13*, 704–711. [CrossRef]
41. Faulkner, G.P.; Pourshahidi, L.K.; Wallace, J.M.; Kerr, M.A.; McCaffrey, T.A.; Livingstone, M.B. Perceived 'healthiness' of foods can influence consumers' estimations of energy density and appropriate portion size. *Int. J. Obes.* **2014**, *38*, 106–112. [CrossRef]
42. De Stefanis, E.; Sgrulletta, D.; Pucciarmati, S.; Ciccoritti, R.; Quaranta, F. Influence of durum wheat-faba bean intercrop on specific quality traits of organic durum wheat. *Biol. Agric. Hortic.* **2017**, *33*, 28–39. [CrossRef]
43. Fagnano, M.; Fiorentino, N.; D'Egidio, M.G.; Quaranta, F.; Ritieni, A.; Ferracane, R.; Raimondi, G. Durum wheat in conventional and organic farming: Yield amount and pasta quality in Southern Italy. *Science* **2012**, *2012*, 973058. [CrossRef]
44. Mazzoncini, M.; Antichi, D.; Silvestri, N.; Ciantelli, G.; Sgherri, C. Organically vs. conventionally grown winter wheat: Effects on grain yield, technological quality, and on phenolic composition and antioxidant properties of bran and refined flour. *Food Chem.* **2015**, *175*, 445–451. [CrossRef]

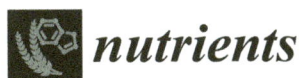

Article

Supermarket Circulars Promoting the Sales of 'Healthy' Foods: Analysis Based on Degree of Processing

Alyne Michelle Botelho [1], Anice Milbratz de Camargo [1], Kharla Janinny Medeiros [1], Gabriella Beatriz Irmão [1], Moira Dean [2] and Giovanna Medeiros Rataichesck Fiates [1,*]

1. Graduate Program in Nutrition, Nutrition in Foodservice Research Centre, Federal University of Santa Catarina, University Campus João David Ferreira Lima-Trindade, Florianópolis, SC 88040-900, Brazil; alyne.botelho@posgrad.ufsc.br (A.M.B.); anice.camargo@posgrad.ufsc.br (A.M.d.C.); kharla.medeiros@ufsc.br (K.J.M.); gabriella.irmao@grad.ufsc.br (G.B.I.)
2. Institute for Global Food Security, School of Biological Sciences, Queen's University Belfast, Belfast BT9 5DL, UK; moira.dean@qub.ac.uk
* Correspondence: giovanna.fiates@ufsc.br

Received: 27 July 2020; Accepted: 27 August 2020; Published: 21 September 2020

Abstract: The health and wellness food sector grew 98% from 2009 to 2014 in Brazil, the world's fourth-biggest market. The trend has reached supermarket circulars, which recently started to feature whole sections advertising health and wellness-enhancing foods. This study identified food items advertised in circulars' specific sections of two Brazilian supermarket chains (one regional, one national) during a 10-week period. Foods were classified according to degree of food processing and presence/type of claims on their front-of-pack (FoP) labels. Comparison between groups of Unprocessed/Minimally Processed foods vs. Ultra-processed foods and presence/type of claims employed Pearson chi-square test. From the 434 alleged health and wellness-enhancing foods advertised, around half (51.4%) were classified as Ultra-processed. Presence of reduced and increased nutrient-content claims was significantly higher in labels of Ultra-processed foods. Most frequent claims addressed sugar and fibre content. Brazilian supermarket circulars were found to be promoting the sale of Ultra-processed foods in their health and wellness sections, leading to a situation that can mislead the consumer and bring negative health outcomes.

Keywords: supermarket circulars; ultra-processed; food label; health claims

1. Introduction

Healthy eating is essential for health promotion and protection, and as a determinant factor in preventing chronic non-transmissible diseases [1]. Nevertheless, the access to a healthy and adequate diet is proving to be a challenge for modern societies, with the eating practices of Brazilians in different stages of life and across all socioeconomic strata being far from what is considered desirable [2]. Consumption of processed and ultra-processed foods has been growing exponentially in the Brazilian population and is considered a contributing factor for the increased prevalence of obesity and non-communicable diseases in the country [3,4]. Consequently, a new version of the Dietary Guidelines for the Brazilian Population was published, instructing individuals to limit the consumption of processed foods, avoid consumption of ultra-processed foods, and choose fresh and minimally processed foods as the core of their diets. According to the Guidelines, a healthy diet is based on the consumption of natural or minimally processed foods; and of dishes and meals containing such foods [1].

Published in 2015, the Dietary Guidelines for the Brazilian Population established specific eating directives based on degree of food processing, employing a classification system later improved and published under the name of NOVA (a name, not an acronym) [5]. According to NOVA, industrial formulations containing little or no fresh ingredients and food additives to add colour, flavour, texture, and additional sensory properties to unprocessed foods and preparations containing them are classified as Ultra-processed foods [1,5]. The nature of the processes and ingredients used in their manufacture, and their displacement of unprocessed or minimally processed foods and freshly prepared dishes and meals, make ultra-processed foods intrinsically unhealthy. In spite of this, as foods typically energy-dense, rich in sugar, fat, and salt, they are hyper-palatable and cheap, which contributes to their high consumption. Ultra-processed foods are poor in dietary fibre, protein, vitamins, and minerals; and additives contained in their formulation increase shelf-life without increasing their cost [1,5,6].

On the other hand, dietary patterns based on dishes and meals made from a variety of unprocessed or minimally processed plant foods, prepared, seasoned, and cooked with processed culinary ingredients and complemented with processed foods are the healthier ones [6]. Examples of ultra-processed foods include but are not limited to cookies, fizzy drinks, confectionery items, cereal bars, bottled sauces, instant noodles, and sweetened milk-based beverages. Their intake is discouraged, while that of unprocessed or minimally processed foods is encouraged to constitute the core items of the population's diet [1]. Unprocessed (or natural) foods are edible parts of plants (seeds, fruits, leaves, stems, roots) or of animals (muscle, offal, eggs, milk), and also fungi, algae and water, after separation from nature [5]. Minimally processed foods, that together with unprocessed foods make up NOVA group 1 are unprocessed foods altered by industrial processes such as removal of inedible or unwanted parts, drying, crushing, grinding, fractionating, roasting, boiling, pasteurisation, refrigeration, freezing, placing in containers, vacuum packaging or non-alcoholic fermentation. None of these processes add salt, sugar, oils or fats, or other food substances to the original food. Their main aim is to extend the life of grains (cereals), legumes (pulses), vegetables, fruits, nuts, milk, meat and other foods, enabling their storage for longer use, and often to make their preparation easier or more diverse [6].

Despite of what is recommended by official guidelines, people have complex and diversified interpretations about the concept of healthy eating, which reflect their personal, social, cultural, and environmental experiences [7]. The concept of healthy eating is frequently unclear for individuals and is not understood and interpreted identically by all [8]. This can lead to the adoption of different practices in the name of healthy eating [9].

A definitive and universally accepted concept of healthy eating does not exist, but its association with better health and disease prevention is largely recognised [10]. During the second half of the last century, the increased availability and diversity of (un)healthy foods considerably modified the concept of what constitutes a healthy diet [11]. As the focus changed from a nutrient-based approach to a food-based one, food classification systems based on degree of processing were proposed [12]. In this context, the higher the processing degree to which a food has been submitted, the lower is the frequency in which it should be ingested as part of a healthy diet [5].

As ultra-processed foods tend to be energy-dense and low-cost, low energy cost could be one mechanism linking ultra-processed foods with high consumption and consequent negative health outcomes [13]. In Brazil however, the total cost of diets based on natural or minimally processed foods is still lower than the cost of diets based on ultra-processed foods. Relatively expensive perishable foods such as some vegetables, fruits, and fish are and should be consumed with other natural or minimally processed foods that have lower prices, such as rice, beans, potatoes, cassava, and other staple traditional Brazilian foods. Calculations based on Brazilian household budget surveys show that diets based on fresh and minimally processed foods, and dishes and meals made with these foods and culinary ingredients, are cheaper than diets made of ultra-processed foods, as well as being healthier [1].

According to Euromonitor International, Brazilian population's interest in healthy foods has increased between 2009 and 2014 [14]. The health and wellness food sector accounts for a US $35 billion market each year and is expected to grow on average 5% per year until 2021. The 'free from' food category presents the largest growth, stimulated by the increased (but unrelated to dietetic intolerance) consumption of gluten and lactose-free foods [14].

Nutrient-content claims are regulated in Brazil as 'Complementary Nutrition Information' (CNI), defined as 'representations which affirm, suggest or imply that a product has particular nutritional properties especially, but not solely restricted to its energy, protein, fat, carbohydrate and fibre content, and also vitamin and mineral content'. CNIs may refer to absolute or relative/comparative nutrient content of food products using terms as: 'without', 'no', 'absence', 'low content', 'does not contain'; and 'presence', 'contains', 'high content', 'rich', 'source of'. Regulation on parameters for the voluntary display of CNI on front-of-pack (FOP) labels of packaged products exist since 2012 [15], but claims are allowed without consideration for foods' whole nutrient composition or degree of processing. Therefore, an ultra-processed food product containing high levels of sugar and/or sodium may display a nutrient-content claim of 'low fat' or 'vitamin rich' on its label.

Health claims are regulated by a resolution published in 1999 and amended in 2004, which determines that a 'health property claim' is one that affirms, suggests or implies a relationship between the food/ingredient and diseases or health-related conditions [16]. It may also describe a physiological role which assists normal growth, development and functions, and contributes to health maintenance and reduced risk of diet-related disease [16].

Nutrition labelling is designed to help consumers make healthier food choices, provided they understand the vocabulary or layout used to display nutritional information. For this reason, the highlight of positive characteristics in food products by means of nutrient or health claims is regarded as a marketing strategy to promote sales [17], as many are found on unhealthy food items [18]. Claims have the potential to both inform and mislead consumers, depending on the information that is highlighted and the kind of product displaying this information [19]. The highlight of positive characteristics as nutrient claims on front-of-pack labels can generate a 'health halo' effect, when consumers' assessment of a single positive characteristic of the food affects their judgment about the quality of the food as a whole [20]. Health halos can be conferred by claims concerning just one nutrient, because consumers often make generalisations about the overall health of a product based on one piece of information found on labels [21].

Notably, the 'free-from' consumption trend has influenced the content of supermarket circulars. Together with images of products' front-of-pack labels, circulars present products' prices to aid consumers to plan their shopping, but also significantly influencing their shopping decisions. National and regional supermarket chains have started to dedicate whole sections of circulars to the promotion of foods designated by them (possibly together with manufacturers), as health and wellness-enhancing [14].

'Wellness' refers to the positive, subjective state that is opposite to illness [22], an evolving process toward achieving one's full potential [23]. Wellness is positive/affirming and holistic, and encompasses lifestyle, spiritual, and environment wellbeing domains; it also accounts for the physical, mental, and social domains implied in health, and thus health is dependent on sufficient wellness [23]. As consumers today are more health conscious than ever before, and the food and beverage industry is driven by consumer demand and popular trends, the health and wellness trend is increasingly prevalent. Health and wellness foods such as energy bars, gluten and dairy-free products, products containing organic/prebiotic ingredients, and fortified/functional foods are significantly more expensive than the regular offering, which makes them an expensive luxury in many emerging markets [14].

Research on the content of supermarket circulars found that most advertised foods are unhealthy and not conducive to the adoption of a diet in line with official recommendations [24–31]. Studies reported that circular offers did not contribute towards an environment that supports healthy eating behaviour, but most only assessed the products advertised on the front pages and not in the entire circulars. Additionally, they were mostly conducted in European countries, North America, and Australia. Only one study was identified reporting the analysis of Latin American (Brazilian) supermarkets' entire circulars [31].

The situation can mislead consumers and negatively impact their health, as supermarket circulars are reportedly used by consumers as planning tools [32,33], and can predict subsequent memory of the advertised product or brand [34]. Foods advertised in circulars are also further promoted in-store and positioned in strategic places such as end-of-aisle or islands located in places of great circulation, in order to significantly influence shopping decisions [35].

The present study seeks to extend this stream of research focusing on circulars not only advertising novel products or promotions, but dedicating sections specifically to the promotion of as health and wellness-enhancing foods.

To our knowledge, no papers about the quality of products advertised in health and wellness-enhancing sections of supermarket circulars have been published. The aim of this study was to analyse, according to degree of food processing, the quality of foods advertised in the health and wellness-enhancing sections of supermarket circulars from Brazilian supermarkets, and identify presence and type claims on the front-of-pack labels of such products.

2. Materials and Methods

This cross-sectional study was undertaken in the capital city of Santa Catarina state (Florianópolis), southern Brazil. The capital was chosen out of convenience (near the university where the research team works), and also because it is the state's second largest city. The supermarket chains for circulars' collection were defined according to the frequency of circular distribution (fortnightly) and the presence of a specific section advertising health and wellness-enhancing foods. Two supermarket chains (one national and one regional) with stores in the capital distributed circulars with the aforementioned characteristics. Both pertain to the group of 50 companies (national chain: 14th position; regional chain: 44th position) with the highest gross sales (R $2,711,219,166.00 and R $928,708,550.00, national and regional chain, respectively) in 2018 according to the ranking of the Brazilian Association of Supermarkets [36]. The national chain has a total of 29 stores in Brazil, of which six are located in Florianópolis; the regional chain has a total of 22 stores in the state and nine are located in Florianópolis.

To collect the circulars, one store from each chain was conveniently chosen, both located in a residential middle-class neighbourhood near two university campuses. A total of 20 circulars (10 from each chain) were collected in situ or downloaded from the supermarket website, between October 2018 and April 2019, at 15-day intervals. Nineteen printed circulars were retrieved; one circular from the regional chain was only available online. Collection was paused between December and February to avoid the influence of seasonal offers in circulars (Christmas and New Years' holiday season and summer vacation).

All images of products advertised in the health and wellness sections from retrieved circulars were analysed. Different package sizes and shapes of the same product from the same brand were counted as one (e.g., spaghetti and penne pasta). Different flavours of the same food item (e.g., grape juice and orange juice from the same brand) were counted as different items. The same happened to similar products by different brands.

Manufacturers' websites and supermarket stores were then visited to retrieve the ingredient lists of all products (except for unprocessed foods items) in order to proceed with the categorisation according to degree of processing. Foods were categorised into one of four groups as (a) unprocessed and minimally processed foods (U/MP); (b) processed culinary ingredients (PCI); (c) processed foods (P); and (d) ultra-processed foods (UP) (Table S1) [5,6]. A decision flowchart specifically developed to guide the categorisation was used [37]. Whenever the flowchart was not applicable, a conservative criterion [38] was applied (i.e., product categorised in the lower degree of processing).

Products' images on circulars' pages (examples in Figures S1 and S2) were analysed to identify the claims on the 'front-of-pack' (FoP) food labels. Illegible content was further investigated on manufacturers' websites, or in situ at the supermarket stores. Identified claims were further classified as 'Complementary Nutritional Information—CNI' or 'Additional Claims'. CNIs referred to 'reduced amount or absence' and 'increased amount or presence' of determined nutrients and energy value [39]. The terms identified and types of nutrient-content claims are presented in Table 1.

Table 1. Types of claims, terms, and content/nutrients identified as regulated Complementary Nutritional Information—CNI.

Types of Claim	Terms Used	Content/Nutrient
'Reduced amount or absence'	Low, reduced, light, free, very low, not added, zero, 0, 0%	Energy, total fat, saturated fat, trans-fat, cholesterol, sugar, sodium and salt
'Increased amount or presence'	High, rich, with, contains, increased	n-3, n-6, and n-9 fatty acids, proteins, fibre, vitamins and minerals

Reference: elaborated by the authors based on Brazilian Legislation [39].

Claims on FoP labels that did not meet the criteria to be considered CNIs (i.e., 'whole', 'organic', 'healthy', 'natural' [40], were categorised as Additional Claims—AC. In Brazil, legislation determines that the presence of lactose and gluten in foods must be reported in the package labelling section containing the product's ingredient list (usually on the back of the package) [41,42], to alert consumers who are allergic or intolerant. Therefore, the presence of such claims on FoP labels was characterised in the present study as AC.

Due to the large number of different CNIs and ACs identified on FoP labels, they were grouped into similar themes defined by two of the researchers and independently checked by a third researcher. Inconsistencies were discussed and resolved (Table S2).

Information on the description of products was organised in a Microsoft Excel® spreadsheet. Descriptive statistic was used to present data as absolute and relative frequencies, means, standard deviations (SD) or median, interquartile range (IQR) (depending on normality of distribution, assessed with Shapiro-Wilk test). Pearson chi-square test was used to compare the presence of increased and reduced nutrient-content CNIs and ACs in Unprocessed/Minimally Processed vs. Ultra-processed foods. Significance was established at $p < 0.05$. Stata version 13.0 (StataCorp, College Station, TX, USA) was used for data analysis. A post-hoc effect size analysis (w) of Pearson's chi-square tests was conducted with G*power 3.1.9.2 considering an alpha of 0.05 [43].

Review by a Research Ethics Committee was not required for the study, as it did not involve human subjects.

3. Results

3.1. Health and Wellness Food Sections' Characteristics and Degree of Processing of Advertised Food Items

Analysis of the 20 circulars obtained from the two supermarket chains (10 for each chain) led to the identification of 434 food items, with an average number of 21.7 (5.88 SD) foods per health and wellness section. Just over half (51.4%, $n = 223$) of the foods advertised were categorised as ultra-processed, followed by unprocessed/minimally Processed foods at 32.5% ($n = 141$), P foods at 8.7% ($n = 38$), and PCI at 7.4% ($n = 32$).

The three most frequently advertised ultra-processed foods were biscuits (21.1%, $n = 47$), processed cheese (10.8%, $n = 24$), and flavoured yoghurts (8.5%, $n = 19$), followed by vegetable-based beverages, granola, popcorn, ready-to-drink tea, and breads. The three most featured unprocessed/minimally processed food products were fruit juice (15%, $n = 21$), milk (13.6%, $n = 19$), and fish (14%, $n = 10$), followed by tapioca, fresh fruits, and ground coffee.

3.2. Complementary Nutritional Information—Reduced Amount/Absence

A total of 48 different CNIs were identified on the products' FoP labels. From all the foods classified as unprocessed/minimally processed, and ultra-processed, 155 (43%) presented at least one CNI of reduced content or absence. Presence of this type of CNI was significantly higher ($\chi^2 = 28.67$,

$p < 0.001$, effect size = 0.35) in the ultra-processed food group (77%, $n = 120$) when compared with the unprocessed/minimally processed group (23%, $n = 35$). The most frequent CNI of reduced content/absence was about sugar. Only foods from the ultra-processed group presented claims of 'reduced content or absence of saturated fat', 'reduced energy content', and 'light' (Figure 1).

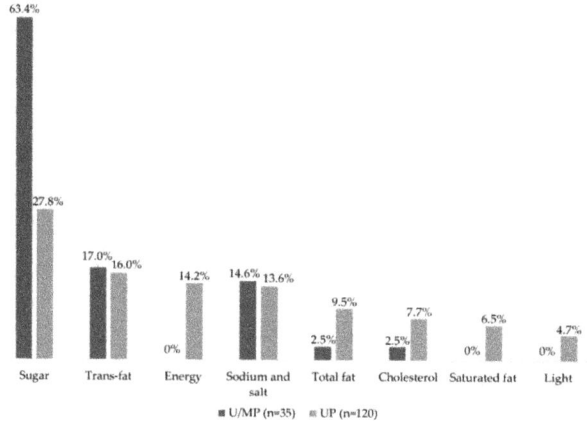

Figure 1. Distribution of Complementary Nutritional Information about 'reduced content' or 'absence' of different nutrients in the analysed products. Legend: U/MP = Unprocessed/Minimally Processed foods. UP = Ultra-processed foods.

3.3. Complementary Nutritional Information—Increased Content/Presence

From the foods classified as unprocessed/minimally processed and ultra-processed, 79 (22%) products presented at least one CNI of increased content or presence of a nutrient. This type of CNI was significantly more common ($\chi^2 = 18.78$, $p < 0.001$, effect size = 0.60) in the ultra-processed food group (82%, $n = 65$) when compared to the unprocessed/minimally processed group (18%, $n = 14$). The most frequent CNI was related to fibre content, which corresponded to more than 50% of the CNIs in both groups (Figure 2).

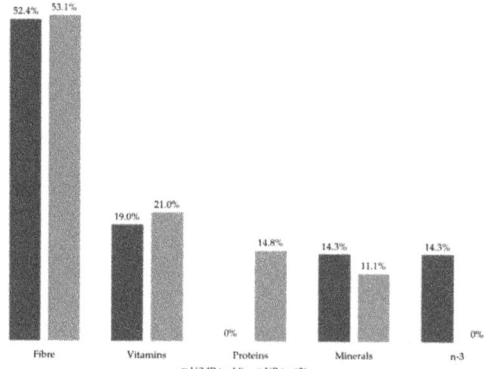

Figure 2. Distribution of Complementary Nutritional Information about 'increased content' or 'presence' of different nutrients in the analysed products. Legend: U/MP = Unprocessed/Minimally Processed foods. UP = Ultra-processed foods.

3.4. Additional Claims

A total of 136 claims classified as Additional Claims were identified on the FoP labels of foods advertised in the circulars. From the foods classified as unprocessed/minimally processed and ultra-processed, 269 (74%) presented at least one AC. The presence of ACs was not statistically different ($\chi^2 = 0.29$, $p = 0.590$) between unprocessed/minimally processed (38%, $n = 102$) and ultra-processed (62%, $n = 167$) groups. In the ultra-processed group, the most frequent ACs were 'whole grain and fibre' (21.7%, $n = 36$), 'free-from' or 'low in lactose' (15.1%, $n = 25$), 'highlight on the presence of ingredients' (10.1%; $n = 17$), and, 'free-from gluten' or 'wheat-free' (9.8%; $n = 16$) (Figure 3).

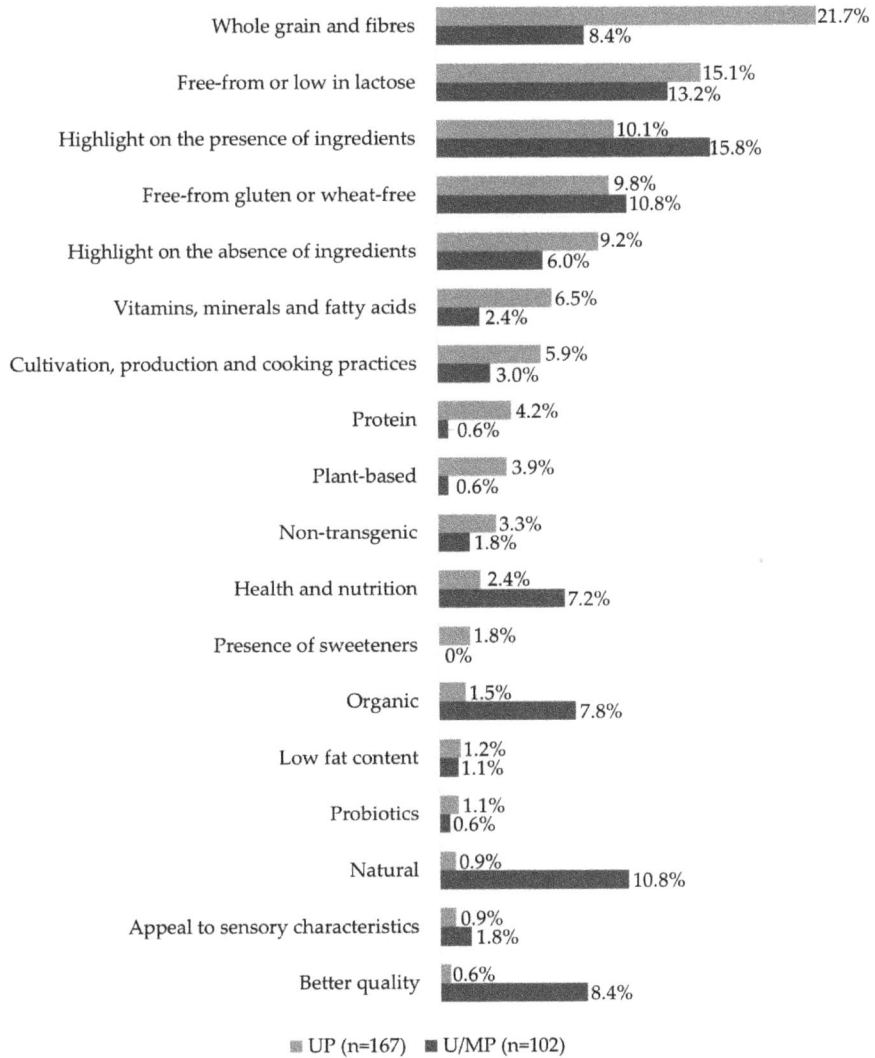

Figure 3. Distribution of Additional Claims in the analysed products, classified by themes (more information available in Supplementary Materials—Table S2). Legend: U/MP = Unprocessed/Minimally Processed foods. UP = Ultra-processed foods.

4. Discussion

This study identified and categorised food products advertised in health and wellness sections of supermarket circulars according to degree of processing, and identified claims on the front-of-pack labels of such products.

Firstly, we found that the most advertised group was of ultra-processed foods. The fact that the present research was limited to the health and wellness sections of supermarket circulars means that such materials may be negatively influencing consumers' food purchases, contributing to the divergence of their diets from the recommendations of the Dietary Guidelines for the Brazilian Population [1]. In Brazilian supermarkets, as in many countries, circulars are made available to consumers online, in-store and also posted into their letter boxes with the intention to promote new products and present special offers [44]. Price affects consumers' choices [45] and most purchases influenced by promotions are unhealthy, as reported in a systematic review [46]. Advertised products are further promoted in-store and positioned in strategic places such as end-of-aisle or islands located in places of great circulation, in order to influence shopping decisions [35]. In addition, circulars are reportedly used by consumers as planning tools [32,33] and can predict subsequent memory of the advertised product or brand [34]. One Brazilian study found that ultra-processed foods were three times more frequently advertised in supermarket circulars than unprocessed/minimally processed foods [31]. Another study analysed circulars from 12 Latin-American countries and reported that in six countries unhealthy foods were more advertised than healthy foods [24]. Our findings are supported by the aforementioned studies about supermarket circulars, but by focusing on the sections dedicated to the promotion of health and wellness-enhancing foods, we extend this stream of research to the phenomenon of increase in the population's interest for healthy foods, reflected in selling strategies [14].

Another important finding was that ultra-processed foods presented significantly more CNIs than unprocessed/minimally processed foods. The most frequent CNIs in ultra-processed food packages were the increased content/presence of fibre and the reduction/absence of sugar. It is quite concerning from a public health point of view that ultra-processed foods are regarded as providers of fibre, because despite fibre content and absence of sugar, other undesirable ingredients such as hydrogenated vegetable fat, modified starch, food additives, artificial sweeteners or other formulations exclusively for industrial use which characterise these foods may also be present. The latter are responsible for increasing the palatability and shelf-life of ultra-processed foods [5,6]. Frequently, the presence of a CNI on labels of ultra-processed foods highlights a positive quality (usually a single nutrient), while negative aspects are not so visibly disclosed. In this sense, CNIs act as advertising strategies to promote sales instead of fulfilling their objective to provide more accessible information to the consumer [17,18]. Additionally, the term 'premium' is often used by the food manufacturing industry to refer to ultra-processed foods that, compared with 'regular' products, contain less 'bad' ingredients such as trans fats, sugar and salt, and more 'good' ingredients such as vitamins, minerals or whole foods such as fruits and nuts. While some of these modifications are positive, others may be harmful, as they will not make these products healthy, but mislead the consumer to think that they are [47]. The influence of nutrient claims on food products' FoP over consumers' perception has been established [48–50]. As Brazil does not have a nutrient profile system in place to evaluate the composition of foods, CNIs that highlight positive qualities of a food (e.g., high fibre content) can mislead the consumer when placed on products whose intake should be limited, such as ultra-processed foods. Brazilian researchers have already suggested that regulations on the use of nutrient claims in products bearing marketing strategies directed to children should be revised, so that only products with appropriate nutrient profiles should be allowed to display nutrient claims [51]. The same can be argued here, where foods advertised as healthy and wellness-enhancing are actually classified as ultra-processed due to their high degree of processing. These findings are cause for concern, as the consumption of ultra-processed foods is associated with higher body mass index and greater prevalence of both excess weight and obesity, as well as other non-communicable diseases [6,52].

Lastly, more than two-thirds of ultra-processed and unprocessed/minimally processed products advertised presented at least one additional claim (AC). Regarding ultra-processed foods, the most frequent ACs identified were related to whole grain, lactose and gluten content. All these claims may induce the consumer to perceive the products as healthier than they are. In spite of the information indeed being relevant to consumers with health issues, the ever-increasing interest by the industry to highlight the absence of lactose and gluten, for example, is not due to increased prevalence of celiac or lactose-intolerant individuals. What informs this strategy is the recent trend in the health and wellness sector to associate the free-from gluten and lactose products with a healthier lifestyle [53,54]. The study by Hartmann et al., (2018) evaluated the effect of free-from labels (including gluten and lactose) on consumers' perception in four European countries, and discovered that consumers evaluated such products in a simplistic way and considered the ones labelled as free-from to be healthier [54]. In another recent study, individuals perceived products labelled as gluten-free as less energy-dense and less processed than similar ones containing gluten [55]. In respect to whole grain products, research revealed that consumers perceive whole grain foods as healthier, and more nutritionally balanced and natural than the refined ones [56] and although the innovative added-fibre to refined grain products may present a solution to increase fibre intakes [57], the mere addition of soluble or insoluble fibre to a product turns it into a ultra-processed food [6]. The ample use of health-related information on food labels and in the media can confuse the consumer [58] and trigger halo effects, in which a consumer thinks a product is healthier than it actually is [59,60] and lead to indulgence when eating them [61,62].

Educational level appears to influence the perception of free-from gluten and lactose products [63], as well as the concern with healthy eating and the practice of unhealthy weight loss strategies [21]. Up to today, no evidence of benefits for healthy individuals to avoid gluten has been obtained, but the idea is so common among certain social strata that the Brazilian Society for Food and Nutrition published a position paper stating that there is no evidence to support the fact that a gluten-free diet would be beneficial for a healthy individual [64]. The benefits attributed by healthy individuals to a lactose-free diet also remain unproven [54].

This study has some limitations. We were able to analyse circulars from only two supermarket chains in the city where the study was conducted, but this was due to the fact that only these two chains featured the health and wellness-enhancing section in their circulars. Additionally, there may be slight differences between circulars from distinct stores from the same chain, but as we collected circulars from only one store from each supermarket chain, we were not able to point those differences out. Regarding the higher presence of CNI of reduced content/absence and of increased content/presence of a nutrient in ultra-processed foods, the results were significant, but with small (0.35) and medium (0.60) effect sizes [65], respectively. Interpretation should be cautious, but amplifying data collection time would most likely not improve size effect as circulars were very similar to each other throughout the months. As we analysed claims present only on the FoP (and not on the other sides of packages) an underestimation of claims may have happened. However, it should be noticed that the FoP is also the first contact the consumer has with products.

To our knowledge, this is the first paper that evaluates the health and wellness-enhancing foods advertised in supermarket circulars. Our findings have important implications to promote healthy eating environments in Brazil. Results highlight to public policy-makers a scenario where food industry places CNIs and additional claims in ultra-processed foods' FoP, which are further promoted by supermarkets as 'healthy' in circulars. Ideally, Brazilian legislation should be revised so that only information truly informing healthy choices to the consumer can be present in FoP labels of products. This is important because using successful advertising practices to promote healthy choices has the potential to enhance the health and well-being of consumers and reduce the expanding healthcare costs [66]. Attention should also be given by health professionals when guiding the population to healthier food choices within the supermarket environment, by disclosing this type of selling strategy.

Further research can be directed at exploring how consumers perceive the advertising of ultra-processed foods in health and wellness-enhancing sections of supermarket circulars and if, how do they shop in these sections. More studies aiming to identify the influence of health claims on FoP over consumer choices are needed, as a systematic review has demonstrated that although those claims are tested in healthy foods, they are mostly used in unhealthy foods [67]. Another potentially interesting area for future research is to investigate whether supermarket circulars in other countries use a similar strategy as in Brazil to promote ultra-processed foods as 'healthy or wellness-enhancing'.

5. Conclusions

Results indicate that supermarket chains included in this study are promoting the sales of ultra-processed foods in the health and wellness-enhancing sections of their promotion circulars. This can lead consumers to inadvertently choose unhealthy foods when trying to adopt a healthy diet, which suggests a need for revision of Brazilian legislation regarding FoP labelling.

Supplementary Materials: The following are available online at http://www.mdpi.com/2072-6643/12/9/2877/s1, Figure S1. Examples of circulars' health and wellness sections (page 1); Figure S2. Examples of circulars' health and wellness sections (page 2); Table S1. NOVA food groups: definition according to the extent and purpose of food processing, and examples; Table S2. Additional Claims (AC) on FoP labels of foods advertised in 'health and wellness' sections of supermarket circulars, classified by themes.

Author Contributions: Conceptualisation, M.D. and G.M.R.F.; data curation, G.M.R.F.; formal analysis, A.M.B., A.M.d.C. and G.B.I.; funding acquisition, M.D. and G.M.R.F.; project administration, M.D. and G.M.R.F.; supervision, K.J.M. and G.M.R.F.; writing—original draft, A.M.B., K.J.M. and G.B.I.; writing—review and editing, A.M.d.C. and M.D. All authors have read and agreed to the published version of the manuscript.

Funding: This work was supported by Newton Mobility Grant Scheme 2015 (Award Reference NG150026 to M.D. and G.M.R.F.), the UK Academies Fellowships Research Mobility, and Young Investigator Awards for UK Researchers in Brazil FAPESC/CONFAP/FUNDO NEWTON (Call N° 02/2017 to M.D. and G.M.R.F.). Coordination for the Improvement of Higher Education Personnel (CAPES) and the National Council for Scientific and Technological Development (CNPq) provided funding in the form of scholarships to A.M.B.; A.M.d.C.; K.J.M. and G.B.I.

Conflicts of Interest: The authors declare no conflict of interest.

References

1. Ministry of Health of Brazil. *Dietary Guidelines for the Brazilian Population*; Ministry of Health of Brazil: Brasilia, Brazil, 2015.
2. De Castro, I.R.R. Challenges and perspectives for the promotion of adequate and healthy food in Brazil. *Cad. Saúde Pública* **2015**, *31*, 7–9. [CrossRef] [PubMed]
3. Martins, A.P.B.; Levy, R.B.; Claro, R.M.; Moubarac, J.C.; Monteiro, C.A.; Martins, A.P.B.; Levy, R.B.; Claro, R.M.; Moubarac, J.C.; Monteiro, C.A. Participacao crescente de produtos ultraprocessados na dieta brasileira (1987–2009). *Revista de Saúde Pública* **2013**, *47*, 656–665. [CrossRef] [PubMed]
4. Louzada, M.L.D.C.; Martins, A.P.B.; Canella, D.S.; Baraldi, L.G.; Levy, R.B.; Claro, R.M.; Moubarac, J.C.; Cannon, G.; Monteiro, C.A. Ultra-processed foods and the nutritional dietary profile in Brazil. *Revista de Saúde Pública* **2015**, *49*. [CrossRef] [PubMed]
5. Monteiro, C.A.; Cannon, G.; Levy, R.; Moubarac, J.-C.; Jaime, P.; Martins, A.P.; Canella, D.; Louzada, M.; Parra, D. NOVA. The star shines bright. *World Nutr.* **2016**, *7*, 28–38.
6. Monteiro, C.A.; Cannon, G.; Levy, R.B.; Moubarac, J.-C.; Louzada, M.L.; Rauber, F.; Khandpur, N.; Cediel, G.; Neri, D.; Martinez-Steele, E.; et al. Ultra-processed foods: What they are and how to identify them. *Public Health Nutr.* **2019**, *22*, 936–941. [CrossRef]
7. Bisogni, C.A.; Jastran, M.; Seligson, M.; Thompson, A. How People Interpret Healthy Eating: Contributions of Qualitative Research. *J. Nutr. Educ. Behav.* **2012**, *44*, 282–301. [CrossRef]
8. Ronteltap, A.; Sijtsema, S.J.; Dagevos, H.; De Winter, M.A. Construal levels of healthy eating. Exploring consumers' interpretation of health in the food context. *Appetite* **2012**, *59*, 333–340. [CrossRef]
9. Ristovski-Slijepcevic, S.; Chapman, G.E.; Beagan, B.L. Engaging with healthy eating discourse(s): Ways of knowing about food and health in three ethnocultural groups in Canada. *Appetite* **2008**, *50*, 167–178. [CrossRef]

10. Temple, N.J. What Is a healthy diet? From nutritional science to food guides. In *Nutrition Guide for Physicians and Related Healthcare Professionals*; Temple, N.J., Wilson, T., Bray, G.A., Eds.; Springer International Publishing: Cham, Switzerland, 2017.
11. Alkerwi, A.A. Diet quality concept. *Nutrition* **2014**, *30*, 613–618. [CrossRef]
12. Moubarac, J.-C.; Parra, D.C.; Cannon, G.; Monteiro, C.A. Food Classification Systems Based on Food Processing: Significance and Implications for Policies and Actions: A Systematic Literature Review and Assessment. *Curr. Obes. Rep.* **2014**, *3*, 256–272. [CrossRef]
13. Gupta, S.; Hawk, T.; Aggarwal, A.; Drewnowski, A. Characterizing Ultra-Processed Foods by Energy Density, Nutrient Density, and Cost. *Front. Nutr.* **2019**, *6*. [CrossRef] [PubMed]
14. Mascaraque, M. Euromonior International, Marketing Research Blog, Top 5 trends shaping Health and Wellness. Available online: https://go.euromonitor.com/white-paper-health-wellness-2019-top-5-trends.html (accessed on 14 January 2020).
15. Ministry of Health of Brazil; Brazilian Health Surveillance Agency. *Resolution–RDC Number 359*; Ministry of Health of Brazil: Brasilia, Brazil, 2003.
16. Ministry of Health of Brazil; Brazilian Health Surveillance Agency. *Resolution–RDC Number 18*; Ministry of Health of Brazil: Brasilia, Brazil, 1999.
17. Nestle, M.; Ludwig, D.S. Front-of-Package Food Labels: Public Health or Propaganda? *JAMA* **2010**, *303*, 771–772. [CrossRef] [PubMed]
18. Colby, S.E.; Johnson, L.; Scheett, A.; Hoverson, B. Nutrition Marketing on Food Labels. *J. Nutr. Educ. Behav.* **2010**, *42*, 92–98. [CrossRef] [PubMed]
19. Campos, S.; Doxey, J.; Hammond, D. Nutrition labels on pre-packaged foods: A systematic review. *Public Health Nutr.* **2011**, *14*, 1496–1506. [CrossRef]
20. Chandon, P. How Package Design and Packaged-based Marketing Claims Lead to Overeating. *Appl. Econ. Perspect. Policy* **2013**, *35*, 7–31. [CrossRef]
21. Christoph, M.J.; Larson, N.; Hootman, K.C.; Miller, J.M.; Neumark-Sztainer, D. Who Values Gluten-Free? Dietary Intake, Behaviors, and Sociodemographic Characteristics of Young Adults Who Value Gluten-Free Food. *J. Acad. Nutr. Diet.* **2018**, *118*, 1389–1398. [CrossRef] [PubMed]
22. Meiselman, H.L. Quality of life, well-being and wellness: Measuring subjective health for foods and other products. *Food Qual. Prefer.* **2016**, *54*, 101–109. [CrossRef]
23. Hetler, B. *Six Dimensions of Wellness*; National Wellness Institute: Stevens Point, WI, USA, 1976.
24. Charlton, E.L.; Kähkönen, L.A.; Sacks, G.; Cameron, A.J. Supermarkets and unhealthy food marketing: An international comparison of the content of supermarket catalogues/circulars. *Prev. Med.* **2015**, *81*, 168–173. [CrossRef]
25. Ravensbergen, E.A.; Waterlander, W.E.; Kroeze, W.; Steenhuis, I.H. Healthy or Unhealthy on Sale? A cross-sectional study on the proportion of healthy and unhealthy foods promoted through flyer advertising by supermarkets in the Netherlands. *BMC Public Health* **2015**, *15*, 470. [CrossRef]
26. Martin-Biggers, J.; Yorkin, M.; Aljallad, C.; Ciecierski, C.; Akhabue, I.; McKinley, J.; Hernandez, K.; Yablonsky, C.; Jackson, R.; Quick, V.; et al. What foods are US supermarkets promoting? A content analysis of supermarket sales circulars. *Appetite* **2013**, *62*, 160–165. [CrossRef]
27. Ethan, D.; Samuel, L.; Basch, C.H. An Analysis of Bronx-based Online Grocery Store Circulars for Nutritional Content of Food and Beverage Products. *J. Community Health* **2013**, *38*, 521–528. [CrossRef] [PubMed]
28. Ethan, D.; Basch, C.H.; Rajan, S.; Samuel, L.; Hammond, R.N. A Comparison of the Nutritional Quality of Food Products Advertised in Grocery Store Circulars of High- versus Low-Income New York City Zip Codes. *Int. J. Environ. Res. Public Health* **2014**, *11*, 537–547. [CrossRef] [PubMed]
29. Cameron, A.J.; Sayers, S.J.; Sacks, G.; Thornton, L.E. Do the foods advertised in Australian supermarket catalogues reflect national dietary guidelines? *Health Promot. Int.* **2017**, *32*, 113–121. [CrossRef] [PubMed]
30. Jahns, L.; Payne, C.R.; Whigham, L.D.; Johnson, L.K.; Scheett, A.J.; Hoverson, B.S.; Kranz, S. Foods advertised in US weekly supermarket sales circulars over one year: A content analysis. *Nutr. J.* **2014**, *13*, 95. [CrossRef]
31. Camargo, A.M.d.; Farias, J.P.d.; Mazzonetto, A.C.; Dean, M.; Fiates, G.M.R. Content of Brazilian supermarket circulars do not reflect national dietary guidelines. *Health Promot. Int.* **2019**. [CrossRef]
32. Bassett, R.; Beagan, B.; Chapman, G.E. Grocery lists: Connecting family, household and grocery store. *Br. Food J.* **2008**. [CrossRef]

33. Cannuscio, C.C.; Hillier, A.; Karpyn, A.; Glanz, K. The social dynamics of healthy food shopping and store choice in an urban environment. *Soc. Sci. Med.* **2014**, *122*, 13–20. [CrossRef]
34. Higgins, E.; Leinenger, M.; Rayner, K. Eye movements when viewing advertisements. *Front. Psychol.* **2014**, *5*. [CrossRef]
35. Hawkes, C. Dietary Implications of Supermarket Development: A Global Perspective. *Dev. Policy Rev.* **2008**, *26*, 657–692. [CrossRef]
36. Associação Brasileira de Supermercadosa-ABRAS, P.- Ranking ABRAS/SuperHiper 2019. Available online: https://www.abras.com.br/clipping.php?area=20&clipping=67764 (accessed on 15 May 2020).
37. Botelho, A.M.; De Camargo, A.M.; Dean, M.; Fiates, G.M.R. Effect of a health reminder on consumers' selection of ultra-processed foods in a supermarket. *Food Qual. Prefer.* **2019**, *71*, 431–437. [CrossRef]
38. Steele, E.M.; Baraldi, L.G.; da Louzada, M.L.; Moubarac, J.-C.; Mozaffarian, D.; Monteiro, C.A. Ultra-processed foods and added sugars in the US diet: Evidence from a nationally representative cross-sectional study. *BMJ Open* **2016**, *6*, e009892. [CrossRef] [PubMed]
39. Ministry of Health of Brazil; Brazilian Health Surveillance Agency. *Resolution–RDC Number 54*; Ministry of Health of Brazil: Brasilia, Brazil, 2012.
40. Rayner, M.; Wood, A.; Lawrence, M.; Mhurchu, C.N.; Albert, J.; Barquera, S.; Friel, S.; Hawkes, C.; Kelly, B.; Kumanyika, S.; et al. Monitoring the health-related labelling of foods and non-alcoholic beverages in retail settings. *Obes. Rev.* **2013**, *14*, 70–81. [CrossRef] [PubMed]
41. Ministry of Health of Brazil; Brazilian Health Surveillance Agency. *Resolution–RDC Number 26*; Ministry of Health of Brazil: Brasilia, Brazil, 2015.
42. Ministry of Health of Brazil; Brazilian Health Surveillance Agency. *Resolution–RDC Number 136*; Ministry of Health of Brazil: Brasilia, Brazil, 2017.
43. Faul, F.; Erdfelder, E.; Lang, A.-G.; Buchner, A. G* Power 3: A flexible statistical power analysis program for the social, behavioral, and biomedical sciences. *Behav. Res. Methods* **2007**, *39*, 175–191. [CrossRef] [PubMed]
44. Miranda, M.J.; Kónya, L. Directing store flyers to the appropriate audience. *J. Retail. Consum. Serv.* **2007**, *14*, 175–181. [CrossRef]
45. Sobal, J.; Bisogni, C.A. Constructing Food Choice Decisions. *Ann. Behav. Med.* **2009**, *38*, s37–s46. [CrossRef] [PubMed]
46. Bennet, R.; Zorbas, C.; Huse, O.; Peeters, A.; Cameron, A.J.; Sacks, G.; Backholer, K. Prevalence of healthy and unhealthy food and beverage price promotions and their potential influence on shopper purchasing behaviour: A systematic review of the literature. *Obes. Rev. Off. J. Int. Assoc. Study Obes.* **2019**, *21*, e12948. [CrossRef]
47. Monteiro, C.A. Nutrition and health. The issue is not food, nor nutrients, so much as processing. *Public Health Nutr.* **2009**, *12*, 729–731. [CrossRef]
48. Talati, Z.; Pettigrew, S.; Hughes, C.; Dixon, H.; Kelly, B.; Ball, K.; Miller, C. The combined effect of front-of-pack nutrition labels and health claims on consumers' evaluation of food products. *Food Qual. Prefer.* **2016**, *53*, 57–65. [CrossRef]
49. Franco-Arellano, B.; Vanderlee, L.; Ahmed, M.; Oh, A.; L'Abbé, M. Influence of front-of-pack labelling and regulated nutrition claims on consumers' perceptions of product healthfulness and purchase intentions: A randomized controlled trial. *Appetite* **2020**, *149*, 104629. [CrossRef]
50. Biondi, B.; Camanzi, L. Nutrition, hedonic or environmental? The effect of front-of-pack messages on consumers' perception and purchase intention of a novel food product with multiple attributes. *Food Res. Int.* **2020**, *130*, 108962. [CrossRef]
51. Rodrigues, V.M.; Rayner, M.; Fernandes, A.C.; De Oliveira, R.C.; Da Costa Proença, R.P.; Fiates, G.M.R. Comparison of the nutritional content of products, with and without nutrient claims, targeted at children in Brazil. *Br. J. Nutr.* **2016**, *115*, 2047–2056. [CrossRef] [PubMed]
52. Rauber, F.; Steele, E.M.; Louzada, M.L.d.C.; Millett, C.; Monteiro, C.A.; Levy, R.B. Ultra-processed food consumption and indicators of obesity in the United Kingdom population (2008–2016). *PLoS ONE* **2020**, *15*. [CrossRef] [PubMed]
53. Strom, S. New York Times. A Big Bet on Gluten-Free. Available online: http://www.nytimes.com/2014/02/18/business/food-industry-wagers-big-on-gluten-free.html?_r=0 (accessed on 17 February 2014).
54. Hartmann, C.; Hieke, S.; Taper, C.; Siegrist, M. European consumer healthiness evaluation of "Free-from" labelled food products. *Food Qual. Prefer.* **2018**, *68*, 377–388. [CrossRef]

55. Prada, M.; Godinho, C.; Rodrigues, D.L.; Lopes, C.; Garrido, M.V. The impact of a gluten-free claim on the perceived healthfulness, calories, level of processing and expected taste of food products. *Food Qual. Prefer.* **2019**, *73*, 284–287. [CrossRef]
56. Arvola, A.; Lähteenmäki, L.; Dean, M.; Vassallo, M.; Winkelmann, M.; Claupein, E.; Saba, A.; Shepherd, R. Consumers' beliefs about whole and refined grain products in the UK, Italy and Finland. *Contrib. Cereals Healthy Diet.* **2007**, *46*, 197–206. [CrossRef]
57. Barrett, E.M.; Foster, S.I.; Beck, E.J. Whole grain and high-fibre grain foods: How do knowledge, perceptions and attitudes affect food choice? *Appetite* **2020**, *149*, 104630. [CrossRef]
58. Benton, D. Portion Size: What We Know and What We Need to Know. *Crit. Rev. Food Sci. Nutr.* **2015**, *55*, 988–1004. [CrossRef]
59. Schuldt, J.P.; Muller, D.; Schwarz, N. The "Fair Trade" Effect: Health Halos from Social Ethics Claims. *Soc. Psychol. Personal. Sci.* **2012**, *3*, 581–589. [CrossRef]
60. Schwartz, M.B.; Just, D.R.; Chriqui, J.F.; Ammerman, A.S. Appetite self-regulation: Environmental and policy influences on eating behaviors. *Obesity* **2017**, *25*, S26–S38. [CrossRef]
61. Chernev, A. The Dieter's Paradox. *J. Consum. Psychol.* **2011**, *21*, 178–183. [CrossRef]
62. Provencher, V.; Polivy, J.; Herman, C.P. Perceived healthiness of food. If it's healthy, you can eat more! *Appetite* **2009**, *52*, 340–344. [CrossRef] [PubMed]
63. Priven, M.; Baum, J.; Vieira, E.; Fung, T.; Herbold, N. The Influence of a Factitious Free-From Food Product Label on Consumer Perceptions of Healthfulness. *J. Acad. Nutr. Diet.* **2015**, *115*, 1808–1814. [CrossRef] [PubMed]
64. Pantaleão, L.C.; Amancio, O.M.S.; Rogero, M.M. Brasilian Society for Food and Nutrition Position Statement: Gluten-free diet. *Nutr. Rev. Soc. Bras. Aliment. Nutr.* **2016**, *41*, 1–4.
65. Cohen, J. *Statistical Power Analysis for the Behavioral Sciences*, 2nd ed.; Lawrence Erlbaum Associates: Mahwah, NJ, USA, 1988.
66. Bublitz, M.G.; Peracchio, L.A. Applying industry practices to promote healthy foods: An exploration of positive marketing outcomes. *J. Bus. Res.* **2015**, *68*, 2484–2493. [CrossRef]
67. Steinhauser, J.; Hamm, U. Consumer and product-specific characteristics influencing the effect of nutrition, health and risk reduction claims on preferences and purchase behavior—A systematic review. *Appetite* **2018**, *127*, 303–323. [CrossRef]

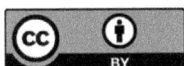

© 2020 by the authors. Licensee MDPI, Basel, Switzerland. This article is an open access article distributed under the terms and conditions of the Creative Commons Attribution (CC BY) license (http://creativecommons.org/licenses/by/4.0/).

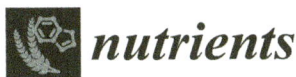

Article

Characteristics of Allergen Labelling and Precautionary Allergen Labelling in Packaged Food Products Available in Latin America

Noé Ontiveros [1], Jesús Aristeo-López Gallardo [2], Jesús Gilberto Arámburo-Gálvez [3], Carlos Eduardo Beltrán-Cárdenas [2], Oscar Gerardo Figueroa-Salcido [3], José Antonio Mora-Melgem [2], Diana María Granda-Restrepo [4], Cecilia Ivonne Rodríguez-Bellegarrigue [5], Marcela de Jesús Vergara-Jiménez [2], Feliznando Isidro Cárdenas-Torres [2], Martina Hilda Gracia-Valenzuela [6,*] and Francisco Cabrera-Chávez [2,*]

[1] Department of Chemical, Biological, and Agricultural Sciences (DC-QB), Division of Sciences and Engineering, Clinical and Research Laboratory (LACIUS, URS), University of Sonora, Navojoa 85880, Sonora, Mexico; noeontiveros@gmail.com

[2] Faculty of Nutrition Sciences, University of Sinaloa, Culiacán 80019, Sinaloa, Mexico; aristeo.lopez37@hotmail.com (J.A.-L.G.); carlos.1.beltran@hotmail.com (C.E.B.-C.); joseantoniomoramelgem@gmail.com (J.A.M.-M.); mjvergara@uas.edu.mx (M.d.J.V.-J.); feliznando@uas.edu.mx (F.I.C.-T.)

[3] Postgraduate in Health Sciences, Division of Biological and Health Sciences, University of Sonora, Hermosillo 83000, Sonora, Mexico; gilberto.aramburo.g@gmail.com (J.G.A.-G.); gerardofs95@hotmail.com (O.G.F.-S.)

[4] Food Department, Faculty of Pharmaceutical and food sciences, University of Antioquia, Antioquia 50010, Medellín, Colombia; diana.granda@udea.edu.co

[5] Luis Edmundo Vasquez School of Health Sciences, Department of Public Health, Dr. José Matías Delgado University, Antiguo Cuscatlán 1502, El Salvador; cirodriguezb@ujmd.edu.sv

[6] Technological Institute of the Yaqui Valley, Bácum 82276, Sonora, Mexico

* Correspondence: mgracia.valenzuela@itvy.edu.mx (M.H.G.-V.); fcabrera@uas.edu.mx (F.C.-C.); Tel.: +52-643-435-7100 (M.H.G.-V.); +52-662-114-6963 (F.C.-C.)

Received: 1 August 2020; Accepted: 30 August 2020; Published: 4 September 2020

Abstract: The characteristics of food allergen labelling are relevant for avoiding accidental exposure to the allergens of interest but no Latin American country has evaluated these characteristics. Our aim was to evaluate the characteristics of food allergen labelling and precautionary allergen labelling (PAL) in six Latin American countries. All data were collected directly from the supermarkets surveyed. A total of 10,254 packaged food products were analyzed, of which 63.3% ($n = 6494$) and 33.2% ($n = 3405$) featured allergen labelling and/or PAL, respectively. Most products complied with local regulations ($\geq 87.4\%$ for both locally produced and imported). Thirty-three types of PAL statements were detected; the most frequent was "may contain traces of … " (35.1%). Countries without regulations on the characteristics of allergen labelling had two-fold more products that contained allergens in their ingredients lists but no food allergen labelling. The use of PAL in countries that regulate it (38.2%) was as high as that in countries without PAL regulations (19.2%–44.7%). The findings suggest that the lack of regulations for the characteristics of allergen labeling increases the risk of accidental exposure to allergens of interest. Our findings also suggest that beyond regulations, a scientific approach is required for minimizing and standardizing the use of PAL.

Keywords: allergen labelling; Latin America; packaged food products

1. Introduction

Food-allergic individuals must avoid the allergen of interest in their diets. Food-allergic reactions can vary from mild symptoms to life-threatening anaphylaxis. Intergovernmental members of the Codex Alimentarius have established mandatory general guidelines for the allergen labelling of packaged food products and countries can adapt these guidelines to their particular needs and regulations [1,2]. Despite this, accidental exposure to the allergen of interest often occur, which sometimes have fatal consequences [3–5]. The prevalence rates of food allergies in children and adults vary between 0.6–10.5% and 3–10%, respectively, but current data suggest that the prevalence of this condition is increasing worldwide [6,7]. This fact represents a challenge for packaged food producers regarding the declaration of allergens. In this context, for allergens used as ingredients in the production of specific foods, allergen labelling must be clear and understandable for the general population and comply with local and overseas regulations for exportation purposes. Conversely, there are no regulations in most countries for packaged food products at risk of cross-contamination with food allergens during the manufacturing process and food producers often use precautionary allergen labelling (PAL) (i.e., "may contain" statements) for filling this gap [8]. Although PAL is not intended to replace allergen risk analysis and management, most food products with PAL do not have detectable levels of the allergen(s) of interest and, therefore, do not represent a risk for the vast majority of food-allergic individuals [9,10]. This fact encourages food-allergic individuals to take the risk of consuming foods with PAL and casts doubts among healthcare professionals about the safe use of foods with PAL in allergen-restricted diets [11–13]. Furthermore, the excessive use of PAL limits the availability of packaged food products for food-allergic individuals and/or parents/caregivers, which could give rise to an additional economic burden [9,12,13]. Developed and emerging countries have evaluated the prevalence and characteristics of food products with PAL [14–16] but in Latin America, no study has addressed either the characteristics of food allergen labelling or PAL. Regulations for food allergen labelling can vary from country to country, with the characteristics of the label and the list of allergens declared on it representing the main sources of variation [2]. The Latin American region has particular characteristics in trade, including food products. There are three major trade blocs in Latin America: the Common Market of the South (MERCOSUR) (encompassing Argentina, Brazil, Paraguay, Uruguay, and Venezuela), the Pacific Alliance (encompassing Chile, Colombia, México, and Peru), and the Secretariat for Central American Economic Integration (SIECA) (encompassing Costa Rica, Guatemala, Honduras, El Salvador, Nicaragua, and Panama) but the harmonization of food regulations remains debated [8,17]. Furthermore, although most Latin American countries regulate the allergens to be declared, the characteristics of food allergen labelling are not regulated in some countries such as México, Panamá, and Colombia, and only Argentina, Brazil, and Chile have regulated the use of PAL [17–20]. Thus, the aim of the present study was to evaluate the characteristics of food allergen labelling and PAL in six Latin American countries.

2. Materials and Methods

2.1. Survey and Data Collection

Cluster sampling was carried out from January to December 2019. Supermarkets were chosen based on information available online and the suggestions of local citizens. At least one local and one multinational supermarket featuring a flow of consumers with different socioeconomic statuses were included in the survey. Three supermarkets were sampled in Culiacán and three in Mexico City (México, North America), three in San Salvador (El Salvador), four in Panama City (Panamá, Central America), four in Medellín (Colombia), three in Quito (Ecuador), and four in Buenos Aires (Argentina, South America). The sample size consisted of all the packaged food products available on the shelves at the time of the survey. For products with multiple package sizes, only one size was included in the analysis to avoid bias [14]. Duplicate products found across the supermarkets in each country were recorded only once. Information was captured via digital images that covered the brands and name of the products as well as ingredients and details of allergen labelling, PAL (when available), and place of manufacture [15]. All images were verified twice to corroborate the match between the label captions and products. The information extracted from the images consisted of the following: product brand and name, place of manufacture, ingredients, food allergen declaration, typography (bold, italics, highlighted, colored, etc.), and PAL statements.

2.2. Food Categories and Allergens

Food products were categorized into twelve groups: baked goods, snacks, confectionaries, baby foods, condiments and sauces, jams and spreads, beverages, powders and pastes, instant foods, chilled and frozen foods, canned foods, and packaged raw foods [15]. The food allergens considered by the Codex Alimentarius guidelines were the focus of the present study (milk and its derivates, egg, soy, wheat, and other cereals containing gluten, peanuts, nuts, fish, and crustaceans) [1].

2.3. Compliance with the Regulations for the Characteristics of Food Allergen Labelling

Both local and imported packaged food products were verified for their compliance with local regulations for the characteristics of allergen labelling regulations or Codex Alimentarius guidelines for this purpose. The following characteristics were verified: for Argentina, allergen labelling statements with the legend "contains . . . " and the use of special typography (capital letters, bold letters, or different colors than the label) as well as the place where the allergen labelling statement appeared on the packaging [18]; for Ecuador, allergen labelling statements with the legend "contains . . . ", the use of capital letters, and the place where the allergen labelling statement appeared on the packaging [21]; for El Salvador, the allergen labelling statement with any legend, the use of any special typography to highlight the allergen labelling statement, and the place where the allergen labelling statement appeared on the packaging [22]; for Colombia, México, and Panamá, the allergen labelling statement with any allergen labelling statement and typography [1,23,24]. Regardless of whether the products featured food allergen labelling, all ingredient lists were inspected to verify that they did not include undeclared allergens, i.e., products without food allergen labelling but containing allergens as ingredients were also recorded. The analyses of compliance with local regulations for the characteristics of food allergen labelling only included products with food allergen labelling.

2.4. Frequency of Food Allergen Labelling, PAL, and the Type of PAL

All products were examined for corroborating the presence of either food-allergic labelling or PAL or both types of allergen labelling. Independently, if the food allergen was declared in the list of ingredients (or not), the products were examined for the presence of PAL. All types of PAL were included in the study.

2.5. Data Analysis

Descriptive statistics was used and the results are shown as percentages. Confidence intervals were calculated (95%) using the OpenEpi software version 3.01.

3. Results

3.1. Frequency of Food Allergen Labelling in Packaged Food Products

Twenty-four supermarkets from six countries (seven cities) were sampled. In total, 10,254 packaged food product labels were analyzed: 71.1% of the products ($n = 7288$; 95% CI, 70.19–71.95) had food allergen labelling and/or PAL. Most of the products without food allergen labelling or PAL were naturally allergen-free products such as chips, juices, rice cookies, and packaged raw food among others (67.70%; $n = 2008/2966$; 95% CI, 65.98–69.38), while 63.3% ($n = 6494$; 95% CI, 62.39–64.26) of the products featured food allergen labelling (Figure 1). Panamá and Argentina had the lowest ($n = 922$; 52.71%) and the highest ($n = 903$; 71.66%) percentages of products with food allergen labelling, respectively (Figure 1A). The most commonly declared allergens were milk, including its derivatives (n = 3397; 52.32%); wheat and other cereals containing gluten (n = 3335; 51.36%); and soybean, including its derivatives (n = 2696; 41.52%) (Figure 1B). The less frequently declared food allergens were fish and crustaceans (n = 220; 3.38% and n = 58; 0.90%, respectively) (Figure 1B). The most frequent statements used for food allergen labelling were "contains … " (87.2%) followed by "this product contains … " (4.6%), "Allergens: contains … " (2.9%), and "contains ingredients from … " (2.8%) (Figure 1C). The most commonly used typography for allergen labelling statements was bold letters (70.52%), in either lower case or capital letters, and capital letters without bold typography (58.3%) (Figure 1D).

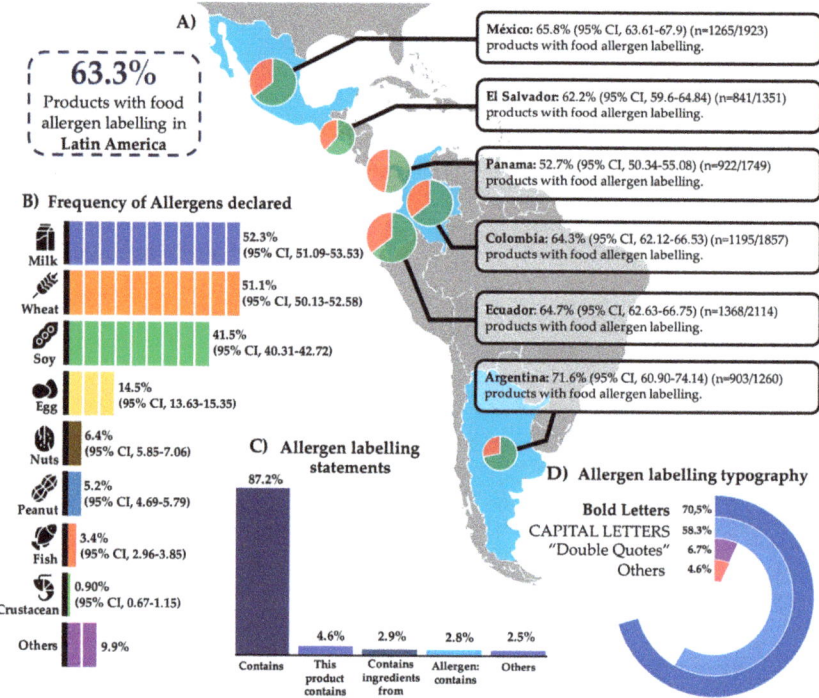

Figure 1. Percentage of products with food allergen labelling and the characteristics of the labelling in commercially available packaged food products in six Latin American countries. (**A**): Percentage of products with food allergen labelling by country (in pie charts: green and red sections; proportions of products with or without food allergen labelling, respectively); (**B**): Percentage of food allergens declared in food allergen labelling; (**C**): Statements used for food allergen labelling; (**D**): Typography used for food allergen labelling (the summation of percentages is greater than 100% due to the use of two or more typographical characteristics in combination).

3.2. Compliance with Local Regulations for the Characteristics of Food Allergen Labelling

Most packaged foods with food allergen labelling were compliant with the local regulations for this purpose (91.0%, n = 5909/6494). Beverages (95.3%), snacks (93.1%), and packaged raw food (92.7%) were the food categories that featured the best compliance with local regulations (Figure 2). The category of baby foods was non-compliant with local regulations to a greater extent than the other categories (15.2%) and was one of the categories with the lowest percentage of allergen labelling (52.27%) (Figure 2). For local or imported food products, 90.67% (range: 77.44%–97.11%) and 87.44% (range: 74.39%–97.92%) of locally produced and imported products complied with local regulations, respectively (Table 1). In total, 6494 products had food allergen labelling and 585 of them (9.0%) were in non-compliance with local regulations. Of these 585 products, 263 (45.0%) had undisclosed allergens in their food allergen labelling, 295 (50.4%) did not use the proper allergen labelling typography, and 76 products (13.0%) used an allergen labelling statement other than those enforced by local regulations (Supplementary Material Table S1). El Salvador, Ecuador, and Argentina were the countries with the highest proportions of products in non-compliance with local regulations (22.00%, 11.47%, and 8.30%, respectively), followed by México, Colombia, and Panamá (6.24%, 5.77%, and 2.16%, respectively) (Table 1). Countries with the highest proportions of products without food allergen labelling but containing allergens as ingredients were Panamá (36.15%, n = 299), Colombia (35.64%, n = 236), and México (35.10%, n = 231), followed by El Salvador (32.74%, n = 167), Argentina (22.12%, n = 79), and Ecuador (15.81%, n = 118) (Table 1). The number of products without food allergen labelling but containing allergens as ingredients was more than two-fold higher, on average, in Colombia, Panamá, and México than in Argentina, Ecuador, and El Salvador (766 vs. 364, respectively) (Table 1). On average, this means that for every 5.7 (1130 out of 6494) products with allergen labelling, there is one product without food allergen labelling but containing allergens as an ingredient in the Latin American countries included in the survey (Table 1).

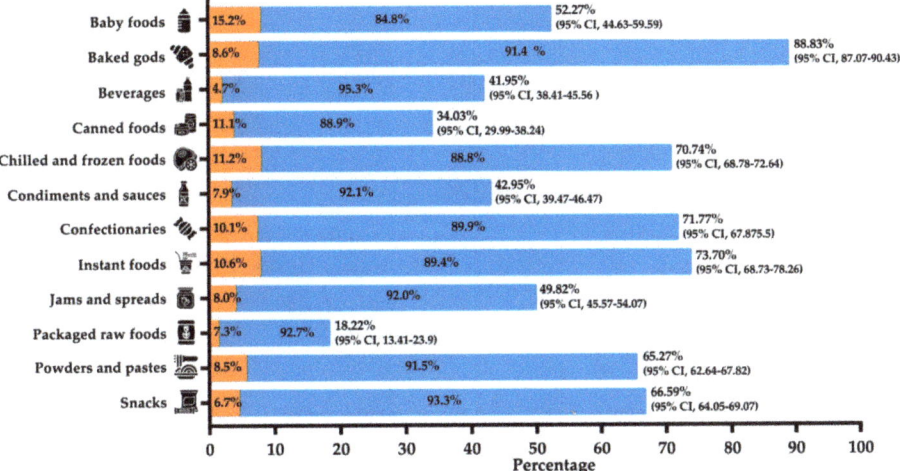

Figure 2. Compliance and non-compliance with local regulations for the characteristics of food allergen labelling by food category. Percentages in orange bars (■): frequency of non-compliance of food products with local regulations for food allergen labelling; Percentages in blue bars (■): frequency of products in compliance with local regulations for food allergen labelling. Percentages at the tops of the bars correspond to the percentages of packaged foods with food allergen labelling.

Table 1. Compliance and non-compliance with local regulations for the characteristics of food allergen labelling.

		Argentina (n = 1260)	Colombia (n = 1857)	Ecuador (n = 2114)	El Salvador (n = 1351)	México (n = 1923)	Panamá (n = 1749)	Total (n = 10,254)
Food allergen labelling	% (n)	71.66 (903)	64.35 (1195)	64.71 (1368)	62.25 (841)	65.78 (1265)	52.71 (922)	63.33 (6494)
	95% CI	69.12–74.09	62.15–66.5	62.65–66.72	59.63–64.8	63.63–67.87	50.37–55.05	62.39–64.26
Compliance with the local regulations	% (n)	91.69 (828)	94.22 (1126)	88.52 (1211)	78.0 (656)	93.75 (1186)	97.83 (902)	90.99 (5909)
	95% CI	89.71–93.32	92.76–95.41	86.73–90.11	75.08–80.67	92.28–94.96	96.67–98.59	90.27–91.66
Non-compliance with the local regulations	% (n)	8.30 (75)	5.77 (69)	11.47 (157)	22.0 (185)	6.24 (79)	2.16 (20)	9.01 (585)
	95% CI	6.67–10.29	4.58–7.24	9.89–13.27	19.33–24.92	5.04–7.71	1.40–3.32	8.33–9.72
No Food allergen labelling	% (n)	28.33 (357)	35.64 (662)	35.28 (746)	37.74 (510)	34.21 (658)	47.28 (827)	36.66 (3760)
	95% CI	25.91–30.88	33.50–37.85	33.28–37.35	35.20–40.37	32.13.36.37	44.95–49.63	35.74–37.61
No Food allergen labelling but allergens in ingredient list	% (n)	22.12 (79)	35.64 (236)	15.81 (118)	32.74 (167)	35.10 (231)	36.15 (299)	30.05 (1130)
	95% CI	18.13–26.72	32.09–39.37	13.38–18.61	28.81–36.93	31.56–38.83	32.95–39.49	28.61–31.54

3.3. Frequency and Characteristics of PAL

The proportion of products with PAL was 33.2% (n = 3405/10,254; 95% CI, 32.29–34.13). This accounts for 46.7% of the total of products with food allergen labelling and/or PAL (3405/7288). PAL was identified in 58.8% (n = 827) of the baked goods, 55.37% (n = 304) of confectionaries, and 47.84% (n = 666) of snacks (Figure 3A). PAL was identified in only 8.5% (n = 45) of the canned foods category (Figure 3A). The most frequently used PAL statements were "may contain traces of . . . " (n= 1195; 35.01%), "may contain . . . " (n = 1004; 29.5%), and "made in plant that processes . . . " (n = 261; 7.7%) (Figure 3B). Thirty more PAL statements were identified in 28.60% (n = 974) of the products evaluated (Table S1). Some products declared two different types of PAL (0.9%; n = 31). The most commonly declared allergens in PAL were nuts (n = 1549; 45.5%), soy (n = 1466; 43%), and milk (n = 1423; 41.8%) (Figure 3B). On average, PAL was identified in 23.6% (n = 622) of naturally allergen-free food products and in 25.5% (n = 2611) of products with food allergen labelling. Ecuador (19.2%; n = 407), Panamá (24.9%; n = 436), and El Salvador (31.7%; n = 428) had the lowest percentages of products with PAL and Argentina (38.2; n = 482), México (42.7%; n = 822), and Colombia (44.7%; n = 482) had the highest percentages.

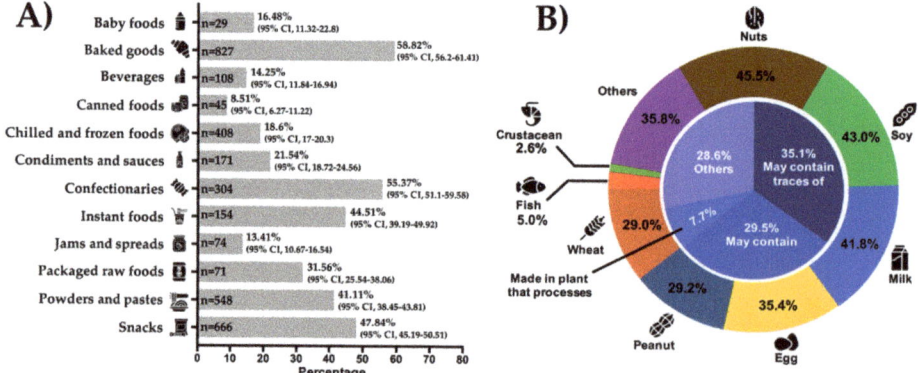

Figure 3. Percentages of packaged foods with precautionary allergen labelling (PAL) and the most frequent types of PAL. (**A**): frequencies of products with PAL by food categories; (**B**): pie center: most frequently used types of PAL in packaged foods; pie periphery: most frequently declared food allergens in PAL (The summation of percentages is more than 100% due to a combination of two or more allergens in PAL).

4. Discussion

The correct allergen labelling of food products is essential to minimize accidental exposure to the allergens of interest among food-allergic individuals and to ameliorate the socioeconomic burden associated with this condition. In the present study, the characteristics of the food allergen labelling and PAL of products available in six Latin American countries were analyzed. The results show that, independently of the country sampled, at least one in two packaged food products available on the shelves of the main supermarkets featured food allergen labelling. This illustrates that food-allergic individuals should analyze the labels of each packaged food product that they choose to buy for the first time or analyze such labels regularly to ensure that food producers have not changed their ingredients or manufacturing processes. Consequently, food-allergic individuals will spend additional time buying foods at the supermarket because they have to identify suitable foods. This extra time can be 39% greater than the time spent by non-food-allergic individuals [9]. The most commonly declared food allergens in the six Latin American counties surveyed were the eight foods considered for allergen labelling in the Codex Alimentarius guidelines (milk, wheat, soy, egg, nuts, peanuts, fish, and crustaceans) [1]. These major food allergens declared in the allergen labelling analyzed were reported to be the main triggers of immediate-type food allergy symptoms by the parents of 11,277 Latin American children with different nationalities [25–28]. Certainly, as per the opinions of others [17], the scientific evidence is still insufficient to state that food allergens other than those considered by the Codex Alimentarius guidelines should be added to the food allergen labelling regulations in Latin American countries. The method for stating food allergens in allergen labelling is important to avoid misinterpretations and to easily identify the presence of the allergen of interest. In the present study, the most common allergen labelling statements were "contains", "this product contains", "contains ingredients from", and "allergen: contains", either in bold or capital letters or a combination of these typographies. These results are consistent with the current regulations of Argentina and Ecuador, which enforce the use of the statement "contains" in capital letters (Ecuador) or special typography (capital letters, bold letters, or different colors than the label (Argentina) [18,21]. Although previous studies highlighted that using symbols in combination with word-based allergen labelling statements can be more effective for communicating with food-allergic individuals than using word-based labelling only [29,30], no Latin American regulations for food allergen labelling enforce the use of symbols for such a purpose. The use of symbols in food allergen labelling could, perhaps, reduce the extra time that food-allergic individuals spend identifying suitable foods.

Regulations for food allergen labelling are mainly intended to protect food-allergic individuals from accidental exposure to the allergen of interest and establish the characteristics of the labels. Non-compliance with local regulations entails sanctions ranging from financial penalties to partial or total closure of the responsible company. In general, 91.0% of the food allergen labelling analyzed complied with local regulations. The food category of baked goods had the highest percentage of allergen labelling (88.8%) and was also one of the food categories with the highest and lowest percentages of compliance (91.4%) and non-compliance (8.6%) with local regulations for allergen labelling. Wheat is the major allergenic ingredient in most conventional formulations of baked goods so its declaration in food allergen labelling is mandatory across all Latin American countries [17]. Furthermore, wheat-based baked goods trigger symptoms not only in wheat-allergic individuals but also in some individuals with celiac disease or irritable bowel syndrome as well as in all those with non-celiac gluten sensitivity [31]. Conversely, baby food was one of the categories with the lowest percentage of allergen labelling (52.3%). Most of the baby foods without allergen labelling had no allergens in their ingredient lists but 6.52% of them had undisclosed allergens. This is intriguing because the target population of these foods is particularly vulnerable for developing food allergies [31]. Although food allergen labelling regulations can vary from one country to another, on average, the percentages of locally produced (90.7%) and imported (87.4%) packaged foods that complied with local food allergen labelling regulations were quite similar. This suggests that beyond differences in country to country regulations, most packaged food products comply with the local food allergen labelling regulations where they are sold. Argentina, Ecuador, and El Salvador established the typography to be used for the food allergen labelling statement and the place where the statement has to be located on the food packaging, with differences in typography between Ecuador and the other two countries [18,21,22]. Furthermore, Argentina and Ecuador have regulated the use of "contains" as their allergen labelling statement [18,22]. Colombia and México have also established food allergen labelling regulations but the allergen labelling statement, typography of the statement, and place where the statement has to be located on the food packaging remain to be established [23,24]. Panamá has not yet established regulations for food labelling [17] but the Codex Alimentarius guidelines are enforced [32,33]. As expected, the countries with "weak" allergen labelling regulations (Colombia, México, and Panamá) had the highest percentage (92.2%, on average) of packaged food products that complied with local allergen labelling regulations. Although this compliance could facilitate the trading of foods among countries, it could also have serious consequences for food-allergic individuals. In this context, our findings show that some products without allergen labelling contained allergens as ingredients and that, on average, the number of products with this peculiarity was two-fold higher in countries that have not yet established the characteristics for their food allergen labelling statements compared with those that have already done so (766 vs. 364). Thus, the risk of choosing a food product at the supermarket without allergen labelling when that food contains allergens is two-fold higher in countries that have not yet regulated the characteristics for food allergen labelling. Others have reported undisclosed allergens in packaged food products using analytical methods [34–36]. Overall, our results suggest that regulations should consider all the characteristics of food allergen labelling to avoid putting food-allergic individuals at increased risk of accidental exposure to their allergens of interest.

PAL is used in food products at the risk of cross-contamination with food allergens during the manufacturing process but there are no regulations for its use in most countries. The present study shows that PAL is widely used in Latin America (33.2% of food products) and that even the proportion of naturally allergen-free products with PAL is considerable (23.6%). Others have reported similar percentages of PAL (28.6%–39.9%) [14,15,37] or even higher (65%) [38]. The PAL statement "may contain traces of ... " was the most commonly utilized statement, which agrees with other studies [15,38] but 32 other types of PAL were also identified in the present study. It should be noted that PAL generates anxiety and confusion among food-allergic individuals and/or parents/caregivers [39] as its excessive use could contribute to increasing the socioeconomic disease burden [12]. Furthermore, both healthcare professionals and food-allergic individuals are facing a dilemma regarding what to do with PAL products [11–13] as most food products with PAL have undetectable levels of allergens and are not risky for most food-allergic individuals [9,10]. Argentina had one of the highest percentage of products with PAL (38.2%) although this country was also the only one that has regulated the use of PAL among the countries surveyed [9,18]. These findings suggest that the regulation of PAL may not be enough to limit its use or to ameliorate the negative impact that the excessive use of PAL has on food-allergic individuals and/or their parents/caregivers. In addition to Argentina, other countries such as South Africa, Brazil, and Chile have regulated the use of PAL. Legislation in these countries allows the use of PAL as long as its use is substantiated by a documented risk assessment demonstrating adherence to good manufacturing practices [9,19,20]. Alternatively, a scientific approach called voluntary incidental trace allergen labelling (VITAL) was developed by the Australian manufacturing industry in 2007 [39]. This approach is based on the reference doses (thresholds) for specific allergens [12,40]. An allergen dose that is likely to trigger allergic reactions in 1% or 5% of the food-allergic population is called ED01 or ED05, respectively [12]. This promising proposal has not been yet endorsed by public health agencies [12] but it seems to have the approval of the majority of the scientific community. Undoubtedly, the endorsement of VITAL by public health agencies, its regulation by countries, and its implementation by food producers will strongly contribute to ameliorating the socioeconomic burden of food allergies and solving the dilemma on how to govern foods products with PAL.

The main strengths of the study are its large number of labels analyzed and its inclusion of countries with different regulations for the characteristics of food allergen labelling including a country that has regulated the use of PAL. These strengths allowed us to draw deeper conclusions than previous studies that have been carried out in only one country. The main limitations of this study include not addressing consumer understandings, perceptions, and interpretations of food allergen labelling and the lack of laboratory tests for confirming the presence or absence of food allergens in products with PAL or in products without food allergen labelling but containing allergens as ingredients. Despite these limitations, the present study provides groundwork for future studies based on immunological methods for detecting food allergens in packaged food products and increases our knowledge about the characteristics of food allergen labelling in the Latin American region.

5. Conclusions

This is the first study carried out in Latin America to evaluate the characteristics of food allergen labelling in commercially available packaged foods. The packaged food products available with food allergen labelling accounted for 63.3% and the vast majority of those products, both locally produced and imported, complied with local regulations. The countries (Colombia, México, and Panamá) that have not yet regulated the characteristics of their food allergen labelling had more than two-fold greater number of products without labelling when those products contained allergens as ingredients compared with the countries that have already done so (Argentina, Ecuador, and El Salvador), putting their food-allergic populations at increased risk of accidental exposure to their allergens of interest. The use of PAL was high in all of the countries surveyed including one country that has regulated the use of PAL. Furthermore, there were many types of PAL (33), with the most common being "may contain traces of ... ". Additional strategies for PAL regulations should be implemented to minimize and standardize the use of PAL.

Supplementary Materials: The following are available online at http://www.mdpi.com/2072-6643/12/9/2698/s1, Table S1: Variations of precautionary allergen labelling (PAL).

Author Contributions: Conceptualization, N.O. and F.C.-C.; methodology, D.M.G.-R., C.I.R.-B., and M.H.G.-V.; formal analysis, J.A.-L.G., J.G.A.-G., C.E.B.-C., O.G.F.-S., J.A.M.-M., F.I.C.-T., and M.d.J.V.-J.; investigation, J.A.-L.G., D.M.G.-R., and C.I.R.-B.; resources, N.O., F.C.-C., D.M.G.-R., and C.I.R.-B.; data curation, J.A.-L.G., J.G.A.-G., C.E.B.-C., O.G.F.-S., J.A.M.-M., and F.I.C.-T.; writing—original draft preparation, N.O., F.C.-C., and J.A.-L.G.; writing—review and editing, M.d.J.V.-J. and M.H.G.-V.; supervision, D.M.G.-R. and C.I.R.-B.; project administration, N.O. and F.C.C. All authors have read and agreed to the published version of the manuscript.

Funding: This research received no external funding.

Acknowledgments: The authors wish to thank CONACyT for the post-graduate fellowship given to J.A.L.-G. and J.G.A.-G., as well as INAPI Sinaloa (Young Scientific Talents, 2019 program) for the financial support given to C.E.B.-C. and J.A.L.-G.

Conflicts of Interest: The authors declare no conflict of interest.

References

1. Codex Alimentarius Commission Joint FAO/WHO Food Standards Programme World Health Organization. *Codex Alimentarius Commission: Procedural Manual*; Food & Agriculture Org.: Rome, Italy, 2007.
2. Gendel, S.M. Comparison of international food allergen labeling regulations. *Regul. Toxicol. Pharmacol.* **2012**, *63*, 279–285. [CrossRef]
3. Dorris, S. Fatal food anaphylaxis: Registering a rare outcome. *Ann. Allergy Asthma Immunol.* **2020**, *124*, 445–446. [CrossRef] [PubMed]
4. Muñoz-Furlong, A.; Weiss, C.C. Characteristics of food-allergic patients placing them at risk for a fatal anaphylactic episode. *Curr. Allergy Asthma Rep.* **2009**, *9*, 57–63. [CrossRef] [PubMed]
5. Poirot, E.; He, F.; Gould, L.H.; Hadler, J.L. Deaths, hospitalizations, and emergency department visits from food-related anaphylaxis, New York city, 2000–2014: Implications for fatality prevention. *J. Public Health Manag. Pract.* **2020**. [CrossRef] [PubMed]

6. Jiang, J.; Warren, C.M.; Gupta, R.S. Epidemiology and racial/ethnic differences in food Allergy. In *Pediatric Food Allergy*; Springer: Cham, Switzerland, 2020; pp. 3–16.
7. Messina, M.; Venter, C. Recent surveys on food allergy prevalence. *Nutr. Today* **2020**, *55*, 22–29. [CrossRef]
8. de Kock, T.; van Niekerk, E.; Steinman, H. Precautionary allergy labelling: 'may contain' some weaknesses but 'contains' great opportunities: Literature review. *Curr. Allergy Clin. Immunol.* **2020**, *33*, 18–22.
9. Allen, K.J.; Turner, P.J.; Pawankar, R.; Taylor, S.; Sicherer, S.; Lack, G.; Rosario, N.; Ebisawa, M.; Wong, G.; Mills, E.C. Precautionary labelling of foods for allergen content: Are we ready for a global framework? *World Allergy Organ. J.* **2014**, *7*, 1–14. [CrossRef]
10. DunnGalvin, A.; Chan, C.H.; Crevel, R.; Grimshaw, K.; Poms, R.; Schnadt, S.; Taylor, S.; Turner, P.; Allen, K.; Austin, M. Precautionary allergen labelling: Perspectives from key stakeholder groups. *Allergy* **2015**, *70*, 1039–1051. [CrossRef]
11. Allen, K.J.; Taylor, S.L. The consequences of precautionary allergen labeling: Safe haven or unjustifiable burden? *J. Allergy Clin. Immunol. Pract.* **2018**, *6*, 400–407. [CrossRef]
12. Graham, F.; Caubet, J.C.; Eigenmann, P.A. Can my child with IgE-mediated peanut allergy introduce foods labeled with "may contain traces"? *Pediatr. Allergy Immunol.* **2020**. [CrossRef]
13. Turner, P.J.; Skypala, I.J.; Fox, A.T. Advice provided by health professionals regarding precautionary allergen labelling. *Pediatr. Allergy Immunol.* **2014**, *25*, 290–292. [CrossRef] [PubMed]
14. Battisti, C.; Chambefort, A.; Digaud, O.; Duplessis, B.; Perrin, C.; Volatier, J.L.; Gauvreau-Béziat, J.; Menard, C. Allergens labeling on French processed foods—An Oqali study. *Food Sci. Nutr.* **2017**, *5*, 881–888. [CrossRef] [PubMed]
15. Soon, J.M. Food allergen labelling:"May contain" evidence from Malaysia. *Food Res. Int.* **2018**, *108*, 455–464. [CrossRef] [PubMed]
16. Zurzolo, G.A.; Mathai, M.L.; Koplin, J.J.; Allen, K.J. Precautionary allergen labelling following new labelling practice in Australia. *J. Paediatr. Child Health* **2013**, *49*, E306–E310. [CrossRef]
17. Lopez, M.C. Food allergen labeling: A Latin American approach. *J. AOAC Int.* **2018**, *101*, 14–16. [CrossRef]
18. Código Alimentario Argentino Capítulo V: Normas Para La Rotulación y Publicidad De Los Alimentos. Available online: http://www.anmat.gov.ar/alimentos/normativas_alimentos_caa.asp (accessed on 17 August 2020).
19. Ministerio De Salud. Republica De Chile. Reglamento Sanitario De Los Alimentos. Available online: http://extwprlegs1.fao.org/docs/pdf/chi9315.pdf (accessed on 17 August 2020).
20. Agência Nacional de Vigilância Sanitária. Aprova o Regulamento Técnico sobre Rotulagem de Alimentos Embalados. Available online: http://grupobeteanblog.com/wp-content/uploads/2015/09/RDC_259.pdf (accessed on 17 August 2020).
21. Instituto Ecuatoriano De Normalización, Norma Técnica Ecuatoriana 1334-1: 2011. Rotulado De Productos Alimenticios Para Consumo Humano. Available online: https://www.controlsanitario.gob.ec/wp-content/uploads/downloads/2014/07/ec.nte_.1334.1.2011.pdf (accessed on 17 August 2020).
22. Reglamento Técnico Centroamericano. Etiquetado General de Alimentos Previamente Envasados. Available online: http://asp.salud.gob.sv/regulacion/pdf/rtca/rtca_67_01_07_10_etiquetado_general_alimentos_preenvasados.pdf (accessed on 17 August 2020).
23. Norma Oficial Mexicana Nom-051-Scfi/Ssa1-2010, Especificaciones Generales De Etiquetado Para Alimentos Y Bebidas No Alcoholicas Preenvasados-Informacion Comercial Y Sanitaria. Available online: https://www.dof.gob.mx/2020/SEECO/NOM_051.pdf (accessed on 17 August 2020).
24. Ministerio de la Protección Social. Resolucion Numero 005109 De 2005. Available online: https://fenavi.org/wp-content/uploads/2019/02/Resolucion_5109-2005.pdf (accessed on 17 August 2020).
25. Cabrera-Chávez, F.; Rodríguez-Bellegarrigue, C.I.; Figueroa-Salcido, O.G.; Lopez-Gallardo, J.A.; Arámburo-Gálvez, J.G.; Vergara-Jiménez, M.d.J.; Castro-Acosta, M.L.; Sotelo-Cruz, N.; Gracia-Valenzuela, M.H.; Ontiveros, N. Food allergy prevalence in Salvadoran schoolchildren estimated by parent-report. *Int. J. Environ. Res. Public Health* **2018**, *15*, 2446. [CrossRef]
26. Gonçalves, L.; Guimarães, T.; Silva, R.; Cheik, M.; de Ramos Napolis, A.; e Silva, G.B.; Segundo, G. Prevalence of food allergy in infants and pre-schoolers in Brazil. *Allergol. Immunopathol.* **2016**, *44*, 497–503. [CrossRef]
27. Hoyos-Bachiloglu, R.; Ivanovic-Zuvic, D.; Álvarez, J.; Linn, K.; Thöne, N.; de Los Ángeles Paul, M.; Borzutzky, A. Prevalence of parent-reported immediate hypersensitivity food allergy in Chilean school-aged children. *Allergol. Immunopathol.* **2014**, *42*, 527–532. [CrossRef]

28. Ontiveros, N.; Valdez-Meza, E.; Vergara-Jiménez, M.; Canizalez-Román, A.; Borzutzky, A.; Cabrera-Chávez, F. Parent-reported prevalence of food allergy in Mexican schoolchildren: A population-based study. *Allergol. Immunopathol.* **2016**, *44*, 563–570. [CrossRef]
29. Cornelisse-Vermaat, J.R.; Voordouw, J.; Yiakoumaki, V.; Theodoridis, G.; Frewer, L.J. Food-allergic consumers' labelling preferences: A cross-cultural comparison. *Eur. J. Public Health* **2008**, *18*, 115–120. [CrossRef]
30. Marra, C.A.; Harvard, S.; Grubisic, M.; Galo, J.; Clarke, A.; Elliott, S.; Lynd, L.D. Consumer preferences for food allergen labeling. *Allergy Asthma Clin. Immunol.* **2017**, *13*, 19. [CrossRef] [PubMed]
31. Ontiveros, N.; Flores-Mendoza, L.; Canizalez-Román, V.; Cabrera-Chavez, F. Food allergy: Prevalence and food technology approaches for the control of IgE-mediated food allergy. *Austin J. Nutr. Food Sci.* **2014**, *2*, 1029.
32. Autoridad Panameña De Seguridad De Alimentos. Instructivos o Guías Para el Registro De Alimentos Pre-Envasados Para Su Posterior Importación Al Territorio De La República De Panamá, Para Estados Unidos De América Y Territorios De Su Jurisdicción. Available online: https://www.aupsa.gob.pa/index.php/descarga/guiainstructivo-para-el-registro-de-alimentos-pre-envasadosprocesados-originarios-de-estados-unidos-de-america-y-territorios-de-su-jurisdiccion/ (accessed on 17 August 2020).
33. Ministerio De Comercio E Industrias. Resolución N° 393. Available online: https://www.gacetaoficial.gob.pa/pdfTemp/26097/GacetaNo_26097_20080804.pdf (accessed on 17 August 2020).
34. Sheridan, M.J.; Koeberl, M.; Hedges, C.E.; Biros, E.; Ruethers, T.; Clarke, D.; Buddhadasa, S.; Kamath, S.; Lopata, A.L. Undeclared allergens in imported packaged food for retail in Australia. *Food Addit. Contam. Part A* **2020**, *37*, 183–192. [CrossRef] [PubMed]
35. Khuda, S.E.; Sharma, G.M.; Gaines, D.; Do, A.B.; Pereira, M.; Chang, M.; Ferguson, M.; Williams, K.M. Survey of undeclared egg allergen levels in the most frequently recalled food types (including products bearing precautionary labelling). *Food Addit. Contam. Part A* **2016**, *33*, 1265–1273. [CrossRef] [PubMed]
36. Surojanametakul, V.; Khaiprapai, P.; Jithan, P.; Varanyanond, W.; Shoji, M.; Ito, T.; Tamura, H. Investigation of undeclared food allergens in commercial Thai food products. *Food Control* **2012**, *23*, 1–6. [CrossRef]
37. Mfueni, E.; Gama, A.P.; Kabambe, P.; Chimbaza, M.; Matita, G.; Matumba, L. Food allergen labeling in developing countries: Insights based on current allergen labeling practices in Malawi. *Food Control* **2018**, *84*, 263–267. [CrossRef]
38. Zurzolo, G.A.; Mathai, M.L.; Koplin, J.J.; Allen, K.J. Hidden allergens in foods and implications for labelling and clinical care of food allergic patients. *Curr. Allergy Asthma Rep.* **2012**, *12*, 292–296. [CrossRef]
39. Zurzolo, G.A.; Peters, R.L.; Koplin, J.J.; de Courten, M.; Mathai, M.L.; Allen, K.J. Are food allergic consumers ready for informative precautionary allergen labelling? *Allergy Asthma Clin. Immunol.* **2017**, *13*, 42. [CrossRef]
40. Yeung, J.; Robert, M.-C. Challenges and path forward on mandatory allergen labeling and voluntary precautionary allergen labeling for a global company. *J. AOAC Int.* **2018**, *101*, 70–76. [CrossRef]

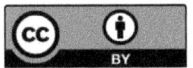

© 2020 by the authors. Licensee MDPI, Basel, Switzerland. This article is an open access article distributed under the terms and conditions of the Creative Commons Attribution (CC BY) license (http://creativecommons.org/licenses/by/4.0/).

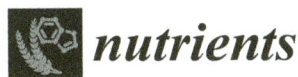

Article

Consumers' Preferences and Willingness to Pay for Fish Products with Health and Environmental Labels: Evidence from Five European Countries

Davide Menozzi [1], **Thong Tien Nguyen** [2,*], **Giovanni Sogari** [1], **Dimitar Taskov** [3], **Sterenn Lucas** [4], **José Luis Santiago Castro-Rial** [5] **and Cristina Mora** [1]

1. Department of Food and Drug, University of Parma, 43124 Parma, Italy; davide.menozzi@unipr.it (D.M.); giovanni.sogari@unipr.it (G.S.); cristina.mora@unipr.it (C.M.)
2. Truong Dai Hoc Nha Trang, Nr. 02, Nguyen Dinh Chieu, Nha Trang, Khánh Hòa 650000, Vietnam
3. Institute of Aquaculture University of Stirling, Stirling FK9 4LA, UK; dimitar.taskov@stir.ac.uk
4. SMART-LERECO AO-INRAE, 35042 Rennes CEDEX, France; sterenn.lucas@agrocampus-ouest.fr
5. Centro Tecnológico del Mar-Fundación CETMAR, Fisheries Socioeconomic Department, 36208 Vigo, Spain; jsantiago@cetmar.org
* Correspondence: thongtiennguyen@gmail.com

Received: 28 July 2020; Accepted: 27 August 2020; Published: 31 August 2020

Abstract: Seafood products are important sources of protein and components of a healthy and sustainable diet. Understanding consumers' preferences for fish products is crucial for increasing fish consumption. This article reports the consumer preferences and willingness to pay (WTP) for different fish species and attributes on representative samples in five European countries (n = 2509): France, Germany, Italy, Spain, and the UK. Consumer choices were investigated for fresh fish in a retail market under hypothetical situations arranged by a labelled choice experiment conducted for seven fish species: Cod, herring, seabass, seabream, salmon, trout, and pangasius. The results show the highest premiums for wild-caught fish than farm-raised alternatives. Ready-to-cook products are generally preferred to whole fish, whereas fish fillet preference is more species-specific. The results show positive premiums for a sustainability label and nutrition and health claims, with high heterogeneity across countries and species. With consumers' preferences and WTP being largely country- and fish-dependent, businesses (fish companies, retailers, and others) should consider the specific market context and adapt their labelling strategies accordingly. Public authorities campaigns should inform consumers about the tangible benefits related with health and environmental labels.

Keywords: choice experiment; willingness to pay (WTP); consumers' preferences; sustainability label; nutrition and health claim; fish species

1. Introduction

Due to the increasing number of diet-related chronic diseases and the impactful environmental damage related to food production and consumption, the concept of healthier and more sustainable dietary habits has been strongly promoted both by public authorities and the private sector [1–3]. Food policy makers have especially tried to promote such behavior through information on the food label like nutrition and sustainable claims. However, the effectiveness of food policies and labelling strongly depends on the understanding of the complexity of consumer choices and the associated elements [4]. For instance, even if fisheries and aquaculture products are an important source of protein and other beneficial components for human health, such as nutrients and essential long-chain polyunsaturated fatty acids (omega-3 fatty acids), their consumption varies greatly across countries. In the EU, fish and seafood consumption has risen over the past 10 years up to the current 24.3 kg per capita per year, with wide differences between countries, ranging from 5.6 kg in Hungary to 56.8 kg in Portugal [5]. Moreover, dietary recommendations and guidelines for fish consumption differ between the EU countries, both in qualitative and quantitative terms [6]. This might be due to inappropriate and broadly-oriented communication strategies [7], as information campaigns toward a specific target of consumers showed higher impact on food choices [8]. Therefore, in a fish market driven by demand, a better understanding of consumers' preferences across the European Union (EU) countries for fish species and product attributes is paramount to sustain this sector.

The role of sustainability and nutrition certification and labelling is transmitting information about an intrinsic quality of a product, e.g., relating to public benefits such as environmental integrity, which is not obvious to consumers when choosing a product. The incentive of producers occurs in the form of a premium received from the final consumer and transmitted up the value chain to the producer to cover the increased operating costs of the augmented practices. For evaluating the profitability of newly designed seafood products, a growing number of studies have focused on consumer preferences and attitude toward fish and seafood, as well as on their willingness to pay a premium price for innovative product features.

The nutritional aspects of fish and the related health effects are among the most important factors affecting consumer choices. Concerning the health benefits, the high omega-3 fatty acid and protein contents, as well as the low fat content, are generally associated with the consumer's perception of fish and seafood as healthy foods [9]. In the past, both qualitative [10] and quantitative [11] studies highlighted the increasing interest in information on the nutritional aspects of fish. However, knowledge about specific nutritional and health benefits of fish consumption does not appear to be strong among the population [9]. Pieniak et al. [7] identified and profiled consumers based on fish consumption, attitudes and knowledge about the health benefits of fish, and the socio-demographic characteristics in three EU countries (France, Poland and Spain). Their results showed that positive health enthusiasts, accounting for only 28% of the sample, have a strong involvement in healthy eating and a higher fish consumption. They also reported the highest subjective knowledge and a higher factual knowledge about fish than consumer segments with a lower interest in healthy eating.

Myrland et al. [12] found that the perception of fish as "difficult to prepare" negatively affected the purchase of whole fish. In this context, new processed fish products (e.g., burgers and ready-to-cook meals) represent an opportunity for producers and retailers to reach those consumers who normally do not buy seafood due to its smell and long preparation time [13]. The importance of the product presentation format is species-related too; for instance, Portuguese consumers seem to prefer whole fish products than fish steaks or fillets, in particular for species like sardine and mackerel that are most often served whole in culinary conventions [14]. Similarly, Thong et al. [15] showed that French consumers are willing to pay a price premium for fillets of pangasius, saithe, and salmon, but not for seabream, sole, tuna, and monkfish. Therefore, the socio-demographic characteristics of consumers and cultural traditions in seafood consumption are likely to influence the ready-meal market development.

The production method, whether wild-caught or farm-raised, is another factor that has been widely investigated. Many studies [16–18] indicated that consumers generally prefer wild-caught fish, as they are perceived as being superior in terms of taste, safety, and nutritional value [9,19]. However, other studies reported that preferences for wild-caught or farm-raised alternatives vary across species [15] or combined with other relevant attributes, such as sustainability labels [20–22].

Although increasing aquaculture may assist with preventing depletion of wild fish stocks, both wild-caught and farmed fish have substantial environmental impacts [23]. Sustainability labelling is a market-based instrument promoting sustainable fisheries [24,25], considered an incentive for a responsible management of fisheries [26,27] as it decreases the information gap between producers and consumers [28]. Specifically, eco-labels are becoming an important attribute of fish choice, and preferences over eco-labelled seafood products have been studied for wild [20,29–40] and farmed species [20,41–44]. Other authors showed that most consumers associate sustainability labels on food products with aspects of environmental protection rather than ethical issues [4]; this also translates to a lower willingness to pay (WTP) for social benefits of sustainability rather than for ecological benefits [45]. Therefore, as also noticed by Carlucci et al. [9], new insights into consumers' preferences for sustainable-labelled fish products, and their interaction with other product features, would be useful for producers (fisherpersons, fish mongers, and processors), retailers, and policy makers.

The objective of this study was to investigate consumer demand and choice behavior for fish products in five European countries (France, Germany, Italy, Spain, and the UK). In particular, consumer preferences were examined for different fish species and different attributes, i.e., sustainability label, nutrition and health claims, products presentation, production system and price. A discrete choice experiment (DCE) was applied to accomplish this objective; this method is strongly consistent with the economic demand theory and, in particular, with multi-attribute demand studies based on the Lancastrian consumer theory [46]. The outcomes allowed us to elicit consumers' preferences and WTP, providing valuable insights into developing targeted food marketing and policies strategies.

2. Materials and Methods

2.1. Econometric Models

2.1.1. Fish Choice Model

According to Lancaster's consumer theory [46], consumer utility stems from product attributes, not the products themselves. In other words, consumer utility can be separated into part-worth utilities. The part-worth utilities equal consumers' preference for corresponding attributes. In marketing research, the product attributes are classified into extrinsic and intrinsic attributes [47,48]. Regardless of whether consumers are exposed to these attributes, they may be important signals of product quality and determinants of consumer preference. The overall utility that a consumer obtains from consuming a fish species j (u_{ij}) can be decomposed into two parts: Observable (v_{ij}) and unobservable (ε_{ij}). In turn, the observable component of the utility is determined by the consumers' valuation on products attributes. The utility (u_{ij}) can be formulated as:

$$u_{ij} = v_{ij} + \varepsilon_{ij} = x'_{ij}\beta + \varepsilon_{ij} \qquad (1)$$

where $i = 1, \ldots, N$ is the individual consumer i; $j = 1, \ldots, J$, which is the product j among J products, u_{ij} is the utility obtained by individual i from product j; x'_{ij} is the product attributes; β is the vector of part-worth utility; and ε_{ij} is the random effect.

It is generally assumed that an individual i chooses a product alternative j (y_{ij}) if the utility derived from this alternative is maximized compared to the other alternatives:

$$y_{ij} = \begin{cases} 1, if\ u_{ij} \geq max(u_i) \\ 0\ otherwise \end{cases} \qquad (2)$$

When facing a choice of fish products, consumers assign a random utility to each product alternatives, and select the one with the highest derived utility. Assuming that the stochastic components ε_j have independent and identical distributed (*iid*) forms, the probability of a consumer i choosing a fish product j ($P(y_{ij} = 1)$) given by the Multinomial Logit (MNL) model [49,50] is expressed:

$$P(y_{ij} = 1) = \frac{exp(x'_{ij}\beta)}{\sum_{j=1}^{J} exp(x'_{ij}\beta)}. \qquad (3)$$

The MNL model presented in Equation (3) is the basic choice model and was proven to have several disadvantages, such as assuming the *iid* of the error and assuming the homogeneity of consumers preference. To overcome the limitations of MNL, many advanced discrete choice models have been suggested such as the Mixed Logit (ML) models (random coefficient, scaled-multinomial logit, and generalized-multinomial logit) and the Latent Class model [51,52]. We extended the basic model to mitigate the disadvantages and take advantage of our experimental data. For instance, we applied the Random Price Effect model (i.e., ML model) to evaluate the individual consumer's preference for the quality attributes of fish. The Mixed Logit (ML) model, in which price is set as a random effect parameter, can be formulated as:

$$P(y_{ij} = 1) = \int_\beta \frac{exp(x'_{ij}\beta)}{\sum_{j=1}^{J} exp(x'_{ij}\beta)} f(\beta|\theta) d\beta. \quad (4)$$

In the unconditional probability in Equation (4), the random parameter (e.g., price) β is the individual-specific parameter that has the density function $f(\beta|\theta)$, given the distributional parameter θ. In contrast to the MNL in Equation (3), the ML model is not a closed-form function, so it is unable to be solved. Simulation was used to obtain the parameter coefficients.

2.1.2. Model Specifications

We collected data via a choice experiment, in which each choice set includes several fish products described by commercial fish species name (e.g., cod, salmon, pangasius), production method (i.e., wild-caught vs. farmed fish), presentation (i.e., whole fish/round cut, fillet, or ready-to-cook), nutrition and health claims (i.e., with/without nutrition and health claims), and sustainability label (i.e., with/without sustainability label). The determined component of the utility function v_{ij} in Equation (1) can therefore be elaborated as:

$$v_{ij} = \alpha_j \, Species_j + \beta_1 Method_{ij} + \beta_2 Presentation_{ij} + \beta_3 Health_{ij} + \beta_4 Sustain_{ij} + \beta_{5i} Price_{ij}. \quad (5)$$

Notice that the random price effect model is estimated so that the price coefficient is an individual specific parameter (β_{5i}).

We used a labelled choice experiment [15,53] to collect data, which enabled us to estimate a Fish-Species-Specific Effect (FSSE) model to elicit the consumers' WTP for fish attributes that are specific to particular fish species. The FSSE model (fish j) is expressed as:

$$v_{ij} = \alpha_j \, Species_{ij} + \beta_{1j} Method_{ij} + \beta_{2j} Presentation_{ij} + \beta_{3j} Health_{ij} + \beta_{4j} Sustain_{ij} + \beta_{5j} Price_{ij}, \quad (6)$$

where β parameters are estimated for part-worth utility of the regarding attribute of the j-th fish species. The difference between the models in Equations (5) and (6) is that β parameters are estimated specifically for the j-th fish species (β_j). The specification of FSSE allowed us to calculate the WTP for considered attributes specific to each of the seven fish species in the choice experiment. We estimated the WTP specific to fish species with expectation that consumers' preference for fish quality attributes depends on specific species [9].

2.1.3. WTP Estimates

The WTP for a non-monetary attribute is the price premium that consumers are willing to pay for obtaining a desired attribute level. In other words, WTP is a marginal rate of substitution between specific attributes of interest (quality and price attribute). The marginal WTP is calculated by taking the ratio of the derivatives of both the attribute of interest (say an attribute level A, e.g., health) and price/cost. In the case of linearity in the attributes, indirect utility specification is given by:

$$WTP_A = \frac{\Delta x_A}{\Delta x_p} = \frac{\frac{\partial v_{ijA}}{\partial x_A}}{\frac{\partial v_{ijA}}{\partial x_p}} = -\frac{\beta_A}{\beta_p}. \quad (7)$$

When the random parameter model is applied in which one or two random parameter follows a distribution, the WTP will also follow a distribution and the calculation in Equation (7) is inaccurate. We applied the Delta method [54] to calculate the WTP for each simulation with assumption of normal distribution of the price coefficient. The individual WTP was then calculated as a mean of the sample. Bayesian statistics use the standard error of the mean, also known as the Monte Carlo standard error (MCSE), which takes into account the autocorrelation and correct the standard error by using effective sample size. Assuming that we have n iid samples, the mean estimate is $\overline{\mu}$, and $\rho_k(\mu)$ is the lag k autocorrelation for μ, the MSCE is calculated by:

$$MCSE(\overline{\mu}) = \frac{1 + 2\sum_{k=1}^{\infty} \rho_k(\mu_i)}{n} \cdot \frac{\sum_{t=1}^{n}(\mu_i^t - \overline{\mu}_t)^2}{(n-1)}. \tag{8}$$

The MCSE provides a measurement of the accuracy of the posterior estimates, and small values do not necessarily indicate that you have recovered the true posterior mean [49].

In addition, the MNL with fish-species-specific effect (i.e., the FSSE model) allowed us to calculate the WTP for each of the seven fish species in the choice experiment. We estimated the WTP specific to fish species considering consumers' preference for fish quality attributes depends in specific species [15]. For instance, consumers may prefer filleted cod to whole fish cod, but they may prefer whole-fish herring to filleted herring. The WTP for an attribute level A from the FSSE model in Equation (6) is calculated as:

$$WTP_{Aj} = -\frac{\beta_{Aj}}{\beta_{5j}} \tag{9}$$

where WTP_{Aj} is the price premium paid for obtaining a desired level of attribute A (i.e., product with health claim) of fish j, and β_{Aj} and β_{5j} are the estimated coefficients of attribute A and price attributes of fish j, respectively The WTP for species-specific attribute is calculated straightforward by the ratio of estimated coefficient of species-specific attributes and species-specific price.

We used the SAS procedure BCHOICE to estimate the fish choice models [55]. The procedure is built up by using Bayesian statistics. We estimated different fish choice models and selected those having the convergence of all estimated parameters [55].

2.2. Label Choice Experiment

A previous qualitative study was performed with approx. 90 individual in-depth interviews conducted in five countries (France, Germany, Italy, Spain, and the UK) to identify the positive or negative motives, perceptions, associations, and attitudes toward fish/seafood consumption, with a focus on the chosen species: Salmon, trout, seabass, seabream, pangasius, herring and cod [56]. The seven fish species were selected within the EU's Horizon 2020 Primefish Project, aiming at analyzing the economic sustainability of the European fisheries and aquaculture sectors. The findings of this qualitative work regarding consumers' perception of the main fish attributes were considered in the development of the choice experiment survey [56]. The final experimental design consisted of five attributes, defined for the seven fish alternatives: Price, production method, presentation, sustainability label, nutrition and health claim (Table 1).

We considered a yearly average market price level (at the retail stage) from official data sources (e.g., governmental agencies, etc.), for the year 2016. The price is indicated in €/kg potentially paid by consumers (£/kg in the U.K.) for the average product/format (fresh product). The production method attribute (wild-caught or farm-raised) was included in the experimental design considering the real availability on the market; in particular, the wild-caught fish level was not applicable for trout and pangasius, whereas the farm-raised fish level was not applicable for herring. The presentation attribute was provided as a picture to consumers. The sustainability label attribute was based on a definition, provided to respondents during the choice experiment as a pop-up linked with the label, based from the available market standards (e.g., Marine Stewardship Council (MSC) and Aquaculture Stewardship

Council (ASC); Table 2). Finally, a nutrition and health claim considering the omega-3 fatty acids content and the relative health benefits was used in the experiment (Table 2) [57]. The experimental design resulted in 9 blocks of 8 choice sets with 7 product profiles plus the "no choice" option (Figure 1). Respondents were randomly assigned to 1 of the 9 blocks. We only considered prepacked chilled fresh fish products, and not, e.g., frozen or canned products, to provide respondents with a unique and realistic, although hypothetical, retail context. Chilled fresh fish products are sold separately from, e.g., frozen fish products, which are sold in retail display cabinet used for the sale of frozen foods. The choice experiment was preceded by a cheap talk explaining the rationale behind the experiment and the need to respond carefully to the questions. Cheap talk strategies have been proved to eliminate or reduce hypothetical bias in several estimates [58].

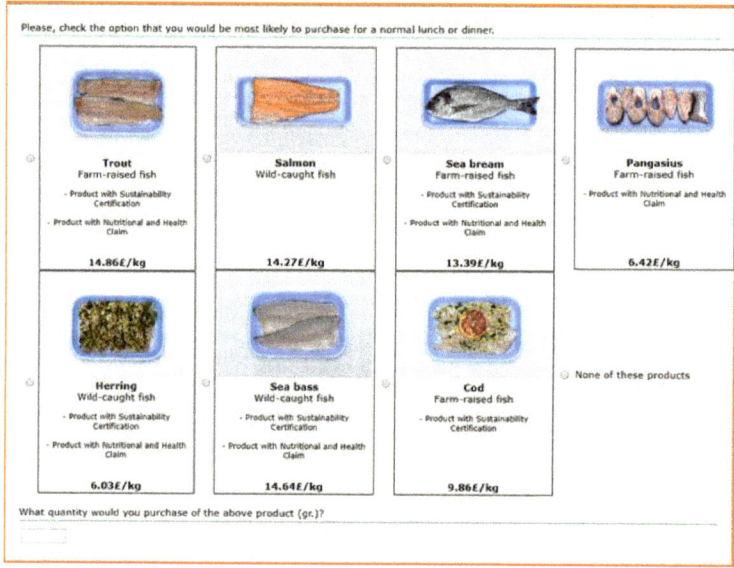

Figure 1. Example of a choice set.

Table 1. Attributes and levels for the choice experiment in the five countries and for the seven fish species (trout, herring, salmon, sea bass, sea bream, cod, and pangasius).

Attributes	Levels
Price	Average market price [1] −30% +30%
Production method	Wild-caught fish [2] Farm-raised fish [3]
Presentation (picture)	Whole fish/Round cut [4] Fillet Ready to cook
Sustainability label	No Yes
Nutrition and Health Claim	No Yes

[1] The average market prices are provided in Table A1; [2] The wild-caught fish level was not applicable for trout and pangasius; [3] The farm-raised fish level was not applicable for herring; [4] Round-cut was applied for salmon and pangasius, whole fish for the other species.

Table 2. Sustainability label and Nutrition and Health Claim used in the experiment.

Sustainability Label	Nutrition and Health Claim
When labelled according to a sustainability scheme, any fish can be traced back to a fishery or to a fish farm that meets principles reflecting the maintenance and re-establishment of healthy populations of targeted species, the maintenance of the integrity of ecosystems, the use of feed and other inputs that are sourced responsibly, and the social responsibility for workers and communities impacted by fishing and fish farming. This standard is intended to be used on a global basis by accredited third party certifiers to undertake the certification of fisheries and fish farmers to the above mentioned principles and criteria.	Product high in omega-3 fatty acids which contribute to maintenance of normal function of the heart and normal blood pressure, with the following condition of use: The beneficial effect is obtained with a daily intake of 250 mg of omega-3 fatty acids. Such amount can be consumed as part of a balanced diet [57].

2.3. Survey and Data Collection

Data for this study were collected in June 2017 through a nationwide online survey administered in the five countries (France, Germany, Italy, Spain, and the UK) by a third-party contractor using its consumer panel database (the survey questionnaire is available upon request). These five countries represent approx. 73% of the household expenditure on fishery and aquaculture products in Europe [1]. The sample in each country consisted of approximately 500 fish consumers (2509 in total), representative of the national populations in at least three of the following criteria: Age, gender, educational level, and geographical macro-areas (e.g., Italy: North, Center, South). We asked the frequency of fish consumption at the beginning of the questionnaire; answering "never" to this question ended the survey. After removing incomplete questionnaire, a final sample of 2433 consumers was analyzed. The main sample characteristics are reported in Table 3. The regions considered in each country are provided in Table A2.

Table 3. Sample (S) and national census (C) socio-demographic characteristics.

	France		Germany		Italy		Spain		UK		Total
	S	C[1]	S	C	S	C	S	C	S	C	S
Number	485	66.6	485	82.8	494	60.7	496	46.6	473	65.7	2433
Gender (%)											
Male	50.7	50.8	52.8	50.7	49.6	49.7	52.2	50.2	50.7	49.8	51.2
Female	49.3	49.2	47.2	49.3	50.4	50.3	47.8	49.8	49.3	50.2	48.8
Age in years (%)											
18–24	12.6	13.4	10.9	12.1	10.3	11.0	11.3	10.5	10.4	14.5	11.1
25–34	18.1	20.1	20.2	20.1	19.2	17.9	19.6	19.0	24.1	21.9	20.2
35–44	22.5	21.4	18.8	18.9	23.1	23.3	26.0	26.0	21.4	20.6	22.4
45–54	23.1	22.4	26.4	25.7	25.3	25.5	22.6	24.0	23.0	22.7	24.1
55+	23.7	22.8	23.7	23.3	22.1	22.3	20.6	20.5	21.1	20.3	22.2
Education (%)											
Less than lower secondary education	17.9	21.2	16.7	16.0	39.3	38.9	36.1	41.0	15.4	19.8	25.2
Upper secondary, non-tertiary education	47.2	46.0	56.9	58.4	44.4	44.7	27.8	25.4	43.4	40.5	43.8
Tertiary education	34.8	32.8	26.4	25.6	16.4	16.4	36.1	33.7	41.3	39.7	31.0

[1] Country population in million residents (Eurostat statistics 2016).

3. Results

Table 4 reports the choice probability of the seven fish species. In general, the results consistently revealed that salmon and cod have the largest market share, exceeding 10% of choice probability in all countries. Salmon and cod are among the most consumed species at the European level and in the surveyed countries [1]. These are followed by seabream and seabass, in particular in Italy, France, and Spain; trout is more likely chosen in Germany and Spain. Even in these countries, the choices expressed in the choice experiment are in line with the actual purchase data [1]. The least frequently chosen fish species were herring and pangasius.

Table 4. Choice probability obtained by Mixed Logit (ML) models (M, mean; SE, Monte Carlo standard error).

	All Countries		France		Germany		Italy		Spain		UK	
	M	SE	M	SE	M	SE	M	SE	M	SE	M	SE
Cod	0.154	0.001	0.150	0.002	0.235	0.004	0.158	0.001	0.130	0.002	0.235	0.004
Herring	0.088	0.001	0.086	0.001	0.112	0.003	0.070	0.001	0.053	0.001	0.112	0.003
Pangasius	0.082	0.001	0.062	0.001	0.032	0.000	0.076	0.002	0.095	0.002	0.032	0.000
Salmon	0.230	0.002	0.252	0.004	0.280	0.004	0.174	0.004	0.189	0.004	0.280	0.004
Seabass	0.113	0.001	0.107	0.001	0.075	0.003	0.174	0.001	0.136	0.001	0.075	0.003
Seabream	0.119	0.001	0.125	0.001	0.042	0.001	0.198	0.001	0.169	0.001	0.042	0.001
Trout	0.109	0.001	0.104	0.001	0.048	0.001	0.082	0.001	0.156	0.003	0.048	0.001
No choice	0.105	0.003	0.114	0.007	0.176	0.009	0.067	0.005	0.073	0.005	0.176	0.009

In the Sections 3.1 and 3.2 we present, respectively, the results of the Mixed Logit (ML) models and the WTP estimates for the considered attributes and levels. In addition, the results of the Fish Species-Specific Effect (FSSE) models and the relative WTP are presented in Tables A1 and A2, and commented in Sections 3.1 and 3.2.

3.1. Model Estimates

Table 5 reports the mean estimates in all countries for ML models and Monte Carlo standard error (SE); Table A3 provides the results of the FSSE models.

The first relevant observation from the ML model results is the significance of all the coefficients estimated, which led us to conclude that all the selected attributes and levels are relevant to consumers when choosing these fish products. The high β coefficient reported in Table 5 for salmon, cod, seabass, and seabream indicated that these fish species are generally preferred by the consumers in the five countries. The results reflected the choices in Table 4, where seabream and seabass were relatively more appreciated in Italy (3.290 and 3.332, respectively) and Spain (3.153 and 3.239, respectively), and trout carried higher utility in Germany (2.877). Salmon showed relatively higher β coefficients in all counties. The least preferred species were pangasius and herring. In this latter case, only German and Spanish consumers exhibited a higher coefficient for this species (2.207 and 2.192, respectively). Germany is the only market among those studied where herring is on the top 10 consumed species [1]. In the UK pangasius carried a low but significant effect (0.285), indicating a low utility associated with this fish.

Wild-caught alternatives were generally preferred compared to the farm-raised fish species, as indicated by positive and significant β coefficients across all countries, with relatively higher values in France and Italy. When single-species effects were considered (Table A3), a relatively stronger effect was found for seabass (0.406). In single countries, wild seabass and cod were more preferred in Italy (0.449 and 0.482, respectively; Table A3), whereas in France, wild seabream, cod and salmon were more appreciated (0.520, 0.436, and 0.436, respectively). The effect was significant for wild salmon and seabass in the UK (0.284 and 0.431, respectively), and for wild salmon (0.237), seabass (0.569) and seabream (0.269) in Germany; in Spain wild seabass positively affected consumer utility (0.267).

The negative β estimates on the presentation row in Table 5 show that ready-to-cook alternatives (the baseline) are generally preferred compared to whole or round-cut fish (−0.118, overall). This was true for almost all countries, with the only exception of Spain, and for all fish species (Table A3). When considering the fish species, round cut salmon was an exception, where a positive estimate (0.253) indicated that this format is preferred over the ready-to-cook alternative; this was also found for whole seabream in Spain (0.238) and Italy (0.179). The fresh fillet was preferred over the ready-to-cook alternative, as indicated in Table 5 by the positive β estimate in the first column (0.092), although with heterogeneity across countries. A higher preference for fillets compared to ready-to-cook alternatives was found in France (0.167) and the UK (0.145), whereas lower effects were found in Italy and Germany. When considering species-specific effects, salmon fillet was generally preferred over the ready-to-cook alternative in all countries (0.414; Table A3). This was also noted for cod fillets in France (0.243) and for seabream fillets Spain (0.222) and Italy (0.192). A negative coefficient indicated that ready-to-cook trout was preferred than the fillet format in all countries (−0.191).

Table 5. β coefficients estimates of Mixed Logit (ML) models (Mean; SE, Monte Carlo standard error).

Species and Attributes	All Countries (n = 2433)		France (n = 485)		Germany (n = 485)		Italy (n = 494)		Spain (n = 496)		UK (n = 473)	
	Mean	SE	Mean	SE	Mean	SE	Mean	SE	Mean	SE	Mean	SE
Cod	2.791	0.002	2.897	0.006	2.641	0.006	3.223	0.005	3.197	0.005	2.774	0.007
Herring	1.381	0.002	1.582	0.005	2.207	0.005	1.963	0.005	2.192	0.006	0.524	0.003
Pangasius	1.285	0.001	1.477	0.004	1.791	0.003	1.643	0.004	1.841	0.004	0.285	0.005
Salmon	3.274	0.002	3.458	0.006	3.626	0.006	3.491	0.005	3.653	0.006	2.979	0.007
Seabass	2.505	0.002	2.505	0.006	2.306	0.006	3.290	0.005	3.153	0.005	1.892	0.008
Seabream	2.437	0.002	2.400	0.005	2.140	0.006	3.332	0.005	3.239	0.005	1.259	0.008
Trout	2.228	0.002	2.586	0.005	2.877	0.005	2.598	0.005	2.552	0.004	1.322	0.007
Wild-Caught vs. Farm-Raised	0.301	0.000	0.455	0.001	0.299	0.001	0.386	0.001	0.157	0.001	0.226	0.001
Presentation: Whole [1] vs. Ready-to-Cook	−0.118	0.000	−0.131	0.001	−0.346	0.001	−0.033	0.001	0.052	0.001	−0.174	0.001
Presentation: Fillet vs. Ready-to-Cook	0.092	0.000	0.167	0.001	−0.006	0.001	0.074	0.001	0.108	0.001	0.145	0.001
Sustainability Label	0.154	0.000	0.138	0.001	0.221	0.001	0.198	0.001	0.121	0.001	0.112	0.001
Nutrition and Health Claim	0.142	0.000	0.067	0.001	0.162	0.001	0.189	0.001	0.186	0.001	0.097	0.001
Price (mean)	−0.240	0.003	−0.259	0.004	−0.236	0.007	−0.278	0.008	−0.308	0.010	−0.256	0.009
Price (variance)	0.027	0.000	0.039	0.000	0.036	0.000	0.044	0.000	0.049	0.000	0.039	0.000
Mean of Log-Likelihood	−34,300.30		−6808.12		−6704.31		−7011.89		−7121.84		−5863.98	
Accepted Rate	0.96		0.89		0.92		0.91		0.93		0.89	
Hit probability	0.22		0.23		0.24		0.22		0.21		0.30	
Average Efficiency	0.57		0.56		0.55		0.56		0.57		0.49	

Note: All estimates are significant at $p < 0.001$. [1] Round cut for salmon and pangasius, whole fish for the other species.

The sustainability label was appreciated in all countries considering all species together (0.154; Table 5). This attribute was associated with a higher utility in Germany (0.221) and Italy (0.198). Considering the species-specific effects model, more significant coefficients were found for seabass carrying sustainability label in France and Germany (0.389 and 0.473, respectively; Table A3) and for cod in Italy (0.336). Lower although significant effects were found for seabream in Italy and Germany (0.222 and 0.447, respectively), and for herring in the UK and Germany (0.249 and 0.223, respectively).

The nutrition and health claim estimates indicated a positive effect on consumers' utility (0.142), with relatively higher values in Italy and Spain (0.189 and 0.186, respectively). When considering inter-species variability of the estimates, the nutrition and health claim associated with seabass carried higher utility in France and Spain (0.258 and 0.189, respectively; Table A3), whereas seabream with this claim was more appreciated in Italy (0.363) and Germany (0.255). The presence of a nutrition and health claim carried high utility for pangasius in Spain (0.349); for salmon in the UK, Germany, and Spain (0.178, 0.165, and 0.181, respectively); for herring in Germany (0.242); and for trout in Spain (0.198).

3.2. WTP Estimates

The WTP results for fish product attributes are shown in Table 6, where the price premiums, expressed in €/kg, obtained from the ML models are reported. Table A4 shows the price premium (in €/kg) per fish species obtained by FSSE Models applying the Equation (9). The WTP values should be interpreted as the maximum amount of money that consumers are willing to pay for obtaining a desired attribute level or, in other words, as the premium that would induce a consumer to be exactly indifferent to buying and not buying fish products with the specified attribute level.

Overall, the highest premium among the attributes proposed was estimated for production method; the ML model for all countries suggested a mean WTP for wild-caught fish relative to farm-raised of €1.29 per kg. The highest premium among the studied countries was found in Italy with €2.03/kg, followed by France (€1.62/kg) and UK (€1.40/kg), whereas the lowest was reported in the Spain (€0.78/kg). A negative premium was found for whole vs. ready-to-cook alternatives, indicating that consumers, on average, were willing to pay an extra premium of €0.50 per kg for a product with convenience (ready-to-cook) over whole format. In this case, the highest premiums were found in Germany (€1.31/kg), and the UK (€1.15/kg). Only Spanish consumers were willing to pay, on average, a €0.25 per kg premium for whole fish species over ready-to-cook alternatives. Considering the product presentation, overall, consumers were willing to pay a €0.43 per kg premium for fillet over ready-to-cook products. The British and French consumers were willing to pay the highest premiums for fish fillets (the estimates were €0.93 and €0.58 per kg, respectively), whereas only German consumers were indifferent (€0.09/kg premium for ready-to-cook over fish fillets).

Table 6. Willingness to pay (WTP) estimates in €/kg (mean values, Monte Carlo standard error in parenthesis) of Mixed Logit (ML) models.

Species and Attributes	All Countries (n = 2433)	France (n = 485)	Germany (n = 485)	Italy (n = 494)	Spain (n = 496)	UK [1] (n = 473)
Wild-Caught vs. Farm-Raised	1.29 (0.006)	1.62 (0.005)	1.10 (0.007)	2.03 (0.003)	0.78 (0.001)	1.40 (0.002)
Presentation (Whole vs. Ready-to-Cook)	−0.50 (0.002)	−0.43 (0.002)	−1.31 (0.008)	−0.13 (0.001)	0.25 (0.001)	−1.15 (0.002)
Presentation (Fillet vs. Ready-to-Cook)	0.43 (0.002)	0.58 (0.002)	−0.09 (0.001)	0.40 (0.001)	0.50 (0.001)	0.93 (0.002)
Sustainability Label	0.69 (0.003)	0.43 (0.002)	0.60 (0.008)	1.02 (0.002)	0.59 (0.001)	0.75 (0.002)
Nutrition and Health Claim	0.51 (0.003)	0.18 (0.001)	0.42 (0.006)	0.96 (0.002)	0.92 (0.001)	0.65 (0.001)

Note: All estimates are significant at $p < 0.001$. [1] The exchange rate used in the UK case was £1 GB = €1.16.

Considering all countries and all fish species, the consumers were willing to pay a €0.69 per kg premium for fish species with a sustainability label, as estimated by the ML model. This premium was relatively higher in Italy (an average €1.02/kg premium); French and Spanish consumers had lower estimates (€0.43/kg and €0.59/kg, respectively). Finally, consumers were willing to pay a €0.51 per kg premium for fish with nutrition and health claims. Italian and Spanish consumers reported higher premiums in this case, being willing to pay on average €0.96 and €0.92 premiums per kg, respectively.

The WTP estimates from the FSSE models in the different countries revealed the high heterogeneity of the consumers estimates and across different species (Table A4). Focusing on the sustainability label, the highest premiums taking the countries all together were found for herrings and salmon (€2.93 and €1.95 per kg, respectively), whereas lower WTP values were estimated for trout and pangasius (€1.05 and €0.75 per kg, respectively). Considering individual countries, the premiums for the sustainability labels were more relevant for herrings in the UK and Germany; for seabass in Germany and France; and for seabream in Germany and Italy. Other significant effects of the sustainability label attribute were found in Italy for cod, and in France for salmon.

Overall, the highest premiums for the nutrition and health claim were estimated for salmon (€2.65/kg), seabream (€1.21/kg), seabass (€1.15/kg), and cod (€1.12/kg). Lower premiums were found for trout (€0.95/kg) and pangasius (€0.90/kg). The consumer WTP for nutrition and health claim was more relevant in Spain for several species, including pangasius, salmon and trout. The WTP for labelled salmon was also relevant in Germany and the UK Other effects of the nutrition and health label attribute were found in Italy for seabream, in France for seabass and in Germany for herring.

4. Discussion and Conclusions

In this study, we investigated consumer choices in five European countries for selected fish attributes: Price, production method, presentation, sustainability label, and nutrition and health claims. Using a labelled hypothetical choice experiment, we estimated their WTP for these attributes across different countries and species, considering consumers' preferences and willingness to pay for single attributes, e.g., production method, may vary across different cultures and fish species.

First, considering the intrinsic value of the fish species, the model results showed that salmon, cod, seabass, and seabream have highly rank-ordered values in the studied markets, whereas herring, pangasius, and trout received lower evaluations. A familiarity with Mediterranean fish species, such as seabass and seabream, may justify the higher estimates in Italy, Spain, and France [41,42], whereas in Germany and the UK cod and salmon were scored relatively higher. Trout carried higher utility in Germany. These results are consistent with actual consumption data: Salmon and cod are among the most consumed species in the surveyed countries; Italy, Greece, Spain, France, and Portugal have the highest seabass and seabream per capita consumption; herring and trout are among the most consumed fish species in Germany [5]. This data triangulation supports our empirical results.

Our results indicated that respondents are willing to pay more for wild-caught than farm-raised fish. This was verified across all countries and fish species. This result aligns with those of several studies carried out in different countries where wild fish was reported as being perceived as superior to farm-raised fish in terms of taste, safety, and nutritional value [15–17,59]. In particular, it was found that when information about the production method was provided to consumers the hedonic evaluation of farmed fish does not change significantly, whereas the liking of wild fish significantly increased [14].

Ready-to-cook products are generally preferred than whole (or round-cut) fish in all countries, with the only exception of Spain. Considering different species, we found consumer preferences for round-cut salmon in France, the UK, and Spain, and whole seabream in Italy and Spain. Salmon and seabream showed the highest choice probability in Spain, and this might have inflated the general preference of Spanish consumers for whole (or round-cut) fish products. Increased familiarity with seabream for Italian and Spanish consumers, increased use with small/medium sized whole products (portion size), and increased familiarity with the cooking skills required for gastronomic preparations might justify the higher WTP for the whole fish. The premiums consumers were willing to pay were generally higher for ready-to-cook pangasius and cod compared to, respectively, round-cut and whole alternatives; ready-to-cook seabass was appreciated in Germany and the UK In this case, the preference for ready-to-cook products might be strictly connected with the desire to save time and effort in food preparation. Convenience perception of meal options is considered an important driver of fish consumption, whereas the difficulty of preparation and manipulation of fish, such as the presence of bones, the lack of cooking skills, and knowledge of recipes for specific fish species, is a strong barrier to the frequency of fish consumption [9,41]. Not surprisingly, round-cut salmon is preferred to the ready-to-cook product since this format is used in several gastronomic preparations.

Fish fillets are generally more appreciated than ready-to-cook alternatives in all countries, with the only exception of Germany where more elaborated products were preferred across fish species. Despite the decline in fish and seafood consumption in Germany in recent years [5], the share of easy-to-cook and convenience fish on the German market is increasing, following a global trend as a consequence of changing lifestyles [60,61]. In the other countries the stated preferences seem more species-specific: Salmon, seabream, and cod fillets are generally preferred to ready-to-cook alternatives, whereas ready-to-cook trout is more appreciated than fillet presentation. In this case, consumers were shown to appreciate new convenient fish products when the original fish characteristics are not significantly altered [14,15]. A French study on seafood showed that increasing the level of processing leads consumers to perceive a decrease in the original quality features like taste, healthiness, and nutritional quality [62]. In Greece, consumers with a high degree of knowledge and expertise in selecting and preparing fish preferred whole or unprocessed fish, whereas younger and less experienced consumers were more willing to consume highly processed and ready-to-cook fish [63].

The results showed positive premiums for a sustainability label, and nutrition and health claims, with high heterogeneity across species and countries. Other studies observed a positive perception and WTP for fish eco-labelling, including specific standards for fishing such as MSC [45], and organic aquaculture [41,42]. However, for sustainability to become a purchase criterion, consumers must have enough information and knowledge about the standard and the requirements, such as resource conservation and depletion of natural fish stocks [20], and trust in the certification system, control mechanisms, and independence of the guarantee body [43]. The WTP estimates are in line with revealed preferences. MSC is the most-studied scheme in fish and seafood using revealed preference methods, and the majority of studies cover the UK retail market for white fish. Sogn-Grundvåg et al. [64] discovered a 10% premium for chilled MSC haddock and 13% premium for MSC cod and haddock in retail market in Glasgow, UK A price premium of 10% was estimated for MSC-certified cod in Sweden [65]. The highest premium for MSC white fish found was 14.2% for frozen Alaska pollock in the London metropolitan area [66]. Similarly, other studies demonstrated consumer interest in the health-related attributes of fish [67], evidencing similarities and differences with those more interested in eco-labelled products [68]. Our results indicated that fish producers could gain significant premiums for sustainability labels as long as they associate benefits to the environment and society with these products [69]. Similarly, the premium that consumers are willing to pay for fish with nutrition and health claims (i.e., an average €0.51 per kg) confirmed the interest in information on the nutritional aspects of fish. However, as noted by other scholars, knowledge about the specific nutritional and health benefits of fish consumption does not appear to be strong among the population [9]. Thus, more evidence of the confidence that consumers attach to the real health benefits provided by fish consumption would help with understanding the real effect of these claims on consumer behavior. The results have also shown different premiums consumers are willing to pay for species with nutrition and health claims, ranging from €0.90/kg (pangasius) to €2.65/kg (salmon). On the one hand, these differences should be considered in relation to the species-specific average prices in the studied countries, as shown in Table A1. For instance, in Italy the premium consumers are willing to pay for pangasius with nutrition and health claims is €0.96/kg, whereas for salmon is €3.19/kg, resulting in a percentage premium above the average market price of, respectively, 17.1% and 21.1%. In France the relative premiums are, respectively, 27.2% and 27.5%. On the other hand, the species-specific variability of the estimates may depend on differences in health benefits perception across species and countries, as also evidenced in other studies [11,18].

The hypothetical nature of the experiment is the main limitation of this study since WTP estimates could have been overestimated; however, the introduction of a cheap talk at the beginning of the choice experiment should have minimized the hypothetical bias [58]. The consistency of our results with the actual consumption patterns in the European countries [5] and with the estimates of revealed preference studies for the sustainability labels indicate the good reliability of the results. Other attributes could have been considered, e.g., country of origin, freshness, and brands, which might have explained consumer choices of fish species and products. For instance, several studies already documented the strong role of domestic origin on consumer choices, which is often perceived as an indicator of the healthfulness and safety of the product [15,41]. Therefore, in this study we decided to focus more on the less-investigated features of fish consumption, at least at the European level, such as sustainability and health-related attributes. The results, obtained in five countries from seven fish species, represent a significant advancement in the understanding of European fish consumer preferences and choices.

In this paper, we provided a wide range of evidence of consumers interest in fish products features from cross-national and cross-species perspectives. Since fish preferences and WTP, for instance for sustainability and production methods, proved to be heterogeneous across countries and species, the results presented in this paper have relevant implications for the success of labelling programs, such as environmental and health-related labelling, applied in different marketing contexts. In other words, businesses (e.g., fish companies and retailers) should consider the specific market context (e.g., familiarity with Mediterranean fish species in Southern EU countries) and adapt their labelling strategies according to country- and species-specific needs. The positive premiums that consumers were willing to pay for eco-friendly and healthy-related labels are promising for public authorities, demonstrating the interest of part of the population in following healthier and more sustainable dietary patterns. The relatively low values of WTP for these attributes in some countries and for some fish species could be due to consumers' perception of the effectiveness of these attributes, and not by the low interest or value per se. Therefore, the results may also suggest the need to implement homogeneous strategies, within EU countries, for educating consumers about the product labelling and the different claims and certifications which can be found on the pack, and about the tangible benefits to consumers' related with health and sustainability labels. From the methodological side, further efforts should be devoted to including a measure of beliefs in the choice modelling for improving the understanding of consumers behavior and WTP [69], or by applying other models, such as the Latent Class model, to gather information about different market segments carrying different patterns of preferences and willingness to pay for attributes and fish species.

Author Contributions: Conceptualization, D.M., T.T.N. and G.S.; methodology, T.T.N., D.M. and G.S.; software, T.T.N.; formal analysis, T.T.N. and D.M.; investigation, D.M., G.S., D.T., S.L. and J.L.S.C.-R.; data curation, T.T.N. and D.M.; writing—original draft preparation, D.M. and T.T.N.; writing—review and editing, D.M., T.T.N., G.S., D.T., S.L., J.L.S.C.-R. and C.M.; visualization, D.M.; supervision, C.M.; project administration, C.M.; funding acquisition, C.M. All authors have read and agreed to the published version of the manuscript.

Funding: This research is part of the activities of the Primefish Project, which is a project that has received funding from the European Union's Horizon 2020 research and innovation program under grant agreement No 635761. For more information, visit http://www.primefish.eu/.

Acknowledgments: The authors would like to thank the Primefish project coordinator Gudmundur Stefansson (MATIS), the WP4 leader Prof. Stéphane Ganassali (Université de Savoie), and all the project partners for their fruitful collaboration. Thanks also to the reviewers for their constructive feedback on an earlier draft of this paper.

Conflicts of Interest: The authors declare no conflict of interest.

Appendix A

Table A1. Average price levels (€/kg, and £/kg for the UK) by fish species in each country.

Country	Trout	Herring	Salmon	Seabream	Seabass	Cod	Pangasius
France	12.80	9.90	14.90	11.50	14.30	14.90	8.50
Germany	11.58	10.86	16.84	16.70	16.80	16.75	5.25
Italy	10.51	9.90	15.10	10.82	11.82	12.21	5.60
Spain	5.97	11.90	12.87	9.87	11.04	12.00	5.23
UK (€/kg)	16.79	5.24	16.13	21.61	23.64	15.91	10.37
UK (£/kg) [1]	14.86	4.64	14.27	19.12	20.92	14.08	9.18

[1] The figure in €/kg was translated in £/kg in the UK. The exchange rate used was £1 GB = €1.16.

Table A2. Sample (S) and national census (C) by Region (in %).

France			Germany			Italy			Spain			UK		
Regions	S	C	Regions	S	C	Regions	S	C	Regions	S	C	Regions	S	C
Île de France	19.8	19.7	Baden-Württemb.	14.3	13.7	Nord-Ovest	20.0	26.2	Noroeste	10.8	9.7	North East	4.2	4.0
Bassin Parisien	9.6	16.5	Bayern	16.1	16.2	Nord-Est	23.8	19.0	Noreste	11.2	9.8	North West	11.0	10.9
Nord-Pas-de-Calais	7.0	6.4	Berlin	4.8	4.5	Centro	26.0	19.8	Comunidad de Madrid	16.6	14.7	Yorkshire and The Humber	8.2	8.2
Est	10.2	8.5	Brandenburg	2.6	3.1	Sud	18.8	23.7	Centro	13.2	12.4	East Midlands	7.8	7.1
Ouest	15.2	13.3	Bremen	0.6	0.8	Isole	11.3	11.3	Este	24.4	30.4	West Midlands	8.6	8.7
Sud-Ouest	11.8	11.0	Hamburg	2.4	2.3				Sur	24.0	23.0	East of England	8.2	9.1
Centre-Est	14.0	12.3	Hessen	7.0	7.8							London	16.4	14.4
Méditerranée	12.6	12.3	Mecklenburg-Vorpommern	2.2	2.0							South East	14.0	13.5
			Niedersachsen	10.2	9.8							South West	8.2	8.1
			Nordrhein-Westf.	23.3	22.3							Wales	4.4	4.6
			Rheinland-Pfalz	4.2	5.1							Scotland	7.4	8.4
			Saarland	1.0	1.2							Northern Ireland	1.8	2.8
			Sachsen	5.0	4.9									
			Sachsen-Anhalt	3.0	2.7									
			Schleswig-Holstein	3.4	3.5									

Table A3. β coefficients estimates (M, mean; SD, standard deviation) of the Fish-Species-Specific Effect (FSSE) model per country.

Attributes/Species Effects	All Countries (n = 2433)		France (n = 485)		Germany (n = 485)		Italy (n = 494)		Spain (n = 496)		UK (n = 473)	
	M	SD	M	SD	M	SD	M	SD	M	SD	M	SD
Species												
Cod	2.073	0.105	2.176	0.244	1.919	0.286	2.558	0.249	2.144	0.262	1.469	0.216
Herring	0.255	0.089	0.600	0.273	1.396	0.237	0.660	0.295	1.099	0.337	−0.064	0.244
Pangasius	1.097	0.097	0.814	0.296	0.812	0.215	1.006	0.278	0.615	0.256	−0.938	0.411
Salmon	1.609	0.095	1.823	0.214	1.761	0.215	1.765	0.239	1.597	0.237	1.569	0.209
Seabass	2.246	0.117	2.040	0.297	1.576	0.360	2.831	0.243	2.325	0.268	0.751	0.359
Seabream	2.303	0.110	2.279	0.273	0.473	0.378	2.367	0.227	2.249	0.241	−0.316	0.433
Trout	1.394	0.083	1.406	0.249	1.613	0.209	1.543	0.267	1.192	0.209	0.245	0.346

Table A3. Cont.

Attributes/Species Effects	All Countries (n = 2433) M	SD	France (n = 485) M	SD	Germany (n = 485) M	SD	Italy (n = 494) M	SD	Spain (n = 496) M	SD	UK (n = 473) M	SD
Price												
Cod	−0.099	0.005	−0.088	0.013	−0.095	0.013	−0.101	0.015	−0.129	0.017	−0.076	0.011
Herring	−0.053	0.008	−0.082	0.025	−0.123	0.020	−0.071	0.026	−0.137	0.026	−0.086	0.045
Pangasius	−0.213	0.013	−0.150	0.033	−0.068	0.036	−0.188	0.045	−0.099	0.043	−0.073	0.042
Salmon	−0.051	0.005	−0.050	0.011	−0.040	0.009	−0.046	0.012	−0.070	0.013	−0.077	0.011
Seabass	−0.116	0.005	−0.139	0.016	−0.067	0.016	−0.111	0.015	−0.129	0.018	−0.043	0.012
Seabream	−0.164	0.006	−0.132	0.019	−0.051	0.017	−0.125	0.016	−0.164	0.019	−0.055	0.018
Trout	−0.129	0.006	−0.123	0.018	−0.098	0.016	−0.135	0.023	−0.090	0.030	−0.099	0.022
Production Method (Wild-Caught vs. Farm-Raised)												
Cod	0.259	0.041	0.436	0.095	0.205	0.111	0.482	0.091	0.132	0.096	0.084	0.082
Salmon	0.282	0.034	0.436	0.075	0.237	0.075	0.340	0.083	0.105	0.081	0.284	0.075
Seabass	0.406	0.047	0.379	0.105	0.569	0.127	0.449	0.084	0.267	0.093	0.431	0.127
Seabream	0.260	0.046	0.520	0.101	0.269	0.134	0.272	0.081	0.113	0.086	0.111	0.160
Cod	−0.405	0.053	−0.468	0.119	−0.796	0.147	−0.372	0.112	−0.143	0.118	−0.402	0.099
Herring	−0.257	0.064	−0.265	0.151	−0.379	0.127	−0.119	0.159	−0.061	0.185	−0.322	0.129
Pangasius	−0.451	0.068	−0.914	0.187	−0.664	0.120	−0.228	0.154	−0.185	0.135	−0.231	0.228
Salmon	0.253	0.043	0.362	0.094	0.031	0.091	0.266	0.109	0.299	0.104	0.331	0.090
Seabass	−0.150	0.057	−0.078	0.134	−0.506	0.163	−0.041	0.103	0.011	0.115	−0.434	0.157
Seabream	0.041	0.057	−0.127	0.124	−0.213	0.169	0.179	0.101	0.238	0.108	−0.313	0.215
Trout	−0.158	0.056	−0.262	0.132	−0.190	0.110	−0.066	0.136	−0.046	0.104	−0.489	0.194
Presentation (Fillet vs. Ready-to-Cook) [1]												
Cod	0.109	0.047	0.243	0.104	−0.015	0.122	0.118	0.103	0.120	0.114	0.091	0.090
Herring	−0.022	0.061	0.040	0.137	−0.063	0.118	−0.037	0.155	0.136	0.178	−0.087	0.121
Pangasius	−0.106	0.062	−0.205	0.149	−0.071	0.103	−0.037	0.144	−0.164	0.132	−0.142	0.218
Salmon	0.414	0.043	0.434	0.092	0.253	0.090	0.496	0.105	0.472	0.104	0.479	0.089
Seabass	−0.052	0.055	0.063	0.129	−0.102	0.145	−0.171	0.105	0.030	0.114	−0.027	0.141
Seabream	0.149	0.056	0.083	0.120	−0.040	0.162	0.192	0.103	0.222	0.110	0.149	0.193
Trout	−0.191	0.057	−0.011	0.127	−0.178	0.111	−0.393	0.148	−0.253	0.112	−0.165	0.173

Table A3. Cont.

Attributes/Species Effects	All Countries (n = 2433) M	SD	France (n = 485) M	SD	Germany (n = 485) M	SD	Italy (n = 494) M	SD	Spain (n = 496) M	SD	UK (n = 473) M	SD
Sustainability Label												
Cod	0.152	0.041	0.017	0.094	0.153	0.111	0.336	0.092	0.153	0.097	0.124	0.080
Herring	0.154	0.052	−0.068	0.119	0.223	0.105	0.144	0.126	0.174	0.148	0.249	0.108
Pangasius	0.159	0.052	0.220	0.136	0.173	0.094	0.221	0.121	0.156	0.108	−0.204	0.186
Salmon	0.100	0.036	0.171	0.077	0.105	0.077	0.066	0.088	0.064	0.086	0.073	0.076
Seabass	0.148	0.046	0.389	0.105	0.473	0.130	0.095	0.085	−0.069	0.093	0.032	0.120
Seabream	0.192	0.045	0.059	0.099	0.447	0.138	0.222	0.081	0.162	0.086	0.165	0.162
Trout	0.135	0.047	0.162	0.108	0.106	0.092	0.200	0.119	0.176	0.091	−0.018	0.152
Cod	0.111	0.040	0.095	0.093	0.180	0.109	0.173	0.088	0.096	0.096	0.054	0.079
Herring	0.082	0.051	0.014	0.116	0.242	0.102	0.081	0.125	0.023	0.142	0.003	0.108
Pangasius	0.191	0.053	−0.009	0.132	0.157	0.091	0.180	0.120	0.349	0.109	0.176	0.181
Salmon	0.136	0.034	−0.010	0.074	0.165	0.073	0.148	0.084	0.181	0.080	0.178	0.071
Seabass	0.134	0.046	0.258	0.107	−0.052	0.123	0.153	0.087	0.189	0.095	0.034	0.122
Seabream	0.197	0.046	0.036	0.098	0.255	0.136	0.363	0.082	0.174	0.086	0.027	0.166
Trout	0.122	0.048	0.027	0.110	0.105	0.091	0.105	0.120	0.198	0.091	0.139	0.155
Mean of Log-likelihood	−37,851.47		−7509.23		−7529.17		−7666.7		−7820.090		−6818.34	
Accepted Rate	0.82		0.602		0.575		0.626		0.621		0.437	
Hit probability	0.162		0.167		0.164		0.165		0.154		0.201	
Average Efficiency	0.935		0.647		0.598		0.71		0.696		0.372	

[1] Round cut for salmon and pangasius, whole fish for the other species.

Table A4. Willingness to pay (WTP) estimates (mean values, €/kg) of the Fish Species-Specific Effect (FSSE) model per country.

	All Countries (n = 2433)	France (n = 485)	Germany (n = 485)	Italy (n = 494)	Spain (n = 496)	UK (n = 473)
Production Method (Wild-Caught vs. Farm-Raised)	€/kg	€/kg	€/kg	€/kg	€/kg	€/kg
Cod	2.60	4.93	2.15	4.78	1.03	1.10
Salmon	5.50	8.69	5.91	7.33	1.50	3.69
Seabass	3.50	2.72	8.51	4.03	2.06	10.09
Seabream	1.59	3.94	5.29	2.19	0.69	2.03
Presentation (Whole vs. Ready-to-Cook) [1]	€/kg	€/kg	€/kg	€/kg	€/kg	€/kg
Cod	−4.08	−5.29	−8.36	−3.68	−1.11	−5.26
Herring	−4.90	−3.21	−3.08	−1.66	−0.45	−3.75
Pangasius	−2.12	−6.11	−9.77	−1.22	−1.87	−3.15
Salmon	4.93	7.21	0.77	5.72	4.30	4.30
Seabass	−1.29	−0.56	−7.56	−0.37	0.09	−10.16
Seabream	0.25	−0.96	−4.20	1.44	1.45	−5.70
Trout	−1.23	−2.13	−1.93	−0.49	−0.51	−4.94
Presentation (Fillet vs. Ready-to-Cook)	€/kg	€/kg	€/kg	€/kg	€/kg	€/kg
Cod	1.09	2.75	−0.15	1.17	0.93	1.19
Herring	−0.42	0.48	−0.51	−0.52	0.99	−1.01
Pangasius	−0.50	−1.37	−1.04	−0.20	−1.66	−1.94
Salmon	8.07	8.65	6.31	10.69	6.78	6.22
Seabass	−0.45	0.46	−1.53	−1.53	0.23	−0.63
Seabream	0.91	0.63	−0.79	1.54	1.35	2.72
Trout	−1.49	−0.09	−1.81	−2.92	−2.81	−1.67
Sustainability Label	€/kg	€/kg	€/kg	€/kg	€/kg	€/kg
Cod	1.53	0.19	1.61	3.32	1.18	1.62
Herring	2.93	−0.82	1.81	2.02	1.27	2.89
Pangasius	0.75	1.47	2.55	1.18	1.58	−2.79
Salmon	1.95	3.40	2.61	1.42	0.91	0.95
Seabass	1.27	2.80	7.06	0.86	−0.53	0.75
Seabream	1.17	0.44	8.80	1.78	0.99	3.00
Trout	1.05	1.31	1.08	1.49	1.96	−0.19
Nutrition and Health Claim	€/kg	€/kg	€/kg	€/kg	€/kg	€/kg
Cod	1.12	1.07	1.89	1.71	0.74	0.70
Herring	1.56	0.16	1.97	1.14	0.17	0.04
Pangasius	0.90	−0.06	2.31	0.96	3.53	2.41
Salmon	2.65	−0.20	4.10	3.19	2.59	2.31
Seabass	1.15	1.86	−0.78	1.38	1.46	0.80
Seabream	1.21	0.27	5.02	2.91	1.06	0.49
Trout	0.95	0.22	1.06	0.78	2.20	1.40

[1] Round cut for salmon and pangasius, whole fish for the other species.

References

1. McGuire, S. World Cancer Report 2014. Geneva, Switzerland: World Health Organization, International Agency for Research on Cancer, WHO Press, 2015. *Adv. Nutr.* **2016**, *7*, 418–419. [CrossRef] [PubMed]
2. Brohm, D.; Domurath, N. The Sustainability Trend. In *Consumer Trends and New Product Opportunities in the Food Sector*; Grunert, K.G., Ed.; Wageningen Academic Publishers: Wageningen, The Netherlands, 2017; pp. 33–42, ISBN 9789086868520.
3. Willett, W.; Rockström, J.; Loken, B.; Springmann, M.; Lang, T.; Vermeulen, S.; Garnett, T.; Tilman, D.; DeClerck, F.; Wood, A.; et al. Food in the anthropocene: The EAT–Lancet Commission on healthy diets from sustainable food systems. *Lancet* **2019**, *393*, 447–492. [CrossRef]

4. Grunert, K.G.; Hieke, S.; Wills, J. Sustainability labels on food products: Consumer motivation, understanding and use. *Food Policy* **2014**, *44*, 177–189. [CrossRef]
5. EUMOFA. *The EU Fish Market*; EUMOFA: Luxemburg, 2019.
6. Hub EU Science. Food-Based Dietary Guidelines in Europe. Available online: https://ec.europa.eu/jrc/en/health-knowledge-gateway/promotion-prevention/nutrition/food-based-dietary-guidelines (accessed on 17 August 2020).
7. Pieniak, Z.; Verbeke, W.; Olsen, S.O.; Hansen, K.B.; Brunsø, K. Health-related attitudes as a basis for segmenting European fish consumers. *Food Policy* **2010**, *35*, 448–455. [CrossRef]
8. Verbeke, W. Impact of communication on consumers' food choices. *Proc. Nutr. Soc.* **2008**, *67*, 281–288. [CrossRef]
9. Carlucci, D.; Nocella, G.; De Devitiis, B.; Viscecchia, R.; Bimbo, F.; Nardone, G. Consumer purchasing behaviour towards fish and seafood products. Patterns and insights from a sample of international studies. *Appetite* **2015**, *84*, 212–227. [CrossRef]
10. Pieniak, Z.; Verbeke, W.; Vermeir, I.; Bruns, K.; Olsen, S.O. Consumer interest in fish information and labelling. *J. Int. Foof Agribus. Mark.* **2007**, *19*, 53–75. [CrossRef]
11. Marette, S.; Roosen, J.; Blanchemanche, S. Health information and substitution between fish: Lessons from laboratory and field experiments. *Food Policy* **2008**, *33*, 197–208. [CrossRef]
12. Myrland, Ø.; Trondsen, T.; Johnston, R.S.; Lund, E. Determinants of seafood consumption in Norway: Lifestyle, revealed preferences, and barriers to consumption. *Food Qual. Prefer.* **2000**, *11*, 169–188. [CrossRef]
13. Gaviglio, A.; Demartini, E.; Mauracher, C.; Pirani, A. Consumer perception of different species and presentation forms of fish: An empirical analysis in Italy. *Food Qual. Prefer.* **2014**, *36*, 33–49. [CrossRef]
14. Cardoso, C.; Lourenço, H.; Costa, S.; Gonçalves, S.; Nunes, M.L. Survey into the seafood consumption preferences and patterns in the portuguese population. Gender and regional variability. *Appetite* **2013**, *64*, 20–31. [CrossRef] [PubMed]
15. Nguyen, T.T.; Haider, W.; Solgaard, H.S.; Ravn-Jonsen, L.; Roth, E. Consumer willingness to pay for quality attributes of fresh seafood: A labeled latent class model. *Food Qual. Prefer.* **2015**, *41*, 225–236. [CrossRef]
16. Claret, A.; Guerrero, L.; Gartzia, I.; Garcia-Quiroga, M.; Ginés, R. Does information affect consumer liking of farmed and wild fish? *Aquaculture* **2016**, *454*, 157–162. [CrossRef]
17. Verbeke, W.; Sioen, I.; Brunsø, K.; De Henauw, S.; Van Camp, J. Consumer perception versus scientific evidence of farmed and wild fish: Exploratory insights from Belgium. *Aquac. Int.* **2007**, *15*, 121–136. [CrossRef]
18. Pieniak, Z.; Verbeke, W.; Scholderer, J. Health-related beliefs and consumer knowledge as determinants of fish consumption. *J. Hum. Nutr. Diet.* **2010**, *23*, 480–488. [CrossRef]
19. Claret, A.; Guerrero, L.; Ginés, R.; Amàlia, G.; Hernández, M.; Enaitz, A.; José, B.; Carlos, F.-P.; Carmen, R.-R. Consumer beliefs regarding farmed versus wild fish. *Appetite* **2014**, *79*, 25–31. [CrossRef]
20. Uchida, H.; Onozaka, Y.; Morita, T.; Managi, S. Demand for ecolabeled seafood in the Japanese market: A conjoint analysis of the impact of information and interaction with other labels. *Food Policy* **2014**, *44*, 68–76. [CrossRef]
21. Zander, K.; Feucht, Y. Who is prepared to pay for sustainable fish? Evidence from a transnational consumer survey in Europe. In Proceedings of the International European Forum on System Dynamics and Innovation in Food Networks, Innsbruck-Igls, Austria, 5–9 February 2018; pp. 99–112.
22. Bronnmann, J.; Asche, F. Sustainable seafood from aquaculture and wild fisheries: Insights from a discrete choice experiment in Germany. *Ecol. Econ.* **2017**, *142*, 113–119. [CrossRef]
23. Reynolds, C.J.; Buckley, J.D.; Weinstein, P.; Boland, J. Are the dietary guidelines for meat, fat, fruit and vegetable consumption appropriate for environmental sustainability? A review of the literature. *Nutrients* **2014**, *6*, 2251–2265. [CrossRef]
24. Jacquet, J.L.; Pauly, D. The rise of seafood awareness campaigns in an era of collapsing fisheries. *Mar. Policy* **2007**, *31*, 308–313. [CrossRef]
25. Washington, S.; Ababouch, L. *Private Standards and Certification in Fisheries and Aquaculture Current Practice and Emerging Issues*; Food & Agriculture Organization: Rome, Italy, 2011.
26. Salladarré, F.; Guillotreau, P.; Perraudeau, Y.; Monfort, M.-C. The demand for seafood eco-labels in France. *J. Agric. Food Ind. Organ.* **2010**, *8*, 1–24. [CrossRef]

27. Gascuel, D.; Bez, N.; Forest, A.; Guillotreau, P.; Laloë, F.; Lobry, J.; Mahévas, S.; Mesnil, B.; Rivot, E.; Rochette, S.; et al. A future for marine fisheries in Europe (Manifesto of the Association Française d'Halieumétrie). *Fish. Res.* **2011**, *109*, 1–6. [CrossRef]
28. Gutierrez, A.; Thornton, T.F. Can consumers understand sustainability through seafood eco-labels? A U.S. and UK case study. *Sustainability* **2014**, *6*, 8195–8217. [CrossRef]
29. Brécard, D.; Hlaimi, B.; Lucas, S.; Perraudeau, Y.; Salladarré, F. Determinants of demand for green products: An application to eco-label demand for fish in Europe. *Ecol. Econ.* **2009**, *69*, 115–125. [CrossRef]
30. Teisl, M.F.; Roe, B.; Hicks, R.L. Can eco-labels tune a market? Evidence from dolphin-safe labeling. *J. Environ. Econ. Manag.* **2002**, *43*, 339–359. [CrossRef]
31. Jaffry, S.; Pickering, H.; Ghulam, Y.; Whitmarsh, D.; Wattage, P. Consumer choices for quality and sustainability labelled seafood products in the UK. *Food Policy* **2004**, *29*, 215–228. [CrossRef]
32. Johnston, R.J.; Roheim, C.A. A Battle of taste and environmental convictions for ecolabeled seafood: A contingent ranking experiment. *J. Agric. Resour. Econ.* **2006**, *31*, 283–300.
33. Johnston, R.J.; Wessells, C.R.; Donath, H.; Asche, F. Measuring consumer preferences for ecolabeled seafood: An international comparison. *J. Agric. Resour. Econ.* **2001**, *26*, 20–39.
34. Lim, K.H.; Hu, W.; Nayga, R.M. Is Marine Stewardship Council's ecolabel a rising tide for all? Consumers' willingness to pay for origin-differentiated ecolabeled canned tuna. *Mar. Policy* **2018**, *96*, 18–26. [CrossRef]
35. Salladarré, F.; Brécard, D.; Lucas, S.; Ollivier, P. Are French consumers ready to pay a premium for eco-labeled seafood products? A contingent valuation estimation with heterogeneous anchoring. *Agric. Econ.* **2016**, *47*, 247–258. [CrossRef]
36. Fonner, R.; Sylvia, G. Willingness to pay for multiple seafood labels in a niche market. *Mar. Resour. Econ.* **2015**, *30*, 51–70. [CrossRef]
37. Xu, P.; Zeng, Y.; Fong, Q.; Lone, T.; Liu, Y. Chinese consumers' willingness to pay for green- and eco-labeled seafood. *Food Control.* **2012**, *28*, 74–82. [CrossRef]
38. Hallstein, E.; Villas-Boas, S.B. Can household consumers save the wild fish? Lessons from a sustainable seafood advisory. *J. Environ. Econ. Manag.* **2013**, *66*, 52–71. [CrossRef]
39. Ramirez, M.Y.; Hernandez, M.A.; Polanco, G.A.; Morales, L.F. Consumer acceptance of eco-labeled fish: A Mexican case study. *Sustainability* **2015**, 4625–4642. [CrossRef]
40. Vitale, S.; Biondo, F.; Bono, G.; Giosuè, C.; Odilichukwu, C.; Okpala, C.; Piazza, I.; Sprovieri, M.; Pipitone, V. Consumers' perception and willingness to pay for eco-labeled seafood: A case-study. *Sustainability* **2018**, *12*, 1–13.
41. Stefani, G.; Scarpa, R.; Cavicchi, A. Exploring consumer's preferences for farmed sea bream. *Aquac. Int.* **2012**, *20*, 673–691. [CrossRef]
42. Mauracher, C.; Tempesta, T.; Vecchiato, D. Consumer preferences regarding the introduction of new organic products. The case of the Mediterranean sea bass (*Dicentrarchus labrax*) in Italy. *Appetite* **2013**, *63*, 84–91. [CrossRef]
43. Risius, A.; Janssen, M.; Hamm, U. Consumer preferences for sustainable aquaculture products: Evidence from in-depth interviews, think aloud protocols and choice experiments. *Appetite* **2017**, *113*, 246–254. [CrossRef]
44. Olesen, I.; Alfnes, F.; Røra, M.B.; Kolstad, K. Eliciting consumers' willingness to pay for organic and welfare-labelled salmon in a non-hypothetical choice experiment. *Livest. Sci.* **2010**, *127*, 218–226. [CrossRef]
45. McClenachan, L.; Dissanayake, S.T.M.; Chen, X. Fair trade fish: Consumer support for broader seafood sustainability. *Fish Fish.* **2016**, *17*, 825–838. [CrossRef]
46. Lancaster, K.J. A new approach to consumer theory. *J. Polit. Econ.* **1966**, *74*, 132–157. [CrossRef]
47. Zeithaml, V.A. Consumer perceptions of price, quality, and value: A means-end model and synthesis of evidence. *J. Mark.* **1988**, *52*, 2–22. [CrossRef]
48. Olsen, S.O.; Toften, K.; Dopico, D.C.; Tudoran, A.; Kole, A. Consumer Evaluation of Tailor-made Seafood Products. In *Improving Seafood Products for the Consumer*; Børresen, T., Ed.; Woodhead Publishing: Cambridge, UK, 2008; pp. 85–110, ISBN 978-1-84569-019-9.
49. SAS Institute Inc. *SAS/STAT® 14.1 User's Guide*; SAS Institute Inc: Cary, NC, USA, 2014.
50. McFadden, D. Conditional Logit Analysis of Qualitative Choice Behavior. In *Frontiers in Economics*; Zarembka, P., Ed.; Academic Press: New York, NY, USA, 1974; pp. 105–142.
51. Fiebig, D.G.; Keane, M.P.; Louviere, J.; Wasi, N. The generalized multinomial logit model: Accounting for scale and coefficient heterogeneity. *Mark. Sci.* **2010**, *29*, 393–421. [CrossRef]

52. Greene, W.H.; Hensher, D.A. A latent class model for discrete choice analysis: Contrasts with mixed logit. *Transp. Res. Part. B Methodol.* **2003**, *37*, 681–698. [CrossRef]
53. Thong, N.T.; Solgaard, H.S. Consumer's food motives and seafood consumption. *Food Qual. Prefer.* **2017**, *56*, 181–188. [CrossRef]
54. Hensher, D.A.; Rose, J.M.; Greene, W.H. *Applied Choice Analysis: A Primer*; Cambridge University Press: Cambridge, UK, 2005.
55. McDowell, A.; Shi, A. Introducing the BCHOICE Procedure for Bayesian Discrete Choice Models. Technical Report; SAS Institute Inc: Cary, NC, USA, 2014.
56. Sveinsdóttir, K.; Untilov, O.; Dietz, N.; Taskov, D.; Setti, A. Qualitative Research Report: Analysis Interviews Aimed Mainly at Identifying the Main Positive and Negative Drivers of Fish/Seafood Consumption (For the Chosen Species). Primefish Project Report (EU Horizon 2020). 2016. Available online: http://www.primefish.eu/sites/default/files/D4_2_Qualitative_research_report.pdf (accessed on 17 August 2020).
57. EFSA Panel on Dietetic Products, Nutrition and Allergies (NDA). Scientific opinion on the substantiation of health claims related to EPA, DHA, DPA and maintenance of normal blood pressure (ID 502), maintenance of normal HDL-cholesterol concentrations (ID 515), maintenance of normal (fasting) blood concentrations of tr. *EFSA J.* **2009**, *7*, 1263. [CrossRef]
58. Penn, J.M.; Hu, W. Understanding hypothetical bias: An enhanced meta-analysis. *Am. J. Agric. Econ.* **2018**, *100*, 1186–1206. [CrossRef]
59. Kole, A.P.W.; Altintzoglou, T.; Schelvis-Smit, R.A.A.M.; Luten, J.B. The effects of different types of product information on the consumer product evaluation for fresh cod in real life settings. *Food Qual. Prefer.* **2009**, *20*, 187–194. [CrossRef]
60. Katrin, Z.; Yvonne, F. How to increase demand for carp? Consumer attitudes and preferences in Germany and Poland. *Br. Food J.* **2020**. [CrossRef]
61. International Trade Commissioners-Agriculture and Agri-Food Canada Sector Trend Analysis—Fish and Seafood Trends in Germany. Available online: https://www.agr.gc.ca/eng/international-trade/market-intelligence/reports/sector-trend-analysis-fish-and-seafood-trends-in-germany/?id=1557330057050 (accessed on 17 August 2020).
62. Debucquet, G.; Cornet, J.; Adam, I.; Cardinal, M. Perception of oyster-based products by French consumers. The effect of processing and role of social representations. *Appetite* **2012**, *59*, 844–852. [CrossRef]
63. Arvanitoyannis, I.S.; Krystallis, A.; Panagiotaki, P.; Theodorou, A.J. A marketing survey on Greek consumers' attitudes towards fish. *Aquac. Int.* **2004**, *12*, 259–279. [CrossRef]
64. Sogn-Grundvåg, G.; Larsen, T.A.; Young, J.A. Product differentiation with credence attributes and private labels: The case of whitefish in UK supermarkets. *J. Agric. Econ.* **2014**, *65*, 368–382. [CrossRef]
65. Blomquist, J.; Bartolino, V.; Waldo, S. Price premiums for providing eco-labelled seafood: Evidence from msc-certified cod in Sweden. *J. Agric. Econ.* **2015**, *66*, 690–704. [CrossRef]
66. Roheim, C.A.; Asche, F.; Santos, J.I. The elusive price premium for ecolabelled products: Evidence from seafood in the UK market. *J. Agric. Econ.* **2011**, *62*, 655–668. [CrossRef]
67. Jacobs, S.; Sioen, I.; Marques, A.; Verbeke, W. Consumer response to health and environmental sustainability information regarding seafood consumption. *Environ. Res.* **2018**, *161*, 492–504. [CrossRef] [PubMed]
68. Brécard, D.; Lucas, S.; Pichot, N.; Salladarré, F. Consumer preferences for eco, health and fair trade labels. An application to seafood product in France. *J. Agric. Food Ind. Organ.* **2012**, *10*. [CrossRef]
69. Lusk, J.L.; Schroeder, T.C.; Tonsor, G.T. Distinguishing beliefs from preferences in food choice. *Eur. Rev. Agric. Econ.* **2013**, *41*, 627–655. [CrossRef]

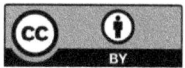

© 2020 by the authors. Licensee MDPI, Basel, Switzerland. This article is an open access article distributed under the terms and conditions of the Creative Commons Attribution (CC BY) license (http://creativecommons.org/licenses/by/4.0/).

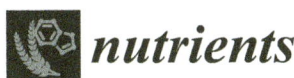

Article

Who Reads Food Labels? Selected Predictors of Consumer Interest in Front-of-Package and Back-of-Package Labels during and after the Purchase

Paweł Bryła

Department of International Marketing and Retailing, Faculty of International and Political Studies, University of Lodz, Narutowicza 59a, 90-131 Lodz, Poland; pawel.bryla@uni.lodz.pl; Tel.: +48-426655830

Received: 13 July 2020; Accepted: 25 August 2020; Published: 27 August 2020

Abstract: The paper aims to identify selected predictors of food label use to extend our knowledge about consumer behavior related to food purchases. Two types of information were examined: front-of-package (FOP) and back-of-package (BOP), and two contexts of reading labels were distinguished: during shopping and at home. Various types of potential predictors were tested, including demographic (e.g., age, gender, household size, place of living), socioeconomic (e.g., education, professional activity, income), behavioral (e.g., purchasing certain types of products), and psychographic (e.g., importance attached to various types of information) criteria. The survey was conducted with the use of the CAWI (Computer-Assisted Web Interviews) methodology in a sample of 1051 Polish consumers. Quota sampling was applied based on sex, age, education, place of living (urban vs. rural), and region. Descriptive statistics, *t*-tests, ANOVAs, Pearson correlation coefficients, and multiple and retrograde step regressions were applied. In retrograde step regression models, only one predictor (self-rated knowledge about nutrition healthiness) turned out to be significant for all four measures of label reading. The remaining predictors were specific to selected measures of reading labels. The importance of the information about the content of fat and that about the health effects of consuming a food product were significant predictors of three types of food label use. This study confirms the necessity to investigate reading labels in fine-grained models, adapted to different types of labels and different contexts of reading. Our results show that demographic or socioeconomic variables are not significant predictors of reading food labels for a large group of Polish consumers.

Keywords: food label use; front-of-package (FOP) labels; back-of-package (BOP) labels; nutrition claims; health claims; nutrition knowledge; consumer behavior

1. Introduction

In previous research, food label use was associated with consumer characteristics, product type, and purchasing context. The following variables were found to affect reading labels: gender [1–5], age [4,6], marital status [7], ethnicity [2], socioeconomic status [2,7], including education level [4,5,7–9], professional activity [9], income [5], place of living—rural or urban areas [2,5], Body Mass Index [2,4], being an athlete [10], food-related motivation [11], nutrition knowledge [4,12,13], self-reported health [4,10], having a special diet [4,9], being concerned with a healthy lifestyle [10], attitude towards the health value of the products [13], health orientation [14], taste [9,13], price [9], product specificity [12], buying the product for the first time [12], the amount of time spent shopping [9], and buying organic food [15]. There are various connections between these predictors, e.g., the gender effect is mainly due to differences in nutrition knowledge levels [12]. Health-related variables were the most important group of predictors of food label use, followed by motivating factors and sociodemographic variables.

Placing importance on health, healthy eating, and nutritional value of food, perceived vulnerability for diet-related diseases, nutrition knowledge, numeracy, and gender were positively associated with the frequency of food label use [16]. Subjective norms and diet-health concern were significant predictors of intention to use food labels [17]. Self-efficacy and health literacy were predictors of food label use among young adults [18]. Consumers' level of nutrition knowledge influenced their ability to process food labels. Experts used the central route processing to scrutinize intrinsic cues and make judgments about food products, while novices used the peripheral route processing to make simple inferences about the extrinsic cues in labels [19]. Nutritional knowledge and attitude toward food label use positively predicted food label use through self-efficacy and trust. However, these mediation effects were moderated by gender such that the indirect relationship was stronger among men than women [20]. In their review [21], Soederberg Miller and Cassady found an overreliance on convenience samples relying on younger adults, limiting our understanding of how knowledge supports food label use in later life. This limitation is overcome in the current study, as it is based on a sample representative by age.

It is also important to distinguish between food label use at the point of purchase and at home. Education has a positive impact on the likelihood of using labels at home but not while shopping. The average amount of time spent on grocery shopping per visit affects label use while shopping but not at home. The same applies to the primary source of nutrition information being books, magazines, radio, TV, or newspapers. Moreover, being on a special diet influenced label reading in the shop but not at home. The importance of price while shopping affected reading labels at home only, and the importance of taste was a significant predictor of reading labels while shopping only [9]. These results support the need to study food label use separately while shopping and at home.

Findings consistently support a relationship between label reading and dietary practices [22,23]. Changes in diet quality due to label use were estimated for different types of label information. Consumer label use increased the average Healthy Eating Index. These improvements differed across label information types that were used. Among nutritional panels, serving sizes, nutrient content claims, a list of ingredients, and health claims, the use of health claims on food labels provided the highest level of improvement in diet quality [24]. Search for total fat, saturated fat, and cholesterol information on food labels was less likely among individuals who consumed more of the three nutrients, respectively. The search was also related to perceived benefits and costs of using the label, the perceived capability of using the label, knowledge of nutrition and fats, perceived efficacy of diets in reducing the risk of illnesses, perceived importance of nutrition in food shopping, perceived importance of a healthy diet, and awareness of a linkage between excessive consumption of the nutrients and health problems [25]. Nutrition knowledge had a strong effect on general label use, degree of use, and on use of nutrient content concerning fat, ingredients, and vitamins/minerals [26]. Subjects with chronic diseases were more aware of nutritional recommendations, checked more often for specific nutrients, and used nutrition information on food labels more often than did participants without such diseases. However, label use behavior was inconsistently associated with dietary guideline compliance [27]. The odds of healthy weight loss behaviors were two to four times higher when food labels were used frequently to seek information on calories and nutrients such as total fat, saturated fat, or cholesterol [28]. A recent review [29], by Anastasiou, Miller, and Dickinson, demonstrated that results were inconsistent in reporting a relationship between diet and food label use but indicated that reading the nutrition facts label was associated with healthier diets, measured by food frequency questionnaires and 24 h recalls. However, there is insufficient research on the association between dietary consumption and the use of ingredients lists, serving size information, and front-of-package (FOP) labels. Nutrition label use decreased the risk of poor dietary quality regardless of poverty status [30]. General food label use was the main determinant of diet quality and partly mediated the association between eating behavior traits and diet quality. The stronger mediating effect observed in men suggested they relied more on food labeling when attempting to restrain themselves, which translated into better diet quality [31].

It is also important to recognize that various food label types have different effects on consumer behavior. Compared with individual characteristics, nutrition label types had an increased impact on food product ranking ability [32]. Different food label formats differed in the understanding of consumers. The multiple traffic light (MTL) labels influenced the perceived healthiness of foods most often [33]. In an international, large-scale survey, viewing the MTL provided the most favorable ratings out of five FOP nutrition label formats (health star rating, MTL, Nutri-Score, reference intakes, and warning label) [34]. The perceived usefulness and public support of mandatory implementation were higher for the MTL than for the Nutri-Score label [35]. Nutri-Score, which is a summary, interpretive, polychromatic FOP label, emerged as the most effective in the Bulgarian context [36]. FOP nutrition labels were more likely to be viewed than Nutrition Facts labels [37]. Different degrees of health-orientation were reflected in the diverse use of labeled information. Highly health-oriented consumers were more likely to refer to the extensive information reported on the nutrition facts panel, whereas claims were of main interest for consumers with a low orientation to health [14]. Furthermore, 52.5% of consumers did not read the ingredients' list written on the food label [38]. Simplified FOP labels can induce healthier purchases compared with when only back-of-package (BOP) nutrition information is available [39]. Clearer BOP labeling is also needed [40]. Nutritional warnings cause a salience bias that makes excessive nutrient content and its negative health consequences more salient in consumers' minds, especially in the case of products with a particular health-related connotation [41]. Although FOP labels may help shoppers make healthier food choices, those advocating for effective labels must resist opposition from food corporations [42]. Future opportunities for FOP labeling include the potential for integrating nutritional profiles with non-nutrient factors affecting health such as food processing and environmental sustainability [43]. Although FOP labels help consumers to identify healthier products, their ability to nudge consumers toward healthier choices is more limited. Importantly, FOP labels may lead to halo effects, positively influencing not only virtue but also vice products, e.g., interpretive nutrient-specific labels improve health perceptions of both vice and virtue products, yet they influence only the purchase intention of virtues [44].

The paper aims to identify selected predictors of reading food labels with the distinction of the label type (FOP and BOP), and the context of food label use (during shopping and afterward, at home). Therefore, four measures of reading labels were considered in this study: FOP in the shop, BOP in the shop, FOP at home, and BOP at home. The main contribution of this paper lies in systematically analyzing predictors of reading labels from the perspective of two major label types (FOP and BOP) and two main reading contexts (in the shop and at home) based on a survey in a large, representative, nation-wide sample of consumers.

2. Materials and Methods

The survey was conducted with the use of the CAWI (Computer Assisted Web Interviews) methodology. The execution of the survey was commissioned to a specialized market research agency. The respondents were informed that the results would be used only for scientific purposes, respecting the anonymity principle. The sample size amounted to 1051 consumers. The target sample size was set at a comparable level with previous consumer studies conducted at the national level in Poland [45–47]. It was aimed to obtain a sample resembling the general population of Polish adults, regarding four criteria: age, sex, education level, and the size of the city of origin (in particular, the urban/rural divide). Quota sampling was applied based on five criteria: sex (men and women), age (the following age intervals: 15–24, 25–34, 35–44, 45–54, 55–64, 65 and more), education (primary, secondary and tertiary), place of living (urban and rural areas), and region (all 16 Polish regions). Thanks to this approach, the sample structure was similar to the general population of Polish consumers according to the above-mentioned criteria (Table A1).

The questionnaire was created by the author of this study. It was composed of elements adapted from previous research using validated tools [14,48–59]. It consisted of 38 questions. The full questionnaire is included in a book in Polish [60]. The operationalization of the key variables used in this study is provided in Table A2. Reading labels was investigated in 4 configurations: (1) FOP in the point of purchase (FOP shop), (2) BOP in the point of purchase (BOP shop), (3) FOP after purchase (FOP home), (4) BOP after purchase (BOP home). It was operationalized as a percentage share of food products the respondent buys. Some more difficult terms were explained in the questionnaire, in particular health claims, nutrition claims, and quality signs. The research examined general food labels. My dependent variables referred to FOP and BOP labels without specifying which information was put on which label. However, in some questions, I examined the importance attached to particular types of information placed on the labels, such as health claims, nutrition claims, list of ingredients, expiry date, country of origin, cooking recipes, brand, organic certificate, quality signs, recommendations of scientific institutes, price, as well as selected types of nutritional information (energy value, the content of fat, sugar, salt, protein, vitamins, dietary fiber, Omega-3 fatty acids) and health information (lowering cholesterol, reducing the risk of heart diseases, strengthening bones, impact on the digestive system, reducing tiredness and fatigue, maintaining proper vision, proper development of children, and proper functioning of the heart). Various types of potential predictors were tested, including demographic (e.g., age, gender, household size, place of living), socioeconomic (e.g., education, professional activity, income), behavioral (e.g., purchasing certain types of products), and psychographic (e.g., importance attached to various types of information) criteria. For most of the questions, 5-point Likert scales were used.

First, I tested the differences in reading food labels depending on selected demographic and socioeconomic criteria: sex, age, place of living, education, professional activity, income, household size, and the number of children. Second, I checked whether reading labels differed depending on some purchasing habits: buying dietary supplements, organic food, functional food, and fair trade products. Third, I examined label use according to selected criteria related to one's health and diet. Fourth, I examined the correlations of food label use with the evaluation of the quantity, understandability, and credibility of selected information on the food packaging.

Next, I tested the associations between food label use and the importance attached to selected types of information placed on the labels. Four questions were devoted to this issue. The first one concerned general food labels. Second, I focused on the importance of information at the first purchase of a given product. This question referred to a product that was new to the consumer and not necessarily to the entire market Third, I took into consideration typical types of nutritional information. Last, I examined the correlations with selected types of health-related information.

Furthermore, the associations between food label use and the importance attached to marketing communication instruments were identified. The following marketing communication options were put forward for the respondents' evaluation: TV commercials, producer website, retailer website, producer social media profile, retailer social media profile, consumer opinions in social media, mobile applications, recommendations of family or friends, recommendations of a dietician, outdoor advertising (e.g., billboards), advertising newsletters of retailers, articles in press and magazines, TV culinary programs, culinary blogs, product packaging, and shop assistant.

Regarding information used in the marketing communication for food products, the following options were considered: health effects of consuming a given product, care for the natural environment, supporting producers (e.g., farmers), low price, national origin of the product, the utility of the product in a certain diet, above-average quality of the product, and traditional method of production.

Based on statistical differences revealed in *t*-tests and ANOVAs as well as the most significant Pearson correlations, 32 independent variables were selected to be analyzed in multiple regressions. Separate regression models were constructed for each type of reading labels.

In the data analysis, descriptive statistics, *t*-tests, analyses of variance (ANOVAs), Pearson correlation coefficients, and multiple and retrograde step regressions were applied. T-tests were used to compare two quantitative results, ANOVAs were used to compare multiple quantitative results, Pearson correlation coefficients were used to examine the linear correlations between quantitative variables, the multiple regression models were used to examine the simultaneous influence of all independent variables separately on the 4 types of reading labels, and the retrograde step regressions were used to narrow down the set of independent variables to those that remained significant at the $p < 0.05$ level. Independent variables that differentiated any measure of reading labels in a statistically significant way were included in separate multiple regression models for FOP shop, BOP shop, FOP home, and BOP home. To obtain more parsimonious models, only those predictors that reached statistical significance at the level of $p < 0.05$ were accepted in retrograde step regressions. The analyses were conducted in Statistica 12 (TIBCO Software Inc., Palo Alto, CA, USA). I report continuous p-values instead of thresholds, following the recent guidelines of statisticians [61]. Results that are statistically significant at $p < 0.05$ are boldfaced to increase their visibility.

3. Results

Women read food labels more often than men, but the sex differences reached statistical significance only for reading BOP labels at the point of purchase (BOP shop) and FOP labels after the purchase at home (FOP home) (Table 1).

Table 1. Reading food labels by sex.

Reading Labels (%)	Women	Men	t	p
FOP shop	56.72	53.77	1.726	0.085
BOP shop	52.59	47.69	2.888	**0.004**
FOP home	51.49	46.29	2.763	**0.006**
BOP home	52.86	50.04	1.502	0.133

A series of ANOVAs demonstrated that age (measured in 10-year intervals) did not differentiate any measure of reading labels (Table 2).

Table 2. Reading food labels by age.

Reading Labels (%)	Age Intervals					ANOVA	
	15–24	25–34	35–44	45–54	55–64	≥65	F	p
FOP shop	59.75	55.15	53.17	53.87	54.50	55.81	1.160	0.327
BOP shop	51.94	50.57	50.34	47.75	50.70	50.24	0.372	0.868
FOP home	48.80	49.17	47.55	47.26	51.84	49.57	0.479	0.792
BOP home	53.63	51.99	51.38	48.10	53.68	50.46	0.746	0.589

Reading labels was not affected by the place of living (defined as rural areas, towns up to 50,000, cities of 50–500,000, and cities of more than 500,000) either (Table 3).

Table 3. Reading food labels by the place of living.

Reading Labels (%)	Place of Living				ANOVA	
	Rural Areas	<50,000	50,000–500,000	>500,000	F	p
FOP shop	54.20	58.34	55.30	54.66	1.016	0.385
BOP shop	48.89	51.78	51.16	50.45	0.639	0.590
FOP home	48.91	51.13	48.57	47.81	0.409	0.746
BOP home	50.87	54.08	50.75	51.67	0.581	0.627

As far as the education level is concerned, only the FOP shop was influenced in a significant way (Table 4). Respondents who had tertiary education read food labels in shops more often than the other education groups.

Table 4. Reading food labels by education.

Reading Labels (%)	Education				ANOVA	
	Primary	Vocational	Secondary	Tertiary	F	p
FOP shop	55.89	52.50	55.96	59.08	2.750	**0.042**
BOP shop	51.16	48.21	51.21	52.11	1.209	0.305
FOP home	48.77	48.31	50.38	48.51	0.310	0.818
BOP home	51.72	49.19	54.45	51.15	1.787	0.148

As far as the professional activity is concerned, it affected reading labels at the point of purchase—both FOP and BOP—but not after the purchase at home. White-collar workers read food labels most frequently in-store (both FOP and BOP) (Table 5).

Table 5. Reading food labels by professional activity.

Reading Labels (%)	Professional Activity						ANOVA	
	1	2	3	4	5	6	F	p
FOP shop	61.16	52.52	48.49	57.98	54.05	55.68	2.725	**0.019**
BOP shop	56.15	48.03	40.80	51.93	49.57	50.58	2.924	**0.013**
FOP home	51.44	48.34	43.73	47.15	47.72	50.73	0.820	0.535
BOP home	55.81	50.34	45.41	53.95	50.55	51.31	1.209	0.303

Notes: 1—white-collar worker, 2—blue-collar worker, 3—unemployed, 4—student, 5—not working and taking care of one's family, 6—old age pensioner or disability pensioner; the category "other" was excluded from the ANOVA.

Reading food labels was associated with household income only for the FOP shop. It was highest among respondents living in households with middle income (3001–4000 PLN) and the highest income (over 6000 PLN per month) (Table 6).

Table 6. Reading food labels by income.

Reading Labels (%)	Income Intervals						ANOVA	
	1	2	3	4	5	6	F	p
FOP shop	48.92	55.33	58.52	55.58	55.01	57.83	2.509	**0.029**
BOP shop	46.66	50.50	50.65	49.49	52.43	53.53	1.034	0.396
FOP home	48.15	49.38	51.31	44.96	50.93	50.15	1.081	0.369
BOP home	47.96	51.54	52.87	52.03	51.56	53.03	0.586	0.711

Notes: the average monthly disposable income of one's household; 1—below 2000 PLN, 2—2001–3000 PLN, 3—3001–4000 PLN, 4—4001–5000 PLN, 5—5001–6000 PLN, 6—over 6000 PLN.

Only FOP label reading (in the shop and at home) correlated positively and significantly with the size of one's household (Table 7).

Table 7. Pearson correlation coefficients of reading food labels with the size of one's household and the number of children.

Number of Persons	FOP Shop		BOP Shop		FOP Home		BOP Home	
	r	p	r	p	r	p	r	p
Household	0.076	**0.013**	0.043	0.164	0.066	**0.031**	0.031	0.320
Children	0.043	0.164	0.054	0.081	0.039	0.211	0.040	0.199

Notes: household—the number of people in one's household, children—the number of children in one's household.

Reading food labels was associated with purchasing certain types of products, namely dietary supplements, organic food, functional food, and fair trade products (Table 8). Buying dietary supplements increased the frequency of reading labels on the front of the package in the shop and at home as well as on the back of the package at home only. Buying organic food affected all measures of reading labels in a highly significant way. Buying functional food influenced all kinds of reading labels except for the FOP shop. Buying fair trade products differentiated significantly reading only the BOP information.

Table 8. Reading food labels by purchasing certain products.

Reading Labels (%)	Yes	No	t	p
Buying dietary supplements				
FOP shop	57.71	53.11	2.698	**0.007**
BOP shop	51.84	48.85	1.759	0.079
FOP home	51.40	46.86	2.410	**0.016**
BOP home	54.17	49.08	2.716	**0.007**
Buying organic food				
FOP shop	58.41	51.73	3.926	**<0.001**
BOP shop	54.71	45.11	5.715	**<0.001**
FOP home	52.92	44.52	4.486	**<0.001**
BOP home	56.05	46.24	5.273	**<0.001**
Buying functional food				
FOP shop	56.41	54.75	0.930	0.353
BOP shop	54.15	48.18	3.385	**0.001**
FOP home	52.03	47.43	2.341	**0.019**
BOP home	57.11	48.48	4.434	**<0.001**
Buying fair trade products				
FOP shop	57.80	54.41	1.769	0.077
BOP shop	54.31	48.78	2.913	**0.004**
FOP home	50.35	48.57	0.840	0.401
BOP home	56.80	49.56	3.454	**0.001**

Note: the category "No" includes direct "No" answers and "I don't know" answers.

Reading food labels was correlated with self-rated healthiness of one's diet, one's knowledge about healthy nutrition, and self-rated health but not BMI (Body Mass Index) (Table 9).

Table 9. Pearson correlation coefficients of reading food labels with the self-rated healthiness of one's diet, self-rated knowledge about healthy nutrition, self-rated health, and BMI.

Self-Rated Measures	FOP Shop		BOP Shop		FOP Home		BOP Home	
	r	p	r	p	r	p	r	p
Diet	0.072	**0.019**	0.104	**0.001**	0.075	**0.014**	0.091	**0.003**
Knowledge	0.089	**0.004**	0.118	**<0.001**	0.087	**0.005**	0.097	**0.002**
Health	0.072	**0.020**	0.088	**0.004**	0.063	**0.042**	0.076	**0.014**
BMI	−0.029	0.344	−0.049	0.109	0.026	0.401	−0.020	0.512

Note: BMI—Body Mass Index (kg/m^2).

However, none of the investigated measures of reading labels depended on being on a special diet for health reasons (Table 10).

Table 10. Reading food labels by being on a special diet for health reasons.

Reading Labels (%)	Yes	No	t	p
FOP shop	52.71	55.87	−1.378	0.168
BOP shop	50.83	50.19	0.279	0.780
FOP home	48.55	49.16	−0.242	0.809
BOP home	53.13	51.23	0.753	0.452

Reading BOP labels was related to the evaluation of the quantity of selected information (health claims, nutrition claims, and quality signs) on food labels (Table 11). Those who considered that there was too little such information tended to read food labels more often. Moreover, all measures of reading labels were associated with the self-evaluated understandability of information put on the labels (namely health claims, nutrition claims, quality signs, functional food, and organic food). Finally, reading labels correlated with the perceived credibility of such information (health claims, nutrition claims, list of ingredients, expiry date, organic certificate, and quality signs). Those who trusted information placed on the labels more tended to read them more often both in the shop and at home.

Table 11. Pearson coefficients of reading food labels with the evaluation of the quantity, understandability, and credibility of selected information on food packaging.

Reading Labels (%)	Quantity		Understandability		Credibility	
	r	p	r	p	r	p
FOP shop	0.033	0.287	0.080	0.009	0.083	0.007
BOP shop	0.143	<0.001	0.079	0.010	0.072	0.019
FOP home	0.051	0.098	0.073	0.018	0.080	0.010
BOP home	0.125	<0.001	0.080	0.010	0.074	0.017

Reading food labels depended on the importance attached to selected information put on them (Table 12). The subjective importance of almost all types of information correlated positively and significantly with reading FOP and BOP food labels both at the point of purchase and at home, except cooking recipes, the importance of which was correlated significantly only with the FOP home.

Table 12. Pearson correlation coefficients of reading food labels with the subjective importance of selected information on labels.

Types of Information	FOP Shop		BOP Shop		FOP Home		BOP Home	
	r	p	r	p	r	p	r	p
Health claims	0.078	0.011	0.103	0.001	0.076	0.013	0.102	0.001
Nutrition claims	0.081	0.009	0.111	<0.001	0.088	0.004	0.104	0.001
List of ingredients	0.091	0.003	0.141	<0.001	0.084	0.007	0.122	<0.001
Expiry date	0.093	0.002	0.087	0.005	0.070	0.024	0.081	0.009
Country of origin	0.067	0.029	0.095	0.002	0.080	0.009	0.088	0.004
Cooking recipes	0.045	0.147	0.053	0.088	0.082	0.008	0.059	0.055
Brand	0.070	0.024	0.072	0.020	0.080	0.009	0.074	0.016
Organic certificate	0.081	0.008	0.102	0.001	0.090	0.003	0.088	0.004
Quality signs	0.084	0.006	0.086	0.005	0.088	0.004	0.094	0.002
Recommendations *	0.081	0.009	0.092	0.003	0.097	0.002	0.092	0.003
Price	0.075	0.015	0.070	0.023	0.074	0.016	0.078	0.011
Average**	0.079	0.010	0.095	0.002	0.085	0.006	0.092	0.003

Notes: * of scientific institutes; ** average evaluation of the importance of all types of information mentioned in this column of the table.

As far as the importance of information at the first purchase of a food product (excluding price) is concerned, it differentiated only BOP label reading, both in the shop and at home. The respondents indicating the list of ingredients read the highest share of BOP labels in both contexts (Table 13).

Table 13. Reading food labels by the most important information on the food label at the first purchase (excluding price).

Reading Labels (%)	Most Important at First Purchase					ANOVA	
	COO	NI	HI	LI	ED	F	p
FOP shop	53.52	53.94	54.25	58.68	55.84	1.260	0.284
BOP shop	47.04	53.80	44.34	56.82	47.67	7.257	<0.001
FOP home	52.08	47.30	54.56	49.61	48.33	1.145	0.334
BOP home	52.18	54.49	49.47	56.64	47.93	3.878	0.004

Notes: COO—the country of origin, NI—nutritional information (e.g., about the content of fat or dietary fiber), HI—information on health effects (e.g., good for the bones, lowering cholesterol), LI—list of ingredients, ED—expiry date; the reading labels indicators were measured in percentages of food products the consumer bought; the responses "other" and "I don't know" were excluded from the ANOVAs.

All the investigated nutritional information types correlated significantly with all four measures of reading labels (Table 14).

Table 14. Pearson correlation coefficients of reading food labels with the subjective importance of selected nutritional information on labels.

Types of Information	FOP Shop		BOP Shop		FOP Home		BOP Home	
	r	p	r	p	r	p	r	p
Energy value (calories)	0.078	0.011	0.120	<0.001	0.093	0.003	0.111	<0.001
Content of fat	0.090	0.004	0.128	<0.001	0.106	0.001	0.130	<0.001
Content of sugar	0.088	0.004	0.135	<0.001	0.097	0.002	0.127	<0.001
Content of salt	0.071	0.022	0.118	<0.001	0.104	0.001	0.116	<0.001
Content of protein	0.095	0.002	0.127	<0.001	0.100	0.001	0.120	<0.001
Content of vitamins	0.088	0.004	0.123	<0.001	0.102	0.001	0.123	<0.001
Content of dietary fiber	0.096	0.002	0.123	<0.001	0.106	0.001	0.116	<0.001
Content of Omega-3 fatty acids	0.082	0.008	0.120	<0.001	0.104	0.001	0.116	<0.001

All of the investigated health information types correlated significantly with all the measures of reading labels (Table 15).

Table 15. Pearson correlation coefficients of reading food labels with the subjective importance of selected health information on labels.

Information about the Impact of the Product on:	FOP Shop		BOP Shop		FOP Home		BOP Home	
	r	p	r	p	r	p	r	p
Lowering cholesterol	0.071	0.021	0.084	0.007	0.109	<0.001	0.100	0.001
Reducing the risk of heart diseases	0.079	0.010	0.084	0.006	0.100	0.001	0.094	0.002
Strengthening bones	0.088	0.004	0.097	0.002	0.099	0.001	0.099	0.001
The digestive system	0.082	0.008	0.101	0.001	0.094	0.002	0.103	0.001
Reducing tiredness and fatigue	0.091	0.003	0.097	0.002	0.105	0.001	0.100	0.001
Maintaining proper vision	0.084	0.007	0.094	0.002	0.104	0.001	0.102	0.001
Proper development of children	0.075	0.016	0.080	0.009	0.093	0.002	0.085	0.006
Proper functioning of the heart	0.080	0.009	0.090	0.004	0.096	0.002	0.100	0.001

Furthermore, reading food labels was associated with the importance attached to all investigated promotion instruments for food products with health and nutrition claims, with some minor exceptions for particular food label use measures (Table 16).

Table 16. Pearson correlation coefficients of reading food labels with the evaluation of the importance of selected promotion instruments for food products with health and nutrition claims.

Promotion Instruments	FOP Shop		BOP Shop		FOP Home		BOP Home	
	r	p	r	p	r	p	r	p
TV commercials	0.068	**0.028**	0.055	0.073	0.075	**0.015**	0.056	0.072
Producer website	0.071	**0.020**	0.070	**0.023**	0.088	**0.004**	0.077	**0.012**
Retailer website	0.064	**0.038**	0.064	**0.038**	0.078	**0.012**	0.067	**0.029**
Producer social media profile	0.067	**0.031**	0.055	0.073	0.084	**0.007**	0.067	**0.029**
Retailer social media profile	0.071	**0.022**	0.061	**0.048**	0.086	**0.005**	0.068	**0.028**
Consumer opinions in social media	0.077	**0.012**	0.076	**0.014**	0.083	**0.007**	0.083	**0.007**
Mobile applications	0.059	0.058	0.062	**0.043**	0.080	**0.010**	0.067	**0.031**
Recommendations of family or friends	0.081	**0.009**	0.090	**0.004**	0.080	**0.010**	0.092	**0.003**
Recommendations of a dietician	0.074	**0.016**	0.095	**0.002**	0.073	**0.018**	0.093	**0.002**
Outdoor advertising (e.g., billboards)	0.076	**0.014**	0.063	**0.040**	0.090	**0.004**	0.073	**0.018**
Advertising newsletters of retailers	0.062	**0.045**	0.064	**0.039**	0.063	**0.040**	0.062	**0.043**
Articles in press and magazines	0.068	**0.027**	0.066	**0.032**	0.081	**0.009**	0.069	**0.025**
TV culinary programs	0.085	**0.006**	0.065	**0.034**	0.095	**0.002**	0.072	**0.019**
Culinary blogs	0.075	**0.015**	0.087	**0.005**	0.095	**0.002**	0.089	**0.004**
Product packaging	0.087	**0.005**	0.077	**0.013**	0.078	**0.012**	0.084	**0.007**
Shop assistant	0.076	**0.014**	0.053	0.087	0.077	**0.012**	0.057	0.065

All kinds of reading labels were associated the most strongly with the importance attached to the health effects of consuming a given product (Table 17).

Table 17. Pearson correlation coefficients of reading food labels with the subjective importance of selected information types in the marketing communication for food products.

Information Type	FOP Shop		BOP Shop		FOP Home		BOP Home	
	r	p	r	p	r	p	r	p
Health effects of consuming a given product	0.099	**0.001**	0.109	**<0.001**	0.101	**0.001**	0.116	**<0.001**
Care for the natural environment	0.087	**0.005**	0.098	**0.001**	0.092	**0.003**	0.088	**0.004**
Supporting producers (e.g., farmers)	0.067	**0.031**	0.073	**0.018**	0.092	**0.003**	0.082	**0.008**
Low price	0.083	**0.007**	0.059	0.056	0.085	**0.006**	0.062	**0.043**
Polish origin of the product	0.057	0.064	0.077	**0.012**	0.088	**0.004**	0.084	**0.007**
Utility of the product in a certain diet	0.087	**0.005**	0.097	**0.002**	0.099	**0.001**	0.085	**0.006**
Above average quality of the product	0.088	**0.004**	0.096	**0.002**	0.083	**0.007**	0.094	**0.002**
Traditional method of production	0.071	**0.021**	0.099	**0.001**	0.089	**0.004**	0.099	**0.001**

It is also worth noting that all the analyzed types of reading labels correlated significantly with the willingness to pay (WTP) a higher price for food products with health claims and nutrition claims compared to conventional products (Table 18). The strongest correlation was observed between the BOP shop and the WTP for nutrition claims.

Table 18. Pearson correlation coefficients of reading food labels with the willingness to pay more for food products with health and nutrition claims compared to conventional products.

WTP	FOP Shop		BOP Shop		FOP Home		BOP Home	
	r	p	r	p	r	p	r	p
WTP HC	0.073	**0.018**	0.079	**0.011**	0.077	**0.012**	0.091	**0.003**
WTP NC	0.075	**0.015**	0.087	**0.005**	0.077	**0.012**	0.096	**0.002**

The multiple regression models explained better reading BOP labels (BOP shop $R^2 = 0.173$, BOP home $R^2 = 0.143$) than FOP labels (FOP shop $R^2 = 0.091$, FOP home $R^2 = 0.089$) (Table 19). In the full multiple regression model, reading FOP labels at the point of purchase was determined by only three predictors: self-rated knowledge about healthy nutrition, the importance of the expiry date information on the food packaging, and the importance of the information about the health effects of consuming a given product. Second, reading BOP information in the shop turned out to depend on five variables. It was positively associated with the importance attached to the list of ingredients, self-rated nutrition knowledge, indicating the list of ingredients as the most important information at the first purchase, and average assessment of the quantity of selected information on the food packaging: health claims, nutrition claims, and quality signs. It was negatively related to the consumer education level. The third regression model reported in this table refers to reading FOP labels at home. Six variables had a significant impact on this measure, four out of which were positively related: self-rated nutrition knowledge, the importance attached to culinary blogs, the importance of information about the health effects of consuming the product, and the importance of the information that the product reduces tiredness and fatigue. On the other hand, it was negatively associated with the information about the impact of the product on the digestive system and the importance attached to the recommendations of a dietician. The last regression model concerned the predictors of reading BOP information after the purchase. It was found to depend on five variables, all of which contributed positively: the importance of the information about the content of fat, the importance of the list of ingredients, the importance of the information about the health effects of consuming a product, the evaluation of the quantity of information on the label, and the importance of the list of ingredients when one buys a food product for the first time.

Table 19. Selected predictors of reading food labels—full multiple regression models.

Independent Variables	FOP Shop		BOP Shop		FOP Home		BOP Home	
	β	p	β	p	β	p	β	p
Woman	−0.004	0.899	0.020	0.525	0.045	0.161	−0.020	0.515
Education	0.031	0.362	−0.070	**0.033**	−0.024	0.490	−0.042	0.205
White-collar	0.050	0.131	0.045	0.149	0.012	0.706	0.029	0.358
Student	0.020	0.556	−0.039	0.222	−0.022	0.521	−0.003	0.924
Income	0.041	0.208	0.042	0.175	0.024	0.462	0.026	0.405
Household	−0.009	0.776	−0.032	0.306	−0.041	0.218	−0.054	0.092
Dietary suppl.	0.035	0.259	−0.001	0.961	0.021	0.507	0.027	0.365
Organic	0.036	0.298	0.039	0.237	0.065	0.060	0.011	0.747
Functional	−0.034	0.304	0.018	0.562	0.012	0.712	0.042	0.193
Fair trade	0.010	0.763	0.032	0.314	−0.025	0.453	0.043	0.183
Diet	−0.041	0.292	0.035	0.347	−0.029	0.454	0.030	0.420
Knowledge	0.117	**0.002**	0.131	**<0.001**	0.110	**0.004**	0.062	0.094
Health	−0.002	0.955	0.060	0.067	−0.005	0.879	0.044	0.180
Quantity	0.025	0.459	0.067	**0.037**	0.021	0.523	0.069	**0.034**
Understandability	0.042	0.253	0.026	0.452	0.011	0.760	0.054	0.127
Credibility	0.056	0.144	−0.063	0.088	0.037	0.336	−0.033	0.380
List of ingredients	−0.022	0.565	0.170	**<0.001**	−0.033	0.400	0.103	**0.006**
Expiry date	0.112	**0.001**	−0.002	0.956	0.003	0.941	0.012	0.727
Institutes	0.017	0.643	−0.014	0.690	0.053	0.147	−0.005	0.890
First-time LI	0.048	0.124	0.085	**0.004**	−0.006	0.852	0.060	**0.048**
Sugar	−0.049	0.318	0.056	0.228	−0.037	0.455	0.045	0.344
Fat	0.038	0.466	0.055	0.266	0.091	0.079	0.108	**0.031**
Dietary fiber	0.043	0.338	0.016	0.701	0.033	0.462	−0.031	0.481
Cholesterol	−0.045	0.325	−0.071	0.098	0.077	0.089	0.010	0.813
Digestive system	−0.070	0.172	0.008	0.865	−0.108	**0.037**	−0.027	0.590
Fatigue	0.070	0.128	0.018	0.685	0.091	**0.046**	−0.001	0.988
Dietician	−0.058	0.130	0.003	0.933	−0.107	**0.005**	−0.018	0.628
Blogs	0.028	0.461	0.033	0.364	0.099	**0.010**	0.039	0.293
Packaging	0.055	0.116	−0.035	0.296	0.020	0.574	0.008	0.814

Table 19. Cont.

Independent Variables	FOP Shop		BOP Shop		FOP Home		BOP Home	
	β	p	β	p	β	p	β	p
Health effects	0.110	**0.009**	0.055	0.166	0.094	**0.025**	0.104	**0.010**
WTP HC	−0.004	0.941	−0.029	0.594	−0.011	0.847	−0.007	0.900
WTP NC	−0.027	0.640	−0.006	0.907	−0.071	0.214	0.000	0.994
R^2	0.091		0.173		0.089		0.143	

According to the final retrograde step regression models (Table 20), the FOP shop increased with being a white-collar worker, having better (self-rated) knowledge about healthy nutrition, evaluating the credibility of information on labels higher, attaching importance to the expiry date, and health effects in the marketing communication for food products. Second, the BOP shop increased with one's knowledge about a healthy diet, better self-rated health, evaluating the quantity of information on labels as insufficient, attaching importance to the list of ingredients in general and during first-time purchases, and attaching importance to the content of fat. Third, reading FOP labels at home increased with the knowledge about a healthy diet, attaching importance to the content of fat and to the impact of the product on lowering cholesterol, attaching importance to culinary blogs, and to health effects in the marketing communications but decreased with the importance attached to the recommendations of a dietician. Finally, reading BOP labels at home depended on buying functional food, one's knowledge about a healthy diet, evaluation of the quantity of information on food labels, the importance attached to the list of ingredients, to the content of fat, and to health effects in the marketing communication.

Table 20. Selected predictors of reading food labels—retrograde step regression models.

Independent Variables	FOP Shop		BOP Shop		FOP Home		BOP Home	
	β	p	β	p	β	p	β	p
White-collar	0.072	**0.017**	x	x	x	x	x	x
Functional	x	x	x	x	x	x	0.062	**0.039**
Knowledge	0.115	**<0.001**	0.168	**0.031**	0.105	**0.031**	0.107	**0.001**
Health	x	x	0.065	**0.030**	x	x	x	x
Quantity	x	x	0.076	**0.029**	x	x	0.062	**0.037**
Credibility	0.066	**0.040**	x	x	x	x	x	x
List of ingredients	x	x	0.175	**0.033**	x	x	0.120	**<0.001**
Expiry date	0.116	**<0.001**	x	x	x	x	x	x
First-time LI	x	x	0.086	**0.029**	x	x	x	x
Fat	x	x	0.094	**0.033**	0.081	**0.036**	0.113	**0.001**
Cholesterol	x	x	x	x	0.086	**0.036**	x	x
Dietician	x	x	x	x	−0.092	**0.037**	x	x
Blogs	x	x	x	x	0.107	**0.035**	x	x
Health effects	0.096	**0.003**	x	x	0.081	**0.037**	0.106	**0.002**
R^2	0.066		0.152		0.068		0.124	

Note: only predictors significant at $p < 0.05$ are included in these models.

4. Discussion

The main contribution of this paper is the identification of variables that influence food label use in four configurations: FOP in the shop, BOP in the shop, FOP at home, and BOP at home, based on a survey in a large, representative, nation-wide sample of consumers. In retrograde step regression models, only one predictor (self-rated knowledge about healthy diet) turned out to be significant for all four measures of label reading. Two more predictors (importance attached to the content of fat and health effects in marketing communication) were significant in three out of the four investigated forms of reading labels. The remaining independent variables were specific to one or two forms only. It confirms the necessity to study reading labels in fine-grained models, adapted to different types of labels and different contexts of reading. Moreover, this study demonstrated that sociodemographic and behavioral characteristics have limited power of explaining reading labels in multivariate models (except being a white-collar worker for FOP shop and buying functional food for BOP home). Most of the relevant predictors were psychographic, as they concerned the importance attached to selected information types put on the labels or used in the marketing communication as well as the evaluation of the quantity and credibility of information placed on the labels. It is also worth noting that most of the predictors were related to the nutrition and health aspects of communication.

My results differed from some previous findings. In a sample of US adults, significant differences in food label use were observed across all demographic characteristics examined [62]. This difference may stem from: (1) international differences in food label use, (2) a different operationalization of food label use as well as (3) the inclusion of a wide set of psychographic criteria in my multivariate models, which turned out to be better predictors. In another study, determinants of food label use differed by sex. Age and diet quality perception were significant predictors of food label use for both men and women, but ethnicity was significant for males only. Similar to my findings, women checked food label components more often than men [63], but the current study distinguishes various forms and contexts of food label use. Significant differences between men and women were observed for reading BOP labels in the shop and FOP labels at home. Reading food labels has different predictors than the importance attached to some types of information placed on the labels. For instance, another study based on the same dataset demonstrated that the importance attached to salt content information depended on sex and age [64]. Following most previous studies, my results confirmed the impact of nutrition knowledge on food label use. However, interestingly, this relationship may be treated as bidirectional. Cavaliere et al. found that food label use increased the nutritional knowledge of consumers, which in turn favored a healthy diet [65]. It is also important to realize that the valuation of information on the labels is heterogeneous across consumer segments. For instance, Ballco and De Magistris [66] identified three consumer segments: "health-claims oriented", "nutritional- and health-claim oriented", and "indifferent". There is a complexity of targeting nutrition labels because a nonlinear effect of health attitude on the selection of products with increased nutrients content was revealed in previous research [67].

Information may not always be effective in improving food choices. One explanation is that nutrition information is complex and difficult to convey in a clear, actionable manner. In addition, knowledge, while necessary, may not be sufficient to motivate behavior change [68]. The online shopping environment offers new promising tools, such as dynamic food labels with real-time feedback [69], which are not available offline. Even though food label use was associated with improved dietary factors, it was not sufficient alone to modify behavior ultimately leading to improved health outcomes [62]. The perceived credibility of nutrition claims, agreeing that the availability of health-related information is not sufficient for the vast majority of consumers to change their food preferences, and believing that foods carry an excessive number of nutrition claims affected the importance of nutrition claims among food processors and distributors [70]. There is also evidence of mistrust in health claims, as indicated by the negative relationship between the consideration of such claims and the stated importance of "quality" and perceived need to "change dietary quality"—the more discerning shoppers were the least likely to consider health claims [71].

There are a few limitations to this study. The first one is that it is based on self-reported data only. A known limitation of self-report instruments such as surveys and questionnaires is their susceptibility to socially desirable responding. Socially desirable responding is the tendency to give answers that make the respondent look good, or the tendency "to stretch the truth in an effort to make a good impression" [72]. In my survey, I minimized this bias by ensuring the survey anonymity and confidentiality of answers. At the beginning of the questionnaire, the respondents were informed that the survey was anonymous and the results would be used for scientific purposes only. Both self-reported and objective measures of food label use were positively associated with dietary quality. However, self-reported measures appeared to capture a greater motivational component of food label use than did more objective measures [73]. Second, the determination coefficients in my regression models were relatively low, especially for reading FOP labels. This means that there may be other important predictors, which were not included in my study. Nevertheless, taking into consideration the wide range of potential predictors that were examined in my models, it may be also due to the difficulty of assessing the percentage of products the labels of which are read by the given respondent. I opted for the percentage measure rather than a Likert-type scale of frequency because of its higher objectivity. Responses such as "often" or "seldom" can be understood by different consumers differently, e.g., for some people reading 30% of labels may mean "often" and for others "seldom". That is why I preferred the percentage measures, bearing in mind also the weakness of this measure related to the different numerical skills of respondents. This shortcoming of my study may be overcome by applying a combination of observational methods (ethnography) and surveys in future research.

There are several implications of my results. First, nutrition knowledge improvement programs should be developed, as higher nutrition knowledge was found to translate into a higher interest in reading all kinds of food labels (FOP and BOP) in both contexts (during the purchase and after the purchase), and food label use leads to more favorable food choices for public health. Second, food processors and retailers should more often consider the possibility of emphasizing the health effects of a given product alongside or even instead of other attributes. Third, consumers are particularly sensitive to information about the content of fat. Therefore, the use of nutrition claims and graphical designs of the packaging pointing to the low-fat or zero-fat properties of a product is encouraged. Fourth, retailers should encourage their customers to read the labels at the point of purchase, which may be achieved by allocating special space and offering tools to obtain additional information about the products. Fifth, smartphone apps should be developed to facilitate consumer understanding of information placed on the labels and to facilitate comparisons across products in a given category. Sixth, it is important to pay attention not only to the type of information placed on the labels but also its quantity, and last but not least, credibility. The manufacturers should be selective and focus on the consumer-friendly design of labels. Public authorities should facilitate the use of official nutrition claims and health claims, at the same time keeping high standards of awarding such claims. Public information campaigns should be organized to explain the transparency of the procedures of obtaining health and nutrition claims and the credibility of other types of information on the labels. Finally, public authorities should increase their effort in monitoring the industry so that it adheres to high standards of labeling, including the accuracy, completeness, and visibility of information sought by consumers.

Funding: This research was funded by the National Science Centre, Opus grant numbers 2017/25/B/HS4/00031 and 2015/17/B/HS4/00253. The APC was funded by the National Science Centre, Opus grant number 2017/25/B/HS4/00031.

Conflicts of Interest: The author declares no conflict of interest. The funder had no role in the design of the study; in the collection, analyses, or interpretation of data; in the writing of the manuscript, or in the decision to publish the results.

Appendix A

Table A1. A comparison of the sample with the general population (%).

Characteristics	Categories	General Population	Study Sample
Sex	Women	52.1	53.3
	Men	47.9	46.7

Table A1. Cont.

Characteristics	Categories	General Population	Study Sample
Age	15–24	12.5	15
	25–34	17.8	17.3
	35–44	18.7	17.9
	45–54	14.5	13.9
	55–64	16.5	15.7
	65 and more	20	20.2
Education	Primary	49.4	47.7
	Secondary	31.9	31.6
	Tertiary	18.7	20.7
Place of living	Urban areas	60.7	61.7
	Rural areas	39.3	38.3
Region	Dolnośląskie	7.6	7.6
	Kujawsko-pomorskie	5.4	5.6
	Lubelskie	5.6	5.6
	Lubuskie	2.6	2.7
	Łódzkie	6.5	6.7
	Małopolskie	8.7	8.6
	Mazowieckie	13.9	13.5
	Opolskie	2.6	2.8
	Podkarpackie	5.5	5.6
	Podlaskie	3.2	3.3
	Pomorskie	5.9	6
	Śląskie	11.9	11.4
	Świętokrzyskie	3.4	3.4
	Warmińsko-mazurskie	3.7	3.8
	Wielkopolskie	9	9
	Zachodniopomorskie	4.5	4.4

Note: general population refers to the inhabitants of Poland aged 15 and more.

Table A2. The operationalization of key variables used in this study.

Variable	Operationalization	Measurement Scale and Coding
FOP shop	While shopping, you read the information on the front of the packaging for what share of food products you buy?	%
BOP shop	While shopping, you read the information on the back of the packaging for what share of food products you buy?	%
FOP home	At home, you read the information on the front of the packaging for what share of food products you have bought?	%
BOP home	At home, you read the information on the back of the packaging for what share of food products you have bought?	%
Woman	Sex	Woman—1, Man - 0
Education	Education level	Primary—1, Vocational—2, Secondary—3, Tertiary—4
White-collar	Professional activity—a single-choice question with the following catalog of answers: (a) white-collar worker, (b) blue-collar worker, (c) unemployed, (d) student, (e) I don't work and I take care of the family, (f) old age pensioner/disability pensioner, (g) other. What?	White-collar worker selected—1, White-collar worker not selected—0
Student	Professional activity—a single-choice question with the following catalog of answers: (a) white-collar worker, (b) blue-collar worker, (c) unemployed, (d) student, (e) I don't work and I take care of the family, (f) old age pensioner/disability pensioner, (g) other. What?	Student selected—1, Student not selected—0
Income	What is the total monthly net, i.e., disposable, income of all members of your household? A single-choice question with the following catalogue of answers: (a) below 2000 PLN, (b) 2001–3000 PLN, (c) 3001–4000 PLN, (d) 4001–5000 PLN, (e) 5001–6000 PLN, (f) over 6000 PLN	(a) below 2000 PLN—1, (b) 2001–3000 PLN—2, (c) 3001–4000 PLN—3, (d) 4001–5000 PLN—4, (e) 5001–6000 PLN—5, (f) over 6000 PLN—6

Table A2. Cont.

Variable	Operationalization	Measurement Scale and Coding
Household	Size of your household	Number of persons
Dietary suppl.	Do you buy the following products? Dietary supplements	Yes—1, No—0, I don't know—0
Organic	Do you buy the following products? Organic food	Yes—1, No—0, I don't know—0
Functional	Do you buy the following products? Functional food	Yes—1, No—0, I don't know—0
Fair trade	Do you buy the following products? Fair trade products	Yes—1, No—0, I don't know—0
Diet	How do you evaluate your diet?	Very healthy—5, Rather healthy—4, Average—3, Rather unhealthy—2, Very unhealthy—1
Knowledge	How do you evaluate your knowledge about healthy nutrition?	Very big—5, Rather big—4, Average—3, Rather small—2, Very small—1
Health	How do you evaluate your health status?	Very good—5, rather good—4, average—3, rather poor—2, very poor—1
Quantity	How do you assess the quantity of the following information on food product packages?	Measured separately for health claims, nutrition claims, and quality signs. Too much—1, Appropriate—2, Too little—3. The arithmetical mean
Understandability	How understandable for you is the following information on food product packages?	Measured separately for health claims, nutrition claims, quality signs, functional food, and organic food. Very understandable—5, Rather understandable—4, Average—3, Rather not understandable—2, Completely not understandable—1. The arithmetical mean
Credibility	How credible for you is the following information on food product packaging?	Measured separately for health claims, nutrition claims, list of ingredients, expiry date, organic certificate, and quality signs. Very credible—5, Rather credible—4, Average—3, Rather not credible—2, Definitely not credible—1. The arithmetical mean
List of ingredients	How important for you is the following information on food product packages? List of ingredients	Very important—5, Rather important—4, Average—3, Rather not important—2, Without any importance—1
Expiry date	How important for you is the following information on food product packages? Expiry date	Very important—5, Rather important—4, Average—3, Rather not important—2, Without any importance—1
Institutes	How important for you is the following information on food product packages? Recommendations of scientific institutes	Very important—5, Rather important—4, Average—3, Rather not important—2, Without any importance—1
First-time LI	What constitutes the most important information on a food product label when you buy it for the first time (excluding price)? A single-choice question with the following answer options: (a) country of origin, (b) nutritional information (e.g., about the content of fat or dietary fiber), (c) information about health effects (e.g., good for the bones, lowering cholesterol), (d) list of ingredients, (e) expiry date, (f) other, (g) I don't know	List of ingredients selected—1, List of ingredients not selected—0
Sugar	How important for you is the following information on food product packages? Content of sugars	Very important—5, Rather important—4, Average—3, Rather not important—2, Without any importance—1
Fat	How important for you is the following information on food product packages? Content of fats	Very important—5, Rather important—4, Average—3, Rather not important—2, Without any importance—1
Dietary fiber	How important for you is the following information on food product packages? Dietary fiber	Very important—5, Rather important—4, Average—3, Rather not important—2, Without any importance—1

Table A2. Cont.

Variable	Operationalization	Measurement Scale and Coding
Cholesterol	How important for you is the following information on food product packages? Impact of the product on lowering cholesterol	Very important—5, Rather important—4, Average—3, Rather not important—2, Without any importance—1
Digestive system	How important for you is the following information on food product packages? Impact of the product on the digestive system	Very important—5, Rather important—4, Average—3, Rather not important—2, Without any importance—1
Fatigue	How important for you is the following information on food product packages? Impact of the product reducing tiredness and fatigue	Very important—5, Rather important—4, Average—3, Rather not important—2, Without any importance—1
Dietician	In your opinion, how important are the following ways of promoting food products with health and nutrition claims? Recommendations of a dietician	Very important—5, Rather important—4, Average—3, Rather not important—2, Without any importance—1
Blogs	In your opinion, how important are the following ways of promoting food products with health and nutrition claims? Culinary blogs	Very important—5, Rather important—4, Average—3, Rather not important—2, Without any importance—1
Packaging	In your opinion, how important are the following ways of promoting food products with health and nutrition claims? Food packages	Very important—5, Rather important—4, Average—3, Rather not important—2, Without any importance—1
Health effects	How important for you is the following information concerning food products? Health effects of consuming a given product	Very important—5, Rather important—4, Average—3, Rather not important—2, Without any importance—1
WTP HC	Are you willing to pay more for products with health claims (compared to similar products without such claims)?	Definitely yes—5, Rather yes—4, I don't know—3, Rather not—2, Definitely not—1
WTP NC	Are you willing to pay more for products with nutrition claims (compared to similar products without such claims)?	Definitely yes—5, Rather yes—4, I don't know—3, Rather not—2, Definitely not—1

References

1. Mandal, B. Use of food labels as a weight loss behaviour. *J. Consum. Aff.* **2010**, *44*, 516–527. [CrossRef]
2. Chen, X.; Jahns, L.; Gittelsohn, J.; Wang, Y. Who is missing the message? Targeting strategies to increase food label use among US adults. *Public Health Nutr.* **2012**, *15*, 760–772. [CrossRef] [PubMed]
3. Smith, S.; Taylor, J.; Stephen, A. Use of food labels and beliefs about diet-disease relationships among university students. *Public Health Nutr.* **2000**, *3*, 175–182. [CrossRef] [PubMed]
4. Ozimek, I.; Tomaszewska-Pielacha, M. Czynniki wpływające na czytanie przez konsumentów informacji zamieszczanych na opakowaniach produktów żywnościowych. *Studies Proc. Polish Assoc. Knowl. Manag.* **2011**, *52*, 26–35.
5. Niewczas, M. Kryteria wyboru żywności. *Żywność. Nauka. Technologia. Jakość* **2013**, *6*, 204–219.
6. Macon, J.; Oakland, M.; Jensen, H.; Kissack, P. Food label use by older Americans. *J. Nutr. Elderly* **2004**, *24*, 35–52. [CrossRef] [PubMed]
7. Besler, H.; Buyuktuncer, Z.; Uyar, M. Consumer understanding and use of food and nutrition labeling in Turkey. *J. Nutr. Educ. Behav.* **2012**, *44*, 584–591. [CrossRef]
8. Vemula, S.; Gavaravarapu, S.; Mendu, V.; Mathur, P.; Avula, L. Use of food label information by urban consumers in India – a study among supermarket shoppers. *Public Health Nutr.* **2014**, *17*, 2104–2114. [CrossRef]
9. Nayga, R.; Lipinski, D.; Savur, N. Consumers' use of nutritional labels while food shopping and at home. *J. Consum. Aff.* **1998**, *32*, 106–120. [CrossRef]
10. Moreira, M.; García-Díez, J.; de Almeida, J.; Saraiva, C. Evaluation of food labelling usefulness for consumers. *Int. J. Consum. Stud.* **2019**, *43*, 327–334. [CrossRef]
11. Mulders, M.; Corneille, O.; Klein, O. Label reading, numeracy and food & nutrition involvement. *Appetite* **2018**, *128*, 214–222. [CrossRef] [PubMed]
12. Nayga, R. Nutrition knowledge, gender, and food label use. *J. Consum. Aff.* **2005**, *34*, 97–112. [CrossRef]

13. Al-Barqi, R.; Al-Salem, Y.; Mahrous, L.; Abu Abat, E.; Al-Quraishi, R.; Benajiba, N. Understanding barriers towards the use of food labels among Saudi female college students. *Mal J Nutr* **2020**, *26*, 19–30. [CrossRef]
14. Cavaliere, A.; De Marchi, E.; Banterle, A. Does consumer health-orientation affect the use of nutrition facts panel and claims? An empirical analysis in Italy. *Food Qual. Prefer.* **2016**, *54*, 110–116. [CrossRef]
15. Nestorowicz, R.; Pilarczyk, B. Wyzwania wobec komunikacji marketingowej na rynku żywności ekologicznej w Polsce – w świetle badań konsumentów. *Marketing i Rynek* **2014**, *8*, 583–589.
16. Hess, R.; Visschers, V.; Siegrist, M. The role of health-related, motivational and sociodemographic aspects in predicting food label use: A comprehensive study. *Public Health Nutr.* **2012**, *15*, 407–414. [CrossRef]
17. Vijaykumar, S.; Lwin, M.; Chao, J.; Au, C. Determinants of food label use among supermarket shoppers: A Singaporean perspective. *J. Nutr. Educ. Behav.* **2013**, *45*, 204–212. [CrossRef]
18. Cha, E.; Kim, K.; Lerner, H.; Dawkins, C.; Bello, M.; Umpierrez, G.; Dunbar, S. Health literacy, self-efficacy, food label use, and diet in young adults. *Am. J. Health Behav.* **2014**, *38*, 331–339. [CrossRef]
19. Walters, A.; Long, M. The effect of food label cues on perceptions of quality and purchase intentions among high-involvement consumers with varying levels of nutrition knowledge. *J. Nutr. Educ. Behav.* **2012**, *44*, 350–354. [CrossRef]
20. Limbu, Y.; McKinley, C.; Gautam, R.; Ahirwar, A.; Dubey, P.; Jayachandran, C. Nutritional knowledge, attitude, and use of food labels among Indian adults with multiple chronic conditions: A moderated mediation model. *Brit. Food J.* **2019**, *121*, 1480–1494. [CrossRef]
21. Soederberg Miller, L.; Cassady, D. The effects of nutrition knowledge on food label use. A review of the literature. *Appetite* **2015**, *92*, 207–216. [CrossRef] [PubMed]
22. Kreuter, M.; Brennan, L.; Scharff, D.; Lukwago, S. Do nutrition label readers eat healthier diets? Behavioral correlates of adults' use of food labels. *Am. J. Prev. Med.* **1997**, *13*, 277–283. [CrossRef]
23. Amuta-Jimenez, A.; Lo, C.; Talwar, D.; Khan, N.; Barry, A. Food label literacy and use among US adults diagnosed with cancer: Results from a national representative study. *J. Cancer Educ.* **2019**, *34*, 1000–1009. [CrossRef] [PubMed]
24. Kim, S.; Nayga, R.; Capps, O. Food label use, self-selectivity, and diet quality. *J. Consum. Aff.* **2005**, *35*, 346–363. [CrossRef]
25. Lin, C.; Lee, J.; Yen, S. Do dietary intakes affect search for nutrient information on food labels? *Soc. Sci. Med.* **2004**, *59*, 1955–1967. [CrossRef]
26. Drichoutis, A.; Lazaridis, P.; Nayga, R. Nutrition knowledge and consumer use of nutritional food labels. *Eur. Rev. Agric. Econ.* **2005**, *32*, 93–118. [CrossRef]
27. Lewis, J.; Arheart, K.; LeBlanc, W.; Fleming, L.; Lee, D.; Davila, E.; Cabán-Martinez, A.; Dietz, N.; McCollister, K.; Bandiera, F.; et al. Food label use and awareness of nutritional information and recommendations among persons with chronic disease. *Am. J. Clin. Nutr.* **2009**, *90*, 1351–1357. [CrossRef]
28. Laz, T.; Rahman, M.; Berenson, A. Association of frequent use of food labels with weight loss behaviors among low-income reproductive-age women. *J. Am. Coll. Nutr.* **2015**, *34*, 73–79. [CrossRef]
29. Anastasiou, K.; Miller, M.; Dickinson, K. The relationship between food label use and dietary intake in adults: A systematic review. *Appetite* **2019**, *138*, 280–291. [CrossRef]
30. Wilson, M.; Ramírez, A.; Arsenault, J.; Miller, L. Nutrition label use and its association with dietary quality among Latinos: The roles of poverty and acculturation. *J. Nutr. Educ. Behav.* **2018**, *50*, 876–887. [CrossRef]
31. Jacob, R.; Drapeau, V.; Lamarche, B.; Doucet, É.; Pomerleau, S.; Provencher, V. Associations among eating behaviour traits, diet quality and food labelling: A mediation model. *Public Health Nutr.* **2020**, *23*, 631–641. [CrossRef] [PubMed]
32. Ducrot, P.; Méjean, C.; Julia, C.; Kesse-Guyot, E.; Touvier, M.; Fezeu, L.; Hercberg, S.; Péneau, S. Objective understanding of front-of-package nutrition labels among nutritionally at-risk individuals. *Nutrients* **2015**, *7*, 7106–7125. [CrossRef] [PubMed]
33. Borgmeier, I.; Westenhoefer, J. Impact of different food label formats on healthiness evaluation and food choice of consumers: A randomized-controlled study. *BMC Public Health* **2009**, *9*, 184. [CrossRef] [PubMed]
34. Talati, Z.; Egnell, M.; Hercberg, S.; Julia, C.; Pettigrew, S. Consumers' perceptions of five front-of-package nutrition labels: An experimental study across 12 countries. *Nutrients* **2019**, *11*, 1934. [CrossRef]
35. Hagmann, D.; Siegrist, M. Nutri-Score, multiple traffic light and incomplete nutrition labelling on food packages: Effects on consumers' accuracy in identifying healthier snack options. *Food Qual. Prefer.* **2020**, *83*, 103894. [CrossRef]

36. Andreeva, V.; Egnell, M.; Handjieva-Darlenska, T.; Talati, Z.; Touvier, M.; Galan, P.; Hercberg, S.; Pettigrew, S.; Julia, C. Bulgarian consumers' objective understanding of front-of-package nutrition labels: A comparative randomized study. *Arch. Public Health* **2020**, *78*, 35. [CrossRef]
37. Graham, D.; Heidrick, C.; Hodgin, K. Nutrition label viewing during a food-selection task: Front-of-package labels vs. Nutrition Facts labels. *J. Acad. Nutr. Diet.* **2015**, *115*, 1636–1646. [CrossRef]
38. Goyal, R.; Deshmukh, N. Food label reading: Read before you eat. *J. of Education and Health Promotion* **2018**, *7*, 56. [CrossRef]
39. Elshiewy, O.; Boztug, Y. When back of pack meets front of pack: How salient and simplified nutrition labels affect food sales in supermarkets. *J. Public Policy Mark.* **2018**, *37*, 55–67. [CrossRef]
40. Temple, N.; Fraser, J. Food labels: A critical assessment. *Nutrition* **2014**, *30*, 257–260. [CrossRef]
41. Ares, G.; Antúnez, L.; Ottrbring, T.; Curutchet, M.; Galicia, L.; Moratorio, X.; Bove, I. Sick, salient and full of salt, sugar and fat: Understanding the impact of nutritional warnings on consumers' associations through the salience bias. *Food Qual. Prefer.* **2020**, *86*, 103991. [CrossRef]
42. Temple, N. Front-of-package food labels: A narrative review. *Appetite* **2020**, *144*, 104485. [CrossRef] [PubMed]
43. El-Abbadi, N.; Taylor, S.; Micha, R.; Blumberg, J. Nutrient profiling systems, front of pack labeling and consumer behavior. *Curr. Atheroscler. Rep.* **2020**, *22*, 36. [CrossRef] [PubMed]
44. Ikonen, I.; Sotgiu, F.; Aydinli, A.; Verlegh, P. Consumer effects of front-of-package nutrition labeling: An interdisciplinary meta-analysis. *J. Acad. Market. Sci.* **2020**, *48*, 360–383. [CrossRef]
45. Ozimek, I.; Żakowska-Biemans, S.; Gutkowska, K. Polish consumers' perception of food-related risks. *Pol. J. Food Nutr. Sci.* **2009**, *59*, 189–192.
46. Jeżewska-Zychowicz, M.; Jeznach, M.; Kosicka-Gębska, M. Consumers' interests in sweets with health-promoting properties and their selected determinants. *Pol. J. Food Nutr. Sci.* **2013**, *63*, 43–48. [CrossRef]
47. Bryła, P. Organic food consumption in Poland: Motives and barriers. *Appetite* **2016**, *105*, 737–746. [CrossRef]
48. Bryła, P. *Marketing Regionalnych I Ekologicznych Produktów Żywnościowych. Perspektywa Sprzedawcy I Konsumenta*; Lodz University Press: Lodz, Poland, 2015. [CrossRef]
49. Cavaliere, A.; Ricci, E.; Banterle, A. Nutrition and health claims: Who is interested? An empirical analysis of consumer preferences in Italy. *Food Qual. Prefer.* **2015**, *41*, 44–51. [CrossRef]
50. Grunert, K.; Scholderer, J.; Rogeaux, M. Determinants of consumer understanding of health claims. *Appetite* **2011**, *56*, 269–277. [CrossRef]
51. Hung, Y.; Grunert, K.; Hoefkens, C.; Hieke, S.; Verbeke, W. Motivation outweighs ability in explaining European consumers' use of health claims. *Food Qual. Prefer.* **2017**, *58*, 34–44. [CrossRef]
52. Kozirok, W.; Marciszewicz, E.; Babicz-Zielińska, E. Postawy i zachowania kobiet wobec żywności prozdrowotnej. *Studia i Prace WNEiZ US* **2016**, *43*, 199–208. [CrossRef]
53. Mackison, D.; Wrieden, W.; Anderson, A. Validity and reliability testing of a short questionnaire developed to assess consumers' use, understanding and perception of food labels. *Eur. J. Clin. Nutr.* **2010**, *64*, 210–217. [CrossRef] [PubMed]
54. Menrad, K.; Sparke, K. *Consumers' Attitudes And Expectations Concerning Functional Food*; University of Applied Sciences of Weihenstephan: Straubing, Germany, 2006.
55. Nestorowicz, R. *Asymetria Wiedzy A Aktywność Informacyjna Konsumentów Na Rynku Produktów Żywnościowych*; University of Economics in Poznan: Poznan, Poland, 2017.
56. Ravoniarison, A.; Gollety, M. L'effet «I can do it!»: Rôle du sentiment d'efficacité personnelle dans la satisfaction à l'égard des aliments santé à orientation fonctionnelle. *Décisions Marketing* **2017**, *85*, 29–47. [CrossRef]
57. Riley, M.; Bowen, J.; Krause, D.; Jones, D.; Stonehouse, W. A survey of consumer attitude towards nutrition and health statements on food labels in South Australia. *Funct. Foods in Health Dis.* **2016**, *6*, 809–821. [CrossRef]
58. Strijbos, C.; Schluck, M.; Bisschop, J.; Bui, T.; de Jong, I.; van Leeuwen, M.; von Tottleben, M.; van Breda, S. Consumer awareness and credibility factors of health claims on innovative meat products in a cross-sectional population study in the Netherlands. *Food Qual. Prefer.* **2016**, *54*, 13–22. [CrossRef]
59. Van Trijp, H.; van der Lans, I. Consumer perceptions of nutrition and health claims. *Appetite* **2007**, *48*, 305–324. [CrossRef]
60. Bryła, P. *Oświadczenia Zdrowotne I Żywieniowe na Rynku Produktów Żywnościowych*; Lodz University Press: Lodz, Poland, 2020. [CrossRef]

61. Wasserstein, R.; Schirm, A.; Lazar, N. Moving to a world beyond "p<0.05". *Am. Stat.* **2019**, *73*, 1–19. [CrossRef]
62. Ollberding, N.; Wolf, R.; Contento, I. Food label use and its relation to dietary intake among US adults. *J. Am. Diet. Assoc.* **2011**, *111*, S47–S51. [CrossRef]
63. Stran, K.; Knol, L. Determinants of food label use differ by sex. *J. Acad. Nutr. Diet.* **2013**, *113*, 673–679. [CrossRef]
64. Bryła, P. Selected predictors of the importance attached to salt content information on the food packaging (a study among Polish consumers). *Nutrients* **2020**, *12*, 293. [CrossRef]
65. Cavaliere, A.; Siletti, E.; Banterle, A. Nutrition information, Mediterranean diet, and weight: A structural equation approach. *Agric. Econ. Czech* **2020**, *66*, 10–18. [CrossRef]
66. Ballco, P.; De Magistris, T. Spanish consumer purchase behaviour and stated preferences for yoghurts with nutritional and health claims. *Nutrients* **2019**, *11*, 2742. [CrossRef]
67. Almli, V.; Asioli, D.; Rocha, C. Organic consumer choices for nutrient labels on dried strawberries among different health attitude segments in Norway, Romania, and Turkey. *Nutrients* **2019**, *11*, 2951. [CrossRef] [PubMed]
68. Guthrie, J.; Mancino, L.; Lin, C. Nudging consumers toward better food choices: Policy approaches to changing food consumption behaviors. *Psychol. Market.* **2015**, *32*, 501–511. [CrossRef]
69. Shin, S. The effects of dynamic food labels with real-time feedback on diet quality: Results from a randomized controlled trial. *Nutrients* **2020**, *12*, 2158. [CrossRef] [PubMed]
70. Bryła, P. Selected antecedents of the importance of nutrition claims for food processors and distributors. *J. Agribus. Rural Dev.* **2019**, *52*, 103–110. [CrossRef]
71. Petrovici, D.; Fearne, A.; Nayga, R.; Drolias, D. Nutritional knowledge, nutritional labels, and health claims on food: A study of supermarket shoppers in the South East of England. *Brit. Food J.* **2012**, *114*, 768–783. [CrossRef]
72. Martin, C.; Nagao, D. Some effects of computerized interviewing on job applicant responses. *J. Appl. Psychol.* **1989**, *74*, 72–80. [CrossRef]
73. Soederberg Miller, L.; Cassady, D.; Applegate, E.; Beckett, L.; Wilson, M.; Gibson, T.; Ellwood, K. Relationships among food label use, motivation, and dietary quality. *Nutrients* **2015**, *7*, 1068–1080. [CrossRef]

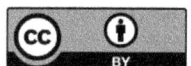

© 2020 by the author. Licensee MDPI, Basel, Switzerland. This article is an open access article distributed under the terms and conditions of the Creative Commons Attribution (CC BY) license (http://creativecommons.org/licenses/by/4.0/).

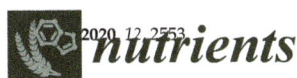
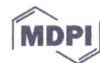

Communication

Dietary Fibre Consensus from the International Carbohydrate Quality Consortium (ICQC)

Livia S. A. Augustin [1,*], Anne-Marie Aas [2,3], Arnie Astrup [4], Fiona S. Atkinson [5,6], Sara Baer-Sinnott [7], Alan W. Barclay [8], Jennie C. Brand-Miller [5,6], Furio Brighenti [9], Monica Bullo [10,11,12], Anette E. Buyken [13], Antonio Ceriello [14], Peter R. Ellis [15], Marie-Ann Ha [16], Jeyakumar C. Henry [17], Cyril W. C. Kendall [18,19,20], Carlo La Vecchia [21], Simin Liu [22], Geoffrey Livesey [23], Andrea Poli [24], Jordi Salas-Salvadó [10,11], Gabriele Riccardi [25], Ulf Riserus [26], Salwa W. Rizkalla [27], John L. Sievenpiper [18,19,28,29], Antonia Trichopoulou [30], Kathy Usic [31], Thomas M. S. Wolever [18,19,28], Walter C. Willett [32] and David J. A. Jenkins [18,19,28,29]

1. Epidemiology and Biostatistics Unit, Istituto Nazionale Tumori-IRCCS-"Fondazione G. Pascale", 80131 Napoli, Italy
2. Section of Nutrition and Dietetics, Division of Medicine, Department of Clinical Service, Oslo University Hospital, 0424 Oslo, Norway; a.m.aas@medisin.uio.no
3. Institute of Clinical Medicine, University of Oslo, 0318 Oslo, Norway
4. Department of Nutrition, Exercise and Sports (NEXS) Faculty of Science, University of Copenhagen, 2200 Copenhagen, Denmark; ast@nexs.ku.dk
5. School of Life and Environmental Sciences, The University of Sydney, 2006 Sydney, Australia; fiona.atkinson@sydney.edu.au (F.S.A.); jennie.brandmiller@sydney.edu.au (J.C.B.-M.)
6. Charles Perkins Centre, The University of Sydney, 2006 Sydney, Australia
7. Oldways, Boston, MA 02116, USA; sara@oldwayspt.org
8. Accredited Practising Dietitian, 2006 Sydney, Australia; alan@dralanbarclay.com
9. Department of Food and Drug, University of Parma, 43120 Parma, Italy; furio.brighenti@unipr.it
10. Departament de Bioquímica i Biotecnologia, Unitat de Nutrició, Universitat Rovira i Virgili, 43201 Reus, Spain; monica.bullo@urv.cat (M.B.); jordi.salas@urv.cat (J.S.-S.)
11. Human Nutrition Unit, University Hospital of Sant Joan de Reus, Institut d'Investigació Sanitària Pere Virgili (IISPV), 43201 Reus, Spain
12. Centro de Investigación Biomédica en Red Fisiopatología de la Obesidad y la Nutrición (CIBEROBN), Institute of Health Carlos III, 28029 Madrid, Spain
13. Institute of Nutrition, Consumption and Health, Faculty of Natural Sciences, Paderborn University, 33098 Paderborn, Germany; anette.buyken@uni-paderborn.de
14. IRCCS MultiMedica, Diabetes Department, Sesto San Giovanni, 20099 Milan, Italy; antonio.ceriello@hotmail.it
15. Biopolymers Group, Departments of Biochemistry and Nutritional Sciences, Faculty of Life Sciences & Medicine, King's College London, Franklin-Wilkins Building, 150 Stamford Street, London SE1 9NH, UK; peter.r.ellis@kcl.ac.uk
16. Spinney Nutrition, Shirwell, Barnstaple, Devon EX31 4JR, UK; nutrition@thespinney.co.uk
17. Clinical Nutrition Research Centre, Singapore Institute for Clinical Sciences, Singapore 637551, Singapore; jeya_henry@sics.a-star.edu.sg
18. Departments of Nutritional Science and Medicine, Faculty of Medicine, University of Toronto, Toronto, ON M5S 1A8, Canada; cyril.kendall@utoronto.ca (C.W.C.K.); john.sievenpiper@utoronto.ca (J.L.S.); thomas.wolever@utoronto.ca (T.M.S.W.); david.jenkins@utoronto.ca (D.J.A.J.)
19. Clinical Nutrition and Risk Factor Modification Centre, St. Michael's Hospital, Toronto, ON M5C 2T2, Canada
20. College of Pharmacy and Nutrition, University of Saskatchewan, Saskatoon, SK S7N 5B5, Canada
21. Department of Clinical Sciences and Community Health, Università degli Studi di Milano, 201330 Milan, Italy; carlo.lavecchia@unimi.it
22. Department of Epidemiology and Medicine, Brown University, Providence, RI 02912, USA; simin_liu@brown.edu
23. Independent Nutrition Logic Ltd., 21 Bellrope Lane, Wymondham NR180QX, UK; glivesey@inlogic.co.uk

24 Nutrition Foundation of Italy, Viale Tunisia 38, I-20124 Milan, Italy; poli@nutrition-foundation.it
25 Department of Clinical Medicine and Surgery, Federico II University, 80147 Naples, Italy; riccardi@unina.it
26 Department of Public Health and Caring Sciences, Clinical Nutrition and Metabolism, Uppsala University, 751 22 Uppsala, Sweden; ulf.riserus@pubcare.uu.se
27 Institute of Cardiometabolism and Nutrition, ICAN, Pitié Salpêtrière Hospital, F75013 Paris, France; salwa.rizkalla@psl.aphp.fr
28 Division of Endocrinology and Metabolism, Department of Medicine, St. Michael's Hospital, Toronto, ON M5C 2T2, Canada
29 Li Ka Shing Knowledge Institute, St. Michael's Hospital, Toronto, ON M5C 2T2, Canada
30 Hellenic Health Foundation, Alexandroupoleos 23, 11527 Athens, Greece; atrichopoulou@hhf-greece.gr
31 Glycemic Index Foundation, 2037 Sydney, Australia; kathyu@gifoundation.org.au
32 Departments of Nutrition and Epidemiology, Harvard T. H. Chan School of Public Health and Harvard Medical School, Boston, MA 02115, USA; wwillett@hsph.harvard.edu
* Correspondence: l.augustin@istitutotumori.na.it

Received: 17 July 2020; Accepted: 19 August 2020; Published: 24 August 2020

Abstract: Dietary fibre is a generic term describing non-absorbed plant carbohydrates and small amounts of associated non-carbohydrate components. The main contributors of fibre to the diet are the cell walls of plant tissues, which are supramolecular polymer networks containing variable proportions of cellulose, hemicelluloses, pectic substances, and non-carbohydrate components, such as lignin. Other contributors of fibre are the intracellular storage oligosaccharides, such as fructans. A distinction needs to be made between intrinsic sources of dietary fibre and purified forms of fibre, given that the three-dimensional matrix of the plant cell wall confers benefits beyond fibre isolates. Movement through the digestive tract modifies the cell wall structure and may affect the interactions with the colonic microbes (e.g., small intestinally non-absorbed carbohydrates are broken down by bacteria to short-chain fatty acids, absorbed by colonocytes). These aspects, combined with the fibre associated components (e.g., micronutrients, polyphenols, phytosterols, and phytoestrogens), may contribute to the health outcomes seen with the consumption of dietary fibre. Therefore, where possible, processing should minimise the degradation of the plant cell wall structures to preserve some of its benefits. Food labelling should include dietary fibre values and distinguish between intrinsic and added fibre. Labelling may also help achieve the recommended intake of 14 g/1000 kcal/day.

Keywords: dietary fibre; labelling; carbohydrate quality; ICQC; consensus

1. Introduction

Conceptually, dietary fibre is a generic term describing non-absorbed plant carbohydrates and relatively small amounts of associated non-carbohydrate components (e.g., phenolic compounds, waxes, and proteins) that are not digested by endogenous enzymes or absorbed in the human small intestine [1,2]. Some forms of dietary fibre are digested by intestinal bacterial enzymes and utilised as substrates for growth and metabolism. The main contributors of fibre to the diet are the cell walls of plant tissues, which are supramolecular polymer networks containing variable proportions of cellulose, hemicelluloses, pectic substances, and the non-carbohydrate components, such as the phenolic compound lignin (Figure 1). Other sources of fibre in the diet include fructans (e.g., inulins), which are not part of the plant cell walls but are synthesised and stored in the cell vacuole [3,4].

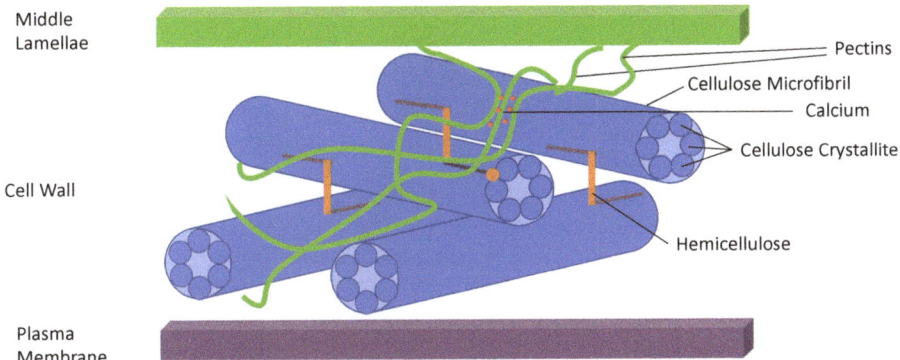

Figure 1. Carbohydrate components of a primary plant cell wall. A cartoon of the carbohydrate components of a primary plant cell wall demonstrating the supramolecular nature of the wall and the diversity of the cell wall constituents which contribute to dietary fibre. The cellulose microfibrils are composed of crystallites which are further composed of cellulose chains. The cellulose microfibrils are stacked upon one another to give strength as the skeleton of the wall. Hemicellulose is thought to keep the microfibrils apart. The nature of hemicellulose present varies considerably between plants. Pectin is a mega molecule, used for water transport throughout the plant. There are various different sections within pectin, the proportions vary between plants. The egg box region is shown here where different strands of pectin are bound together by calcium. There is a high concentration of pectins in the middle lamellae which interact with the neighbouring cell walls [4].

However, there is much that is not known about dietary fibre, in part because the structure of the plant cell wall, which makes up the majority of our dietary fibre, has not been fully elucidated. In turn, the overall structure of the polymers, and how they interact with each other within the plant cell wall, is not yet fully understood [3,4]. Added to this, what occurs to the matrix of the cell wall during chewing (Figure 2) and movement through the digestive tract is not clear [5], and a substantial percentage of dietary fibre is digested by the microbes in the colon. The nature and actions of the microbiome are just beginning to be explored [6].

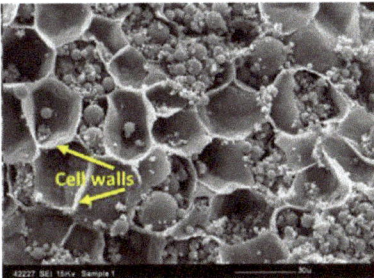

Figure 2. Surface of an almond seed post-mastication showing ruptured cell walls (dietary fibre). Micrograph, produced by scanning electron microscopy, of the surface of a masticated particle of almond seed. The cell walls (dietary fibre) have been ruptured (as marked by arrows) by chewing, exposing the nutrients inside the cells of the almond cotyledon tissue. Many of these cells still contain protein and lipid (oil bodies and coalesced oil droplets), which are potentially available for digestion (i.e., bioaccessible). Nutrients in intact cells below the fractured surface are not bioaccessible because the dietary fibre acts as a physical barrier to digestion. The scale bar is 30 µm.

2. Definitions

There is still disagreement about the definition of dietary fibre and how this very complex array of plant materials should be analysed. Current definitions are typically based around descriptions provided by national and international bodies for food standards, such as CODEX Alimentarius, and have focused on fibre being the non-digested and/or non-absorbed fraction of food carbohydrates derived from plants [7–11]. Dietary fibre definitions around the world have been summarised (10), and countries adopting the CODEX definition include Australia, Canada, China, the European Union, Malaysia, New Zealand, and the USA, among others. The US Food and Drug Administration issued a position paper in 2018 on what constitutes dietary fibre for food labelling purposes [11].

It may be useful to distinguish between dietary fibre, as plant cell walls (the main source of fibre) that are part of the plant food matrix, and fibre supplements that are added to food products for a specific physiological/health outcome (e.g., laxation, cholesterol-lowering, and prebiotic activity) [5]. The term natural fibre may be better described as dietary fibre that is intrinsically part of the cell wall material in edible plants such as fruits, vegetables, cereals, nuts, pulses, and even seaweed in some diets (from now on defined as intrinsic fibre). The intrinsic fibre may be modified when processed commercially and/or domestically and may not have the same physiological and metabolic effects of the original intrinsic fibre. These include the purified fibres derived from cereals (e.g., mixed-linkage β-glucans from barley and oats, among others). Some commercially available types of fibre are semi-synthetic, such as hydroxypropyl methylcellulose, which is a chemically modified cellulose. These may also be called novel types of dietary fibre in certain countries (e.g., Canada).

Another distinction seen in the literature is insoluble versus soluble fractions of fibre, which are classified by chemical analysis but not based on their functional behaviour in vivo [5]. These fractions are based on early attempts to classify fibre according to their dissolution properties in aqueous media in the laboratory. There are different chemical methods used for determining dietary fibre (e.g., the gravimetric AOAC method and GC analysis of non-starch polysaccharides) and values do vary significantly, as do the values for 'soluble' and 'insoluble' fractions. These broad classifications continue to be used in nutrition and public health literature, despite their limited use in providing information about functional properties in the gut, and their specific effects on metabolism. Solubility and viscosity are terms often used interchangeably to describe the same type of fibre; however, a soluble fibre that dissolves in aqueous media may not be viscous. Water-soluble types of fibre have the ability to lower fasting blood cholesterol and postprandial glycaemia [12]. These metabolic effects are linked to the capacity of soluble fibre to increase digesta viscosity and slow down the digestion of starch and other macronutrients. The viscosity-enhancing property of a soluble fibre is highly dependent on its polymer concentration and molecular weight, assuming it has solubilised in the gut.

3. Health Benefits

Dietary fibre can modify gastrointestinal function from the mouth to the anus. The specific physiological effects depend, crucially, on the physico-chemical properties of individual plant polysaccharides and oligosaccharides, and also on the structural integrity of fibre as cell walls, which is an important part of the architecture of the plant tissue [5]. These effects may include increasing or decreasing salivation, luminal viscosity, the gastric emptying rate, nutrient digestion and absorption, transit time, faecal bulking, laxation, fermentation, colonic pH, microbiota amount and composition, and binding of mucus, enzymes, bile acids and other metabolites, which may also be bioactive [13].

Beyond the gut, the established metabolic effects include the lowering of blood cholesterol and postprandial blood glucose, and fasting blood glucose in patients with diabetes [12]. In particular, these effects have been observed with isolated viscous fibres, such as psyllium, mixed-linkage β-glucans, guar gum (galactomannan), glucomannan, and pectic polysaccharides [14]. Another plant isolate, inulin-type fructans, though non-viscous, can lower fasting glucose and insulin and fasting LDL-cholesterol while increasing HDL-cholesterol in patients with diabetes, and to a lesser extent in overweight and obese persons [15]. A manufactured low-viscosity, digestion-resistant maltodextrin also lowers postprandial and fasting blood glucose from drinks and solid foods [16]. The molecular weight of the extracted viscous polysaccharide influences the effectiveness of the metabolic responses [9]. These observations implicate fibre as capable of modifying metabolism. Moreover, fibre-rich sources of edible plants—such as pulses, nuts, barley, oats, and some vegetables and fruits—have been shown to improve long-term control of established cardio-metabolic risk factors, i.e., blood lipids, blood glucose, blood pressure, and body weight. Many of these beneficial health effects have been attributed to the presence of fibre in these foods.

Prospective cohort studies have reported inverse associations between total dietary fibre intake and body weight, risk of type 2 diabetes, cardiovascular disease, stroke, some types of cancer, and total mortality. These associations have been shown with fibre intake from grains, legumes, nuts, fruit, and vegetables. The associations are independent of the dietary glycaemic index and glycaemic load, the effects of which are additive, at least for reducing the risk of diabetes from both observational and interventional studies [17,18]. However, despite the intensive research on nutritional epidemiology, many questions on the role of fibre in disease remain unanswered, and the contribution of associated substances to causality has been difficult to prove. Thus, the associations with fibre seen in epidemiological studies may be partially due to associated components, such as some amino acids, unsaturated fat, minerals, vitamins, and some phytochemicals, such as polyphenols, phytosterols, and phytoestrogens. In nutrition, a distinction needs to be made between intrinsic sources of dietary fibre and purified or chemically/physically modified forms of fibre, given that the three-dimensional (3D) matrix of the plant cell wall confers benefits above fibre isolates. This is because cell walls, and the 3D matrix of the plant cell walls, affect the functional properties of 'fibre' impacting on the digestibility of the cell contents [5]. This may be part of the reason for the strong benefits seen in wheat fibre in cohort studies, despite the lack of effect seen in the short-term clinical trials for cardiovascular risk factors [19–22]. In randomised controlled trials comparing refined and wholegrain cereal foods, when the particle size of the fibre is made too small, the plant cell wall integrity and tissue architecture may be lost. When tissue and the cell wall 3D matrix are sufficiently intact, it can lead to nutrients being slowly absorbed or even not absorbed. For example, cereal foods with a substantially intact tissue structure can also contribute starch as a source of a slowly and/or non-digestible food carbohydrate [23–25].

Fibre in wholefoods, isolates, and modified forms can be sources of substrate for micro-organisms in the large intestine, affecting the amount and species composition of the microbiota and their collective functional capacity to improve the health of the gut and other organs via modulation of the immune system, production of bioactive metabolites (e.g., short-chain fatty acids), and the reduction of intracolonic pH, with beneficial effects on the colonic mucosa and blood lipid levels [26].

At the population level, we suggest replacing some animal foods, and high glycaemic index foods containing refined starches and sugars, with slowly digestible carbohydrate foods with a low glycaemic index that are rich in fibre. This would have a favourable impact on glycaemic control and, hence, diabetes, cardio-metabolic risk, and possibly some diabetes-related cancers [27]. Minimising the degradation of the plant cell wall structures and tissue architecture is important where slow digestibility of macronutrients, such as starch, is required for the production of healthy foods, and also in the development of low glycaemic index foods. These issues are important, especially in some parts of the world with a high risk of cardio-metabolic disease, where dietary fibre intake tends to be below the recommended intake levels. However, it is recognised that in foods where mineral bioavailability needs to be increased, the rupture of the cell walls may provide a way to improve mineral status, e.g., a higher iron bioavailability through the micro-milling of wheat aleurone [28].

Much research is still required to fully understand the physiological and nutritional effects of dietary fibre. We need to further understand the interaction of fibre with the microbiota, and we also need to understand more about the structure, physico-chemical properties, and composition of dietary fibre. Additionally, we require an improved mechanistic insight into how the components associated with dietary fibre interact with fibre, and the impact on metabolic outcomes. Furthermore, an improved understanding is required on the role played by the 3D architecture of dietary fibre on nutrient release (i.e., bioaccessibility), fermentability by gut bacteria, prebiotic activity, and the roles these have in human health. When these are better elucidated, there will be a need to communicate to food producers, consumers, and health professionals on how to make better food choices [5].

Certain types of dietary fibre affect the amount and composition of microbiota, which has been studied mostly in regard to fermentative micro-organisms in the large intestine. Inulins, found in plants like chicory root and galacto-oligosaccharides, present in or from milk, are prime examples of non-digestible carbohydrate or dietary fibres that, among others, behave as prebiotics [29–31]. A prebiotic was recently defined by consensus as "a substrate that is selectively utilised by host micro-organisms conferring a health benefit" [32]. Putative health benefits include the inhibition of pathogens reaching the large intestine, immune stimulation, improved cardiometabolic status, improved mental health, and support to bone mineralisation, among others [32]. More long-term randomized controlled trials are needed to establish causality, which appears promising, though prebiotic effects may not be seen in everyone, especially in persons already in good health or having a sufficient amount and composition of beneficial micro-organisms. Moreover, not all dietary fibres are prebiotic, but the effect prebiotic fibre has can depend on the amount of other dietary fibre that is consumed [33].

Many chemical/enzyme methods exist for analysing dietary fibre, but those used for labelling are often different from those used in food composition tables. Current analytical methods reflect a heterogeneous mix of chemical entities, with no information on any subspecies of fibre or any information on the structural characteristics of the fibre present. One example of how dietary fibre is measured is by using the AOAC enzyme-gravimetric method, which is intended to simulate the physiological conditions of digestion, and measures all the components of fibre, as currently defined by CODEX Alimentarius. This kind of analysis is limited when being used to interpret mechanistic data on the functional properties of cell walls, individual cell wall polysaccharides and storage oligosaccharides. More informative methods, notably dissolution kinetics, molecular weight of individual polysaccharides, and cell wall porosity are urgently required for characterising dietary fibre in nutritional and epidemiological studies, if food sources of dietary fibre for health are to be optimised.

4. Recommendations to the Public and to Health Professionals

It is generally agreed that dietary fibre is an important part of a sustainable, balanced, healthy diet [34]. Consumption of dietary fibre is below the recommended intake levels for optimal health in many parts of the world and may be decreasing. We recommend maintaining or increasing dietary fibre intake to the recommended levels.

We support the Institute of Medicine recommendations for the total dietary fibre of 14 g/1000 kcal/day. We suggest that this should mainly come from intrinsic dietary fibre. Data from cohort studies with intakes beyond this amount are limited, but many traditional societies consume larger amounts and have a lower risk of chronic diseases.

5. Recommendations to the Food Industry

The food industry plays an important role in developing new food ingredients and products that have public health benefits and are also highly palatable. In developing new high-fibre foods, the sensory characteristics are important and will strongly influence whether people consume them. At the same time, if these do not have nutritional benefits then such products would be of little nutritional value, regardless of how technologically innovative they may be. It is important to recognise that increasing the fibre content on the food label does not guarantee any enhanced nutritional benefits in a product.

Recommendations to the food industry would depend on the reasons why particular types of fibre are being added, and how they are processed, given that mechanical and hydrothermal processing can affect their properties. For example, in wheat grain there is an advantage in preserving some of the structural integrity of the cell walls of the starch-rich endosperm, in order to produce flour that is digested more slowly and has a beneficial impact on postprandial glycaemia (23). However, if the health outcome is to improve the iron bioavailability in wheat, then there may be advantages to micro-milling (rupturing) the aleurone cell layer, which has a high iron concentration (28). In producing foods for the general population, the first example would be the most appropriate recommendation while, for populations with nutritional deficiencies, the second recommendation may preferentially apply. Therefore, we generally encourage the food industry to preserve many of the benefits of dietary fibre rich foods by minimising the degradation of the plant cell wall structures and tissue architecture, while maintaining palatability, except in situations of special dietary requirements and specific physiological or clinical outcomes (e.g., the use of prebiotic oligosaccharides and viscous polysaccharides).

Currently, labelling the dietary fibre content of foods in certain countries around the world, including Europe, is not mandatory. This represents a problem for consumers, researchers, and medical staff dealing with patient diets. We support the mandatory use of fibre on food labels.

Labelling should distinguish between fibre that is endogenous to foods and that added as a functional supplement because synthetic or purified fibre will not be accompanied by the micronutrients and phytochemicals in foods and, thus, may not predict the same health outcomes. Functional (or other) supplemental fibre, where permitted, should be listed separately among ingredients. The labelling of dietary fibres could be of the form "FIBRE N g PER 100 g, of which X g is SUPPLEMENTAL".

6. Conclusions

Dietary fibre and its associated non-carbohydrate components have been inversely associated with disease outcomes. Food labelling should include dietary fibre, and distinguish between intrinsic and purified added fibre, given that the intact plant cell wall may confer benefits beyond fibre isolates. The labelling of dietary fibre may also help to achieve the recommended intake of 14 g/1000 kcal/day for health benefits. To extend these recommendations, further studies on the interrelation of dietary fibre, prebiotics, and health, which aim to optimise both the health potential of foods and related food processing methods, are advised. This would include how the structures and the 3D matrix, composition, and physico-chemical properties of dietary fibre affect digestion, gastrointestinal function, and the role of the microbiome.

Author Contributions: All authors have made contributions to the statements and various drafts and read and approved the final manuscript. All authors have read and agreed to the published version of the manuscript.

Funding: No funding was received for this consensus statement. The dietary fibre consensus meeting was held as part of the 4th International Carbohydrate Quality Consortium (ICQC) Meeting, Palinuro, Italy, Sept 12–13, 2019, which was funded through unrestricted educational grants from Abbott, Arla Foods, Barilla, Beneo Institute, General Mills, Global Pulse Confederation, Inquis Clinical Research, International Pasta Organization, Nestle' Research and Development, Pulse Canada, McCain, and Quaker. The meeting was co-organized by the Toronto 3D Knowledge Synthesis and Clinical Trials foundation, Nutrition Foundation of Italy, and the Glycemic Index Foundation.

Conflicts of Interest: L.S.A.A. is a founding member of the International Carbohydrate Quality Consortium (ICQC) and has received honoraria from the Nutrition Foundation of Italy (NFI), research grants from LILT (a non-profit organization for the fight against cancer) and in-kind research support from Abiogen Pharma, the Almond Board of California (USA), Barilla (Italy), Consorzio Mandorle di Avola (Italy), DietaDoc (Italy), Ello Frutta (Italy), Panificio Giacomo Luongo (Italy), Perrotta (Italy), Roberto Alimentare (Italy), SunRice (Australia). A.A. is a project director at the Novo Nordisk Foundation, responsible for prevention of childhood obesity. He is in the Scientific Advisory Board/Consultant/Board of Directors of Gelesis, USA; Ferrero, Italy; Groupe Éthique et Santé, France; International Egg Commission/Danske Æg, Denmark; McCain Foods Limited, USA; Novo Nordisk, Denmark; Rituals, USA; and Weight Watchers, USA. A.W.B. is consultant at the University of Sydney and is Honorary Associate of the Glycemic Index Foundation, Allied Pinnacle, Beneo, and Nestle, and has authored/co-authored 5 books about dietary carbohydrate and diabetes. J.C.B.-M. is a co-author of books about the glycemic index of foods. She is President of the GI Foundation Limited, a non-profit company that administers the Australian 'GI Symbol' program and oversees the Sydney University Glycemic Index Research Service (SUGiRS), a non-profit GI testing facility for the food industry. She has received honoraria for speaking engagements on the glycemic index of foods. F.B.: declares no ownership or other investments-including shares-in commercial activities, intellectual property rights and consultancy/advice to private stakeholders. He served as Deputy-Chancellor for Research at the University of Parma from 2013 to 2017 and as representative of University of Parma of the Steering Board of ASTER, an in-house Public Research organization owned by Regione Emilia Romagna and research institutions of the region. Both positions involved coordination of activities with a large number of companies in order to attract European founds and develop Research and Innovation in the Emilia Romagna region. From 2011 to 2016 he served as legal representative (President) of the Italian Nutrition Society SINU–a not-for- profit scientific society. Associates to SINU include companies operating in the fields of nutrition, body composition, nutrition software, meal distribution and food production. Since 2017 he has been a Member of the Board of the Federation of European Nutrition Societies (FENS). He is the spouse of Silvia Valtuena Martinez, MD, PhD, a Scientific Officer at the NDA Unit of the European Food Safety Authority, the agency of the European Union (EU) that provides independent scientific advice and communicates on existing and emerging risks associated with the food chain. A.E.B.: Member of the ILSI Europe Expert Group 'Carbohydrates based recommendations as a basis for public dietary guidelines' (coordinated by the Dietary Carbohydrates Task Force). Member of the Executive Committee of the German Nutrition Society (Guidelines Committee 'Carbohydrate intake and prevention of nutrition-related diseases', Guidelines Committee 'Protein intake and prevention of nutrition-related diseases', Head Section "Public Health Nutrition"). A.C.: is in the advisory board for BD (Beckton Dikinson), Eli Lilly, Mundipharma; gave lectures sponsored by Astra Zeneca, Berlin Chemie, Boehringer Ingelheim, Eli Lilly, Mundipharma, Novo Nordisk and Roche Diagnostics; and received research grants from Mitsubishi. P.R.E.: some of his almond studies were funded by the Almond Board of California. M.-A.H.: Director of East Anglia Food. J.C.H.: his Clinical Nutrition Research Centre conducts food and nutrition research for several companies including Beneo, Roquette, Tate and Lyle, Wilmar and Nestle. D.J.A.J.: has received research grants from Saskatchewan & Alberta Pulse Growers Associations, the Agricultural Bioproducts Innovation Program through the Pulse Research Network, the Advanced Foods and Material Network, Loblaw Companies Ltd., Unilever Canada and Netherlands, Barilla, the Almond Board of California, Agriculture and Agri-food Canada, Pulse Canada, Kellogg's Company, Canada, Quaker Oats, Canada, Procter & Gamble Technical Centre Ltd., Bayer Consumer Care, Springfield, NJ, Pepsi/Quaker, International Nut & Dried Fruit (INC), Soy Foods Association of North America, the Coca-Cola Company (investigator initiated, unrestricted grant), Solae, Haine Celestial, the Sanitarium Company, Orafti, the International Tree Nut Council Nutrition Research and Education Foundation, the Peanut Institute, Soy Nutrition Institute (SNI), the Canola and Flax Councils of Canada, the Calorie Control Council, the Canadian Institutes of Health Research (CIHR), the Canada Foundation for Innovation (CFI)and the Ontario Research Fund (ORF). He has received in-kind supplies for trials as a research support from the Almond board of California, Walnut Council of California, American Peanut Council, Barilla, Unilever, Unico, Primo, Loblaw Companies, Quaker (Pepsico), Pristine Gourmet, Bunge Limited, Kellogg Canada, WhiteWave Foods. He has been on the speaker's panel, served on the scientific advisory board and/or received travel support and/or honoraria from the Almond Board of California, Canadian Agriculture Policy Institute, Loblaw Companies Ltd, the Griffin Hospital (for the development of the NuVal scoring system), the Coca-Cola Company, EPICURE, Danone, Diet Quality Photo Navigation (DQPN), Better Therapeutics (FareWell), Verywell, True Health Initiative (THI), Heali AI Corp, Institute of Food Technologists (IFT), Soy Nutrition Institute (SNI), Herbalife Nutrition Institute (HNI), Saskatchewan & Alberta Pulse Growers Associations, Sanitarium Company, Orafti, the American Peanut Council, the International Tree Nut Council Nutrition Research and Education Foundation, the Peanut Institute, Herbalife International, Pacific Health Laboratories, Nutritional Fundamentals for Health (NFH), Barilla, Metagenics, Bayer Consumer Care, Unilever Canada and Netherlands, Solae, Kellogg, Quaker Oats, Procter & Gamble, Abbott Laboratories, Dean Foods, the California Strawberry Commission, Haine Celestial, PepsiCo, the Alpro Foundation, Pioneer Hi-Bred International, DuPont Nutrition and Health, Spherix Consulting and WhiteWave Foods, the Advanced Foods and Material Network, the Canola and Flax Councils of Canada, Agri-Culture and Agri-Food Canada, the Canadian Agri-Food Policy Institute, Pulse Canada, the Soy Foods Association of North America, the Nutrition Foundation of Italy (NFI), Nutra-Source Diagnostics, the McDougall Program, the Toronto Knowledge Translation Group (St. Michael's Hospital), the Canadian College of Naturopathic Medicine, The Hospital for Sick Children, the Canadian Nutrition Society (CNS), the American Society of Nutrition (ASN), Arizona State University, Paolo Sorbini Foundation and the Institute of Nutrition, Metabolism and Diabetes. He received an honorarium from the United States Department of Agriculture to present the 2013 W.O. Atwater Memorial Lecture. He received the 2013 Award for Excellence in Research from the International Nut and Dried Fruit Council. He received funding and travel support from the Canadian Society of Endocrinology and Metabolism to produce mini cases for the Canadian Diabetes Association (CDA). He is a member of the International Carbohydrate Quality Consortium (ICQC). His wife, Alexandra L Jenkins, is a director and partner of INQUIS Clinical Research for the Food Industry, his 2 daughters, Wendy Jenkins and Amy Jenkins, have published a vegetarian book that promotes the use of the foods described here, The Portfolio Diet for Cardiovascular Risk Reduction (Academic Press/Elsevier 2020 ISBN:978-0-12-810510-8)and his sister, Caroline Brydson, received funding through a grant from the St. Michael's Hospital Foundation to develop a cookbook for one of his studies. C.W.C.K.: has received grants/research support from Advanced Food Materials Network, Agriculture and Agri-Foods Canada (AAFC), Almond Board of California, Barilla, Canadian Institutes of Health Research (CIHR), Canola Council of Canada, International Nut and Dried Fruit Council, International Tree Nut Council Research and Education Foundation, Loblaw Brands Ltd, National Dried Fruit Trade Association, Pulse Canada, and Unilever; in-kind research support from the Almond Board of California, the American Peanut Council, Barilla, the California Walnut Commission, Danone, Kellogg Canada, Loblaw Companies, Nutrartis, Quaker (Pepsico), Primo, Unico, Unilever and Upfield; travel support/honoraria from the American Peanut Council, the International Nut and Dried Fruit Council, the International Pasta Organization, Lantmannen, Oldways Preservation Trust, and the Peanut Institute. He has served on the scientific advisory board for the International Pasta Organization, McCormick Science Institute, Oldways Preservation Trust. He is a member of the International Carbohydrate Quality Consortium (ICQC), Executive Board Member of the Diabetes and Nutrition Study Group (DNSG) of the European Association for the Study of Diabetes (EASD), is on the Clinical Practice Guidelines Expert Committee for Nutrition Therapy of the EASD and is a Director of the Toronto 3D Knowledge Synthesis and Clinical Trials foundation. C.L.V.: serves on the scientific board of the ISA (International Sweeteners Association) and has received grants from Soremartec. S.L.: has received consulting payments and honoraria for scientific presentations or reviews at numerous venues, including but not limited to Barilla, Johns Hopkins University, Fred Hutchinson Cancer Center, Harvard University, University of Buffalo, Guang Dong General Hospital and Academy of Medical Sciences, and the National Institutes of Health. He is also a member of the Data Safety and Monitoring Board for a trial of pulmonary hypertension in diabetes patients at Massachusetts General Hospital. He receives royalties from UpToDate. Liu receives an honorarium from the American Society of Nutrition for his duties as Associate Editor. G.L.: holds shares in Independent Nutrition Logic Ltd., a consultancy. He and his wife have benefitted from research grants, travel funding, consultant fees, and honoraria from the American Association for the Advancement of Science (USA), the All Party Parliamentary Group for Diabetes (London, UK), Almond Board of California (USA), BENEO GmbH (DE), Biotechnology and Biosciences Research Council (UK), British Nutrition Foundation(UK), Calorie Control Council (USA), Cantox (CA), Colloides Naturel International (FR), Coca Cola (UK), Danisco (UK & Singapore), Diabetes Nutrition Study Group (EASD, EU), DiabetesUK (UK), Elsevier Inc. (USA), European Commission (EU), European Polyol Association (Brussels), Eureka (UK), Food and Agricultural Organization (Rome), Granules India (Ind), General Mills (USA), Health Canada (CA), Institute of Food Research (UK), International Carbohydrate Quality Consortium (CA), Institute of Medicine (Washington, DC), International Life Sciences Institute (EU & USA), Life Sciences Research Office, FASEB (USA), Nutrition Society of Australia, Knights Fitness (UK), Leatherhead Food Research (UK), LitghterLife (UK), Matsutani (JPN), Medical Research Council (UK), MSL Group (UK), Porter Novelli (UK), Sudzuker (DE), Sugar Nutrition/WSRO (UK), Tate & Lyle (UK), The Food Group (USA),WeightWatchers (UK),Wiley-Blackwell (UK).World Health Organization (Geneva). He is a member of the EASD Nutrition Guidelines Committee. PA: is the President of the Nutrition Foundation of Italy (NFI) a non-profit organization partially supported by Italian and non-Italian Food Companies. J.S.-S.: serves on the board of (and receives grant support through his institution from) the International Nut and Dried Fruit Council and the Eroski Foundation. He also serves on the Executive Committee of the Instituto Danone, Spain, and on the Scientific Committee of the Danone International Institute. He has received research support from the Patrimonio Comunal Olivarero, Spain, and Borges S.A., Spain. He receives consulting fees or travel expenses from Danone, the Eroski Foundation, the Instituto Danone, Spain, and Abbot Laboratories. J.L.S.: has received research support from the Canadian Foundation for Innovation, Ontario Research Fund, Province of Ontario Ministry of Research and Innovation and Science, Canadian Institutes of health Research (CIHR), Diabetes Canada, PSI Foundation, Banting and Best Diabetes Centre (BBDC), American Society for Nutrition (ASN), INC International Nut and Dried Fruit Council Foundation, National Dried Fruit Trade Association, National Honey Board, International Life Sciences Institute (ILSI), The Tate and Lyle Nutritional Research Fund at the University of Toronto, The Glycemic Control and Cardiovascular Disease in Type 2 Diabetes Fund at the University of Toronto (a fund established by the Alberta Pulse Growers), and the Nutrition Trialists Fund at the University of Toronto (a fund established by an inaugural donation from the Calorie Control Council). He has received in-kind food donations to support a randomized controlled trial from the Almond Board of California, California Walnut Commission, American Peanut Council, Barilla, Unilever, Upfield, Unico/Primo, Loblaw Companies, Quaker, Kellogg Canada, WhiteWave Foods, and Nutrartis. He has received travel support, speaker fees and/or honoraria from Diabetes Canada, Dairy Farmers of Canada, FoodMinds LLC, International Sweeteners Association, Nestlé, Pulse Canada, Canadian Society for Endocrinology and Metabolism (CSEM), GI Foundation, Abbott, Biofortis, ASN, Northern Ontario School of Medicine, INC Nutrition Research & Education Foundation, European Food Safety Authority (EFSA), Comité Européen des Fabricants de Sucre (CEFS), and Physicians Committee for Responsible Medicine. He has or has had ad hoc consulting arrangements with Perkins Coie LLP, Tate & Lyle, Wirtschaftliche Vereinigung Zucker e.V., and Inquis Clinical Research. He is a member of the European Fruit Juice Association Scientific Expert Panel and Soy Nutrition Institute (SNI) Scientific Advisory Committee. He is on the Clinical Practice Guidelines Expert Committees of Diabetes Canada, European Association for the study of Diabetes (EASD), Canadian Cardiovascular Society (CCS), and Obesity Canada. He serves or has served as an unpaid scientific advisor for the Food, Nutrition, and Safety Program (FNSP) and the Technical Committee on Carbohydrates of ILSI North America. He is a member of the International Carbohydrate Quality Consortium (ICQC), Executive Board Member of the Diabetes and Nutrition Study Group (DNSG) of the EASD, and Director of the Toronto 3D Knowledge Synthesis and Clinical Trials foundation. His wife is an employee of AB InBev. T.M.S.W.: he and his wife are part owners and employees of INQUIS Clinical Research, Ltd. (formerly GI Labs), a contract research organization in Toronto, Canada. He has authored or co-authored several books on the glycemic index for which has received royalties from Philippa Sandall Publishing Services and CABI Publishers. He has received research support, consultant fees or honoraria from or served on the scientific advisory board for Canadian Institutes of Health Research, Canadian Diabetes Association, Dairy Farmers of Canada, Agriculture Agri-Food Canada, Public Health Agency of Canada, GI Labs, GI Testing, Abbott, Proctor and Gamble, Mars Foods, McCain Foods, Bunge, Temasek Polytechnic Singapore, Northwestern University, Royal Society of London, Glycemic Index Symbol program, CreaNutrition AG, McMaster University, University of Manitoba, University of Alberta, Canadian Society for Nutritional Sciences, National Sports and Conditioning Association, Faculty of Public Health and Nutrition and Autonomous University of Nuevo Leon, Diabetes and Nutrition Study Group of the European Association for the Study of Diabetes (EASD). All other authors declare no conflict of interest.

References

1. Burkitt, D.P.; Trowell, H.C. *Refined Carbohydrate Food and Disease*; Academic Press: London, UK, 1975.
2. Trowell, H.C.; Burkitt, D.P. The development of the concept of dietary fibre. *Mol. Asp. Med.* **1987**, *9*, 7–15. [CrossRef]
3. Ha, M.A.; Jarvis, M.C.; Mann, J.I. A definition for dietary fibre. *Eur. J. Clin. Nutr.* **2000**, *54*, 861–864. [CrossRef] [PubMed]
4. Jarvis, M.C. Plant cell walls: Supramolecular assemblies. *Food Hydrocoll.* **2011**, *25*, 257–262. [CrossRef]
5. Grundy, M.M.; Edwards, C.H.; Mackie, A.R.; Gidley, M.J.; Butterworth, P.J.; Ellis, P.R. Re-evaluation of the mechanisms of dietary fibre and implications for macronutrient bioaccessibility, digestion and postprandial metabolism. *Br. J. Nutr.* **2016**, *116*, 816–833. [CrossRef] [PubMed]
6. Rastall, R.F.; Javier Moreno, F.J.; Hernandez-Hernandez, O. Dietary carbohydrate digestibility and metabolic effects in human health. *Front. Nutr.* **2019**. [CrossRef] [PubMed]
7. Food Standards Australia. Available online: http://www.foodstandards.gov.au/code/applications/Documents/A277%20IR(FULL).pdf (accessed on 21 August 2020).
8. FAO. *Food and Agriculture Organization of the United Nations, Codex Alimentarius Commission FAO/WHO Distribution of the Report of the 30th Session of the Codex Committee on Nutrition and Foods for Special Dietary Uses*; (ALINORM 09/32/26); FAO: Rome, Italy, 2009.
9. Scientific Advisory Committee on Nutrition (SACN) 2015. Carbohydrates and Health; London TSO, TSO Norwich NR3 1GN, UK. Available online: https://www.gov.uk/government/publications/sacn-carbohydrates-and-health-report (accessed on 21 August 2020).
10. Jones, J.M. CODEX-aligned dietary fiber definitions help to bridge the 'fiber gap'. *Nutr. J.* **2014**, *13*, 34. [CrossRef]
11. FDA. 2018. The Declaration of Certain Isolated or Synthetic Non-Digestible Carbohydrates as Dietary Fiber on Nutrition and Supplement Facts Labels: Guidance for Industry. Available online: https://www.fda.gov/media/113663/download (accessed on 21 August 2020).
12. Jenkins, D.J.; Kendall, C.W.; Axelsen, M.; Augustin, L.S.; Vuksan, V. Viscous and nonviscous fibres, nonabsorbable and low glycaemic index carbohydrates, blood lipids and coronary heart disease. *Curr. Opin. Lipidol.* **2000**, *11*, 49–56. [CrossRef]
13. Capuano, E. The behavior of dietary fiber in the gastrointestinal tract determines its physiological effect. *Crit. Rev. Food Sci. Nutr.* **2017**, *57*, 3543–3564. [CrossRef]
14. Jenkins, D.J.; Wolever, T.M.; Leeds, A.R.; Gassull, M.A.; Haisman, P.; Dilawari, J.; Goff, D.V.; Metz, G.L.; Alberti, K.G. Dietary fibres, fibre analogues, and glucose tolerance: Importance of viscosity. *Br. Med. J.* **1978**, *1*, 1392–1394. [CrossRef]
15. Liu, F.; Prabhakar, M.; Ju, J.; Long, H.; Zhou, H.W. Effect of inulin-type fructans on blood lipid profile and glucose level: A systematic review and meta-analysis of randomized controlled trials. *Eur. J. Clin. Nutr.* **2017**, *71*, 9–20. [CrossRef]
16. Livesey, G.; Tagami, H. Interventions to lower the glycemic response to carbohydrate foods with a low-viscosity fiber (resistant maltodextrin): Meta-analysis of randomized controlled trials. *Am. J. Clin. Nutr.* **2009**, *89*, 114–125. [CrossRef] [PubMed]
17. Livesey, G.; Taylor, R.; Hulshof, T.; Howlett, J. Glycemic response and health a systematic review and meta-analysis: Relations between dietary glycemic properties and health outcomes. *Am. J. Clin. Nutr.* **2008**, *87*, 258S–268S. [CrossRef] [PubMed]
18. Salmeron, J.; Manson, J.E.; Stampfer, M.J.; Colditz, G.A.; Wing, A.L.; Willett, W.C. Dietary fiber, glycemic load, and risk of non-insulin-dependent diabetes mellitus in women. *JAMA* **1997**, *277*, 472–477. [CrossRef] [PubMed]
19. Hu, Y.; Ding, M.; Sampson, L.; Willett, W.C.; Manson, J.E.; Wang, M.; Rosner, B.; Hu, F.B.; Sun, Q. Intake of whole grain foods and risk of type 2 diabetes: Results from three prospective cohort studies. *BMJ* **2020**, *370*, m2206. [CrossRef] [PubMed]
20. Jenkins, D.J.; Kendall, C.W.; Augustin, L.S.; Martini, M.C.; Axelsen, M.; Faulkner, D.; Vidgen, E.; Parker, T.; Lau, H.; Connelly, P.W.; et al. Effect of wheat bran on glycemic control and risk factors for cardiovascular disease in type 2 diabetes. *Diabetes Care* **2002**, *25*, 1522–1528. [CrossRef]

21. Jenkins, D.J.; Kendall, C.W.; McKeown-Eyssen, G.; Josse, R.G.; Silverberg, J.; Booth, G.L.; Vidgen, E.; Josse, A.R.; Nguyen, T.H.; Corrigan, S.; et al. Effect of a low-glycemic index or a high-cereal fiber diet on type 2 diabetes: A randomized trial. *JAMA* **2008**, *300*, 2742–2753. [CrossRef]
22. Jenkins, D.J.; Jones, P.J.; Lamarche, B.; Kendall, C.W.; Faulkner, D.; Cermakova, L.; Gigleux, I.; Ramprasath, V.; de Souza, R.; Ireland, C.; et al. Effect of a dietary portfolio of cholesterol-lowering foods given at 2 levels of intensity of dietary advice on serum lipids in hyperlipidemia: A randomized controlled trial. *JAMA* **2011**, *306*, 831–839. [CrossRef]
23. Edwards, C.H.; Grundy, M.M.L.; Grassby, T.; Vasilopoulou, D.; Frost, G.S.; Butterworth, P.J.; Berry, S.E.E.; Sanderson, J.; Ellis, P.R. Manipulation of starch bioaccessibility in wheat endosperm to regulate starch digestion, postprandial glycemia, insulinemia, and gut hormone responses: A randomized controlled trial in healthy ileostomy participants. *Am. J. Clin. Nutr.* **2015**, *102*, 791–800. [CrossRef]
24. Livesey, G.; Wilkinson, J.A.; Roe, M.; Faulks, R.; Clark, S.; Brown, J.C.; Kennedy, H.; Elia, M. Influence of the physical form of barley grain on the digestion of its starch in the human small intestine and implications for health. *Am. J. Clin. Nutr.* **1995**, *61*, 75–81. [CrossRef]
25. Jenkins, D.J.; Wesson, V.; Wolever, T.M.; Jenkins, A.L.; Kalmusky, J.; Guidici, S.; Csima, A.; Josse, R.G.; Wong, G.S. Wholemeal versus wholegrain breads: Proportion of whole or cracked grain and the glycaemic response. *BMJ* **1988**, *297*, 958–960. [CrossRef]
26. Wolever, T.M.; Schrade, K.B.; Vogt, J.A.; Tsihlias, E.B.; McBurney, M.I. Do colonic short-chain fatty acids contribute to the long-term adaptation of blood lipids in subjects with type 2 diabetes consuming a high-fiber diet? *Am. J. Clin. Nutr.* **2002**, *75*, 1023–1030. [CrossRef]
27. Augustin, L.S.; Kendall, C.W.; Jenkins, D.J.; Willett, W.C.; Astrup, A.; Barclay, A.W.; Björck, I.; Brand-Miller, J.C.; Brighenti, F.; Buyken, A.E.; et al. Glycemic index, glycemic load and glycemic response: An International Scientific Consensus Summit from the International Carbohydrate Quality Consortium (ICQC). *Nutr. Metab. Cardiovasc. Dis.* **2015**, *25*, 795–815. [CrossRef]
28. Aslam, M.F.; Ellis, P.; Berry, S.E.; Latunde-Dada, G.O.; Sharp, P.A. Enhancing mineral bioavailability from cereals: Current strategies and future perspectives. *Nutr. Bull.* **2018**, *43*, 184–188. [CrossRef] [PubMed]
29. Delcour, J.A.; Aman, P.; Courtin, C.M.; Hamaker, B.R.; Verbeke, K. Prebiotics, Fermentable Dietary Fiber, and Health Claims. *Adv. Nutr.* **2016**, *7*, 1–4. [CrossRef] [PubMed]
30. Mills, S.; Stanton, C.; Lane, J.A.; Smith, G.J.; Ross, R.P. Precision Nutrition and the Microbiome, Part I: Current State of the Science. *Nutrients* **2019**, *11*, 923. [CrossRef] [PubMed]
31. Mills, S.; Lane, J.A.; Smith, G.J.; Grimaldi, K.A.; Ross, R.P.; Stanton, C. Precision Nutrition and the Microbiome Part II: Potential Opportunities and Pathways to Commercialisation. *Nutrients* **2019**, *11*, 1468. [CrossRef]
32. Gibson, G.R.; Hutkins, R.; Sanders, M.E.; Prescott, S.L.; Reimer, R.A.; Salminen, S.J.; Scott, K.; Stanton, C.; Swanson, K.S.; Cani, P.D.; et al. Expert consensus document: The International Scientific Association for Probiotics and Prebiotics (ISAPP) consensus statement on the definition and scope of prebiotics. *Nat. Rev. Gastroenterol. Hepatol.* **2017**, *14*, 491–502. [CrossRef]
33. Holscher, H.D. Dietary fiber and prebiotics and the gastrointestinal microbiota. *Gut Microbes* **2017**, *8*, 172–184. [CrossRef]
34. Willett, W.C.; Rockström, J.; Loken, B.; Springmann, M.; Lang, T.; Vermeulen, S.; Garnett, T.; Tilman, D.; DeClerck, F.; Wood, A.; et al. Food in the Anthropocene: The EAT-Lancet Commission on healthy diets from sustainable food systems. *Lancet* **2019**, *393*, 447–492. [CrossRef]

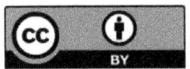 © 2020 by the authors. Licensee MDPI, Basel, Switzerland. This article is an open access article distributed under the terms and conditions of the Creative Commons Attribution (CC BY) license (http://creativecommons.org/licenses/by/4.0/).

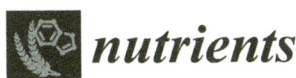

Article

The Effect of Labelling and Visual Properties on the Acceptance of Foods Containing Insects

Klaudia Modlinska [1,*], Dominika Adamczyk [2], Katarzyna Goncikowska [2], Dominika Maison [2] and Wojciech Pisula [1]

1. Institute of Psychology, Polish Academy of Sciences, 1 Jaracza St., 00-378 Warsaw, Poland; wojciech.pisula@wp.pl
2. Faculty of Psychology, University of Warsaw, 5/6 Stawki St., 00-183 Warsaw, Poland; dominika.adamczyk@psych.uw.edu.pl (D.A.); katarzyna.goncikowska@gmail.com (K.G.); dominika@psych.uw.edu.pl (D.M.)
* Correspondence: kmodlinska@wp.pl

Received: 27 July 2020; Accepted: 17 August 2020; Published: 19 August 2020

Abstract: Introducing insects as a source of nutrients (e.g., protein) plays a key role in many countries' environmental policies. However, westerners generally reject insects as an ingredient of food products and meals. The aim of our study was to assess if explicitly labelling food as containing insects and/or implying it by manipulating the appearance of food influences the participants' perception of food products or their behavioral reaction to such products. Participants were asked to try a range of foods, none of which contained ingredients derived from insects. However, the experimental conditions varied with regard to food labelling (insect content) and appearance (traces of insect-like ingredients). We observed the participants' non-verbal behavioral reactions to the foods. Next, the respondents filled in a questionnaire evaluating the food's properties. Additionally, we asked the participants to fill in a set of questionnaires measuring other variables (food neophobia, disgust, variety seeking, etc.) The results showed that products labelled as containing insects are consumed with reluctance and in lower quantities despite their appearance. In addition, people with lower general neophobia and a higher tendency to seek variety tried the insect-labelled samples sooner than people from the other groups. Recommendations for marketing strategies are provided.

Keywords: food labelling; entomophagy; insect-based foods; edible insects; food sustainability; perception of food; novel food; disgust; neophobia; variety seeking; food technology neophobia; consumer studies; behavior

1. Introduction

While food shortages mainly affect developing countries, where malnutrition is a problem for millions [1], in highly developed countries the conventional methods of food production burden the environment and pose a threat to animal welfare. Introducing insect-based food products could contribute to solving both issues [2].

Entomophagy is present in many cultures and is the main source of nutritious food for many communities [3]. Insects are a source of protein (and amino acids), fats, vitamins (e.g., vitamin B12), beta-carotene, several minerals, fiber and other valuable substances [4–8]. Insect production requires less space [9] and leaves a significantly smaller ecological footprint than livestock farming, and is more ecologically sustainable [10,11]. Moreover, as insects are evolutionarily distant from humans, they are less likely to carry pathogens that could pose a risk to human health [7,12].

Although nowadays the consumption of insects by humans is regularly discussed in the media, attempts at changing people's eating habits and introducing these new types of food have so far generally met with individual and social rejection. Although some recent studies show a positive effect of information on the willingness to try insect-based foods (e.g., [13–16]), it seems that, in general, rational arguments stressing the advantages of insect production and consumption are not sufficient to change our eating habits [17,18] (see also [19]). In general, westerners are largely opposed to eating insects, as they are an unfamiliar food source that deviates from cultural norms and are expected to have undesirable sensory properties [20] (cf. [21]).

It seems that the main psychological barriers to consuming this kind of novel food are disgust and fear [22–24]. Most people object not only to eating insects, but also to the very idea of eating insects [22,23], and their negative reactions to insects may be very deeply rooted and automatic [25]. The first explanation for this reaction is disgust. Disgust is an emotion that elicits thoughts and behaviors that result in avoiding the objects that trigger it [26]. Things that elicit disgust differ largely from one culture to another; they are acquired in the learning process and are deeply rooted in social norms. Disgust correlates with the evolutionary need to avoid infection, dirt and disease, and may lead to fear [23]. In the case of food, this fear is manifested in anxious hesitation to consume unknown items, which is called food neophobia [27]. Food neophobia correlates positively with general neophobia [27], which may increase reluctance towards unfamiliarity. Therefore, it is likely that persons with a high level of food neophobia, as well as a high level of general neophobia, would be prone to the feeling of disgust (see [28–30]). Persons who fit this profile are very likely to be the least willing to include insects in their diet [18]. Moreover, in the case of such new commercially available products as insects and insect flour, and their mostly unknown production processes, Food Technology Neophobia [31] may also play a crucial part. On the other hand, it is possible that other characteristics such as the Variety Seeking Tendency [32], which involves an intrinsic desire for variety in many aspects of life, including food consumption, may increase the willingness to try new food products [33].

Although the main psychological variables influencing the acceptance/rejection of insect-based foods seem to have been identified, the problem of a limited willingness to incorporate such foods into everyday diet has not been resolved. Over the past few decades, researchers have been trying to devise a strategy to convince people that insects are indeed edible, safe, and tasty. It may be hypothesized that one such strategy could involve adapting foods containing insects to the consumers' general eating preferences. It is clear, for instance, that consumers prefer fatty and sweet products (e.g., [34,35]). Serving insects in the form of, or as an ingredient of, snacks or sweet foods may increase their acceptance and create positive associations with such types of food, facilitating habituation to insect-based foods. On the other hand, studies by Tan et al. [36] showed that sweet-flavored insects were considered less appropriate than savory insect-based meals, especially when the entire insect body or insect body parts were easily discernible.

Another way of reducing the level of food neophobia may be to add insects to familiar dishes [14] (cf. [37]). However, the form in which they are added also plays a part. It seems that adding ground insects to a meal could reduce reluctance to consume it by reducing exposure to the visual stimulus (e.g., [20]). In the case of unconventional animal-derived foods, evoking the image of the entire animal often elicits strong objection to the food offered and is connected with strong negative emotions [38]. When eating animals, we usually consume pieces that do not resemble living individuals; we are reluctant to eat animal heads, entire limbs, etc. Perhaps in the case of insects, the fact that they are often served whole elicits similar reactions in humans by making it clear what they are about to consume. Moreover, adding entire insects to meals may give the impression that a food is polluted or rotten. Evidence to support this claim has been provided in a study by Gmuer et al. [39], which showed that potato chips which contained insect flour or insect elements were assessed less negatively than chips mixed with whole insects (see also [29,40,41]). Other studies, however, show no such correlation (e.g., [42,43]). In addition, the widely applied marketing strategy of presenting insects as sustainable substitutes for animal protein is also problematic, as it gives rise to an expectation that the products will be similar to meat in texture and taste, as is the case with plant-based products made to look similar to their meat-based counterparts [17] (cf. [30]).

Nevertheless, it seems that the reluctance to eat insects is so strong that the very awareness of consuming them elicits an aversive reaction, which may then be generalized to other accompanying products. This hypothesis seems to have been confirmed by Rozin et al. [44] in a study where participants assessed a drink more negatively if the cup they drank from had been in contact with a sterile insect before it was used. Such a reaction may be explained by the participants' feeling that the cup had been contaminated during contact with the insect, and the disgust triggered by that perception was generalized to the drink. In the case of commercially available products, information on insect content is provided in visual form on packaging or it is provided in the product name, which may have a similar effect. Studies carried out to date have shown that both verbal and visual information on packaging has a significant impact on how consumers evaluate the taste and smell of the substances they ingest (e.g., [45–48]). The very indication of insect content on the packaging may affect consumers' assessment of the product quality. Moreover, it may be assumed that ingredients whose appearance suggests the presence of traces of insects in a product may additionally reinforce the label effect by reinforcing the impression that the product has been contaminated (cf. [23]).

Based on the above, we are convinced that more research is needed to further explore the factors influencing peoples' attitude to eating insect-based foods and to identify marketing strategies and educational campaigns. We would like to propose the study protocol involving an assessment of several variables that have been identified in other studies (the results of which, however, are in some cases inconclusive) or that stem from our predictions. In our study, we intended to check, first of all, whether the mere fact of providing information about insect content (label) would influence the sensory evaluation and acceptance of different foods. In this way, we wanted to replicate the findings obtained by Mancini and colleagues [14]. However, we decided to use sweet foods (pastry, sweets), as we hypothesized that snacks would be more likely to encourage people to try this kind of food, especially bearing in mind the general preference for sweetness among consumers. Secondly, we hoped to broaden the scope of the study by evaluating the effect of visibility of insect parts on the level of acceptance of insect-based foods, as studies that have analyzed these aspects have been inconclusive. We expected that the differences in the results obtained by other researchers could have arisen from a specific "presentation" of insects, but also from an interactive effect of the information on insect content and the appearance of food. In addition, we planned to control the mediating effect of commonly studied psychological variables, such as food neophobia and disgust. However, we also incorporated other measures in the study; we used the food technology neophobia scale and the variety-seeking tendency scale to further explore the mechanism underlying the acceptance of insect-based food.

We intended to analyze these aspects by checking experimentally reactions to food products depending on (a) the information about insect content provided on product labelling, and (b) the appearance of products suggestive of traces of insect-like ingredients. To address these issues, we conducted an experiment whereby we observed participants' reactions to specific products: a cookie, a muffin, and a date ball. The experiment resembled a classic product test in which the consumers tried and assessed three products in terms of taste, smell, appearance, etc. Depending on the experimental conditions (2 × 2), the products differed either (a) with regard to the information about the presence or absence of insect content, or (b) in appearance: they are artificially "dotted" to suggest insect content or not. In reality, none of the products used in the experiment contained insects or insect-derived ingredients.

Another important novel element of our experiment, when compared to many previous studies, was the fact that we not only measured participant reactions in qualitative scale-based terms (declaration of willingness to taste a specific product), but we also observed several non-verbal behavioral indicators (e.g., we measured the time and frequency of sampling products and how much of the product was ingested). What is more, after the experiment, we conducted interviews with the participants, which served as a source of additional information to enrich the discussion section of the paper and allow us to suggest possible marketing strategies.

Based on the results of previous studies, we formulated the following hypotheses:

Hypothesis 1 (H1). *Information about insect-based ingredients on the product label will translate into lower product evaluation scores and will have an impact on the behavioral reactions to the product (cf. [44–48]).*

Hypothesis 2 (H2). *Product appearance (traces of ingredients suggesting insect content) will translate into lower product evaluation scores and will have an impact on the behavioral reactions to a product (e.g., [20,29,39,41]).*

Hypothesis 3 (H3). *The perception of the product and behavioral indicators will be controlled by different psychological features. People with higher food neophobia, sensitivity to disgust, food technology neophobia, and general neophobia are expected to be less willing to try products described as containing insect-derived ingredients (product evaluation and behavioral reactions to the products), while people with a high level of variety-seeking tendency will be more open to this kind of novel food (e.g., [22,23,32,43]).*

2. Methods

2.1. Participants

The participants were recruited by means of announcements posted online, on website panels, and individual personal requests. All participants gave their oral consent to participate in the study. They also confirmed that they did not suffer from any form of food allergy or intolerance. One person was excluded from the study after having a strong emotional reaction to the food samples and after disclosing an existing psychiatric condition. The final sample comprised 99 participants (81 females and 18 males). The participants were aged between 18 and 45 years old, while the average age was 22. They were mostly university students who came from big cities (>50,000 inhabitants).

The participants were randomly assigned to four experimental groups. In each group, the male to female ratio was comparable. They were told that the purpose of the experiment was to study food preferences. Before the experiment, they were not informed that the experiment involved tasting insect-based products, so their attitudes and expectations did not affect the answers given in the questionnaires and the participants who tasted products with no indication of insects did not feel they were being misled, or that the products they were supposed to try contained hidden insect parts. The data was collected anonymously. Each person was assigned an individual number to allow the data from all parts of the experiment to be linked.

2.2. Procedure and Methods

The study consisted of three parts. In Part 1 the participants were asked to fill in a set of questionnaires. In Part 2 a behavioral experiment was conducted. Part 3 involved conducting a short interview with the participants.

Part 1—Questionnaires

The participants answered a set of questionnaires preceded by socio-demographic questions. They were also asked about their diet preferences (whether they followed a meat or non-meat diet). This information was collected to control the characteristics of the experimental groups and to avoid any possible impact of this variable on the behavioral data collected in Part 2. All questionnaires were administered in a paper-and-pen form. The time to complete the questionnaires was not limited.

Part 2—Behavioral assessment

After completing the questionnaires, the participants were asked to move to another room, where behavioral assessment was conducted. They were seated at a small table and received instructions about the experimental procedure. The participants were randomly assigned to one of four experimental set-ups (Table 1). Each person received a set of three food products (A—a cookie, B—a muffin, C—a date ball). The products were placed on a paper plate, and a label with the name of the product was placed above each item (Figure 1). In two of the four groups, the labels explicitly stated that the products contained insects and in the two other groups, there was no information about insect content. In addition, half of the participants were given samples that could suggest the presence of mildly processed insects in the food (e.g., chunks of cranberries or nuts easily discernible in the products), while the other half were served "smooth" products. The experimental group set-up followed the ANOVA 2 × 2 procedure (Table 1).

Table 1. Experimental group set-up. The products in groups 1A and 2A (no visual clues suggestive of insect content) and in groups 1B and 2B (presence of visual clues suggestive of insect content) looked identical, but differed in the information provided on the labels.

		Label—Explicit Information about the Presence or Absence of Insect Content	
		No Insect Content "1"	Insect Content "2"
Appearance—presence or absence of visual features of the product suggestive of insect content	No visual clues suggestive of insect content "A"	Condition 1A	Condition 2A
	Visual clues suggestive of insect content "B"	Condition 1B	Condition 2B

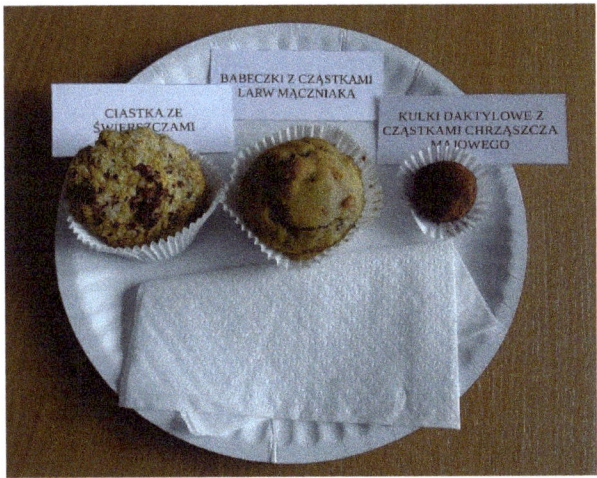

Figure 1. A set of three food products: (from left to right:) a cookie, a muffin, a date ball. Labels attached to food products: **Group 1A:** Rice flour cookie; amaranth flour cupcakes; plain date balls—products labelled as not containing insects. **Group 2A:** Cricket flour cookie; mealworm flour cupcakes; beetle flour date balls—products labelled as containing insects. **Group 1B:** cookies with chunks of cranberries; cupcakes with chunks of walnuts; date balls with linseed—products labelled as not containing insects. **Group 2B:** Cookies with crickets; cupcakes with particles of mealworm larvae; date balls with May beetle particles—products labelled as containing insects.

The participants were asked to try the products in a given order. The questionnaires assessing the properties of each of the three products were placed above the plate in front of each participant. The questionnaire concerned the respondents' willingness to try the product; the visual attractiveness of the product; smell; taste; and willingness to eat more of the product. The respondents were asked to indicate their answers on a 10-point linear scale with descriptive explanations provided at the end-points. In addition, each participant received a napkin and a cup filled with water. The participants were told that they were free to eat as much of any of the products as they wanted, and that they were free not to try any of them if they did not want to.

Each participant's behavior during the food-tasting session was recorded with a video camera placed approx. 2 meters in front of the participant.

Part 3—Interview

After the tasting session, the participants moved to an adjacent room for a short qualitative semi-structured individual interview. The interviews were aimed at broadening the scope of data collected in the study and at providing a context for the quantitative data collected. The scenario comprised a few precisely defined thematic areas, but the questions pertaining to those areas were not pre-determined and they were individually adapted to the respondent and interview dynamics.

The aim of the interview was to examine the opinions and experiences of the respondents with respect to entomophagy; to gain a more in-depth knowledge about the participants' experience of the food-tasting session; to understand the motivations behind the (un)willingness to try the products; and to examine the declared readiness to include insects in the daily diet and the participants' view on the social aspects of insect-based diets. The participants were asked about their previous experience with entomophagy (e.g., whether they had ever heard of this phenomenon before, whether they had ever tried insects, whether they believed that insects could be part of a normal human diet and what potential consequences of such a diet could be). Next, the participants were asked about their impressions from the tasting session and the likelihood of including insects in their own diet. The interviewees were encouraged to elaborate on their answers so that a wider range of information could be collected.

The interviews were recorded and transcribed.

2.3. Ethical Statement

All subjects gave their informed consent for inclusion before they participated in the study. The study was conducted in accordance with the Declaration of Helsinki, and the protocol was approved by the Commission of Ethics of Scientific Research of the Faculty of Psychology, University of Warsaw, Poland (No. 21/03/2019). Additionally, the participants signed a consent form agreeing to the processing of their personal data (including audio and video recordings). They were also assured that they could withdraw from the experiment at any point of the procedure and that all the data collected during the study (including the recordings) would only be available to the research team members.

2.4. Questionnaires

All the questionnaires were translated from English into Polish using the back-translation method [49,50]. First, the questionnaires were translated from English into Polish by a professional translator, then a different translator translated the Polish version back into English. The original English and the back-translated versions were compared by a native English speaker. The text was edited according to the native English speakers' comments, following which the reformulated items were translated into English by a translator not familiar with the content of the comments or the original questionnaire; they were then compared with the original by a native English speaker. The final Polish versions of the questionnaires were then consolidated. The internal consistency of the Polish versions of the questionnaires was determined using Cronbach's alpha.

2.4.1. FNS

The Food Neophobia Scale (FNS), developed by Pilner and Hobden [33], is often used to measure the willingness to try new foods [51]. It consists of ten items on a scale from 1 ("strongly disagree") to 7 ("strongly agree"); five statements are positive (indicative of neophilic attitudes) and five are negative (indicative of neophobic attitudes). Examples of statements include: "I don't trust new foods" and "At dinner parties, I will try a new food". The internal consistency of the Polish version of the scale in our study measured using Cronbach's alpha was estimated at 0.87.

2.4.2. GNS

The General Neophobia Scale (GNS) is a scale measuring the general level of neophobia. It was developed by Pliner and Hobden [33] together with the Food Neophobia Scale. It is an eight-item 7-point Likert scale from 1 ("strongly disagree") to 7 ("strongly agree"). Examples of statements include: "I am afraid of the unknown" and "Whenever I am on vacation, I can't wait to get home". The internal consistency of the Polish version of the scale in our study measured using Cronbach's alpha was estimated at 0.91.

2.4.3. FTNS

The Food Technology Neophobia Scale (FTNS; [31]) is a tool suitable for measuring the willingness to try new food products manufactured using new food technologies and attitudes to new food technologies. It consists of thirteen items scaled from 1 ("strongly disagree") to 7 ("strongly agree"). Examples of statements include: "It can be risky to switch to new food technologies too quickly" and "New products produced using new food technologies can help people have a balanced diet". The internal consistency of the Polish version of the scale in our study measured using Cronbach's alpha was estimated at 0.88.

2.4.4. The Disgust Sensitivity Scale

The Disgust Sensitivity Scale (Version 1; [52]) is a measure of individual differences in sensitivity to disgust. It is a scale with thirty-two items: the first sixteen are binary "true" or "false" questions, the rest assess how disgusting a given experience seems on a scale from 0 ("not disgusting at all") to 2 ("very disgusting"). Example items include: "Even if I was hungry, I would not drink a bowl of my favourite soup if it had been stirred by a used but thoroughly washed flyswatter" and "Seeing a cockroach in someone else's house doesn't bother me". The internal consistency of the Polish version of the scales in our study measured using Cronbach's alpha was estimated at 0.825.

2.4.5. VARSEEK-Scale

The Variety Seeking Tendency Scale (VARSEEK-Scale; [32]) is a scale measuring individual variety-seeking tendency in food choices [53]. The respondents assessed eight statements on a five-point Likert scale (from "completely disagree" to "completely agree"). Examples of statements include: "I prefer to eat food products I am used to" and "When I eat out, I like to try the most unusual items, even if I am not sure I would like them". The internal consistency of the Polish version of the scale in our study measured using Cronbach's alpha was estimated at 0.89.

2.5. Data Processing and Statistical Analysis

In addition to using the questionnaires measuring specific psychological traits, we also analyzed the behavioral data collected during the experimental (product tasting) phase. This data was analyzed on the basis of video recordings made during the experiment. We used BORIS software [54] to code behaviors on the basis of the recorded material, which made it possible to define selected behaviors and to assess their duration and frequency. We scored the behaviors the participants engaged in during the entire experimental phase. Consequently, we were able to assign specific scores to the duration of separate bouts of behavior, their frequency, and the total time participants spent engaging in specific behaviors. We measured the following variables: latency to pick up food products from the plate; latency to begin eating; amount of food eaten (for each product separately); time spent eating; time and frequency of sniffing food products, time and frequency of looking at the food products; frequency of drinking water during the tasting session. In addition, we analyzed the scores awarded by the participants for the products tasted.

The measurements of different behaviors taken in the course of the experiment (as a response to the exposure to food products) were analyzed using an analysis of covariance (ANCOVA) with Label

(2) × Appearance (2) as between-subject factors. The behavioral measurements served as dependent variables, while Label and Appearance manipulations stood for independent variables. Scores from the questionnaires served as covariates. For multiple comparisons, the Bonferroni correction was applied to reduce the likelihood of Type I error. Differences were considered significant for p values of <0.05.

For the amount of food eaten, a repeated measures ANOVA was conducted to analyze the effect of possible differences between the three food products (A—cookie, B—muffin, C—date ball) on a given variable. Label (2) × Appearance (2) were used as between-subject factors and Sample as the within-subject factor (3). Scores obtained from the questionnaires served as covariates.

Descriptive statistics are set out in Appendix A.

The audio data collected during the interviews was transcribed and then subjected to the thematic analysis, which is a method for developing qualitative data consisting of identification, analysis and description of thematic areas [55]. In this type of analysis, a thematic unit is treated as an element related to the research problem that includes an important aspect of data. Two interview moderators, i.e., persons responsible for interviewing the respondents, encoded and analyzed the transcriptions. Next, the created codes were cross-checked. An important advantage of thematic analysis is its flexibility, which makes it possible to adopt a research strategy best suited to the phenomenon under examination. In our study, the thematic analysis focused on various aspects of insect consumption and general attitudes towards insects. However, account was taken of the exploratory nature of the study and the novelty of the phenomenon, and thus the low level of the participants' familiarity with the topic.

3. Results

Characteristics of the participants. First, we checked the characteristics of the study participants, especially whether they were distributed equally between the four groups with respect to the demographic variables and the basic psychological measures included in the study (Table 2). Statistical analysis showed no significant differences between the four experimental set-ups with regard to gender balance, age, level of education, and psychological variables. Even though the number of women was four times higher than the number of men, the ratio of men to women was the same in each set-up.

Table 2. Characteristics of the study groups. Abbreviation sd refers to the standard deviation.

Variable	Group 1A $N = 24$	Group 1B $N = 25$	Group 2A $N = 25$	Group 2B $N = 25$	Statistics
Sex (women—F; men—M)	18F/6M	22F/3M	19F/6M	21F/4M	$\chi^2(3) = 1.893$, $p = 0.959$
Age—mean (sd)	22.1 (3.7)	22.5 (5.3)	22.2 (5.4)	23 (6.9)	$F(3; 95) = 0.139$, $p = 0.936$
Education (secondary/student/higher)	0/21/3	2/19/4	1/20/4	1/22/2	$\chi^2(5) = 3.071$, $p = 0.800$
Diets (meat/non-meat)	16/8	13/12	11/14	14/11	$\chi^2(9) = 10.637$, $p = 0.301$
Food Neophobia—mean (sd)	32.3 (8.5)	32.2 (11.4)	30.8 (11.8)	29.2 (12.3)	$F(3; 95) = 0.435$, $p = 0.729$
General Neophobia—mean (sd)	26.0 (10.8)	30.4 (11.0)	32.0 (11.5)	27.6 (10.8)	$F(3; 95) = 1.499$, $p = 0.220$
Food Technology Neophobia—mean (sd)	46.6 (12.7)	46.4 (10.1)	51.3 (13.9)	50.4 (13.5)	$F(3; 95) = 0.980$, $p = 0.405$
Variety Seeking Tendency—mean (sd)	30.8 (5.6)	31.0 (6.4)	31.7 (6.0)	31.2 (7.3)	$F(3; 95) = 0.094$, $p = 0.963$
Disgust—mean (sd)	15.2 (5.6)	16.1 (4.4)	14.1 (4.6)	15.7 (4.8)	$F(3; 95) = 0.777$, $p = 0.510$

3.1. Effect of Label and Appearance on Food Acceptance (Behavioural Data)

Latency to pick up food. The analysis of the latency to pick up the food products from the plate showed a main effect of Label ($F(1, 89) = 6.456$, $p = 0.013$, $eta^2 = 0.068$). Products labelled as containing insects were picked up later than those with labels not indicating any insect content ($t = 2.541$, $p = 0.013$, $d = 0.507$). There was no interactive effect of Label and Appearance, nor a main effect of Appearance. We also found main effects of the covariates General Neophobia ($F(1, 89) = 5.825$, $p = 0.018$, $eta^2 = 0.061$) and Variety Seeking ($F(1, 89) = 6.896$, $p = 0.01$, $eta^2 = 0.072$). There was a positive correlation between the latency to pick up food and General Neophobia scores ($r = 0.206$, $p < 0.05$), while a negative correlation was observed for Variety Seeking Tendency ($r = -0.219$, $p < 0.05$). This may suggest that participants with a higher level of general neophobia started eating food samples later than those with a lower level of general neophobia. Participants with a higher level of variety seeking tendency started eating sooner than those demonstrating a lower level of this characteristic.

Latency to begin eating. In the case of latency to begin eating, we observed a main effect of Label ($F(1, 88) = 5.570$, $p = 0.020$, $eta^2 = 0.059$). Participants began to digest food samples labelled as containing insects later than those with labels not indicating any insect content ($t = 2.360$, $p = 0.020$, $d = 0.503$). There was no interactive effect of Label and Appearance, nor a main effect of Appearance. There was no effect of covariates.

Sniffing and looking at products. Analyses of the time and frequency of sniffing the food products and the time and frequency of looking at the food products showed no differences between the groups, which means that participants examined olfactory and visual properties of the samples for a comparable amount of time despite their different labels and appearances. No effect of covariates was found.

Amount of food eaten. A repeated measures ANOVA for the amount of food eaten revealed a main effect of Label for all three food samples ($F(1, 90) = 23.918$, $p = 0.001$, $eta^2 = 0.210$), but there was no main effect of Appearance or Sample – Figure 2. There were no interactive effects of Sample and Label, nor an interactive effect of Sample and Appearance. This may indicate that the food samples were found to be equally tasty, and the effect of Label was similar for all the samples. Samples labelled as containing insects were consumed in lower quantities then those with labels not indicating insect content regardless of the type of food (sample A: $t = 6.282$, $p < 0.001$, $d = 0.884$; sample B: $t = 2.637$, $p < 0.001$, $d = 0.551$; sample C: $t = 4.646$, $p < 0.001$, $d = 0.963$). A significant effect of the Food Neophobia covariate was also found ($F(1, 90) = 4.283$, $p = 0.041$, $eta^2 = 0.045$). The correlation between Food Neophobia scores and the amount of food eaten was found to be negative, but only for sample C ($r = -0.21$, $p = 0.037$).

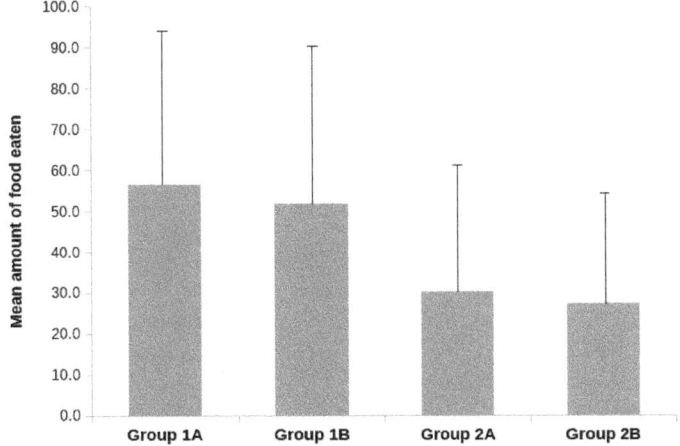

Figure 2. Mean amount of food eaten in each group.

Time spent eating. An ANCOVA analysis conducted for the time spent eating yielded a significant effect for Label (F(1, 89) = 5.922, p = 0.017, eta^2 = 0.062), with participants exposed to meals labelled as containing insects eating for a shorter time than individuals who were offered samples with labels not indicating insect content (t = −2.433, p = 0.017, d = 0.527). There was no main effect of Appearance, nor an interactive effect of Label and Appearance.

A similar effect was observed in the case of the frequency of eating bouts. The analysis showed only a main effect of Label (F(1, 89) = 10.541, p = 0.002, eta^2 = 0.106). Participants who ingested food labelled as containing insects ate less frequently than those who were offered food with labels not indicating insect content. These two results may be correlated, as the shorter consumption time probably involves less frequent bites. No effect of covariates was observed.

Frequency of drinking water. Differences between the groups were observed in the frequency of drinking water when ingesting food. An ANCOVA revealed an interactive effect of Label and Appearance (F(1, 89) = 4.625, p = 0.034, eta^2 = 0.049). A post-hoc analysis showed that participants who ate the samples with labels and appearance not indicating insect content drank water more frequently than those who ate the products labelled as containing insects with a matching appearance (t = 3.214, p = 0.011, d = 0.793) and than those who ate the products labelled as containing insects with a "smooth" appearance (t = 2.906, p = 0.028, d = 0.121). No effect of covariates was observed.

The above results support the first hypothesis. The effect of Label was found in the latency to pick up food, latency to begin eating, amount of food eaten, and time spent eating variations. Food labelled as containing insects was tasted later and in smaller quantities than food labelled as not containing insects.

However, we found no support for the second hypothesis. There were no differences in the behavioral measures between the foods with traces of insect-like parts and those with a smooth appearance.

Additionally, no interactive effect of Label and Appearance was observed.

The third hypothesis was only partially confirmed. The level of food neophobia correlated only with the amount of food eaten for sample C. General neophobia level and variety seeking tendency level correlated with the latency to pick up food. However, we did not find any confounding effect of disgust and food technology neophobia.

3.2. Influence of Label and Appearance on Food Evaluation (Product Questionnaires)

We conducted an ANCOVA analysis of food evaluation scores depending on product information (label) and food appearance. For the first question about the willingness to try the products offered, there was a main effect of Label (F(1, 89) = 5.379, p = 0.023, eta^2 = 0.056) and a main effect of Appearance (F(1, 89) = 4.460, p = 0.037, eta^2 = 0.047), but no interactive effect was observed. Participants declared less willingness to try the products labelled as containing insects (t = 2.319, p = 0.023, d = 0.471) and the "smooth" products with no easily discernible elements (t = 2.112, p = 0.037, d = 0.414). However, there were no differences between the experimental groups with regard to the scores awarded for appearance, smell, taste, and willingness to eat more of the product. There was no effect of covariates.

These findings support the first and second hypotheses, but only as regards the first question of the questionnaire.

3.3. Qualitative Data Analysis—Interviews

Previous experience of eating insects. Prior to the experiment, all respondents had some experience of entomophagy. In most cases, however, this involved observing insect-eating behaviors in other people (on television, the internet) rather than through direct personal experience of ingesting insects. Insects are perceived as exotic and are associated with Asian (particularly Vietnamese, Chinese, Cambodian, Indian) or African food, as shown on travel or survival TV shows. The few persons who had themselves tried dishes containing insects before participating in the experiment, tried insects bought by their friends as "souvenirs" from far-away countries.

"For sure, only not in our culture. In Asia, if I'm not mistaken, Thailand, I think. Chinese markets are what I always associate [with insects], like on travel shows, with tonnes of colourful larvae. It is certainly controversial for Europeans—it would most likely be for me, but [I would be willing to try insects] out of curiosity what that would be like (...)."

Barriers to eating insects. The first reaction to ingesting insects was disgust. In the participants' opinion, insects are slimy and evoke associations with filth, basements, and waste. These associations are further reinforced by the image of insects on TV shows, especially on children's programs.

Because we associate bugs with something disgusting, bugs in food are more often associated with throwing away food and not eating it. Bugs are eaten by wild animals and not by humans.

I would be afraid that I would feel the structure of this thing and that it would simply be disgusting: limbs or feelers or something like that. I think everyone is afraid that an insect can come alive in your mouth. Out of some internal fear—they are so disgusting and unpleasant.

The respondents claimed that in our culture "one does not eat insects—it is as simple as that". Some participants, even though they were unable to specifically identify what makes insects so disgusting, pointed to the cultural aspects and the importance of upbringing: "we are simply not used to [eating insects]".

It is a cultural thing. For us, [insects] are exotic, disgusting, because we have learned to think [about them] this way. [They are] food, as any other type of food, specific for particular regions. And this works this way for us too—we eat pickled cucumbers and sauerkraut, which for some people is simply rotten food. So if we looked at it completely objectively, it seems that eating rotten food is a bigger problem than eating processed insects.

On the other hand, the participants stated it would be sufficient to "get over oneself and try". They claimed to see a potential advantage in the wider availability of insects and in their potential to become something commonplace and therefore not rejected by the society in general.

It is all in your head—we have always been told that an insect is just an insect, it is disgusting, it is a pest. I think this has a huge impact. Insects are not soft and fluffy, but they have hard shells or something, so they don't look too good either, to be perfectly honest.

Perceived advantages of eating insects. Many respondents pointed to insects' high nutritional value as an advantage; they evoked their high protein content and occasionally mentioned other unspecified vitamins and nutrients.

Some respondents mentioned the economic aspects of industrial insect farming. Insects are thought to be inexpensive and easy to produce and transport. Occasionally, the participants described insects as a potential future substitute for meat. Such statements, however, mostly came from vegetarians, who also expressed concerns over the ethical aspects of insect farming. Their answers indicated that they were not certain whether insects were animals. A criterion commonly used for assessing the morality of eating insects was their ability to feel pain. The respondents were not sure whether insects feel pain.

Perhaps also because, for example, when we kill and eat mammals, they certainly feel more pain than insects—it is as simple as that. Maybe it would be more ... humane ... this may be the wrong word here ... but maybe we could follow that path to reduce the number of animals bred for meat.

Experiences from the tasting session. The main reason for which the participants decided to try the cookies with insects was curiosity. After seeing a "normal" looking cookie, they were curious whether it tasted different from what they expected from its appearance.

> No, I was wondering if I was going to get anything from the new technologies and if it was going to look strange and resemble God knows what, but I was positively surprised, because it looked tasty. Yes, at first, yes, to some degree, in general, when I saw the labels I thought 'What did they give me? There is no way I'm trying it.' But when I had a look, all looked good and this encouraged me to try it. If I had got an insect on my plate, I would never have tried it. When I tried the first one, I completely switched off thinking that I was eating insects.

The decision to try the products was also made easier by the fact that the products looked appetizing and nice. Another safeguard encouraging the participants to try the cookies was the scientific setting; participating in a research experiment guaranteed the safety and hygiene of the products ingested ("you would not give me anything poisonous to eat"). According to the study participants, one of the potential barriers could be the lack of hygiene linked to eating insects, resulting from the aforementioned associations with filth.

The study participants were unable to precisely identify their expectations and assumptions with regard to the taste of the cookies. They expected the cookies to taste strange or different, "like a bug", but they were unable to say what they specifically meant. After trying the products, they referred to their own preferences for desserts rather than to the insect content. Their experience was not particularly positive or negative.

Potential for adding insects to everyday diet. The study participants imagined a potential insect consumer to be a young person who is open to new experiences, with a positive attitude, who eats meat but wants to reduce the amount of meat in their diet or to stop eating it completely. In the participants' opinion, insects could become a fashionable "curiosity" in certain social circles.

The respondents suggested that insect-based food may not be a good idea for the elderly or for vegetarians or vegans (due to the unclear status of insects as animals being able to feel pain). Despite the perceived advantages of insects, their market potential and the positive experiences from the tasting session, most participants claimed that insects were not an appropriate food for them. Yet, some answers suggested a willingness to try insects if they were commercially available. The participants thought, however, that it would rather be a one-off experience than a decision to include insects in their diet on a regular basis. They expressed a wish to reduce the amount of meat and not a need to include other types of meat in their diet. They did not see any direct value for themselves resulting from including insects in their everyday diet.

> It can always be a new taste. I'm curious, I must admit. This can always be a new food form. I doubt that I would be eating [insects] in any large quantities—I'm more interested to just try [them]. I doubt I would try the same form. I have eaten a cookie, maybe [I could eat] an entire cricket, but it only happened once, and that's probably enough. Yes, I would most likely not include [insects] in my diet, but I would only try [them], in small amounts, out of curiosity.

The participants believed that the way of serving and the manner of presenting insects could help encourage more people to eat insect-based products. It would be best if insect bodies or parts were not discernible, i.e., if they were added in powder form as a ground protein additive. Some insect types evoke more disgust than others, and the participants stated explicitly that their names should not be provided on product labels or should be indicated in another way that does not elicit negative associations (e.g., larvae). Overcoming the barrier involving associations with filth could be facilitated, in the view of some participants, by the mere presence of products containing insects in grocery shops. They believe that making a product widely available on the market makes people perceive it as being tested and suitable for human consumption. Other respondents pointed to the need to create appropriate insect production safety certificates.

4. Discussion

The analysis of the data collected during the experiment revealed a significant effect of Label on product evaluation. Products labelled as containing insects were ingested in smaller quantities and less frequently, regardless of their appearance. In addition, the latency to pick up and eat products was higher in the case of products labelled as containing insects. The effect of label was also found in a study by Mancini and colleagues [14]. The addition of elements imitating insect parts had no effect on consumption levels. This shows that labelling a product as containing insects is, in itself, sufficient to elicit a reluctance to ingest it and results in a decrease in the amount of food ingested. This effect seems to occur regardless of the form in which the insects are served (insect parts or insect flour). Moreover, the type of insect (larvae, crickets, or cockroaches) specified on the label did not affect the quantity of food ingested, which was comparable for all three products. Additionally, when filling in the food evaluation questionnaires, the respondents stated that they were less willing to try products containing insects regardless of insect type and appearance.

While the effect of Label observed in our study is in line with our expectations and confirms the commonly expressed reluctance and aversion to ingesting insect-based products or products with insect content [22–24], the fact that no effect of appearance was observed raises several questions. It cannot be ruled out that the appearance of the elements imitating insect parts affected the outcome of the evaluation. The elements were sufficiently small that they did not resemble whole insects or discernible insect body parts (limbs, wings, etc.) It seems that the form of the added elements did not elicit associations with contamination or pollution [44]. At the same time, this effect may confirm earlier observations that adding processed insects elicits fewer negative impressions than adding whole insects (e.g., [20,39]). It may be suggested that the required level of processing need not reduce insects to flour—it is sufficient that consumers are unable to discern insect body parts in the product.

It is interesting, however, that although the respondents were less willing to try products containing insects, there was no difference in scores awarded for sensory qualities. All the products received similar scores on the taste, smell, and appearance scales. Moreover, there was no difference between the groups with regard to the respondents' willingness to eat those products again. Possible explanations for this may be found in the interviews carried out after the tasting session. The participants stated that they had expected a specific insect taste, and when it turned out that the products labelled as containing insects did not have a new or an unfamiliar taste, they scored the products in the same way as they would score any other cake or pastry. These results are in line with the findings of Sogari and colleagues [43], who showed that both unprocessed and processed insect-based products generate more positive perceptions after tasting compared to expectations. This may suggest that the absence of an unfamiliar taste decreased the novelty effect, thereby reducing neophobia (cf. [27,56]). This is borne out by the fact that in most of the conducted analyses there was no effect of food neophobia as a covariate (cf. [20,57]). The forms of the products (cookie, muffin) were familiar and their taste did not differ from the taste of regular cakes, which may explain why this factor was not observed in the analysis. The only less-commonly known product was the date ball. In this case, food neophobia was only manifested in the amount of food eaten. Participants scoring higher on the food neophobia scale ingested less of the product labelled as containing insects than persons with lower food neophobia levels. Of the three products used in our study, the date ball is the least common and the least widely available in shops. This reduced availability may have elicited a neophobic reaction to an unfamiliar product in some participants [27,56].

The reluctance to try products labelled as containing insects, measured by the latency to pick up food, revealed an effect of the General Neophobia and Variety Seeking Tendency covariates. Participants scoring high on the GN scale picked up the products labelled as containing insects after a longer time than those with low GN levels. Conversely, respondents with high VST scores picked them up sooner than those scoring low on the VST scale. This suggests that the effect of novelty of the products labelled as containing insects manifested itself immediately when participants came into contact with the products. After the product was assessed as safe, however, this effect decreased. The absence of the novelty effect was also observed in the investigative behavior measurements. There were no differences between the groups with regard to the amount of time spent sniffing and looking at the products.

The frequency of water drinking is difficult to explain. There was an interactive effect of Label and Appearance for this variable. When ingesting products in the case of which no insect content was either explicitly indicated on the label or implied by the additional particles, the participants drank water more frequently than when eating products with explicitly stated or implied insect content. It seems that those respondents who ingested non-insect products ate more of the food and therefore needed to drink more water when ingesting it.

The initial reaction to insect-based food that people commonly express verbally is disgust, as confirmed by previous studies (cf. [20,57,58]) and by the interviews conducted in our study. However, this variable was not observed in the behavioral assessment measures, which may be linked, as mentioned above, to the appearance of the elements added to the products that did not elicit associations with contamination or pollution (cf. [44]) and did not resemble whole animal bodies. Low disgust levels may also stem from the experimental setting; in the interviews, the respondents said that they were convinced that in a scientific experiment they would be given safe and hygienic products. They also mentioned that the products were aesthetically pleasing and their dessert form encouraged the participants to try them. This may indicate that serving insects as ingredients in favorite desserts may be a good strategy (cf. [36]), but it may also depend on the food preferences typical of a specific culture. Moreover, it seems that the feeling of disgust reported when thinking about ingesting insects is replaced by other emotions during contact with an aesthetically pleasing product prepared and served in a safe setting.

This may suggest that it is possible to create such products and eating conditions that could help reduce the effect of disgust. If a product is familiar (cf. [14]), has an aesthetically pleasing form, and if consumers are convinced it is safe, such a product may be accepted despite information on insect content (cf. [58,59]). Outside research settings, product safety is determined on the basis of where it is sold. The respondents stated that a product's widespread commercial availability in shops would encourage them to think that it is safe and that its sales are monitored (cf. [60]). Official safety certificates awarded by appropriate institutions or organizations could have a similar effect. Widespread availability would also convey the impression of a product being widely consumed by others (social proof—[61]). Limited availability, coupled with the fact that they are sold in tourism and pet shops, leads people to still perceive insect-based products to be exotic and foreign.

To conclude, the results of our study confirm the first hypothesis. However, the second hypothesis was not confirmed. The participants, regardless of the appearance of the products, ingested products labelled as containing insects in smaller amounts. In the interviews, the respondents implied that the information about insect content was in itself enough to evoke reluctance and doubts as to whether they should try the product. They pointed out that images of insects on product packaging would also create a negative impression and suggested that certain types of insects (e.g., mealworm larvae) were more disgusting than others.

It seems, however, that it is without consequence whether insects are added in the form of small pieces or flour, as long as whole insects or their body parts are not easily discernible. It is a good strategy to add insects to well-liked products. Insects should be added to familiar products, with familiar taste/smell/texture, and the elements added should not change those properties. The products themselves should have an aesthetically pleasing appearance. All those measures may help convince consumers that such products are safe. In this way, the consumers' preferences for specific products may be generalized to insect-based products.

The study has many implications for management and marketing strategies. First, the results of the study showed that the manner of communicating information on insect-based ingredients has a huge impact on the perception of the product and its future marketing success. The presence of such information is enough to reduce interest in the product. Therefore, placing such products on the market should be preceded by extensive consumer research conducted with a view to selecting the right message and labelling to eliminate that negative effect. Second, to ensure a product's marketing success, it is important to select the right target group. Our research has shown that the group most open to insect-based food are experimenters and variety seekers; on the other hand, the group most reluctant to accept such products are people with high levels of neophobia. This result suggests that an effective positioning strategy of a product containing insect ingredients should refer to "variety seeking" or "experimenting". This study also showed no differences in the evaluation of taste regardless of whether the products had been labelled as containing insects or not. At the same time, unwillingness to try products labelled as containing insects suggests that the problem does not lie in the taste of the product (which has also been confirmed by other studies), but rather in some sort of prejudice against products that contain insects. This is linked to the third implication: it is probably worthwhile to place such products on the market using a "sampling strategy", such as food tasting campaigns in shops, which can help consumers overcome their mental block and try these products.

A very significant aspect of our study is the fact that we used several behavioral measures and not only participants' declarations, as is the case with many studies conducted to date. In doing so, we were able to observe real-life multidimensional reactions to the products used. The interviews conducted after the behavioral assessment phase proved helpful for interpreting the quantitative results and provided ideas for future research and practical solutions.

The study, however, has certain limitations. The study population was characterized by a significant gender imbalance, which prevented us from analyzing the effect of the gender variable. Nevertheless, there was no theoretical basis for assuming such an effect, and we strove to ensure that the gender ratio was identical in each group. The same applied to the remaining demographic data, i.e., level of education and age, as well as dietary preferences—no differences were observed for those variables between the groups. Another limitation was that the majority of participants were students, which may reduce the ability to generalize the results to the general population. However, the participants in our study were full-time as well as evening-course students. The latter represent a broader spectrum of population, as they are often older than full-time students; they often work full-time and have families, which may reduce the effect of the specificity of the study group. Nevertheless, future research should be conducted on a more socio-economically diverse sample to help identify the general mechanisms underlying the phenomenon examined and to ensure the relevance of the findings for marketing strategies. Another important factor that should be considered is personal food preference, especially attitudes towards meat consumption. The results of the interviews show that people following a vegetarian diet are not sure about the appropriateness of consuming insects, as they do not fully understand whether arthropods are able to feel pain, etc.

It is crucial to examine cultural differences between the populations (e.g., participants from different countries), as populations may differ in their food preferences. It is possible that this factor substantially influences acceptance of insects as food and the choice of specific products. Cross-cultural comparative studies (including Asian countries) would also shed light on the universality of the mechanisms underlying the acceptance/rejection of entomophagy.

With regard to the possibility of applying research results in practice, future studies should examine other measures identifying different personal characteristics, such as the tendency to take risks, curiosity, and the need for exploration, as well as variables related to health and moral values.

Author Contributions: Conceptualization, K.M., D.A., K.G., D.M. and W.P.; methodology, K.M., D.A., D.M. and W.P.; validation, K.M., D.M. and W.P.; formal analysis, K.M., D.A., and W.P.; investigation, D.A., K.G.; resources, K.M. and W.P.; data curation, K.M. and W.P.; writing—original draft preparation, K.M., D.A., K.G., D.M. and W.P.; writing—review and editing, K.M., D.A., K.G., D.M. and W.P.; visualization, K.M.; supervision, K.M.; project administration, K.M. and W.P.; funding acquisition, W.P. All authors have read and agreed to the published version of the manuscript.

Funding: This research was funded by the National Science Centre in Poland, grant number UMO-2017/27/B/HS6/01197.

Conflicts of Interest: The authors declare no conflict of interest.

Appendix A

Descriptive Statistics of All Quantitative Measures Registered in This Study.				
	Group	N	Mean	Standard Deviation
Latency to pick up food sample	1A	24	10.743	7.751
	1B	25	20.191	18.22
	2A	25	35.315	43.451
	2B	25	21.604	18.359
Latency to begin eating	1A	24	22.018	15.059
	1B	25	28.31	17.194
	2A	25	33.991	18.752
	2B	25	34.015	19.735
Frequency of sniffing food samples	1A	24	3.708	2.136
	1B	25	4.32	1.52
	2A	25	3.333	2.099
	2B	25	4.08	2.1
Frequency of looking at food samples	1A	24	12	6.386
	1B	25	12.76	9.791
	2A	25	8.375	5.046
	2B	25	11.28	8.503
Time spent sniffing food samples	1A	24	6.21	4.728
	1B	25	5.992	3.505
	2A	25	5.601	5.158
	2B	25	4.596	2.404
Time spent looking at food samples	1A	24	36.309	25.171
	1B	25	44.262	36.747
	2A	25	28.044	20.075
	2B	25	34.713	25.275
Amount of eaten sample A	1A	24	43.681	35.925
	1B	25	39.061	39.095
	2A	25	14.543	19.209
	2B	25	16.305	21.256
Amount of eaten sample B	1A	24	45.169	40.854
	1B	25	39.27	35.224
	2A	25	26.29	30.39
	2B	25	27.511	30.362
Amount of eaten sample C	1A	24	80.306	32.5
	1B	25	77.298	37.458
	2A	25	50.038	44.672
	2B	25	37.981	38.167

Descriptive Statistics of All Quantitative Measures Registered in This Study.				
	Group	N	Mean	Standard Deviation
Time spent eating	1A	24	402.23	153.93
	1B	25	405.18	196.216
	2A	25	316.694	139.009
	2B	25	327.623	131.485
Frequency of the eating bouts	1A	24	9	4.181
	1B	25	8.72	6.724
	2A	25	5.875	4.875
	2B	25	5.84	4.22
Frequency of drinking water	1A	24	36.309	25.171
	1B	25	44.262	36.747
	2A	25	28.044	20.075
	2B	25	34.713	25.275

References

1. FAO UN. *The State of Food Insecurity in the World*; FAO UN: Rome, Italy, 2015.
2. Van Huis, A. Prospects of insects as food and feed. *Org. Agric.* **2020**, *9*, 108. [CrossRef]
3. Ramos-Elorduy, J. Anthropo-entomophagy: Cultures, evolution and sustainability. *Entomol. Res.* **2009**, *39*, 271–288. [CrossRef]
4. Belluco, S.; Losasso, C.; Maggioletti, M.; Alonzi, C.C.; Paoletti, M.G.; Ricci, A. Edible insects in a food safety and nutritional perspective: A critical review. *Compr. Rev. Food Sci. Food Saf.* **2013**, *12*, 296–313. [CrossRef]
5. Bukkens, S.G. The nutritional value of edible insects. *Ecol. Food Nutr.* **1997**, *36*, 287–319. [CrossRef]
6. Looy, H.; Dunkel, F.V.; Wood, J.R. How then shall we eat? Insect-eating attitudes and sustainable foodways. *Agric. Hum. Values* **2014**, *31*, 131–141. [CrossRef]
7. Van Huis, A. Edible insects and research needs. *J. Insects Food Feed* **2013**, *3*, 3–5. [CrossRef]
8. Vane-Wright, R.I. Why not eat insects? *Bull. Entomol. Res.* **1991**, *81*, 1–4. [CrossRef]
9. Oonincx, D.G.; De Boer, I.J. Environmental impact of the production of mealworms as a protein source for humans–a life cycle assessment. *PLoS ONE* **2012**, *7*, e51145. [CrossRef]
10. Rumpold, B.A.; Schlüter, O.K. Potential and challenges of insects as an innovative source for food and feed production. *Innov. Food Sci. Emerg. Technol.* **2013**, *17*, 1–11. [CrossRef]
11. Testa, M.; Stillo, M.; Maffei, G.; Andriolo, V.; Gardois, P.; Zotti, C.M. Ugly but tasty: A systematic review of possible human and animal health risks related to entomophagy. *Crit. Rev. Food Sci. Nutr.* **2017**, *57*, 3747–3759. [CrossRef]
12. Raubenheimer, D.; Rothman, J.M. Nutritional ecology of entomophagy in humans and other primates. *Ann. Rev. Entomol.* **2013**, *58*, 141–160. [CrossRef] [PubMed]
13. Barsics, F.; Megido, R.C.; Brostaux, Y.; Barsics, C.; Blecker, C.; Haubruge, E.; Francis, F. Could new information influence attitudes to foods supplemented with edible insects? *Br. Food J.* **2017**, *119*, 2027–2039. [CrossRef]
14. Mancini, S.; Sogari, G.; Menozzi, D.; Nuvoloni, R.; Torracca, B.; Moruzzo, R.; Paci, G. Factors predicting the intention of eating an insect-based product. *Foods* **2019**, *8*, 270. [CrossRef] [PubMed]
15. Rumpold, B.A.; Langen, N. Potential of enhancing consumer acceptance of edible insects via information. *J. Insects Food Feed* **2019**, *5*, 45–53. [CrossRef]
16. Woolf, E.; Zhu, Y.; Emory, K.; Zhao, J.; Liu, C. Willingness to consume insect-containing foods: A survey in the United States. *LWT* **2019**, *102*, 100–105. [CrossRef]
17. Deroy, O.; Reade, B.; Spence, C. The insectivore's dilemma, and how to take the West out of it. *Food Q. Prefer.* **2015**, *44*, 44–55. [CrossRef]

18. Lammers, P.; Ullmann, L.M.; Fiebelkorn, F. Acceptance of insects as food in Germany: Is it about sensation seeking, sustainability consciousness, or food disgust? *Food Q. Prefer.* **2019**, *77*, 78–88. [CrossRef]
19. Hieke, S.; Taylor, C.R. A critical review of the literature on nutritional labeling. *J. Consum. Aff.* **2012**, *46*, 120–156. [CrossRef]
20. Hartmann, C.; Siegrist, M. Becoming an insectivore: Results of an experiment. *Food Q. Prefer.* **2016**, *51*, 118–122. [CrossRef]
21. Pelchat, M.L.; Pliner, P. "Try it. You'll like it". Effects of information on willingness to try novel foods. *Appetite* **1995**, *24*, 153–165. [CrossRef]
22. Dermody, J.; Chatterjee, I. Food Glorious Food, Fried Bugs and Mustard! Exploring the Radical Idea of Entomophagy in Advancing Sustainable Consumption to Protect the Planet. In Proceedings of the Competitive paper in Conference Proceedings, Academy of Marketing Annual Conference, Newcastle, UK, 4–7 July 2016.
23. Lockwood, J. *The Infested Mind: Why Humans Fear, Loathe, and Love Insects*; Oxford University Press: New York, NY, USA, 2013.
24. Toti, E.; Massaro, L.; Kais, A.; Aiello, P.; Palmery, M.; Peluso, I. Entomophagy: A Narrative Review on Nutritional Value, Safety, Cultural Acceptance and A Focus on the Role of Food Neophobia in Italy. *Eur. J. Investig. Health Psychol. Educ.* **2020**, *10*, 46. [CrossRef]
25. Greenwald, A.G.; McGhee, D.E.; Schwartz, J.L. Measuring individual differences in implicit cognition: The implicit association test. *J. Personal. Soc. Psychol.* **1998**, *74*, 1464–1480. [CrossRef]
26. Rozin, P.; Fallon, A.E. A perspective on disgust. *Psychol. Rev.* **1987**, *94*, 23–41. [CrossRef] [PubMed]
27. Pliner, P.; Hobden, K. Development of a scale to measure the trait of food neophobia in humans. *Appetite* **1992**, *19*, 105–120. [CrossRef]
28. Al-Shawaf, L.; Lewis, D.M.; Alley, T.R.; Buss, D.M. Mating strategy, disgust, and food neophobia. *Appetite* **2015**, *85*, 30–35. [CrossRef] [PubMed]
29. Ruby, M.B.; Rozin, P.; Chan, C. Determinants of willingness to eat insects in the USA and India. *J. Insects Food Feed* **2015**, *1*, 215–225. [CrossRef]
30. Verbeke, W. Profiling consumers who are ready to adopt insects as a meat substitute in a Western society. *Food Q. Prefer.* **2015**, *39*, 147–155. [CrossRef]
31. Cox, D.N.; Evans, G. Construction and validation of a psychometric scale to measure consumer's fears of novel food technologies: The food technology neophobia scale. *Food Q. Prefer.* **2008**, *19*, 704–710. [CrossRef]
32. Van Trijp, H.C.; Steenkamp, J.B.E. Consumers' variety seeking tendency with respect to foods: Measurement and managerial implications. *Eur. Rev. Agric. Econ.* **1992**, *19*, 181–195. [CrossRef]
33. Pliner, P.; Salvy, S. Food neophobia in humans. *Front. Nutr. Sci.* **2006**, *3*, 75.
34. Drewnowski, A. Taste preferences and food intake. *Ann. Rev. Nutr.* **1997**, *17*, 237–253. [CrossRef] [PubMed]
35. Logue, A.W.; Smith, M.E. Predictors of food preferences in adult humans. *Appetite* **1986**, *7*, 109–125. [CrossRef]
36. Tan, H.S.G.; Fischer, A.R.; van Trijp, H.C.; Stieger, M. Tasty but nasty? Exploring the role of sensory-liking and food appropriateness in the willingness to eat unusual novel foods like insects. *Food Q. Prefer.* **2016**, *48*, 293–302. [CrossRef]
37. Caparros Megido, R.; Sablon, L.; Geuens, M.; Brostaux, Y.; Alabi, T.; Blecker, C.; Francis, F. Edible Insects Acceptance by Belgian Consumers: Promising Attitude for Entomophagy Development. *J. Sens. Stud.* **2014**, *29*, 14–20. [CrossRef]
38. Veeck, A. Encounters with extreme foods: Neophilic/neophobic tendencies and novel foods. *J. Food Prod. Mark.* **2010**, *16*, 246–260. [CrossRef]
39. Gmuer, A.; Guth, J.N.; Hartmann, C.; Siegrist, M. Effects of the degree of processing of insect ingredients in snacks on expected emotional experiences and willingness to eat. *Food Q. Prefer.* **2016**, *54*, 117–127. [CrossRef]
40. Megido, R.C.; Gierts, C.; Blecker, C.; Brostaux, Y.; Haubruge, É.; Alabi, T.; Francis, F. Consumer acceptance of insect-based alternative meat products in Western countries. *Food Q. Prefer.* **2016**, *52*, 237–243. [CrossRef]
41. Schösler, H.; De Boer, J.; Boersema, J.J. Can we cut out the meat of the dish? Constructing consumer-oriented pathways towards meat substitution. *Appetite* **2012**, *58*, 39–47. [CrossRef]
42. Alemu, M.H.; Olsen, S.B.; Vedel, S.E.; Pambo, K.O.; Owino, V.O. Combining product attributes with recommendation and shopping location attributes to assess consumer preferences for insect-based food products. *Food Q. Prefer.* **2017**, *55*, 45–57. [CrossRef]

43. Sogari, G.; Menozzi, D.; Mora, C. Sensory-liking expectations and perceptions of processed and unprocessed insect products. *Int. J. Food Syst. Dyn.* **2018**, *9*, 314–320.
44. Rozin, P.; Millman, L.; Nemeroff, C. Operation of the laws of sympathetic magic in disgust and other domains. *J. Personal. Soc. Psychol.* **1986**, *50*, 703–712. [CrossRef]
45. Barnett, A.; Spence, C. Assessing the effect of changing a bottled beer label on taste ratings. *Nutr. Food Technol. Open Access* **2016**, *2*, 2413–2414.
46. Herz, R.S.; von Clef, J. The influence of verbal labeling on the perception of odors: Evidence for olfactory illusions? *Perception* **2001**, *30*, 381–391. [CrossRef] [PubMed]
47. Lee, W.C.J.; Shimizu, M.; Kniffin, K.M.; Wansink, B. You taste what you see: Do organic labels bias taste perceptions? *Food Q. Prefer.* **2013**, *29*, 33–39. [CrossRef]
48. Wansink, B.; Park, S.B.; Sonka, S.; Morganosky, M. How soy labeling influences preference and taste. *Int. Food Agribus. Manag. Rev.* **2000**, *3*, 85–94. [CrossRef]
49. Bradley, C. *Handbook of Psychology and Diabetes: A Guide to Psychological Measurement in Diabetes Research and Practice*; Routledge: London, UK, 2013.
50. Eremenco, S.L.; Cella, D.; Arnold, B.J. A comprehensive method for the translation and cross-cultural validation of health status questionnaires. *Eval. Health Prof.* **2005**, *28*, 212–232. [CrossRef]
51. Ritchey, P.N.; Frank, R.A.; Hursti, U.K.; Tuorila, H. Validation and cross-national comparison of the food neophobia scale (FNS) using confirmatory factor analysis. *Appetite* **2003**, *40*, 163–173. [CrossRef]
52. Haidt, J.; McCauley, C.; Rozin, P. Individual differences in sensitivity to disgust: A scale sampling seven domains of disgust elicitors. *Persnal. Individ. Differ.* **1994**, *16*, 701–713. [CrossRef]
53. Lähteenmäki, L.; Van Trijp, H.C. Hedonic responses, variety-seeking tendency and expressed variety in sandwich choices. *Appetite* **1995**, *24*, 139–151. [CrossRef]
54. Friard, O.; Gamba, M. BORIS: A free, versatile open-source event-logging software for video/audio coding and live observations. *Methods Ecol. Eval.* **2016**, *7*, 1325–1330. [CrossRef]
55. Braun, V.; Clarke, V. Using thematic analysis in psychology. *Qual. Res. Psychol.* **2006**, *3*, 77–101. [CrossRef]
56. Modlinska, K.; Pisula, W. Selected psychological aspects of meat consumption—A short review. *Nutrients* **2018**, *10*, 1301. [CrossRef] [PubMed]
57. La Barbera, F.; Verneau, F.; Amato, M.; Grunert, K. Understanding Westerners' disgust for the eating of insects: The role of food neophobia and implicit associations. *Food Q. Prefer.* **2018**, *64*, 120–125. [CrossRef]
58. Sogari, G.; Bogueva, D.; Marinova, D. Australian consumers' response to insects as food. *Agriculture* **2019**, *9*, 108. [CrossRef]
59. Van Thielen, L.; Vermuyten, S.; Storms, B.; Rumpold, B.; Van Campenhout, L. Consumer acceptance of foods containing edible insects in Belgium two years after their introduction to the market. *J. Insects Food Feed* **2019**, *5*, 35–44. [CrossRef]
60. Sidali, K.L.; Pizzo, S.; Garrido-Pérez, E.I.; Schamel, G. Between food delicacies and food taboos: A structural equation model to assess Western students' acceptance of Amazonian insect food. *Food Res. Int.* **2019**, *115*, 83–89. [CrossRef]
61. Cialdini, R.B. *Influence: The Psychology of Persuasion*; Collins: New York, NY, USA, 1984.

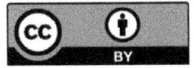

© 2020 by the authors. Licensee MDPI, Basel, Switzerland. This article is an open access article distributed under the terms and conditions of the Creative Commons Attribution (CC BY) license (http://creativecommons.org/licenses/by/4.0/).

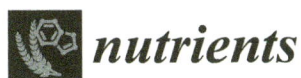

Article

Energy Density of New Food Products Targeted to Children

Danielle J. Azzopardi [1], Kathleen E. Lacy [2,*] and Julie L. Woods [2]

[1] Deakin University, School of Exercise and Nutrition Sciences, Geelong, VIC 3220, Australia; dazzopar@deakin.edu.au
[2] Deakin University, Institute for Physical Activity and Nutrition (IPAN), School of Exercise and Nutrition Sciences, Geelong, VIC 3220, Australia; j.woods@deakin.edu.au
* Correspondence: katie.lacy@deakin.edu.au

Received: 12 June 2020; Accepted: 23 July 2020; Published: 27 July 2020

Abstract: High dietary energy density (ED) is linked to childhood obesity and poor diet quality. The Australian Health Star Rating (HSR) system aims to assist consumers in making healthful food choices. This cross-sectional study used 2014–2018 data from the Mintel Global New Products Database to describe the ED of new food products targeted to children (5–12 years) released after the introduction of HSR and examine relationships between ED and HSR. Products were categorised by ED (low < 630 kJ/100 g, medium 630–950 kJ/100 g, high > 950 kJ/100 g) and HSR (no, HSR < 2.5 low, HSR ≥ 2.5 high). Non-parametric statistics were used to examine ED and HSR. A total of 548 products targeted children: 21% low, 5% medium, 74% high ED. One hundred products displayed an HSR: 24% low, 76% high; 53 products with both high HSR and ED. The EDs of products differed by HSR ($p < 0.05$), but both group's medians (HSR < 2.5: 1850 kJ/100 g, HSR ≥ 2.5: 1507 kJ/100 g) were high. A high proportion of new products had a high ED, and the HSR of these foods did not consistently discriminate between ED levels, particularly for high ED foods. Policies to promote lower ED foods and better alignment between ED and HSR may improve childhood obesity and diet quality.

Keywords: energy density; health star rating; children; food supply; front-of-pack label; discretionary

1. Introduction

Childhood overweight and obesity are global concerns. The worldwide prevalence of overweight and obesity in children and adolescents is just over 18% [1]. In Australia, at least one in four children and adolescents aged 5–17 years are currently considered overweight or obese [2]. Measures of overweight, obesity, and adiposity are positively associated with dietary energy density [3–5].

The energy density (ED) of a food is defined as the amount of energy in a specific weight of that food and is usually expressed as kilojoules per 100 g (kJ/100 g). The macronutrient composition and moisture content of the food determine its ED, with foods higher in fat tending to have higher EDs than other foods and water-rich foods tending to have lower EDs than other foods. Food energy density is potentially modifiable by adjusting the macronutrient and/or moisture content of foods. Multiple within-subject crossover design experimental feeding studies have demonstrated that lowering the ED of foods, while maintaining their palatability, reduces children's energy intake (EI) [6–8]. Dietary energy density can be reduced by adjusting food energy density, incorporating more foods that are lower in energy density into the diet or reducing consumption of energy-dense foods. In children, decreasing the ED of the diet is a way to prevent overconsumption of energy without reducing EI below the child's current needs [7] and could contribute to a reduction in rates of childhood obesity.

Diets that are lower in ED tend to be of higher quality [9–11] and more in line with dietary guidelines [9]. They tend to include plenty of vegetables, fruit, wholegrain cereals, low-fat dairy, lean sources of protein and healthy oils [12]. There is strong evidence that higher ED diets are of lower quality [9–11]. Studies involving children and adolescents in several countries have shown dietary ED to be positively associated with the consumption and availability of discretionary foods high in sugar and fat and inversely associated with the consumption and availability of fruit, vegetables, protein and fibre [13–16].

Several population-based surveys have found that Australian children regularly consume discretionary foods [17–19]. The Australian National Health Survey found that just under 40% of the total energy consumed by 4- to 13-year-old children came from discretionary foods [19]. Children in this age group have considerable input into the food products purchased for them by their carers, initially through "pester power" [20] and then through a more collaborative decision-making process [21]. Understanding the retail food supply targeting this age group is important for developing strategies to improve children's dietary intakes.

The Health Star Rating (HSR) system was introduced in Australia in 2014 as a voluntary, front-of-pack label to assist consumers in making healthy food choices in a discretionary food-flooded environment. This system rates the overall healthiness of a product on a scale from a half to five stars, with a greater number of stars indicating a healthier product [22]. The number of stars is calculated based on an algorithm, which scores 'negative' nutrients (energy, saturated fat, total sugar and salt) and 'positive' attributes (fruit, vegetable, legume and nut content and, in some cases, protein and fibre content). The number of stars a product receives should increase as its ED decreases, giving this system the potential of assisting consumers in choosing lower ED options. Being a voluntary system for food manufacturers, only 40.7% had taken it up in 2019 [23]. It is evident that manufacturers are selectively applying the HSR to foods, which score ≥ 3.0 stars (i.e., healthier choices), and have been reluctant to display it on foods with lower star scores, although supermarket own brands have applied it across all products regardless of the score [24].

Despite the current knowledge of dietary ED and its links with increased EI, lower diet quality and obesity, no studies have examined the ED of new food products targeted to children entering the retail food market in Australia, either long-term or since the introduction of the HSR system. Advertising and supermarkets target children and promote the consumption of discretionary foods [25–27]. The high ED of such foods results in a greater likelihood of excess EI and overweight and obesity. Examining the ED and HSR of these products is vital to provide a greater understanding of the food supply and the potential of the HSR system in being able to distinguish between foods with high and low ED. The results of this study could potentially be used to advocate for change in the HSR system, which, in turn, may influence food manufacturers to release products with lower ED.

The aims of this study were to:

1. Describe the ED of new food products targeted to children that have entered the Australian retail food market since the introduction of the HSR system in 2014.
2. Examine the relationship between the ED and the HSR of new food products targeted to children that have entered the Australian retail food market and display an HSR.
3. Examine the relationship between core and discretionary products, ED and the HSR of new food products targeted to children that have entered the Australian retail food market and display an HSR.

2. Materials and Methods

This cross-sectional study examined the ED and HSR, where available, of all new products targeted to children and launched in Australia from 27th June 2014 to 27th June 2018 recorded in the Mintel Global New Products Database [28].

2.1. The Mintel Global New Products Database

The Mintel Global New Products Database (GNPD) is an online database of consumer-packaged goods from 62 countries, created and maintained by Mintel, a private international market research company [28]. A network of trained Mintel shoppers frequently monitors the release of new products and updates the database at least monthly. The database captures more than 80 fields of information per item for 17 distinct categories of foods: Baby Food, Bakery, Breakfast Cereals, Chocolate Confectionery, Dairy, Desserts and Ice-Creams, Fruits and Vegetables, Meals and Meal Centres, Processed Fish, Meat and Eggs, Sauces and Seasonings, Savoury Spreads, Side Dishes, Snacks, Soups, Sweets and Gum, Sweet Spreads and Sweeteners and Sugar. The dataset consists mainly of packaged foods and does not generally include fresh, non-processed single foods, such as fresh fruit and/or vegetables.

GNPD fields of information include nutrient data, packaging format, claims made and manufacturing details. The GNPD records if a product is targeted to a particular demographic, namely, babies and toddlers (0–4 years), children (5–12 years), teenagers (13–17 years), females, males and seniors (aged 55+ years). The present study used the children (aged 5–12 years) demographic category. As of 27th June 2018, the database listed 62,066 foods and beverages released in Australia since its launch in 1998. A total of 2683 of these are included in the children 5–12 years demographic category, with 579 products added under this demographic since June 2014 [28].

2.1.1. Search for Products in Demographic 5–12 Years

The GNPD was searched using filters that restricted results from June 2014 to June 2018 in Australia, to foods (not beverages) and for children aged 5–12 years. The GNPD defines this demographic category as foods designed for consumption by children and, more specifically, products which are "also dependent on presentation and format, such as child-inspired graphics like cartoon characters, bright colours and/or pictures of children, or particular language like 'great in lunch boxes' [29]. Data from all 17 GNPD food categories were used in this study; however, some sub-categories were excluded. Beverages were excluded because the grouping of beverages and foods together when calculating ED complicates the interpretation of the results, as beverages are relatively low in ED due to their high water content and can have a substantial impact on overall ED values [30].

2.1.2. Additional Product Searches

To ensure no products were missed, further searches were performed without the demographic filter but with the addition of relevant keywords, such as 'children', in the product description. These searches also used filters that restricted results from June 2014 to June 2018 in Australia.

2.1.3. Data Extraction

In this study, data from 10 of the 80 fields available for each product were extracted from the GNPD: date published, company, brand, product name, category, sub-category, energy (kJ/100 g), demographic, packaging pictures and ingredients list. Company and brand fields were extracted to help exclude duplicates and identify products that display an HSR. Packaging images and descriptions of each product were extracted in order to determine the presence of an HSR, as the GNPD does not routinely include information about HSR. Data were downloaded into Microsoft Excel for analysis.

Sorting was used to remove duplicates from multiple searches. Seasonal products, such as Halloween confectionary and Easter chocolates, were also removed as these products are not available all year and so do not make up the typical range of food items available to children. It is possible for a product to lie within multiple demographics; for example, Bellamy's Organic Apple Snacks are listed with both the 0–4 years and 5–12 years demographics. These records were retained, even if the food category was Baby Food. The description and packaging images for such products were examined, and the product was removed if determined unsuitable (e.g. supplement or formula drinks/foods, such as Ensure). Where a product was a variety pack, that is, two or more flavour varieties of the same or similar food in the one pack, the record was duplicated for each variety. The overall total of products was 548.

2.1.4. Data Cleaning

Data were checked for accuracy and completeness, and a total of 23 records were found to be missing the value for ED (kJ/100 g). Thirteen of these were variety packs, and the missing data were found on the nutrition information panels from the product images. For 9 of the remaining records, missing data were retrieved from similar products of the same brand ($n = 2$) or different brands ($n = 7$) in the GNPD. Missing data for the final record (Tic-Tac) were obtained from the product website.

2.2. Determination of Energy Density Category, HSR Presence and Core or Discretionary Classification

Products were categorised into one of three ED categories (low: <630 kJ/100 g; medium: 630–950 kJ/100 g; high: >950 kJ/100 g), according to those defined by the World Cancer Research Fund [31]. Whether a product had an HSR and the number of stars it had was determined by examining packaging images from the GNPD and were added to the relevant record. Each product with an HSR was then classified as discretionary or core, according to the Discretionary Food List produced by the Australian Bureau of Statistics (ABS) in the Australian Health Survey User Guide [32].

2.3. Statistical Analysis

All statistical analyses were conducted in IBM SPSS Statistics version 23 (IBM, St Leonards, NSW, Australia). The ED data were not normally distributed, and so medians and interquartile ranges (IQRs) were reported and used for analysis. Descriptive statistics (frequency, median, IQR, minimum and maximum) for EDs were calculated for each food category, products without an HSR, products with an HSR, products with a low HSR (<2.5 stars) and products with a high HSR (≥2.5 stars). Mann-Whitney U tests were performed to compare the EDs of foods with an HSR to those without, foods that had low (<2.5) and high (≥2.5) HSRs and foods that were classified as core or discretionary. A Chi-square test was performed to compare the proportions of low, medium and high ED products within the groups of products with and without an HSR. The proportion of products with <2.5 stars and ≥2.5 stars in each of the three ED categories was determined, but inferential statistics could not be performed due to violations of assumptions for non-parametric statistical tests.

2.4. Ethics

This study did not include an animal or human participants or existing data collected from them and so, in accordance with Australia's National Statement of Ethical Conduct in Human Research [33], is deemed negligible risk and did not require ethical review.

3. Results

3.1. All Products: GNPD Food Category Distributions and Energy Densities

The 548 food products targeted to children released into the Australian market between 27th June 2014 and 27th June 2018, were from 14 of the 17 food categories in the GNPD. No products were found from the Sauces and Seasonings, Soup and Sweeteners and Sugar food categories. The greatest proportion of foods (30.7%) was from the Snacks category, and almost half (49.3%) were from the Snacks and Bakery categories combined. The additional inclusion of the discretionary categories Chocolate and Confectionary, Desserts and Ice Cream and Sugar and Gum Confectionery represented 76.5% of the entire sample.

The EDs for the sample ranged from 6 kJ/100 g to 2556 kJ/100 g (Table 1). Aside from Fruit and Vegetables (138 kJ/100 g), the categories with the lowest median EDs were Dairy (377 kJ/100 g) and Desserts and Ice Cream (409 kJ/100 g). Nine of the 14 categories had median EDs that were considered high (i.e., >950 kJ/100 g), although three of these categories had low numbers of foods ($n < 3$). There were 117 (21.4%) products that were categorised as low ED, 28 (5.1%) as medium ED, with the vast majority categorised as high ED ($n = 403$, 73.5%). In particular, more than 86% of the Bakery, Breakfast Cereals and Snacks items had high EDs, and more than 98% of the Chocolate Confectionery and Sugar and Gum Confectionery items had high EDs.

3.2. Products With and Without an HSR: GNPD Food Category Distributions and Energy Densities

One hundred (18.2%) of the 548 products in the sample displayed an HSR on the packaging (Table 2). Nine out of the 14 categories of foods targeted to children contained products that displayed an HSR. Three categories (Bakery, Breakfast Cereals and Snacks) made up 80% of all items displaying an HSR and had high median ED. All of the Bakery and Breakfast Cereals items with HSRs had high EDs. Although the median EDs of the group of foods without an HSR and the group of foods with an HSR were similar (1490 kJ/100 g and 1594 kJ/100 g, respectively), the variability of the EDs for the group of foods without an HSR was higher (IQR = 1070) than that for the groups of foods with an HSR (IQR = 774). A Mann-Whitney U test comparing mean ranks for the products with an HSR and those without found that the groups were not statistically significantly different ($U = 21182$, $p = 0.395$). The proportions of low, medium and high ED products within the groups of foods without an HSR and with an HSR are shown in Appendix A. A Chi-square test for independence indicated no significant association between ED category and the presence of an HSR, $\chi^2 (1, n = 548) = 2.695$, $p = 0.26$, Cramer's $V = 0.07$.

3.3. Products with a Low or High HSR: GNPD Food Category Distributions and Energy Densities

The breakdown of products across food categories for items with low (HSR < 2.5 stars) and high (HSR ≥ 2.5 stars) HSRs is shown in Table 3. Only the categories Bakery and Breakfast Cereals contained products with a low HSR, and these two food categories combined made up 24% of all products displaying an HSR. The remaining 76% of products, those with a high HSR, were spread across nine food categories, with the majority falling under Snacks (52.6%) and Breakfast Cereals (14.5%), both of which had high median ED. The median ED of products with a low HSR was 1850 kJ/100 g (IQR = 147) compared with 1507 kJ/100 g (IQR = 1005) for products with a high HSR. Although both of these medians represent high ED, statistically, the median ED of products with a high HSR ($M = 42.26$) was lower than the median of those with a low HSR ($M = 76.58$; $U = 286$, $p < 0.05$).

Table 1. Numbers of products in each Global New Products Database (GNPD) food category classified as low, medium and high energy density (ED) and median ED for each GNPD food category.

GNPD Food Category [1]	n (%) [2]				kJ/100 g or kJ/100 mL			
	Low ED (<630 kJ/100 g)	Medium ED (630–950 kJ/100 g)	High ED (>950 kJ/100 g)	Total Products	Median	IQR [3]	Minimum	Maximum
Baby Food	8 (1.5)	1 (0.2)	10 (1.8)	19 (3.5)	1467	1477	273	2380
Bakery	0 (0)	2 (0.4)	100 (18.2)	102 (18.6)	1845	291	871	2180
Breakfast Cereals	1 (0.2)	0 (0)	29 (5.3)	30 (5.5)	1586	94	411	1711
Chocolate Confectionery	0 (0)	0 (0)	30 (5.5)	30 (5.5)	2265	120	1867	2360
Dairy	37 (6.8)	0 (0)	15 (2.7)	52 (9.5)	377	853	290	1790
Desserts and Ice Cream	41 (7.5)	8 (1.5)	4 (0.7)	53 (9.7)	409	334	6	1300
Fruit and Vegetables	3 (0.5)	0 (0)	0 (0)	3 (0.5)	138	-	60	242
Meals and Meal Centres	7 (1.3)	3 (0.5)	1 (0.2)	11 (2.0)	468	359	260	956
Processed Fish, Meat and Egg Products	0 (0)	9 (1.6)	1 (0.2)	10 (1.8)	806	142	724	975
Savoury Spreads	0 (0)	0 (0)	1 (0.2)	1 (0.2)	1092	-	1092	1092
Side Dishes	0 (0)	1 (0.2)	1 (0.2)	2 (0.4)	1143	-	795	1490
Snacks	20 (3.6)	3 (0.5)	145 (26.5)	168 (30.7)	1613	457	227	2556
Sugar and Gum Confectionery	0 (0)	1 (0.2)	65 (11.9)	66 (12.0)	1462	203	731	2130
Sweet Spreads	0 (0)	0 (0)	1 (0.2)	1 (0.2)	1413	-	1413	1413
Total	117 (21.4)	28 (5.1)	403 (73.5)	548	1514	1006	6	2556

[1] No products found in the Sauces and Seasonings, Soup and Sweeteners and Sugar food categories. [2] Percentages may not equal 100 due to rounding. [3] Indicates not possible to calculate due to a low number of products in the category. IQR, interquartile range.

Table 2. The energy density of products without a Health Star Rating (HSR) and with an HSR by Global New Products Database (GNPD) food category.

GNPD Food Category [1]	Products without HSR					Products with HSR				
	n (%) [2]	kJ/100 g or kJ/100 mL				n (%) [2]	kJ/100 g or kJ/100 mL			
		Median	IQR [3]	Minimum	Maximum		Median	IQR [3]	Minimum	Maximum
Baby Food	19 (4.2)	1467	1477	273	2380	0 (0)	–	–	–	–
Bakery	78 (17.4)	1837	453	871	2180	24 (24.0)	1870	137	986	2110
Breakfast Cereals	14 (3.1)	1575	94	411	1668	16 (16.0)	1586	107	1400	1711
Chocolate Confectionery	30 (6.7)	2265	120	1867	2360	0 (0)	–	–	–	–
Dairy	48 (10.7)	379	970	290	1790	4 (4.0)	372	27	363	399
Desserts and Ice Cream	47 (10.5)	409	335	6	1300	6 (6.0)	389	451	181	737
Fruit and Vegetables	1 (0.2)	60	–	60	60	2 (2.0)	190	–	138	242
Meals and Meal Centres	5 (1.1)	290	113	260	474	6 (6.0)	645	474	279	956
Processed Fish, Meat and Egg Products	9 (2.0)	788	130	724	975	1 (1.0)	927	–	927	927
Savoury Spreads	1 (0.2)	1092	–	1092	1092	0 (0)	–	–	–	–
Side Dishes	1 (0.2)	1490	–	1490	1490	1 (1.0)	795	–	795	795
Snacks	128 (28.6)	1613	467	229	2556	40 (40.0)	1607	454	227	2200
Sugar and Gum Confectionery	66 (14.7)	1462	203	731	2130	0 (0)	–	–	–	–
Sweet Spreads	1 (0.2)	1413	–	1413	1413	0 (0)	–	–	–	–
Total	448	1490	1070	6	2556	100	1594	774	138	2200

[1] No products found in the Sauces and Seasonings, Soup and Sweeteners and Sugar food categories. [2] Percentages may not equal 100 due to rounding. [3] Indicates not possible to calculate due to a low number of products in the category.

Table 3. The energy density of products with a Health Star Rating (HSR) <2.5 and with an HSR≥2.5 by Global New Products Database (GNPD) food category.

GNPD Food Category [1]	Products with HSR < 2.5					Products with HSR ≥ 2.5				
	n (%)	kJ/100 g or kJ/100 mL				n (%)	kJ/100 g or kJ/100 mL			
		Median	IQR	Minimum	Maximum		Median	IQR [2]	Minimum	Maximum
Bakery	19 (79.2)	1880	160	1800	2110	5 (6.6)	1860	677	986	1961
Breakfast Cereals	5 (20.8)	1600	58	1600	1667	11 (14.5)	1533	178	1400	1711
Dairy	0 (0)	–	–	–	–	4 (5.3)	372	27	363	399
Desserts and Ice Cream	0 (0)	–	–	–	–	6 (7.9)	389	451	181	737
Fruit and Vegetables	0 (0)	–	–	–	–	2 (2.6)	190	–	138	242
Meals and Meal Centers	0 (0)	–	–	–	–	6 (7.9)	645	474	279	956
Processed Fish, Meat and Egg Products	0 (0)	–	–	–	–	1 (1.3)	927	–	927	927
Side Dishes	0 (0)	–	–	–	–	1 (1.3)	795	–	795	795
Snacks	0 (0)	–	–	–	–	40 (52.6)	1607	454	227	2200
Total	24 (100)	1850	147	1600	2110	76 (100)	1507	1005	138	2200

[1] No products found in the Baby Food, Chocolate Confectionery, Sauces and Seasonings, Savoury Spreads, Soup, Sugar and Gum Confectionery, Sweet Spreads and Sweeteners and Sugar food categories. [2] Indicates not possible to calculate due to a low number of products in the category.

The median HSR for all 100 products with an HSR was 3.5 stars (IQR=1.5), with a range of 0.5 to 5 stars. A total of 16 of the 100 products with an HSR were from the low ED category, and all scored a high HSR (median 4 stars (IQR = 1.4); range 3 to 5 stars). All seven of the products in the medium ED category scored a high HSR (median 3.5 stars (IQR = 1); range 2.5 to 4.5 stars). The median HSR for the high ED category was also 3.5 stars (IQR=2) but with the full range of 0.5 to 5 stars represented. Figure 1 shows the scatterplot of HSRs by low, medium and high ED categories. Among the 77 products from the high ED category, only 24 (31%) scored a low HSR. However, 53 (69%) of the products, categorised as high ED, also scored a high HSR, with the majority of these categorised as Snacks. The breakdown of all 100 products by ED and HSR categories is shown in Appendix B.

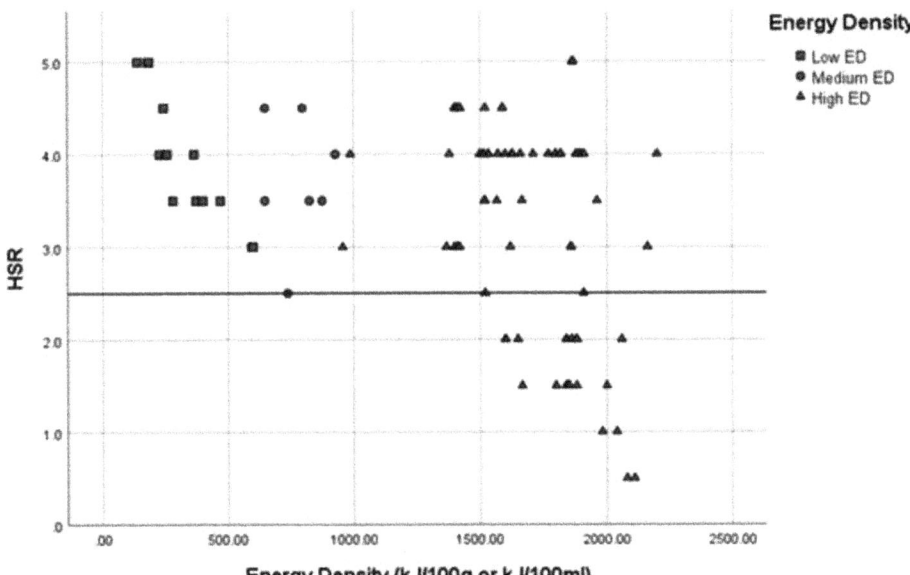

Figure 1. Scatterplot of product Health Star Rating (HSR) by low, medium and high energy density (ED).

3.4. Core vs. Discretionary Products: Category Distributions, Energy Densities and HSRs

The breakdown of products with HSRs as core or discretionary foods across food categories is shown in Table 4. Overall, 30% of products displaying an HSR were classified as core and 70% as discretionary. The categories Bakery and Snacks combined accounted for 81.5% of all discretionary products. The median ED of core products was 971 kJ/100 g (IQR = 1164) compared with 1800 kJ/100 g (IQR = 355) for discretionary products, with both medians in the high ED range. The EDs of core products (M = 28.72) were significantly lower than those of discretionary products (M = 59.84; U = 1703.5, $p < 0.05$). The distribution of core and discretionary products across the three categories of ED is shown in Appendix C.

The median HSR for core products was 4 stars (IQR = 0.5) and ranged from 2 to 5 stars. For discretionary products, the median was 3.5 stars (IQR = 2.0), with the full range of 0.5 to 5.0 stars. Only 3% of core foods displayed a low HSR and 97% a high HSR. On the other hand, only 33% of discretionary foods displayed a low HSR, whereas the majority (67%) of discretionary foods displayed a high HSR. The distribution of core and discretionary products across the two categories of HSR is shown in Appendix D.

Table 4. The energy density of the core and discretionary products displaying the Health Star Ratings (HSRs) by Global New Products Database (GNPD) food category.

GNPD Food Category [1]	Core					Discretionary				
	n (%)	kJ/100 g or kJ/100 mL				n (%)	kJ/100 g or kJ/100 mL			
		Median	IQR [2]	Minimum	Maximum		Median	IQR [2]	Minimum	Maximum
Bakery	1 (3.3)	986	–	986	986	23 (32.9)	1880	142	1520	2110
Breakfast Cereals	11 (36.7)	1533	198	1400	1711	5 (7.1)	1600	50	1567	1667
Dairy	4 (13.3)	372	27	363	399	0 (0)	–	–	–	–
Desserts and Ice Cream	0 (0)	–	–	–	–	6 (8.6)	389	451	181	737
Fruit and Vegetables	2 (6.7)	190	–	138	242	0 (0)	–	–	–	–
Meals and Meal Centers	6 (20.0)	645	474	279	956	0 (0)	–	–	–	–
Processed Fish, Meat and Egg Products	0 (0)	–	–	–	–	1 (1.4)	927	–	927	927
Side Dishes	0 (0)	–	–	–	–	1 (1.4)	795	–	795	795
Snacks	6 (20.0)	828	1296	227	1908	34 (48.6)	1645	378	823	2200
Total	30 (100)	971	1164	138	1908	70 (100)	1800	355	181	2200

[1] No products found in the Baby Food, Chocolate Confectionery, Sauces and Seasonings, Savoury Spreads, Soup, Sugar and Gum Confectionery, Sweet Spreads and Sweeteners and Sugar food categories. [2] Indicates not possible to calculate due to a low number of products in the category.

4. Discussion

Between June 2014 and June 2018, the majority of new food products targeted to Australian children had high ED. Less than 20% of products displayed an HSR, and the HSR system did not consistently distinguish between low ED and high ED products. About three-quarters of products with an HSR were categorised as having a high HSR, and the majority of products with an HSR (70%) were categorised as discretionary foods.

These findings are consistent with previous Australian and New Zealand research, which found that the majority of food products available for sale [34] and directed at children [35] were considered 'less healthy' using nutrient profiling criteria. Additionally, several population-based surveys have found that Australian children regularly consume high ED, nutrient-poor foods [17–19]. While it is important to encourage children to meet dietary recommendations and energy needs through healthful food intake and limited intake of high ED, nutrient-poor foods, additional strategies targeting the retail food market have the potential to assist in moderating children's dietary energy density and energy intake. For example, a recent study showed that total and saturated fat reformulation of some UK supermarket bakery items (cakes and biscuits) could result in substantial reductions in product energy density [36]. In the present study, a large proportion (18%) of the products that entered the retail food market during the four years of interest were bakery items, suggesting a large segment of the market that could also be reformulated in Australia. While food reformulation of processed foods is potentially useful to reduce the energy density of the food supply, it must not be used as a way to increase the perceived healthfulness of discretionary processed foods.

An HSR was displayed on 18.2% of products examined in this study. This result is higher than that obtained in a study by Lawrence et al., who found that 10.5% of new products (using Mintel's GNPD) released between 27th June 2014 and 27th June 2017 displayed an HSR, and a study by Dickie et al. using the same database but for the time period 6 June 2014–30 June 2019, who found an HSR on 17.6% of products [37,38]. Differences in the database dates used, target sample and/or the product sample size could explain these differing proportions of foods displaying an HSR. Bakery and Snacks categories were the most prevalent products displaying an HSR, as also found by Lawrence et al. and Dickie et al. [37,38]. The food categories in this study that did not have any products displaying an HSR were mostly discretionary foods, for example, Chocolate Confectionary and Sugar and Gum Confectionery. As the HSR system is currently voluntary, manufacturers can selectively apply the HSR to products receiving higher ratings. For example, Shahid et al. reported that for a number of manufacturers, there was a 1.9 to 2.5-star difference between mean HSR displayed on their products compared with their other products that did not display the HSR [23]. This is also supported by the finding that just over three-quarters of products in this study had an HSR ≥ 2.5 stars with a median across the whole sample at an HSR of 3.5 stars.

Despite the voluntary nature of the HSR and the propensity of manufacturers to apply the HSR to higher scoring foods, there was no significant difference between numbers of products with and without HSRs in each of the three ED categories. It could be hypothesised that if the HSR system was better aligned with ED, there would be a greater proportion of products with an HSR in the low ED category [23]. This is the first study to look at ED and HSRs, so it is not possible to compare this finding to the existing literature.

Among the foods displaying an HSR, all low and medium ED foods displayed a high HSR, as would be expected. However, only 31% of high ED foods displayed a low HSR, with the remaining 69% displaying a high HSR. Some high ED products may deserve high HSR. For example, The Happy Snack Company's Roasted Fav-va Beans in four different flavours have an ED of 1867 kJ/100 g, yet score highly on the HSR algorithm for being high in protein and fibre and containing more than 80% legume. However, there are also products that are clearly discretionary, such as Messy Monkey Strawberry and Apple Snack Bars by Freedom Foods. This snack item has 4.5 stars, yet has an ED of 1410 kJ/100 g, is one-third sugar, and contains mostly dried fruit, which is recommended as occasional by the Australian Dietary Guidelines [39]. If the HSR was classifying foods correctly on the basis of ED, then we would expect a much lower percentage of high ED foods displaying a high HSR. This further adds to the body of literature, demonstrating the shortcomings of the HSR system [23,37,38,40–43], and shows that it does not consistently discriminate between levels of ED, especially when considering high ED foods. The median ED of products with a high HSR was 1507 kJ/100 g, well above the cut-off (950 kJ/100 g), signifying the beginning of the high ED range [31].

The classification of food products into core and discretionary groups seemed to align more accurately with the ED categories, with increasing proportions of discretionary foods in each increasing ED category. This supports previous studies that have shown that high ED is associated with discretionary foods [9,13,15,44]. The results relating to core foods (only 3% displaying a low HSR) indicated good concordance between core foods and HSR. However, the same could not be concluded with regard to discretionary foods, with 67% displaying a high HSR. Consistent with this study, Lawrence et al. found that 57% of discretionary foods had an HSR ≥ 2.5, and Pulker et al. found that 55% of ultra-processed foods carried HSRs ≥ 3 [27,37]. These findings are concerning in that they show that the HSR is likely to have the opposite effect to what Hawkes et al. posit the role of front-of-pack nutrition labels should be—to decrease the perceived healthiness of discretionary products rather than increase the perceived healthiness of healthy products [45]. By not accurately discriminating amongst discretionary and high ED foods, the HSR is effectively allowing these foods to be perceived as healthier than they actually are.

Several studies in Australia and New Zealand have found that consumers prefer HSRs over other packaging labels, such as nutrition information panels or daily guide, although product visuals (for example, artificial or natural looking food, pictures of fresh fruit, images of sport, etc.) were found to be the foremost influence on choice [46–49]. Hamlin et al. performed a longitudinal study on the effectiveness of the HSR and, despite heavy advertising campaigns for the HSR system in New Zealand, found it to be ineffective at influencing the customer in their choice between products in a food category [50]. Likewise, Ares et al. found the HSR to be less effective than Nutri-score and a warning symbol in catching attention, healthiness perception and intention to purchase (Comparison of three systems) [51]. An international comparison of a number of different front-of-pack nutrition labels found that most increased consumer ability to rank food healthfulness but that colour coded varieties, such as Nutri-score and traffic lights, were more beneficial than the HSR [52].

In light of the continuing support for the expansion of HSRs, it is imperative that the system provides appropriate guidance for shoppers in making food choices in line with the Australian Dietary Guidelines [39]. We have shown here that when choosing between two products with HSRs, selecting the food with the greater number of health stars will not always be the "healthier" or lowest ED choice [42]. With most new foods marketed to children categorised as high ED and the majority of those with an HSR considered discretionary, consumers need a more consistent measure of healthiness.

This is the first study to examine new food products targeted at children entering the Australian retail food market and assess their ED and discretionary or core grouping with their HSR. The Mintel GNPD is comprehensive, up-to-date and well suited to this study and its aims, as it focuses on new product activity. This is particularly relevant as new food products represent ways in which manufacturers have responded to the introduction of the HSR system. It should also be noted that the GNPD does not reflect a product's market share, only its existence, and so the product's pervasiveness in the diets of Australian children is unclear.

It is difficult to keep up with innovations and developments in food items, making it difficult for the Australian Bureau of Statistics Discretionary Food List to accurately distinguish between discretionary and core foods. Errors may have occurred in classifying the 100 products displaying an HSR into discretionary or core categories. However, to reduce the possibility of error, the coding into categories was checked by both co-researchers.

It would be of benefit to extend the work of the current study to cover all food products on the Australian market targeted to children and not just new foods. This study raises questions regarding the three-way relationship between ED, discretionary foods and HSRs. Future research that combines the analysis of these three measures using a larger sample of foods would further the knowledge in this area. The present study weighted all food products equally and not by market share. Research to analyse EDs of food products and adjust their impact using their prevalence in the supermarket would help deepen the understanding around foods available to children. It would also be of benefit to undertake similar research for seasonal products, that is, analysing their availability in the existing market and their market share, as well as studies to measure the impact of seasonal foods on children's diets. Further research is needed into the effectiveness of the HSR system on whether it is meeting its objectives for consumers at the point of sale and resulting in the purchasing of healthier food products.

The Australian Government acknowledges the need to take action against obesity in children by improving the food environment and, therefore, individual diets through the introduction of initiatives, such as the HSR System [22]. The Australian food industry is also making attempts to improve the food environment by introducing voluntary guidelines to reduce the levels of saturated fat, sodium and energy in foods targeted to children. However, these initiatives by the food industry and the Government to get children eating healthier foods will likely have difficulty translating into positive results while they remain voluntary and unenforced [53].

5. Conclusions

A high proportion of new food products targeted to children is of high ED, and the HSR of these foods, when displayed, does not consistently discriminate between levels of ED or between core and discretionary foods. Most new products for children that display HSR are discretionary foods, which are likely contributing to lower diet quality and excess EI. There exist potential opportunities (prompted by food manufacturers wanting to achieve higher HSRs) to reduce the ED of some of these foods to help curb excess EI and improve diet quality. The results of this study support the need to advocate for a food policy change that will result in lower ED foods and improvements to the accuracy and consistency of the HSR system, with the aim to improve the diet quality of Australian children and reduce rates of childhood obesity.

Author Contributions: Conceptualisation, D.J.A., K.E.L. and J.W.; methodology, D.J.A., K.E.L. and J.L.W.; formal analysis, D.J.A.; data curation, D.J.A.; writing—original draft preparation, D.J.A.; writing—review and editing, D.J.A., K.E.L. and J.L.W.; supervision, K.E.L and J.L.W. All authors have read and agreed to the published version of the manuscript.

Funding: This research received no external funding.

Conflicts of Interest: The authors declare no conflict of interest.

Appendix A

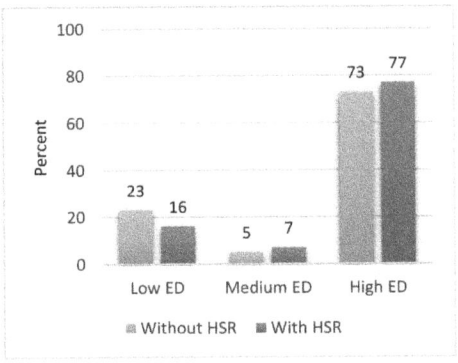

Figure A1. Proportions of low, medium and high energy density (ED) products without and with a Health Star Rating (HSR).

Appendix B

Table A1. Number of products by energy density (ED) and Health Star Rating (HSR) categories.

GNPD Food Category [1]	Energy Density							Total
	Low ED		Medium ED		High ED			
	Low HSR	High HSR	Low HSR	High HSR	Low HSR	High HSR		
Bakery	0	0	0	0	19	5		24
Breakfast Cereals	0	0	0	0	5	11		16
Dairy	0	4	0	0	0	0		4
Desserts and Ice Cream	0	5	0	1	0	0		6
Fruit and Vegetables	0	2	0	0	0	0		2
Meals and Meal Centers	0	2	0	3	0	1		6
Processed Fish, Meat and Egg Products	0	0	0	1	0	0		1
Side Dishes	0	0	0	1	0	0		1
Snacks	0	3	0	1	0	36		40
Totals	0	16	0	7	24	53		100

[1] No products found in the Baby Food, Chocolate Confectionery, Sauces and Seasonings, Savoury Spreads, Soup, Sugar and Gum Confectionery, Sweet Spreads and Sweeteners and Sugar food categories.

Appendix C

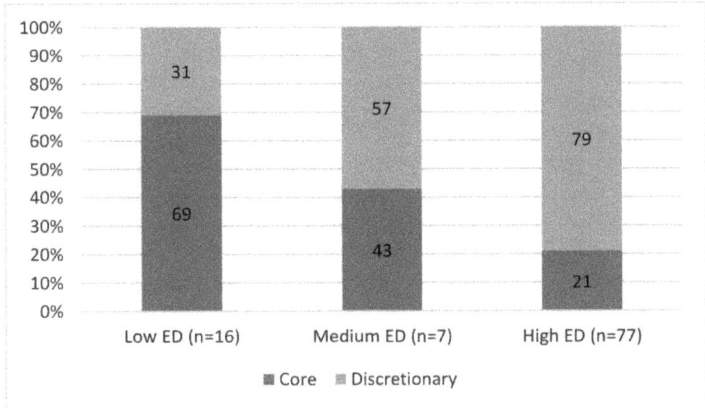

Figure A2. Core and discretionary products displaying the Health Star Ratings (HSRs) by energy density (ED) category.

Appendix D

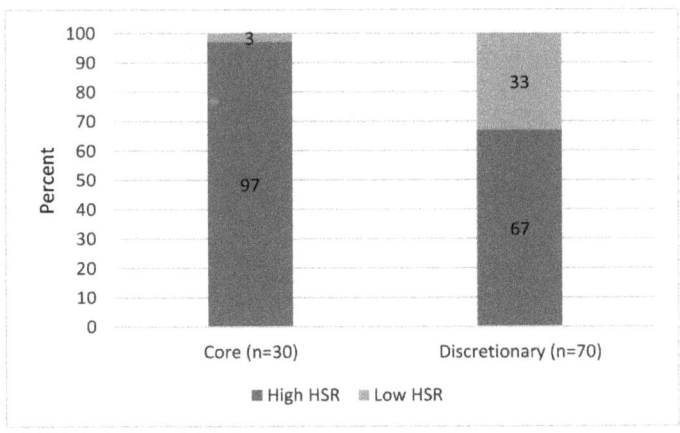

Figure A3. Core and discretionary foods by Health Star Rating (HSR) category ($n = 100$).

References

1. NCD Risk Factor Collaboration (NCD-RisC). Worldwide trends in body-mass index, underweight, overweight, and obesity from 1975 to 2016: A pooled analysis of 2416 population-based measurement studies in 128·9 million children, adolescents, and adults. *Lancet* **2017**, *390*, 2627–2642. [CrossRef]
2. Australian Bureau of Statistics. National Health Survey 2014–2015: Children's Risk Factors. Available online: http://www.abs.gov.au/ausstats/abs@.nsf/Lookup/by%20Subject/4364.0.55.001~{}2014-15~{}Main%20Features~{}Children\T1\textquoterights%20risk%20factors~{}31 (accessed on 20 September 2018).
3. Pérez-Escamilla, R.; Obbagy, J.E.; Altman, J.M.; Essery, E.V.; McGrane, M.M.; Wong, Y.P.; Spahn, J.M.; Williams, C.L. Dietary energy density and body weight in adults and children: A systematic review. *J. Acad. Nutr. Diet* **2012**, *112*, 671–684. [CrossRef] [PubMed]

4. Rouhani, M.H.; Haghighatdoost, F.; Surkan, P.J.; Azadbakht, L. Associations between dietary energy density and obesity: A systematic review and meta-analysis of observational studies. *Nutrition* **2016**, *32*, 1037–1047. [CrossRef] [PubMed]
5. Aburto, T.C.; Cantoral, A.; Hernandez-Barrera, L.; Carriquiry, A.L.; Rivera, J.A. Usual dietary energy density distribution is positively associated with excess body weight in Mexican children. *J. Nutr.* **2015**, *145*, 1524–1530. [CrossRef]
6. Leahy, K.E.; Birch, L.L.; Rolls, B.J. Reducing the energy density of multiple meals decreases the energy intake of preschool-age children. *Am. J. Clin. Nutr.* **2008**, *88*, 1459–1468. [CrossRef]
7. Smethers, A.D.; Roe, L.S.; Sanchez, C.E.; Zuraikat, F.M.; Keller, K.L.; Rolls, B.J. Both increases and decreases in energy density lead to sustained changes in preschool children's energy intake over 5 days. *Physiol. Behav.* **2019**, *204*, 210–218. [CrossRef]
8. Fisher, J.; Liu, Y.; Birch, L.L.; Rolls, B.J. Effects of portion size and energy density on young children's intake at a meal. *Am. J. Clin. Nutr.* **2007**, *86*, 174–179. [CrossRef]
9. Poole, S.; Hart, C.; Jelalian, E.; Raynor, H. Relationship between dietary energy density and dietary quality in overweight young children: A cross-sectional analysis. *Pediatr. Obes.* **2016**, *11*, 128–135. [CrossRef]
10. Schroder, H.; Mendez, M.A.; Gomez, S.F.; Fito, M.; Ribas, L.; Aranceta, J.; Serra-Majem, L. Energy density, diet quality, and central body fat in a nationwide survey of young Spaniards. *Nutrition* **2013**, *29*, 1350–1355. [CrossRef]
11. Thompson, D.; Ferry, R., Jr.; Cullen, K.; Liu, Y. Improvement in fruit and vegetable consumption associated with more favorable energy density and nutrient and food group intake, but not kilocalories. *J. Acad. Nutr. Diet* **2016**, *116*, 1443–1449. [CrossRef]
12. National Health and Medical Research Council. Australian Guide to Healthy Eating. Available online: https://www.eatforhealth.gov.au/guidelines/australian-guide-healthy-eating (accessed on 2 August 2018).
13. Vernarelli, J.A.; Mitchell, D.C.; Hartman, T.J.; Rolls, B.J. Dietary energy density is associated with body weight status and vegetable intake in U.S. Children. *J. Nutr.* **2011**, *141*, 2204–2210. [CrossRef] [PubMed]
14. Murakami, K.; Livingstone, M.B. Associations between energy density of meals and snacks and overall diet quality and adiposity measures in British children and adolescents: The National Diet and Nutrition Survey. *Br. J. Nutr.* **2016**, *116*, 1633–1645. [CrossRef] [PubMed]
15. Moubarac, J.C.; Batal, M.; Louzada, M.L.; Martinez Steele, E.; Monteiro, C.A. Consumption of ultra-processed foods predicts diet quality in Canada. *Appetite* **2017**, *108*, 512–520. [CrossRef] [PubMed]
16. Kachurak, A.; Bailey, R.L.; Davey, A.; Dabritz, L.; Fisher, J.O. Daily snacking occasions, snack size, and snack energy density as predictors of diet quality among US children aged 2 to 5 years. *Nutrients* **2019**, *11*, 1440. [CrossRef]
17. Innes-Hughes, C.; Hardy, L.L.; Venugopal, K.; King, L.A.; Wolfenden, L.; Rangan, A. Children's consumption of energy-dense nutrient-poor foods, fruit and vegetables: Are they related? An analysis of data from a cross sectional survey. *Health Promot. J. Austr.* **2011**, *22*, 210–216. [CrossRef]
18. CSIRO. *2007 Australian National Children's Nutrition and Physical Activity Survey: Main Findings*; Department of Health and Ageing: Canberra, Australia, 2008.
19. Australian Bureau of Statistics. Australian Health Survey: Nutrition First Results—Foods and Nutrients, 2011–12. Available online: http://www.ausstats.abs.gov.au/ausstats/subscriber.nsf/0/4683FD7315DFDFDBCA257D080014F9E0/$File/australian%20health%20survey%20nutrition%20first%20results%20-%20food%20and%20nutrients,%202011-12.pdf (accessed on 19 August 2018).
20. Papoutsi, G.S.; Nayga, R.M.; Lazaridis, P.; Drichoutis, A.C. Fat tax, subsidy or both? The role of information and children's pester power in food choice. *J. Econ. Behav. Organ.* **2015**, *117*, 196–208. [CrossRef]
21. Baldassarre, F.; Campo, R.; Falcone, A. Food for kids: How children influence their parents purchasing decisions. *J. Food Prod. Market* **2016**, *22*, 596–609. [CrossRef]
22. Health Star Rating Advisory Committee. About Health Star Ratings. Available online: http://healthstarrating.gov.au/internet/healthstarrating/publishing.nsf/Content/About-health-stars (accessed on 18 August 2018).
23. Shahid, M.; Neal, B.; Jones, A. Uptake of Australia's Health Star Rating System 2014–2019. *Nutrients* **2020**, *12*, 1791. [CrossRef]
24. Pulker, C.; Trapp, G.; Scott, J.; Pollard, C. Alignment of supermarket own brand foods' front-of-pack nutrition labelling with measures of nutritional quality: An Australian Perspective. *Nutrients* **2018**, *10*, 1465. [CrossRef]

25. Sadeghirad, B.; Duhaney, T.; Motaghipisheh, S.; Campbell, N.R.; Johnston, B.C. Influence of unhealthy food and beverage marketing on children's dietary intake and preference: A systematic review and meta-analysis of randomized trials. *Obes. Rev.* **2016**, *17*, 945–959. [CrossRef]
26. Cameron, A.J. The shelf space and strategic placement of healthy and discretionary foods in urban, urban-fringe and rural/non-metropolitan Australian supermarkets. *Public Health Nutr.* **2018**, *21*, 593–600. [CrossRef]
27. Pulker, C.E.; Scott, J.A.; Pollard, C.M. Ultra-processed family foods in Australia: Nutrition claims, health claims and marketing techniques. *Public Health Nutr.* **2017**, *21*, 38–48. [CrossRef] [PubMed]
28. Mintel. Mintel GNPD—Global New Products Database. Available online: http://www.mintel.com/global-new-products-database (accessed on 23 May 2018).
29. Mintel. GNPD Glossary. Available online: https://downloads.mintel.com/private/dfKio/files/556573/ (accessed on 6 June 2018).
30. Johnson, L.; Wilks, D.C.; Lindroos, A.K.; Jebb, S.A. Reflections from a systematic review of dietary energy density and weight gain: Is the inclusion of drinks valid? *Obes. Rev.* **2009**, *10*, 681–692. [CrossRef]
31. World Cancer Research Fund/American Institute for Cancer Research. *Food, Nutrition, Physical Activity, and the Prevention of Cancer: A Global Perspective*; American Institute for Cancer Research: Washington, DC, USA, 2007.
32. Australian Bureau of Statistics. Australian Health Survey: Users' Guide, 2011–2013 Discretionary Foods. In *Australian Bureau of Statistics*. Available online: http://www.abs.gov.au/ausstats/abs@.nsf/Lookup/4363.0.55.001Chapter65062011-13 (accessed on 20 September 2018).
33. National Health and Medical Research Council. *National Statement on Ethical Conduct in Human Research (Updated 2018)*; National Health and Medical Research Council: Canberra, Australia, 2007.
34. Mhurchu, C.N.; Brown, R.; Jiang, Y.; Eyles, H.; Dunford, E.; Neal, B. Nutrient profile of 23,596 packaged supermarket foods and non-alcoholic beverages in Australia and New Zealand. *Public Health Nutr.* **2016**, *19*, 401–408. [CrossRef] [PubMed]
35. Meloncelli, N.J.L.; Pelly, F.E.; Cooper, S.L. Nutritional quality of a selection of children's packaged food available in Australia. *Nutr. Diet* **2016**, *73*, 88–94. [CrossRef]
36. Alessandrini, R.; He, F.J.; Hashem, K.M.; Tan, M.; MacGregor, G.A. Reformulation and priorities for reducing energy density; Results from a cross-sectional survey on fat content in pre-packed cakes and biscuits sold in British supermarkets. *Nutrients* **2019**, *11*, 1216. [CrossRef]
37. Lawrence, M.A.; Dickie, S.; Woods, J.L. Do nutrient-based front-of-pack labelling schemes support or undermine food-based dietary guideline recommendations? Lessons from the Australian Health Star Rating system. *Nutrients* **2018**, *10*, 32. [CrossRef]
38. Dickie, S.; Woods, J.L.; Baker, P.; Elizabeth, L.; Lawrence, M.A. Evaluating nutrient-based indices against food- and diet-based indices to assess the health potential of foods: How does the Australian Health Star Rating System perform after five years? *Nutrients* **2020**, *12*, 1463. [CrossRef]
39. Department of Health and Ageing. *Australian Dietary Guidelines*; Commonwealth of Australia: Canberra, Australia, 2013.
40. Cooper, S.L.; Pelly, F.E.; Lowe, J.B. Assessment of the construct validity of the Australian Health Star Rating: A nutrient profiling diagnostic accuracy study. *Eur. J. Clin. Nutr.* **2017**, *71*, 1353–1359. [CrossRef]
41. Hamlin, R.; McNeill, L. Does the Australasian "Health Star Rating" front of pack nutritional label system work? *Nutrients* **2016**, *8*, 327. [CrossRef]
42. Peters, S.; Dunford, E.; Jones, A.; Mhurchu, C.N.; Crino, M.; Taylor, F.; Woodward, M.; Neal, B. Incorporating added sugar improves the performance of the Health Star Rating front-of-pack labelling system in Australia. *Nutrients* **2017**, *9*, 701. [CrossRef] [PubMed]
43. Vandevijvere, S.; Mackay, S.; D'Souza, E.; Swinburn, B. *How Healthy are New Zealand Food Environments? A Comprehensive Assessment 2014–2017*; The University of Auckland: Auckland, New Zealand, 2018.
44. O'Connor, L.; Walton, J.; Flynn, A. Dietary energy density and its association with the nutritional quality of the diet of children and teenagers. *J. Nutr. Sci.* **2013**, *2*, e10. [CrossRef] [PubMed]
45. Hawkes, C.; Smith, T.G.; Jewell, J.; Wardle, J.; Hammond, R.A.; Friel, S.; Thow, A.M.; Kain, J. Smart food policies for obesity prevention. *Lancet* **2015**, *385*, 2410–2421. [CrossRef]
46. Russell, C.G.; Burke, P.F.; Waller, D.S.; Wei, E. The impact of front-of-pack marketing attributes versus nutrition and health information on parents' food choices. *Appetite* **2017**, *116*, 323–338. [CrossRef]

47. Neal, B.; Crino, M.; Dunford, E.; Gao, A.; Greenland, R.; Li, N.; Ngai, J.; Mhurchu, C.N.; Pettigrew, S.; Sacks, G.; et al. Effects of different types of front-of-pack labelling information on the healthiness of food purchases—A randomised controlled trial. *Nutrients* **2017**, *9*, 1284. [CrossRef]
48. Pettigrew, S.; Talati, Z.; Miller, C.; Dixon, H.; Kelly, B.; Ball, K. The types and aspects of front-of-pack food labelling schemes preferred by adults and children. *Appetite* **2017**, *109*, 115–123. [CrossRef]
49. Talati, Z.; Pettigrew, S.; Kelly, B.; Ball, K.; Dixon, H.; Shilton, T. Consumers' responses to front-of-pack labels that vary by interpretive content. *Appetite* **2016**, *101*, 205–213. [CrossRef]
50. Hamlin, R.; McNeill, L. The impact of the Australasian 'Health Star Rating', front-of-pack nutritional label, on consumer choice: A longitudinal study. *Nutrients* **2018**, *10*, 906. [CrossRef]
51. Ares, G.; Varela, F.; Machin, L.; Antúnez, L.; Giménez, A.; Curutchet, M.R.; Aschemann-Witzeld, J. Comparative performance of three interpretative front-of-pack nutrition labelling schemes: Insights for policy making. *Food Qual. Prefer.* **2018**, *68*, 215–225. [CrossRef]
52. Egnell, M.; Hercberg, S.; Julia, C.; Talati, Z.; Pettigrew, S.; Julia, C. Objective understanding of front-of-package nutrition labels: An international comparative experimental study across 12 countries. *Nutrients* **2018**, *10*, 1542. [CrossRef]
53. Spiteri, S.A.; Olstad, D.L.; Woods, J.L. Nutritional quality of new food products released into the Australian retail food market in 2015—Is the food industry part of the solution? *BMC Public Health* **2018**, *18*, 222. [CrossRef] [PubMed]

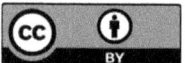

© 2020 by the authors. Licensee MDPI, Basel, Switzerland. This article is an open access article distributed under the terms and conditions of the Creative Commons Attribution (CC BY) license (http://creativecommons.org/licenses/by/4.0/).

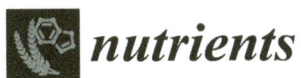 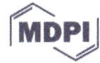

Article

Consumer Misuse of Country-of-Origin Label: Insights from the Italian Extra-Virgin Olive Oil Market

Francesco Bimbo, Luigi Roselli *, Domenico Carlucci and Bernardo Corrado de Gennaro

Department of Agricultural and Environmental Sciences, University of Bari Aldo Moro, 70126 Bari, Italy; francesco.bimbo@uniba.it (F.B.); domenico.carlucci@uniba.it (D.C.); bernardocorrado.degennaro@uniba.it (B.C.d.G.)
* Correspondence: luigi.roselli@uniba.it

Received: 23 June 2020; Accepted: 17 July 2020; Published: 19 July 2020

Abstract: Providing information to consumers through the label is a means for food companies to inform consumers about product's attributes, including the country of origin (COO). In the EU, COO labeling has been made mandatory for several categories of food products, to enable consumers to make informed choices at the point of sale. In particular, Regulation (EU) No 29/2012 has introduced a mandatory country-of-origin labeling system for extra virgin olive oil (EVOO). In the present study, conducted in Italy, we test whether there is a price differential associated with the COO information for EVOO. To this end, we employ a hedonic price model and data about the purchase of EVOO products collected from 982 consumers at the supermarket checkout. Having interviewed these consumers, we also assess the share of EVOO consumers that correctly identify the country of origin of the product purchased. Our findings point out that, in Italy, the EVOO with domestic origin, indicated on the label, benefits of a premium price equal to +35% compared to the product labeled as blend of European EVOOs, while a discount of −10.8% is attached to EVOOs from a non-European origin. A significant share of consumers in our sample (19.04%) is, however, unable to correctly identify the origin of the EVOO purchased. This label misuse mostly occurs among consumers who report that they had purchased Italian EVOO, while they had actually purchased a blend of European EVOOs. Female and more highly educated consumers are less likely to misuse label information about the product's origins.

Keywords: consumer choice; food labeling; extra virgin olive oil; hedonic price model; country of origin

1. Introduction

Extra-virgin olive oil (EVOO) is the superior olive oil category extracted from olives by the mechanical extraction process. EVOO is one of the main components of the Mediterranean diet and it is considered worldwide as one of the healthiest oils. The European Union (EU) is the largest EVOO producer worldwide, and production is concentrated in three Mediterranean countries: Spain produces about 57.5% of EU EVOO output, Italy over 19.5%, and Greece about 15.8% [1]. Due to increasing consumption in non-producing countries, both within the EU (e.g., UK and Germany) and outside Europe (e.g., China, Japan, Russia, Australia, Brazil, Canada, and the US), demand for European EVOO is expected to rise until 2030 [2,3]. Rising EVOO consumption in non-producing countries leads Mediterranean EVOO producers to export their EVOO to other markets [2,3]. The steadily increasing demand for EVOO in non-producing countries has led Italy to export a large share of domestically produced EVOO, which is no longer sufficient to satisfy the domestic market. Such supply imbalance is constantly re-balanced by importing EVOO from Spain and non-European Mediterranean countries, such as Tunisia and Turkey. This EVOO is usually priced lower than Italian EVOO. Compared to Italian EVOO producers, the Spanish benefit from economies of scale and non-European producers with lower labor costs [3]. Production costs at farm level for a liter of Italian EVOO are, on average, 30% higher than the production costs recorded for Spanish and non-European Mediterranean producers [1]. As a result, Italian EVOO sold on the Italian market competes with EVOO imported from other countries.

Over the last three decades, consumers have placed increasing importance on the product's origin. However, the latter cannot be verified either ex-ante or ex-post consumption and asymmetric information about the products' origins arises between producers and consumers. Providing information about products' origins through the label has become a widely adopted tool to mitigate the information gap between consumers and producers. Country of origin labeling policies, by informing consumers about a product's origin, transform information about the origin of the product, that is a credence attribute, into a searchable characteristic and so alleviate the problem of asymmetric information [4,5] Generally speaking, labeling policies address a market failure, asymmetric information, through costly expenditures borne by a combination of consumers, firms, and taxpayers. First, the industry bear costs of labeling, which likely pass on consumers at higher prices. Second, the government's costs of label monitoring and enforcement system are borne by taxpayers via higher taxes. Third, mandatory label exacerbates other market distortions such as decrease competition or encourage rent-seeking and gaming, as well as introduces trade distortions across countries [6].

In the case of the EVOO market, EU policymakers have introduced Regulation (EU) No 29/2012, a mandatory labeling information system requiring producers to indicate on the label the country of origin (COO) of the EVOO. This Regulation establishes that the labeling of extra virgin olive oil and virgin olive oil must bear a designation of origin. Bottlers can use, on the label, one of the following claims relating to origin: (a) in the case of olive oils originating from one Member State or third country, a reference to the Member State, to the Union, or to the third country, as appropriate; (b) in the case of blends of olive oils originating from more than one Member State or third country; or one of the following statements, as appropriate: (i) 'blend of olive oils of European Union origin' or a reference to the Union; (ii) 'blend of olive oils not of European Union origin' or a reference to origin outside the Union; (iii) 'blend of olive oils of European Union origin and not of European Union origin' or a reference to origin within the Union and outside the Union; or (c) a protected designation of origin or a protected geographical indication referred to in Regulation (EU) No 1151/2012, in accordance with the provisions relating to the product specification concerned [7]).

On the one hand, the introduction of Regulation No (EU) 29/2012, by informing consumers about the origin of EVOO, is potentially beneficial to Italian EVOO producers. Since Italian consumers strongly prefer domestic EVOO over non-Italian alternatives and are willing to pay a premium price for it [3,8–11], the regulation would support Italian producers to ensure fair revenues for their product. In other words, by informing consumers about the COO of EVOO, Italian producers are able to differentiate their products and add value to these.

On the other hand, the measures based on informing consumers through the label implicitly assume that information on the label eliminates asymmetric information by fully informing consumers about the product's features, and so restoring information symmetry between consumers and producers. The existing literature points, however, to many instances where the labeling policy is not be able to restore full information. This occurs because consumers either do not make full use of the label, or the label's information is not clear, or consumers are not fully aware of the information's availability [12]. Furthermore, consumers may not fully trust label information due to the risk of incurring food fraud. Frauds are more likely to occur in products that benefit from premium prices. Indeed, the latter work as an incentive for producers to commit fraud [13].

As a result, the aim of the present study is twofold: (i) to test whether there is a price differential associated with COO information for EVOO by using retail level data collected from Italian EVOO consumers purchases; and, (ii) to assess in what measure consumers correctly use the information about the origin of the EVOO they purchased. To the best of our knowledge, no previous studies investigated to what extent consumers correctly identify the origin of the EVOO purchased by using the origin information on the label. We did so by interviewing EVOO shoppers at the supermarket checkout about the origins of the product they have purchased. By inspecting the labeling of the product these shoppers purchased, we assess whether their understanding of the product's origin matches what is reported on the label. We then analyze consumer groups of differing abilities in identifying the COO of the product according to their socio-economic characteristics, as well as their self-declared interest in the product's label information, the origin of the product, and interest in branded products more widely. Indirectly, this allows us to infer the effectiveness of the mandatory COO label in correctly informing consumers and orienting their food choices. The remainder of the paper is structured as follows: the next section presents a description of survey design, the data and the model used; then, we discuss the empirical results. We conclude by providing recommendations for EVOO producers and policymakers.

2. Materials and Methods

2.1. Survey and Data Collection

The survey involved 982 EVOO consumers interviewed at the supermarket checkout counters. Consumers were selected on voluntary basis and did not receive any monetary compensation to participate in the study. Once consumers were approached at supermarket cashiers were asked their willingness to participate in the study or not. For those who accepted to participate, written informed consent according to the national ethical requirement "Italian Personal Data Protection Code" (L.D. 196/2003) was collected. Then, the interviewers asked them to state the origin of the EVOO they had just purchased. Consumers were free to answer by selecting one of the following statements: "I am unaware of the origin of the EVOO I purchased", "It is a blend of non-European EVOOs", "It is a blend of European EVOOs" and "It is a 100% Italian EVOO". The interviewers then inspected the labeling of the product purchased. By comparing consumers' answers and the information on the origin of the EVOO found on the label, they were able to assess the correctness of what consumers stated about the COO of the EVOO purchased. The share of consumers that correctly identified the origins of the product was used as a proxy for the effectiveness of the EU Reg. 29/2012 to inform consumers about such origins.

The interviewers also collected information on the characteristics of the EVOO that consumers purchased, including its COO attribute, used for sizing their monetary value by means of the hedonic price model. Socio-economic information about the consumers, if they shopped for EVOO as a result of price promotion, as well as their interest in labeling information, in the origin of products, and preference for branded products, were also collected. These served as a proxy for consumers' knowledge about the product purchased. To this end, five-point Likert scales were employed, assigning point 1 to "strongly disagree" and 5 to "strongly agree". Table 1 reports the summary statistics and a description of the data collected on both the products and consumers' characteristics. The data collection of was carried out between March and July 2017 and consumers were recruited from a regionally representative sample of 14 hypermarkets and supermarkets, all located in the Apulian region (Italy). The sample of hypermarkets and supermarkets included at least one outlet in each of the six provincial capitals of the region, as well as a selection of the leading retailers in the Apulian region, namely Auchan, Conad, COOP, and Famila.

Table 1. Summary statistics related to product and consumer characteristics (982 observations).

Variables	Description	Mean (St. Dev.) [a]
Product variables		
Dependent Variable		
Price	EVOO price €/l	6.088 (1.7139)
Explanatory Variable		
Organic	1 = EVOO made from organic agricultural practices	0.024
GIs	1 = EVOO sold with Geographical Indications (DOP/PGI)	0.038
Italian Origin	1 = Italian EVOO	0.430
Non-European Origin	1 = Product from Non-European EVOOs	0.321
European Origin	1 = Product from European EVOOs	0.249
Filtered	1 = Filtered Product	0.989
Unfiltered	1 = Unfiltered Product	0.011
Product in Promotion	1 = Product sold in promotion	0.563
Glass Packaging	1 = Product sold in glass packages	0.986
Other Packaging Material	1 = Product sold in other packages (e.g., plastic)	0.014
1 L	1 = Package Size 1liter	0.891
0.75 L	1 = Package Size 0.75 L	0.078
0.5 L	1 = Package Size 0.5 L	0.031
Consumer variables		
Gender	1=Female consumer	0.529
Household size	1–6 = Number of household members	3.089 (1.1311)
Child below 18 years old	1 = Household with child below 18 years old	0.671
Education	1–3 = 1 Middle school education, 2 High school education, 3 University education	2.227 (0.6935)
Income	1–3 = 1 Individual monthly income below 1000€, 2 between 1001€–2000€, 3 above 2001€	2.258 (0.6860)
Shopping EVOO on offer	1 = Purchase an EVOO on promotion	0.562
Interest in label information	1–5 = "I am interested in labeling", where 1 stands for "strongly disagree" and 5 for "strongly agree"	4.220 (0.7075)
Interest in product origin	1–5 = "I am interested in product origins", where 1 stands for "strongly disagree" and 5 for "strongly agree"	3.910 (0.9470)
Interest in branded products	1–5 = "I am interested in branded products", where 1 stands for "strongly disagree" and 5 for "strongly agree"	3.899 (0.9662)

[a] For all binary variables the mean represents the percentage of observations, the value of the standard deviation is omitted.

2.2. Model and Statistical Analysis

To measure the monetary value of the product's features, we used the standard hedonic price model first introduced by Rosen in 1974 [14]. According to hedonic price theory, a product is considered as a bundle of attributes. Each consumer in the market selects the set of features which maximizes his/her utility, subject to a budget constraint. Likewise, manufacturers maximize profits by setting the product's price according to its attributes [14]. In a market for products presenting a unique bundle of attributes, buyers' marginal bids and sellers' marginal offers match at equilibrium and the joint envelope of consumers' bids and sellers' offers generate the hedonic price function [13]. Thus, the price, P, of a product, j, can be described as:

$$P_j = f(Z_j) \qquad (1)$$

where Z is a vector of product attributes belonging to product j and f(.) is an unspecified functional form. Equation (1) implies that the price consumers pay for product P is a function of the marginal monetary values of j's attributes Z [14–16] and can be obtained by partially differentiating (1) with respect to each attribute. Furthermore, the implicit marginal price a consumer pays for the attribute Z corresponds to the marginal cost which the producer incurs in offering that attribute on the market. Equation (1) was estimated by ordinary least squares (OLS).

Then, to measure the share of consumers able to correctly identify the origin of the EVOO products they purchased and infer the effectiveness of the mandatory COO information in correctly orienting consumers' food choices, a cross-tabulation analysis was performed. A Pearson Chi-square test and a Goodman and Kruskal's gamma statistic were used to assess whether the outcomes from the cross-tabulation were statistically significant, so testing the presence of a positive and statistically significant association between consumers' statements about the origins of the product and the verified origins [17,18]. The work ends by profiling consumer groups based on their ability to correctly discriminate the product's origins. Consumers' socioeconomic characteristics, their interest in the information on the product's label, in the origin of the product, as well as in branded products, were used to profile consumer groups. A Tukey test assessed whether consumers differ according to the characteristics listed above [19].

3. Results and Discussion

The estimated parameters of Equation (1), using the logarithmic transformation of the price as the dependent variable, are reported in the first column of Table 2, along with their standard errors in parenthesis. The functional form using the log-linear transformation of the price shows the lowest value of log-likelihood function testing it competitively with the linear and the box-cox transformation of the dependent variable. Marginal prices of each attribute (in percentage terms) are also calculated using Kennedy's (1981) adjustment and reported in the last column [20] In Equation (1), we also control for brand fixed effects. For the sake of brevity, the resulting coefficients are not reported in the manuscript, but are available upon request. The baseline product is a non-organic EVOO from EU countries, filtered, and sold in 1 L glass bottle at an average price of 6.08 €/L. Based on the Ramsey's RESET statistics for omitted variable bias [21], the model does not suffer from misspecification, and, since the null hypothesis of homoscedasticity of the Breusch–Pagan/Cook–Weisberg test cannot be rejected, the error terms are homoscedastic [22,23]. Skewness and Kurtosis test indicates the normality of the error terms distribution [24]. The model shows an adjusted R^2 of 0.9694 and a statistically significant value of the F-statistic, suggesting the join significance of coefficients regressors. These statistics confirm that the semi-logarithmic specification of Equation (1) is the most appropriate among the possible functional forms for $f(.)$.

The first notable finding reported in Table 2 is that the "Italian" origin label has a positive and significant effect on the price of EVOO sold in Italy and amounts to a price premium of +35%, relative to the baseline product, which is equivalent to +2.18€/liter. This result is consistent with other studies that found a willingness of Italian consumers to pay more for domestic EVOO products. Compared to the price of a European EVOO, "Non-European" EVOO is instead sold at a discount of −10.8%, equivalent to −0.70€/liter [6–8].

The geographical indication labels "GIs" show a positive and significant effect on price of +7.12 €/liter, or +112%, relative to the baseline product's price. This attribute records the highest price premium among all the considered EVOO's attributes and the result is consistent with several studies which also found that consumers, including those on the Italian market, prefer GIs products over regular ones and are willing to pay higher prices for such products [25–27]. The higher price of EVOO with GIs may, however, reflect the higher cost of GIs products, since farmers/producers seeking to sell their products with a GI label have to meet costly production standards that are frequently regarded as a barrier for the compliance with GIs standards [28–30].

Interestingly, the "Organic" attribute records a positive and significant impact on the EVOO price of +15.1% over the baseline product price, equivalent to a price premium of 0.91€/liter. The premium price associated with this attribute is likely to be the result of consumers' willingness to pay for a "sustainable" product, which has been reported in several studies [31–33]. Products labeled as organic also are often perceived as healthier than regular ones, and, indeed, consumers' primary reason for buying organic foods is their belief that these products support human health [34]. Thus, the premium price attached to organic EVOO may also be due to consumers' willingness to buy products which they regard as supporting their health.

Table 2. Estimated parameters and percentage of premium price.

Variable	β	Percentage, Premium Price [a]
Organic	0.141 **	+15.1
	(0.0710)	
GIs	0.776 ***	+117.0
	(0.0570)	
Italian Origin	0.301 ***	+35.0
	(0.0830)	
Non-European Origin	−0.114 ***	−10.8
	(0.0210)	
Unfiltered	+0.245 **	+21.6
	(0.1030)	
Product in promotion	−0.001	−0.1
	(0.0060)	
Other Packaging Material	−0.123	−11.5
	(0.1020)	
0.75 L Package Size	0.143 ***	+15.4
	(0.0450)	
0.5 L Package Size	0.115 *	+12.2
	(0.0630)	
Constant	1.726 ***	
	(0.0970)	
Number of Observations	982	
R-square	0.961	
Specification test Ramsey's RESET $F_{(2, 870)}$	1.32	
p-value	0.2672	
Heteroskedasticity Breusch-Pagan/Cook-Weisberg $\chi^2(1)$	0.18	
p-value	0.6731	
Normality Skewness and Kurtosis $\chi^2(2)$	0.1355	
p-value	0.125	

[a] Adjustment made according to Kennedy (1981). *, ** and *** are 10, 5 and 1 percent significance levels.

The marginal prices associated with the unfiltered attribute, "Unfiltered", is positive and statistically significant. Unfiltered EVOO is sold with a markup of +21.6% or +1.28 €/liter. This suggests that the "unfiltered" claim on the label can be used by consumers to infer a higher degree of wholesomeness/naturalness [34], and a premium is thus associated with this attribute.

The marginal prices associated with the packaging variables show positive and statistically significant coefficients. They indicate that premium prices are associated with EVOO products sold in glass packages smaller than 1 L. Products sold in glass bottles of 0.75 L ("Package Size 0.75 L") benefit from a premium price of 0.912 €/liter, while products sold in 0.5 L glass bottles ("Package Size 0.5 L") secure a premium price of 0.742 €/liter. The estimated marginal prices for products sold in other packaging material ("Other Packaging Material"), such as plastic or tin, as well as sold on promotion ("Promotion") are negative, but not statistically significant.

With regard to Table 3, the data on consumers' reports at checkout shows that 13.1% of EVOO consumers (129) in our sample were not aware of the origin of the product purchased, while a minority of 0.2% (2) reports their having purchased non-European EVOO. A larger share of EVOO consumers in the sample, approximately 28.0% (275), report having purchased a European EVOO and the majority of them, 255 out of 275, correctly identified the product's origins. The largest group of EVOO consumers interviewed, 58.7% of the total sample (576), reports the purchase of Italian EVOO. In the latter group, one out of three consumers incorrectly identified the Italian product's origin since they believed that they had purchased an Italian EVOO, but the product purchased actually was a blend of European EVOOs (165 out 576). The misuse about the product COO label then occurs more often when consumers report their having purchased Italian EVOO.

Table 3. Consumer-declared origin of the EVOO products purchased and the actual one.

EVOO's Origin of Actual Purchases	Non-European Countries	European Countries	Italian	Total Respondents [a]
EVOO's origin declared:				
"I am unaware of the origin of the EVOO I purchased"	1 (100%)	112 (20.97%)	16 (3.58%)	129 (13.1%)
"It is a blend of Non-European EVOOs"	0 (0.00)	2 (0.37%)	0 (0.00)	2 (0.20%)
"It is a blend of European EVOOs"	0 (0.00)	**255** (**47.75%**)	20 (4.47%)	275 (28.0%)
"It is 100% Italian EVOO"	0 (0.00)	165 (30.90%)	**411** (**91.95%**)	576 (58.7%)
Total respondents	1	519	462	982
Pearson $\chi^2(6)$ = 373.7349 Pr = 0.000; Gamma = 0.6986 ASE = 0.036				

[a] The share of respondents over the total number of respondents of the column is reported in parenthesis. The number of respondents who correctly indicated the product's origin is in the highlighted in bold.

A potential cause of the erroneous consumers' identification of foreign EVOO as Italian may be related to the fact that consumers may be not aware of, or may not use, the COO information on the label. Another cause can be related to the fact that many non-Italian companies, after multiple mergers and acquisitions, hold in their portfolio several Italian EVOO brands (e.g., Bertolli, Carapelli, Sasso owned by Deoleo S.A.; Sagra and Filippo Berio by the Bright Food Group Co Ltd.). Companies use these brands to market non-Italian EVOO, so increasing the likelihood that consumers mistakenly infer from the brand name that the origin of the EVOO purchased is Italian. The use of a brand name with a more favorable image (in this case an Italian brand-name) to deliberately lead consumers to associate the origins of brand and product is a strategy previously reported for many other consumers goods markets [35]. If consumers use the brand as a clue to the origin of the product and other information on the origin of the product is not taken into account in the purchasing process, this marketing strategy lowers the ability of consumers to correctly identify the product's origins. As proposed by Zhou, Yang, and Hui (2010, p. 204), *"the origin information for most brands may not be readily accessible either because global marketers have the desire to mask the origins of their brands or the globalization of firms and the cross-border acquisition of brands complicate the nature of brand origin"* [36].) Lastly, another hurdle for consumers in correctly identifying the origin of the product may be the fact that several Italian EVOO producers, aiming to offer consumers a greater variety of products, sell both Italian and non-Italian products under the same brand name. Such choice may further lower consumers' ability to correctly identify the country of origin (COO) of the product during their food purchase.

Overall, the data in Table 3, reported in bold, indicates that 666 consumers, 67.8% of the sample, correctly associate the COO of the EVOO purchased. The positive association between the reported and verified origins of the product, and thus the overall ability to correctly associate the product and its origins, is statistically significant. The Goodman and Kruskal's gamma statistic and the Pearson Chi-square test have a low p-values (<0.05). This indicates that the likelihood that consumers' identification of the product's origin corresponds to the correct one is high [17,18].

On the one hand, the results discussed above indicate that, overall, the mandatory COO information on EVOO products (EU Reg. 29/2012) is an effective tool in guiding consumers in the identification and selection of EVOO based on its origins. On the other hand, results show that there is still a consistent number of Italian consumers (187) who do not correctly associate the product with its actual origins and in most of the cases they are consumers who reported, and believed that they had purchased an Italian EVOO. Thus, the misuse of COO label mostly occurs where foreign EVOO products are identified as Italian.

Lastly, Table 4 identifies consumer groups according to their ability to correctly associate the COO of the EVOO purchased, characterizing them in relation to their socio-economic characteristics, as well as their interest in labeling information, in the origin of the product and in branded products more generally.

The first consumer group, reporting that they are unaware of the product's origin, encompasses 13.1% of consumers sampled. These consumers are mostly male, with a lower level of education compared to the average level of EVOO consumers in our sample. Furthermore, consumers unaware of the origins of the product live in a household with less than 3 individuals and their income is lower than in the other groups. These consumers purchase EVOO more often than others when it is sold on promotion at an average price of approximately 5.50 €/liter. Compared to consumers in the other two groups, these consumers also reported less interest in the information on the label, in the product's origins and in brands.

The second group, representing 19.04% of EVOO consumers in the sample, encompasses individuals who incorrectly identify the country of origin of the product at the supermarket checkout. Consumers in this group are mostly male and have a higher level of education than those reporting unawareness of the product's origins. Furthermore, they live in larger households and purchase products on promotion at 5.88 €/liter, which is not statistically different to the 5.50 €/liter paid by consumers that are not aware of the origins of the EVOO purchased. Compared to the previous group, consumers in this group report having a slightly greater interest in branded products.

The third and last consumer group, accounting for 67.82% of the total sample, encompasses consumers who correctly identify the product's country of origin. This consumer group is largely composed of female consumers and has the highest level of education. These consumers purchase EVOO on promotion less frequently and also report their being highly interested in labeling information, as well as in the product's origins and in branded products. On average, they pay 6.24 € for a liter of EVOO, a price that is higher and statistically different from that paid by consumers belonging to the two groups discussed before.

Focusing on consumers who correctly identify Italian EVOO, reported in the last column of Table 4, they are again female EVOO shoppers with a higher level of education, highly interested in labeling information, in the origins of the product, and in branded products. This consumer group pays on average above 6.60 €/liter for an EVOO product. The data in Table 4 shows that consumers who place importance on information reported on the food label, including brand and the origins of the product, are more likely than others to correctly identify the product's origins, if their level of education is higher than the average.

Table 4. Characteristics of consumers groups.

	Full Sample (Obs. = 982)			Subsample (Obs. = 576)	
	Unaware of the Origin of the EVOO	Incorrectly Classify the EVOO Origin.	Correctly State the EVOO Origin.	Incorrectly Classify the Italian EVOO Origin.	Correctly Classify the Italian EVOO Origin.
Share of respondents	13.10%	19.04%	67.82%	28.64%	71.36%
Consumer variables					
Gender	0.380 a	0.460 a	0.577 b	0.461 a	0.604 b
	(0.4872)	(0.4997)	(0.4945)	(0.5003)	(0.4896)
Education	1.791 a	1.930 b	2.332 c	1.985 a	2.360 b
	(0.6334)	(0.7336)	(0.6645)	(0.7170)	(0.6619)
Household size	2.783 a	3.166 b	3.092 b	3.156 a	3.060 a
	(1.1247)	(1.2134)	(1.0992)	(1.1667)	(1.1016)
Child less than 18Y	0.426 a	0.615 ab	0.716 b	0.602 a	0.680 a
	(0.6821)	(0.8369)	(0.8128)	(0.8270)	(0.8046)
Income	2.031 a	2.241 ab	2.251 b	2.283 a	2.367 a
	(0.7340)	(0.6727)	(0.6888)	(0.6473)	(0.6558)
Purchase on promotion	0.605 a	0.572 a	0.520 b	0.680 a	0.375 b
	(0.4908)	(0.4961)	(0.5000)	(0.4678)	(0.4848)
Interest in label information	3.860 a	4.305 ab	4.255 b	4.248 a	4.405 b
	(0.9499)	(0.6625)	(0.6812)	(0.6564)	(0.6430)
Interest in product origin	3.829 a	3.947 ab	3.983 b	3.829 a	4.244 b
	(1.0978)	(0.9601)	(0.9134)	(0.9633)	(0.8518)
Interest in branded products	3.605 a	3.952 b	3.959 b	3.879 a	4.103 b
	(1.0998)	(0.9798)	(0.9354)	(0.9671)	(0.9084)
Price	5.489 a	5.881 ab	6.241 b	5.740 a	6.630 b
	(1.0329)	(1.5327)	(1.8203)	(1.5083)	(2.0618)

a, b, c: values with the same letter as the superscript indicate no statistically significant differences between the groups (columns) based on the pairwise mean comparison across groups using Tukey Kramer test, $p < 0.05$.

Table 4 thus highlights how gender and education is likely to play a role in consumers' ability to identify the origin of the EVOO product. This is consistent with findings from the general psychological theory about consumers and food labels, which identifies female and educated consumers as having greater ability to understand labeling information, as well as being more likely to take informed food choices and pay a higher price for their purchases [37,38].

4. Conclusions

The present study confirms that the COO label is an effective tool to differentiate food products, in this case EVOO. In particular, our findings point out that, in Italy, the EVOO with domestic origin gains a premium price equal to +35% (+2.13 €/liter) compared to a product labeled as a blend of European EVOOs. Thus, on average, the mandatory COO labeling regulation for EVOO (Reg. (EU) No 29/2012) can be an effective tool for consumers to identify the origin of the product and for producers to differentiate their products. There is, however, a share of consumers in our sample, 19.04% (187), that incorrectly identifies the origin of EVOO purchased and this more often occurs among consumers who report having purchased Italian EVOO. On the one hand, this is likely due to producers' branding strategies, which may hinder the effectiveness of COO information on labels in signaling the origin of the product. On the other hand, COO information, while useful for legal purposes, is not necessarily relevant to all consumers of EVOO, since other extrinsic clues like price may sometimes prevail in orienting EVOO choices.

Findings also indicate that education likely plays a role in correctly identifying the origin of the product, since it enhances consumers' ability to process the information reported on the label of the product, including information about the product's origins. Regarding this last point, government bodies, as well as food manufacturers and retailers, could implement signpost colored labeling to more easily communicate the origins of the product. A simple visual symbol to indicate a product's origins may lower the cognitive effort needed to process the information on the label and so facilitate consumers' identification of the country of origin. The use of a visual, color-based symbol has already been identified as a promising policy tool to support consumers in making healthier food choices at the supermarket. Several studies are offering encouraging findings in support of color-based labels as an effective policy approach to guiding consumers' food purchases [39,40].

The present analysis is not, however, free from limitations. First, it does not explain the mechanism preventing consumers from decoding the origin of the product. This can depend on several additional psychological factors as well as on consumer knowledge related aspects, including the individual olive oil knowledge, which are not captured in the present analysis. Second, the study focuses on a consumer sample interviewed in a single Italian region, and on a single product category, EVOO, to test consumers' ability to correctly identify a product's origin. Future research will therefore aim to address these limitations by exploring the psychological mechanism underlying the incorrect association between the product and country of origin as well as exploring to what extent the olive oil knowledge affects such relation. Furthermore, we will expand the list of products against which consumer's ability to correctly identify the country of origin is tested.

Author Contributions: Conceptualization, F.B., L.R. and B.C.d.G.; methodology, L.R. and F.B.; writing—original draft preparation, F.B. and L.R.; writing—review and editing, L.R., D.C. and F.B.; visualization, F.B., D.C. and B.C.d.G.; supervision, B.C.d.G. All authors have read and agreed to the published version of the manuscript.

Funding: This work has been supported by AGER 2 Project, grant n° 2016-0174 and by the EU through the Puglia Region: "Avviso aiuti a sostegno dei Cluster Tecnologici Regionali per l'Innovazione"—Progetto: "T.A.P.A.S.S.—Tecnologie Abilitanti per Produzioni Agroalimentari Sicure e Sostenibili"—codice PELM994.

Conflicts of Interest: The authors declare no conflict of interest.

References

1. International Olive Council (IOC). EU Olive Oil Figures. 2019. Available online: https://www.internationaloliveoil.org/what-we-do/economic-affairs-promotion-unit/#figures (accessed on 5 June 2020).

2. Roselli, L.; Carlucci, D.; De Gennaro, B.C. What Is the Value of Extrinsic Olive Oil Cues in Emerging Markets? Empirical Evidence from the US E-Commerce Retail Market. *Agribusiness* **2016**, *32*, 329–342. [CrossRef]
3. European Commission. *EU agricultural outlook for markets and income, 2018–2030*; European Commission, DG Agriculture and Rural Development: Brussels, Belgium, 2018.
4. Caswell, J.A.; Mojduszka, E.M. Using informational labeling to influence the market for quality in food products. *Am. J. Agric. Econ.* **1996**, *78*, 1248–1253. [CrossRef]
5. Roe, B.; Sheldon, I. Credence good labeling: The efficiency and distributional implications of several policy approaches. *Am. J. Agric. Econ.* **2007**, *89*, 1020–1033. [CrossRef]
6. Roe, B.E.; Teisl, M.F.; Deans, C.R. The economics of voluntary versus mandatory labels. *Annu. Rev. Resour. Econ.* **2014**, *6*, 407–427. [CrossRef]
7. Commission Implementing Regulation (EU) No 29/2012 on Marketing Standards for Olive Oil of 13 January 2012 (Codification). Available online: https://eur-lex.europa.eu/legal-content/EN/TXT/HTML/?uri=CELEX:32012R0029&from=EN (accessed on 27 March 2020).
8. Fotopoulos, C.; Krystallis, A. Purchasing motives and profile of the Greek organic consumer: A countrywide survey. *Br. Food J.* **2002**, *104*, 730–765. [CrossRef]
9. Cicia, G.; Del Giudice, T.; Scarpa, R. Welfare Loss due to lack of traceability in extra-virgin olive oil: A case study. *Cah. Options Mediterr.* **2005**, *64*, 19–27.
10. Bimbo, F.; Bonanno, A.; Viscecchia, R. An empirical framework to study food labelling fraud: An application to the Italian extra-Virgin olive oil market. *Aust. J. Agric. Econ.* **2019**, *63*, 701–725. [CrossRef]
11. Roselli, L.; Cicia, G.; Del Giudice, T.; Cavallo, C.; Vecchio, R.; Carfora, V.; Caso, D.; Sardaro, R.; Carlucci, D.; De Gennaro, B. Testing consumers' acceptance for an extra-virgin olive oil with a naturally increased content in polyphenols: The case of ultrasounds extraction. *J. Funct. Foods* **2020**, *69*, 103940. [CrossRef]
12. Bonroy, O.; Constantatos, C. On the use of labels in credence goods markets. *J. Regul. Econ.* **2008**, *33*, 237–252. [CrossRef]
13. Meerza, S.I.A.; Giannakas, K.; Yiannaka, A. Markets and welfare effects of food fraud. *Aust. J. Agric. Res. Econ.* **2019**, *63*, 759–789. [CrossRef]
14. Rosen, S. Hedonic prices and implicit markets: Product differentiation in pure competition. *J. Political Econ.* **1974**, *82*, 34–55. [CrossRef]
15. Ladd, G.W.; Suvannunt, V. A model of consumer goods characteristics. *Am. J. Agric. Econ.* **1976**, *58*, 504–510. [CrossRef]
16. Szathvary, S.; Trestini, S. A Hedonic Analysis of Nutrition and Health Claims on Fruit Beverage Products. *J. Agric. Econ.* **2014**, *1*, 1–13. [CrossRef]
17. Pearson, K. On the criterion that a given system of deviations from the probable in the case of a correlated system of variables is such that it can be reasonably supposed to have arisen from random sampling. *Lond. Edinb. Dublin Philos. Mag. J. Sci.* **1900**, *50*, 157–175. [CrossRef]
18. Goodman, L.A.; Kruskal, W.H. Measures of association for cross classifications. In *Measures of Association for Cross Classifications*; Springer: New York, NY, USA, 1979.
19. Tukey, J.W. *The Problem of Multiple Comparisons*; Unpublished manuscript; Princeton University: Princeton, NJ, USA, 1953.
20. Kennedy, P.E. Estimation with correctly interpreted dummy variables in semilogarithmic equations. *Am. Econ. Rev.* **1981**, *71*, 801.
21. Ramsey, J.B. Tests for specification errors in classical linear least squares regression analysis. *J. R. Stat. Soc.* **1969**, *31*, 50–371. [CrossRef]
22. Breusch, T.; Pagan, A. A Simple Test of Heteroskedasticity and Random Coefficient Variation. *Econometrica* **1979**, *47*, 1287–1294. [CrossRef]
23. Cook, R.D.; Weisberg, S. Diagnostics for heteroscedasticity in regression. *Biometrika* **1983**, *1*, 1–10. [CrossRef]
24. D'Agostino, R.B.; Balanger, A.; D'Agostino, R.B., Jr. A suggestion for using powerful and informative tests of normality'. *Am. Stat.* **1990**, *44*, 316–321.
25. Carlucci, D.; De Gennaro, B.; Roselli, L.; Seccia, A. E-Commerce retail of extra virgin olive oil: An hedonic analysis of Italian smes supply. *Br. Food J.* **2014**, *116*, 1600–1617. [CrossRef]
26. Vecchio, R.; Annunziata, A. The role of PDO/PGI labelling in Italian consumers' food choices. *Agric. Econ. Res. Rev.* **2011**, *12*, 80–98.

27. Grunert, K.G.; Aachmann, K. Consumer reactions to the use of EU quality labels on food products: A review of the literature. *Food Control* **2016**, *59*, 178–187. [CrossRef]
28. European Commission. Commission Staff Working Paper Summary of the Impact Assessment on Geographical Indicators. 2010. Available online: https://publications.europa.eu/en/publication-detail/-/publication/988e1e61-cdb8-4a99-a005-93863782c6ab/language-en (accessed on 19 March 2020).
29. Aprile, M.C.; Caputo, V.; Nayga, R.M., Jr. Consumers' valuation of food quality labels: The case of the European geographic indication and organic farming labels. *Int. J. Consum.* **2012**, *36*, 158–165. [CrossRef]
30. Menapace, L.; Colson, G.; Grebitus, C.; Facendola, M. Consumers' preferences for geographical origin labels: Evidence from the Canadian olive oil market. *Eur. Rev. Agric. Econ.* **2011**, *38*, 193–212. [CrossRef]
31. Panico, T.; Del Giudice, T.; Caracciolo, F. Quality dimensions and consumer preferences: A choice experiment in the Italian extra-Virgin olive oil market. *Agric. Econ. Res. Rev.* **2014**, *15*, 100–112.
32. Yangui, A.; Costa-Font, M.; Gil, J.M. The effect of personality traits on consumers' preferences for extra virgin olive oil. *Food Qual. Prefer.* **2016**, *51*, 27–38. [CrossRef]
33. Hughner, R.S.; McDonagh, P.; Prothero, A.; Shultz, C.J., II; Stanton, J. Who are organic food consumers? A compilation and review of why people purchase organic food. *J. Consum. Behav.* **2007**, *6*, 94–110. [CrossRef]
34. Grunert, K.G. *Innovation in Agri-food Systems: Product Quality and Consumer Acceptance*; Wageningen Academic Publishers: Wageningen, The Netherlands, 2005.
35. Leclerc, F.; Schmitt, B.H.; Dubé, L. Foreign branding and its effects on product perceptions and attitudes. *J. Mark. Res.* **1994**, *31*, 263–270. [CrossRef]
36. Zhou, L.; Yang, Z.; Hui, M.K. Non-local or local brands? A multi-level investigation into confidence in brand origin identification and its strategic implications. *J. Acad. Mark. Sci.* **2010**, *38*, 202–218. [CrossRef]
37. Rappoport, L.; Peters, G.R.; Downey, R.; McCann, T.; Huff-Corzine, L. Gender and age differences in food cognition. *Appetite* **1993**, *20*, 33–52. [CrossRef]
38. Verbeke, W.; Ward, R.W. Consumer interest in information cues denoting quality, traceability and origin: An application of ordered probit models to beef labels. *Food Qual. Prefer.* **2006**, *17*, 453–467. [CrossRef]
39. Egnell, M.; Talati, Z.; Gombaud, M.; Galan, P.; Hercberg, S.; Pettigrew, S.; Julia, C. Consumers' Responses to Front-of-Pack Nutrition Labelling: Results from a Sample from The Netherlands. *Nutrients* **2019**, *11*, 1817. [CrossRef] [PubMed]
40. Dubois, P.; Albuquerque, P.; Allais, O.; Bonnet, C.; Bertail, P.; Combris, P.; Lahlou, S.; Rigal, N.; Ruffieux, B.; Chandon, P. Effects of front-of-pack labels on the nutritional quality of supermarket food purchases: Evidence from a large-scale randomized controlled trial. *J. Acad. Mark. Sci.* **2019**, *1*, 1–20.

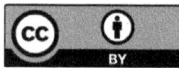

© 2020 by the authors. Licensee MDPI, Basel, Switzerland. This article is an open access article distributed under the terms and conditions of the Creative Commons Attribution (CC BY) license (http://creativecommons.org/licenses/by/4.0/).

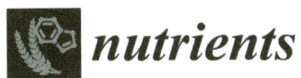

Review

Factors that Influence the Perceived Healthiness of Food—Review

Brigitta Plasek *, Zoltán Lakner and Ágoston Temesi

Department of Food Chain Management, Institute of Agrobusiness, Szent István University, Villányi Str. 29-43, 1118 Budapest, Hungary; lakner.zoltan@etk.szie.hu (Z.L.); temesi.agoston@etk.szie.hu (Á.T.)
* Correspondence: plasek.brigitta@etk.szie.hu; Tel.: +36-1-305-7100 (ext. 6178)

Received: 22 May 2020; Accepted: 22 June 2020; Published: 24 June 2020

Abstract: The interest of consumers is the consumption of healthy food, whereas the interest of food manufacturers is that consumers recognize the produced "healthier" food items on the shelves, so they can satisfy their demands. This way, identifying the factors that influence the perceived healthiness of food products is a mutual interest. What causes consumers to consider one product more beneficial to health than another? In recent years, numerous studies have been published on the topic of the influence of several health-related factors on consumer perception. This analysis collected and categorized the research results related to this question. This review collects 59 articles with the help of the search engines Science Direct, Wiley Online Library, MDPI and Emerald Insight between 1 January 2014 and 31 March 2019. Our paper yielded six separate categories that influence consumers in their perception of the healthiness of food items: the communicated information—like FoP labels and health claims, the product category, the shape and colour of the product packaging, the ingredients of the product, the organic origin of the product, and the taste and other sensory features of the product.

Keywords: perceived healthiness; product attributes; healthy food; consumer perception; food packaging; consumer behavior

1. Introduction

Which food can be considered beneficial to health? Science and consumers answer this question differently. According to certain sources, there is no precise definition of what can be considered healthy food, or else existing definitions are not yet appropriate [1–3]. The understanding of the category of "healthy food" differs even among experts; moreover, some treat the words "healthy" and "nutritious" as synonyms [4,5]. What can be considered healthy for whom depends on gender, age, metabolism, obesity, diseases or sensitivities. A nutritious food product generally considered definitely beneficial to health with several positive effects in case of certain diseases can be harmful for consumers suffering from other diseases [6].

Let us illustrate the effort to define healthy food with two examples. In their article, Zaheer and Bach [7] (p. 1) applied the following definition: "*Per the United States Food & Drug Administration (FDA), Healthy foods are defined as those that are "low in fat, low in saturated fat, contain at least 10% of daily value for vitamins A, C, calcium, iron, protein fiber" and are limited in amount of sodium and cholesterol (USFDA).*" Rodman and his colleagues [5] (p. 83) employed the following definition for their research: "*Foods that provide essential nutrients and energy to sustain growth, health and life while satiating hunger; usually fresh or minimally processed foods, naturally dense in nutrients, that when eaten in moderation and in combination with other foods, sustain growth, repair and maintain vital processes, promote longevity, reduce disease, and strengthen and maintain the body and its functions. Healthy foods do not contain ingredients that contribute* to disease or impede recovery when consumed at normal levels. (University of Washington Center for Public Health Nutrition (UWCPHN) 2013 [8])".

Dieticians argue that there is no such thing as healthy or unhealthy food; instead, there is only appropriate or inappropriate diet (e.g., [1]). However, since consumers consider certain foods healthy, while others unhealthy, it is important for us to know how they make this distinction. Mai and Hoffman [9] (p. 8) use the term perceived healthiness, which, based on Howlett et al. [10], they define as *"Perceived healthiness is a consumer's expectation of a product's influence on his or her state of health"*. The importance of "perceived healthiness" is also supported by the research findings on health claims by Steinhauser and colleagues [11] that the higher the level of perceived healthiness of a product is, the more likely it is that the product will be purchased. All this becomes a factor that also increases the willingness to pay and purchase if it takes into account what influences the credibility of the health benefits of a product [12].

The effects of food on health is a widely researched topic, which gets attention from various aspects, thus our knowledge-base related to its consumer perception is also expanding. In their review, Niebylski and colleagues [13] examined the effects of taxation, subsidies and easy access on the consumption of products considered healthy. According to the results of Provencher and Jacob's review [14] specifically on perceived healthiness, cognitive factors—among them, brand and type of product—have an effect on the perceived healthiness of food, but such features do not influence the choice and intake of food. The reviews of Alba and Williams [15], and Krishna [16] highlight the topic that continues to be researched ever since, namely that the perceived healthiness of food has an effect also on the assessment of the taste of food (e.g., [17,18]). However, research attests that the perception of the healthiness of food is not influenced by one factor only, but by a combination of factors [19,20], so we can state that this topic is highly complex and important both for consumers and companies.

The aim of our literature review is to assemble earlier research and survey the factors that influence consumers in their perception of the healthiness of food.

2. Research Methodology

In an attempt to access the articles related to the perceived healthiness of food, we employed several search engines—Science Direct, MDPI, Emerald Insight, Wiley Online Library—in our literature analysis. In recent years, numerous review-type articles touching on the topic of healthiness have been published (e.g., [12–18,21,22]), but they only fleetingly mention the issue. The present literature review, however, specifically approaches the topic from the consumers' point of view and so examines the factors which, according to research literature, influence consumer perception of the healthiness of food.

Between 2012 and 2016, several review articles touched on the topic of perceived healthiness of food [13,15,16,21,22] or chose it as their main topic [14]. However, it has remained a widely researched area ever since, so we focused on the time period that followed. Articles published between 1 January 2014 and 31 March 2019 were selected using the following terms:

I. "perceived healthiness of food"
II. "evaluating food product healthfulness" OR "evaluation of food healthiness"

We looked for the terms in the title, the abstract or among the key words; naturally, because of the way they work, there were slight differences when using the different search engines.

In the I. case, on the ScienceDirect surface we looked for the exact term "perceived healthiness" in quotation marks in the "title, abstract or keywords" fields, while "food" appeared in the "terms" field. On the MDPI page, a very similar method was used, "perceived healthiness"—again in quotation marks—was searched for in the abstract, while "food" was searched for in "all fields". Between the two terms specified in quotation marks, we used the AND relationship to make sure that the search results include both terms. On the Emerald Insight surface, we looked for the complete terms in the abstract and the title, while with Wiley Online Library, in the abstract only, without quotation marks.

In the II. case, on the ScienceDirect search field first "evaluating healthiness", then "evaluation of healthiness" in quotation marks was in the "title, abstract or keywords" field, while "food" was in the terms field. Very similarly to this and point I, on MDPI, the previously mentioned terms were searched for in the abstract, while the term "foods" was searched for in all fields. Just like in the first case, we ran the search with the AND relationship between the search terms. With Wiley and Emerald Insight, we collected the articles in a similar way, looking for the terms in the abstract only and in the title and the abstract, respectively. The search results and the filtering of hits are illustrated in Figure 1.

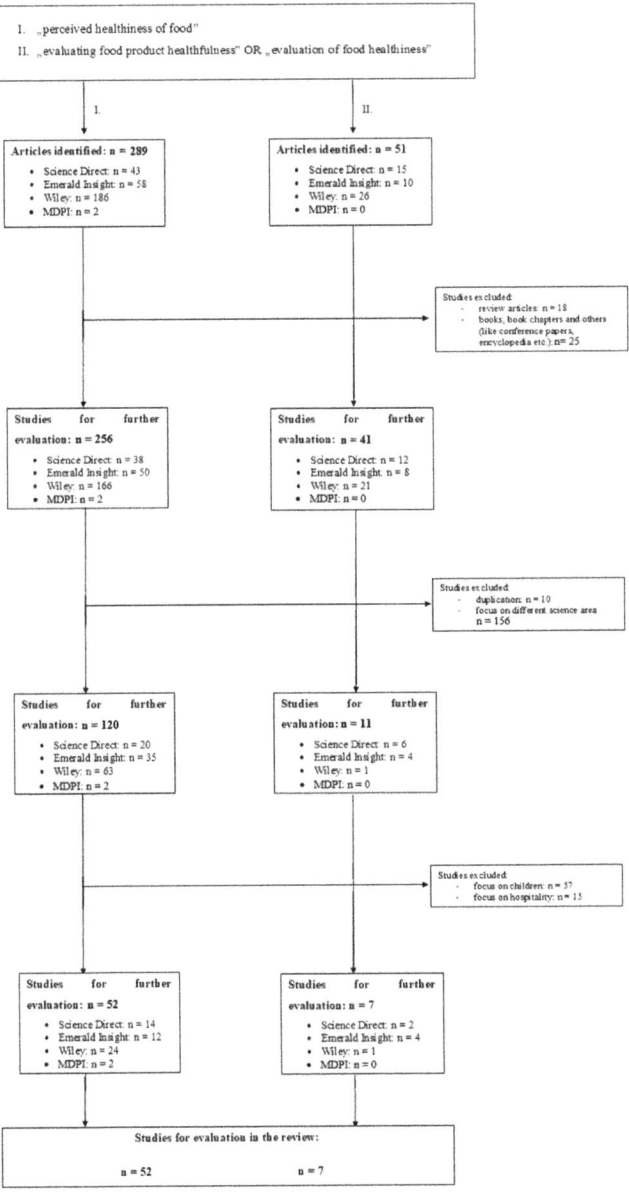

Figure 1. The search hits and the steps of their filtering.

In our analysis, we specifically focused on the products of the food industry, so we did not include research on restaurants, catering establishments, and those on various casseroles, boiled and fried foods served on plates. Moreover, articles on children's dietary habits and on healthy food provision were also not included. The accessed full-length articles were evaluated by two authors (B.P. and Á.T.). Any contested issues were resolved by three authors (B.P., Á.T. and Z.L.).

3. Results

The main question of our research is what influences consumers in their perception of the positive effects of a given product on health, which, for the sake of simplification, we will refer to as the healthiness of the product. We provide a comprehensive display of the main results of the articles on the topic in Table 1, then we analyse them, reviewing the points of agreement and opposition.

Table 1. The articles included in the literature analysis and their main Claims.

Source	Year	Country	Method	Item Number	Main Claims
Marques da Rosa, Spence and Miletto Tonetto [23]	2019	Brazil	2×3 within-groups experimental design; $2 \times 2 \times 2$ intra-groups experiment design	50 + 102	• A buttered product was considered healthier in a round, red and yellow packaging • The colour and shape of the packaging influence perceived healthiness
Pires, de Noronha and Trindade [24]	2019	Brazil	Online survey; focus groups	263 + 16	• In the case of Bolognese sauce, consumers prefer less sodium to omega-3 content
Yarar, Machiels and Orth [25]	2019	Not indicated	One factorial between subject design	78 + 144	• Consumers consider a product in packaging that resembles a slim human figure healthier, especially if they themselves do not have such a figure • The shape of the packaging plays an important role in the perceived healthiness of the product
Machín et al. [26]	2018	Uruguay	shopping situation (on online surface)	1182	• "FOP nutrition labelling schemes effectively improved the average healthfulness of food choice by respondents." (p. 60) • Health motivation can play a key role in the use of FOP (front of package) nutrition information

Table 1. Cont.

Source	Year	Country	Method	Item Number	Main Claims
Hartmann et al. [27]	2018	UK, Sweden, Poland, France	Online survey	1950	• Indicators of perceived healthiness: searching for information, knowledge on nutrition, and the health effects of the nutrients. There was a willingness to pay extra for "Free-from" products among those who look for information and prefer natural products.
Festila and Chrysochou [28]	2018	Denmark, United States	Content analysis	2545 products	• The colour, shape, material of and the illustrations on the packaging differ between the products claimed healthy and those considered "normal" in general and also according to product category • Products considered healthier appear on the market with lighter, matter or more balanced colours and in angular packaging in the examined countries
Polizer Rocha et al. [29]	2018	Brazil	Word association test, EsSense profile, attitudinal questionnaire	120	• The biggest health advantage for consumers of frankfurters can be achieved through a decreased sodium- and fat content. Omega-3 and fibre source are less preferred features in this product
Wijayaratne et al. [30]	2018	Australia	Two stage online survey	756	• Food-literacy has a positive effect on the attitudes of the "dietary-gatekeepers" consumer group towards healthy food • Those with higher food-literacy are more confident in the preparation of a healthier diet
Lee et al. [31]	2018	Taiwan	Survey	122	• Although a bio label influences perceived healthiness, it does not increase the consumption of such products among "health externals"
Vila-López and Küster-Boluda [32]	2018	Spain	Experimental sessions	300	• Younger consumers are more influenced by aesthetic/commercial signs (colours) than by "technical cues" (healthy messages)

Table 1. *Cont.*

Source	Year	Country	Method	Item Number	Main Claims
Lidón et al. [33]	2018	Spain	between-subjects experiment	147	• Placing a picture suggesting healthiness on the packaging may increase willingness to purchase • When perceiving a product, there is a strong positive relationship between healthiness and product quality
Acton and Hammond [34]	2018	Canada	Online survey	1000	• A small group of the respondents (5–10%) said that the "high in … " caption in the front of the packaging (FOP) seemed harsh for them • According to the majority of the respondents, FOP captions help to better control the choice of healthy food products
Carabante et al. [35]	2018	USA	Consumer test, questionnaire	150	• Communicating the health benefits of the fat composition resulting from the diet of grass-fed beef increased overall liking and purchase intent • "Health Benefit Information" (HBI) decreased the effect of juiciness and tenderness on overall liking
Miraballes and Gámbaro [36]	2018	Uruguay	Conjoint analysis	60 + 60	• A product was considered healthier if, in addition to the caption communicating ingredients, there was also a picture/image on it
Wardy et al. [37]	2018	USA	Consumer testing	128	• A 50% and/or 100% decrease of saccharose and the communication of this fact—displaying HBI- had a positive effect on the overall liking of the product
Benson et al. [38]	2018	Ireland	Survey	1039	• Respondents rated the healthiness of the tested products the same regardless of the "nutrition and health claims", there was no significant difference in their assessment
Shan et al. [39]	2017a	Republic of Ireland	Focus groups	40	• The perception of consumers was influenced by the healthiness, taste, and prevalence of the product • To make processed meat products healthier, participants would decrease the sodium- and fat content rather than add health-preserving ingredients

Table 1. Cont.

Source	Year	Country	Method	Item Number	Main Claims
Shan et al. [40]	2017b	Republic of Ireland	Survey	481	• Participants preferred enrichment with omega-3 to the non-enriched product, and the least preferred enriching ingredient was vitamin E.
Labbe et al. [41]	2017	Switzerland	Conjoint	57	• The choice among frozen pre-packaged pizzas was more influenced by the expected taste experience than by perceived health effect and was not influenced by the expected feeling of being sated.
Prada et al. [42]	2017	Portugal	Survey	204 + 85	• Products of organic origin were considered healthier, tastier and less energy-filled than their traditional counterparts—"halo-effect" in case of bio food products
Tijssen et al. [43]	2017	Netherland	Experiment; Implicit Association Test (IAT)	148 + 140	• Participants associated paler coloured packaging with health, whereas regular packaging was considered more striking • Wrapping a 'healthier' product in warmer, fuller, pale coloured packaging improves sensory expectations, and can make the product more attractive
Marino et al. [44]	2017	Italy	Sensory analysis and consumer survey	8 + 250	• When choosing healthy food products, the expected less good taste is the biggest obstacle for consumers not wanting to forgo good taste • If the sensory features of a product are not appropriate, information on nutritional characteristics is not enough for the consumers to choose healthier alternatives
Cavallo and Piqueras-Fiszman [45]	2017	Italy, Netherlands	Consumer survey (online questionnaire)	214	• Italian origin played the biggest role in the perceived healthiness of the examined product (olive oil) • Having a bio origin positively influenced perceived healthiness • For Dutch consumers, hot taste had a negative influence on perceived healthiness, whereas Italian consumers were not influenced by it • In general, a darker glass bottle had a negative effect on the perceived healthiness of the examined product, with some exceptions: it had a positive influence on Italian consumers and on those for whom the origin of the product is important

Table 1. Cont.

Source	Year	Country	Method	Item Number	Main Claims
Gineikiene, Kiudyte and Degutis [46]	2017	Lithuania	Survey; Structural equation modeling	295	• Health-conscious consumers tend to disregard messages related to the health benefits of functional foods, and prefer bio food products • In the case of functional, organic, and traditional products, scepticism towards health claims has a stronger negative effect on the perceived healthiness than the effect of health consciousness
Rebouças et al. [47]	2017	Brazil	Sensory evaluation	96	• Information on the ingredients and nutritional values of cashew- and soy drinks and functional statements related to this information have a positive effect on consumers' perception of healthiness and of nutritional values • The extent of consumer attention paid to a healthy diet and food neophobia did not influence perceived healthiness of the product.
Tleis, Callieris and Roma [48]	2017	Lebanon	Face-to-face survey	320	• Lebanese consumers purchase bio-products because they consider them healthier and safer
Brečić, Mesić, and Cerjak [49]	2017	Croatia	Face-to-face interviews	500	• The dominant factor explaining 18.8% of the sample is "health and sensory characteristics". The factor includes the sensory characteristics (taste, smell) of the product and its composition • One segment is the "healthy and tasty food lovers" who are sensitive to the "inner" characteristics of the food: they are concerned about additives and artificial ingredients and prefer foods rich in vitamins and minerals
Thomson et al. [50]	2017	Melbourne, Shanghai, Vietnam, Indonesia, Singapore	Online survey	3951	• there are differences in the perceived healthiness of a certain product between respondents from different countries • sweetened, higher circulation products and children's drinks were considered healthier in Vietnam, Shanghai and Indonesia than in Singapore and Melbourne
Apaolaza et al. [51]	2017	Spain	one-way between-groups experimental design	90	• "the organic halo effect on hedonic evaluation and purchase intention was totally mediated by increases in sensory ratings and perceived healthiness, providing a process explanation for this effect" • indicating the organic origin of the product significantly increased its perceived healthiness

Table 1. Cont.

Source	Year	Country	Method	Item Number	Main Claims
Anders and Schroeter [52]	2017	Canada	Survey	8114	• Taste, convenience and affordability are more important than information related to healthiness and the resulting benefits
Talati et al. [53].	2016	Australia	Survey	2058	• Testing different FoP labels and their effect on perceived healthiness • "daily intake guide" and "multiple traffic light" had a positive effect on the global perception of the product compared to when no FoP labels were used • Nevertheless, FoP labels only had a weaker effect on perceived healthiness, but a bigger impact on global evaluations
Samoggia [54]	2016	Italy	Face-to-face survey	402	• Health-oriented consumers are open to health-enhancing wine products, and their willingness to pay is also higher. Consumers of wine think that consumption of wine offers protection against hypertension and atherosclerosis. • Consumers consider wine a healthy product
Seegebarth et al. [55]	2016	USA, Germany	Survey	206 + 240	• American consumers appreciated the functional values provided by bio foods more than German consumers did. Moreover, American consumers purchase bio food because they consider them healthier and of better quality.
Puska & Luomala [56]	2016	Finland	Pilot test + online survey	17 + 1081	• Respondents expect different health benefits from two products perceived equally healthy ("physical well-being, outward appearance, energy dimensions" vs. "emotional well-being, self-management and social responsibility")
Larkin and Martin [57]	2016	UK	Experimental sessions	141	• The weight of the consumer influences their perception of the calorie content of a product considered healthy, while this effect is less pronounced in the case of "unhealthy" food • Consumers underestimate the calorie content of foods considered healthy compared to those considered unhealthy
Szocs and Lefebvre [58]	2016	USA	Within subjects experiment, lab study, between subject design,	122 + 111 + 166	• Perceived healthiness and perceived calorie content are not influenced by the physical state of the product (e.g., liquid or solid) • Participants perceived more processed products less healthy and richer in calories • Participants considered the less processed fruit and yoghurt plate healthier than the more processed smoothie

Table 1. Cont.

Source	Year	Country	Method	Item Number	Main Claims
Lazzarini et al. [59]	2016	Switzerland	Experiment	85	• The perceived healthiness and the perceived environmentally friendly nature of a product correlate • The indicators of perceived healthiness: product category, fat content, extent of processing and the indication of organic origin
Jo et al. [60]	2016	France	Framed field experiment	129	• Consumers are willing to pay more for "healthy" products if objective information on the nutritional composition is available • Information on nutritional value increases willingness to pay for "healthy" foods, while decreases it for foods considered unhealthy
Fenko, Lotterman and Galetzka [61]	2016	Netherlands	Questionnaire	165	• Products in angular packaging were perceived healthier than those in rounded packaging • The higher a consumer's general health interest, the less they considered a product healthy • Product category significantly influenced perceived healthiness, while brand name did not
Hipp et al. [62]	2016	USA	Survey	2015	• The examined signs and symbols that were displayed on vending machines and at cafés in order to foster health-conscious food choices did not help consumer decision
Rizk & Treat [63]	2015a	USA	Survey	272	• In the case of products in bigger packaging/portions participants had difficulty in distinguishing their perceived healthiness
Rizk and Treat [64]	2015b	USA	Survey	169	• Single women mostly relied on fat- and fibre content when assessing the healthiness of a product • Displaying protein- and sugar content mitigated reliance on fat- and fibre content
Sütterlin and Siegrist [65]	2015	Switzerland	Experiments	164 + 202 + 251 + 162	• people assess the healthiness of a product with the help of simple heuristics—e.g., in the case of fructose: fruit-healthy—see health halo effect
Wąsowicz et al. [66]	2015	Poland	Focus group, survey	8 + 90	• consumers associate certain colours with the healthiness of the product. yellow, blue, red and green colours may indicate healthiness • blue and yellow colours evoked positive emotions both from the perspective of healthiness and of naturalness

Table 1. Cont.

Source	Year	Country	Method	Item Number	Main Claims
Luomala et al. [67]	2015	Finland	Personal and group interviews	40	• The dieting status and health motivation of consumers as well as the assessment of the benefits offered by the product influence the perceived taste and healthiness of the product • Those who are not on a diet are more critical in their assessment of what is tasty and healthy • Those on a diet consider light salad dressing and light sausage healthy, while those not on a diet consider these products unhealthy
Xie et al. [68]	2015	China	Survey (questionnaire) + in depth interviews	388 + 18	• Health benefits are one of the most important factors that make consumers purchase organic products
Grubor et al. [69]	2015	Serbia	Focus groups, survey	? + 300	• "Consumers' health attitudes" mostly influence the consumption of enriched products the pre-enrichment version of which they had already been familiar with
Vasiljevic, Pechey, and Marteau [70]	2015	UK	Between-subject experiment	955	• Regardless of the label, participants considered chocolate tastier, and a muesli bar healthier • A frowning emoji on a white background had the effect of a muesli bar being considered less tasty and less healthy • Emojis had a stronger influence on the perception of healthiness and tastiness of snacks than did coloured labels • Frowning emojis have a stronger influence than smiley ones on perceived healthiness for products where perception of healthiness is influenced by the health halo effect
Reutner, Genschow and Wänke [71]	2015	Switzerland	Between subject experiment	91 + 143	• The colour red influences the assessment of products considered unhealthy (dangerous) more than that of healthy products • Using red colour mitigated the consumption of foods considered unhealthy, and also influenced the choice of these products
Thomsen and Hansen [72]	2015	Denmark	qualitative pilot study; survey	16 + 599	• Improving consumer knowledge on healthy nutrition could help to make healthy food choices • It is difficult to improve the knowledge of consumers who take less interest in healthy nutrition
Dharni and Gupta [73]	2015	India	Survey	150	• Perceived usefulness of nutritional information is of key importance when making decisions related to healthy nutrition • Understanding information increases perceived usefulness, while the increase of perceived usefulness facilitates choosing better-healthier- food

Table 1. *Cont.*

Source	Year	Country	Method	Item Number	Main Claims
Annunziata, Vecchio and Kraus [74]	2015	Italy	Survey	400	• Consumers over 60 are influenced by health claims in the assessment of the healthiness of functional foods • Consumers over 60 have difficulty verifying the reliability of information • Among the several used symbols, heart was the most valuable for elderly consumers
Maehle et al. [75]	2015	USA	Conjoint analysis	306	• The issue of healthiness is less important in the case of "utilitarian food products" than for hedonic foods • Moreover, in the case of "utilitarian food products", the healthiness of the product is the least important feature compared to the taste and price of the product and the usage of "environmental label"
Bucher, Müller & Siegrist [76]	2015	Switzerland	Survey	85	• Lay consumers assessed the healthiness of a product according to aspects similar to those of experts' • When making decisions, lay consumers ignored the quantity of saturated fat, protein, and sodium in the product • Lay consumers were quite able to assess the nutrition profile of individual food items, but were less able to do so with complete dishes
Kraus [77]	2015	Poland	Survey	200	• The most important health-related features can be ranked the following way: (1) strengthens the immune system (2) lowers the risk of tumour-related diseases (3) lowers the risk of cardiovascular diseases
Rodman et al. [78]	2014	USA (Baltimore, Maryland)	In-depth interview	36	• Organic origin is important for consumers when assessing the healthiness of a product. When communicating the healthiness of the product, organic origin can have effectiveness similar to other health messages.
Orquin [79]	2014	Denmark	Brunswik lens model	1329	• Perceived healthiness mainly depends on two factors: product category and consumer knowledge on individual products • Consumers underestimate the healthiness of milk and yoghurt and overestimate that of butters and cheeses • Consumers are inclined to perceive a product healthier if they are familiar with it

Table 1. Cont.

Source	Year	Country	Method	Item Number	Main Claims
Carrete and Arroyo [80]	2014	Mexico	In-depth interviews, focus groups	8 + 30	• In general, the taste, colour, and texture of a product are more important for consumers than nutritional characteristics, which hinders healthier nutrition
Lin [81]	2014	Taiwan	2 × 2 experimental design	170 + 177	• happier people are more variety seeking in the case of healthful products or products they are not familiar with, while sadder people are more open to variety in the case of hedonic or familiar products • The type of the product "(hedonic vs. Healthful products)" influences the relationship between variety seeking and the mood of the consumer

Table 1 clearly shows that numerous factors influence consumers when assessing the healthiness of a product. In our literature analysis, we categorized these factors as follows:

- Communicated information [26,27,34,35,37,47,60,62,65,73,74,77];
- The shape and colour of the product packaging [23,25,28,32,33,43,61,66,70,71];
- The ingredients of the product [24,29,39,40,49,57,64,76];
- Product category [54,61,69,70,75,78];
- Organic origin of the product [5,31,42,45,46,48,51,55,68];
- The taste and other sensory features of the product [41,44,52,70,79].

The perceived healthiness of a food product is influenced by numerous factors. For bigger clarity, the main points of the research results are summarized in Figure 2.

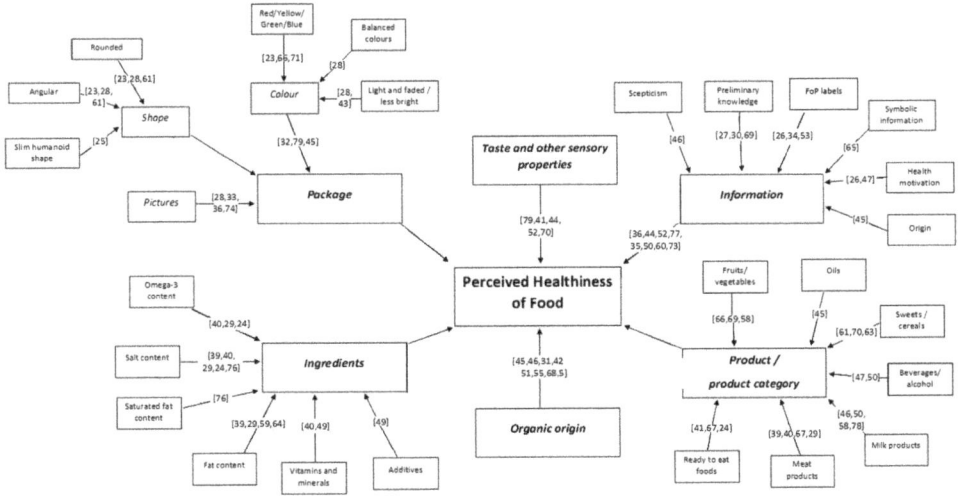

Figure 2. Factors influencing perceived healthiness.

3.1. The Effect of the Communicated Information on the Perceived Healthiness of a Product

When companies provide consumers with information related to nutritional value or to health effects in some way on the product packaging, it has a positive effect on perceived healthiness [26,34–36,47]. At the same time, care must be taken that consumers comprehend this information correctly, so that they do not evoke undesired associations [62], and consumer scepticism related to health claims must also be taken into account [74], as in this case information may even have a negative effect on assessing healthiness.

All this also entails how much of the messages communicated through the product a consumer will comprehend and thus how healthy they will perceive the product. This is supported by the previous knowledge of the consumer, which influences perceived healthiness to a great extent [27,69,78]. Moreover, perceived healthiness of a product is further improved by adding a picture of the product to the communicated information [36] and is also affected by FoP labels and health claims [26,34,38,53]. Although several studies show that FoP labels help consumers choose healthier foods [26,34], due to the diversity of FoP labels, it cannot be clearly stated that their use always helps greatly in increasing the perceived healthiness of the product [53].

The health motivation of the consumer also influences the assessment of the product; Machín et al. [26] maintain that it plays a pivotal role in the way front of package information is used. In contrast, according to the results of Rebouças et al. [47], consumer interest in healthy nutrition does not influence the acceptance and perceived healthiness and nutritional value of the product they examined ("cashew nut beverage").

3.2. The Influence of the Shape and Colour of the Product Packaging

Research results confirm that the shape and colour of the product packaging influence the perceived healthiness of the product, but from certain aspects the results contradict each other. Whereas Marques et al. [23] maintain that a product is perceived to be healthier in a rounded packaging, other researchers [28,61] claim that consumers perceive a product healthier in angular shaped packaging. A further result related to the shape of the packaging is that packaging resembling a slim human figure is perceived healthier [25].

The influence of the colour of the packaging has also been examined by several researchers. According to the results of Marques et al.'s research [23], buttered products were perceived healthier in a red and yellow coloured packaging. The effect of the colour red is mentioned by several other studies. Wąsowicz et al. [66], along with yellow, green and blue, mention the colour red as a colour referring to health. At the same time, Reutner et al. [71] assert that the colour red can have a significant effect on the refusal of unhealthy foods. Certain colours and hues, however, can imply that the product is less healthy: research participants considered dark glass [45] and colours hinting at artificiality ("heather", "pink", "celadon") [66] to be referring to unhealthy or less healthy products.

Contrasts resulting from the perception of colour can be attributed to the variety of products and their different packaging investigated in the studies; so it is possible that in the case of a buttered product, the red & yellow colour combination found by Marques et al. [23] was perceived healthier, while it can be different for other products. Therefore, when discussing the effect of colour, it is important to acknowledge the influence of product category. Differences between countries are also important; so for example, in Denmark, paler, whereas in the United States, balanced colour tones are more standard on healthy products [28]. Moreover, the effect of colour can differ according to the age of the consumer: for example, with young people, colours have a stronger effect than health messages [32].

3.3. The Effect of the Ingredients of a Product on its Perceived Healthiness

Results related to ingredients show that consumers mostly pay attention to the ingredients that nutrition experts emphasize in relation to healthy nutrition. The majority of the research studies we have examined address sodium- and fat content as well as omega-3 content. According to the results of Lazzarini et al.'s [59] research, the fat content of a product is an indicator of perceived healthiness for consumers.

Whether it is Bolognese sauce, frankfurter sausages, or other processed meat products, consumers prefer a reduced sodium- and fat content, so that is how a company can make consumers perceive these products healthier [24,29,39]. Moreover, while there are consumers who rely on the fat- and fibre content of the product for its perceived healthiness [64], others ignore the protein-, sodium-, and saturated fat content when making decisions [76].

The other ingredient featuring in numerous studies was omega-3. In several cases, consumers would choose to change an ingredient other than the fatty acid [24], or they did not consider the product suitable for the addition of omega-3 [29]; at the same time, they prefer if omega-3 fatty acid is added to the product rather than if nothing is added [40].

3.4. The Effect of Product Category on Perceived Healthiness

Perceived healthiness is also influenced by the product or product category [75,78]; in fact, in Orquin's [78] research, product category emerged as one of the two main factors based on which consumers perceived the healthiness of a product. In the studies, products assigned to different categories according to different criteria were compared. Fenko et al. [61] compared consumer perception of cereal- and buttered cookies, of which consumers perceived cereal cookies healthier. Vasiljevic et al. [70] compared muesli bars and chocolate, and their results show that, regardless of label, consumers perceived chocolate tastier and muesli bars healthier. According to Maehle et al.'s [75] surprising result, consumers are less concerned about the healthiness of the product if they consume it for the nutritional value (utilitarian products), than in the case of products consumed for pleasure (hedonic products).

3.5. The Effect of Organic Origin on Perceived Healthiness

Results of numerous studies have confirmed a positive effect of organic origin on the perceived healthiness of a product [42,45,48,51,68]. In addition, organic origin also facilitates the understanding of the communication of "healthy food" [5]. Health-conscious consumers also tend to show openness towards bio foods and generally ignore the health-related messages of functional foods [46].

3.6. The Effect of the Sensory Features of the Product on Perceived Healthiness

The sensory features of the product also play a role in its perceived healthiness. The taste and other sensory features of the product may dominate over the perception of healthiness [41,52,79], and if the sensory features of the product do not satisfy the consumer, then communicating the nutritional value is not enough to make the product accepted [44].

4. Discussion

The aim of our literature analysis was to explore the factors that influence the perceived healthiness of food products. Numerous studies set out to discover what influences the perceived healthiness of individual products in the time period we focused on. In the present article, we only considered research results related to foods.

Based on the research results, we identified six categories that influence perceived healthiness of a product: the effect of the communicated information, product category, the shape and colour of the product packaging, the ingredients of the product, the organic origin of the product and the taste and other sensory features of the product.

The effect of the communicated information clearly influences perceived healthiness; at the same time, previous knowledge clearly affects how this information influences perception. Product category is a main factor in the perceived healthiness of a product. In recent years, a diverse range of product categories has been tested, which makes generalizations difficult.

The most numerous contradictory research results were related to the shape and colour of the product packaging, which calls for further investigation. Research results are ambiguous concerning whether angular or rounded packaging is more suitable to communicate healthiness. One of the most researched colours is the colour red. Nevertheless, results related to the colour red do not point in the same direction.

Research results related to the ingredients of the product confirm that reducing the sodium-, sugar- and fat content increases consumer acceptance of the improved product in terms of health; at the same time, research does not give a definite answer regarding consumer perception of the possible enriching ingredients.

The organic origin of the product positively influences perceived healthiness. Health halo effect emerged in several studies in connection with bio products.

Basically, the taste and other sensory features of the product dominate over perception of healthiness. A common result of the examined studies showed that the unsuitability of sensory features cannot be balanced out by favourable perceived healthiness.

Our collected results and their juxtaposition can help with the proper planning of product development and marketing communication, and they also raise further research questions related to the inconsistent results. Our conclusions can serve as a baseline from several aspects when devising packaging of a new product. They can help with the proper design of the packaging, both in terms of shape and the used colours, and with choosing the right FoP labels. The choice of the labels used on the packaging requires special care. The type of health claim communicated by the company has to be considered carefully, provided that the use of a health claim is effective in the first place. At the same time, it is also important to consider that communicating the different ingredients may be an effective method to reach its goal.

Within the categories, we have found several conflicting results, as well as unanswered research questions, which call for further research. The most important aim of further research may be to gauge the effect of the discovered aspects relative to each other, even comparing all the aspects.

Further research may also aim at clarifying the emerged controversial results, as the research results are not uniform for example in connection with the shape of packaging and colours that evoke a healthy feeling, keeping in mind that these factors may change according to product category. Apart from clarifying discrepancies, further research may take on the task of testing specific features on different food products. Treating the constructed system as a complex entity, it is worth examining whether a different colour and shape of packaging is justified to communicate the health benefits of each food.

5. Limitations

In the course of our literature analysis, we encountered several barriers that have to be taken into account when evaluating the results. There has not been a review article on the topic since 2016, even though several new studies have been published since then. As we reviewed only the 2014–2019 time period, we can only report the results of the most modern research. The surfaces used for data collection are also important to mention: during the research, we had no access to the surfaces covering the whole literature, therefore we chose the above described search surfaces, where we could access the full-length articles. Our options were limited by the year-to-year changes in the agreement between the Hungarian Electronic Information Service National Programme (EISZ) and Elsevier [81].

Author Contributions: Conceptualization, B.P. and Á.T.; methodology, B.P.; writing—original draft preparation, B.P.; writing—review and editing, Á.T.; visualization, B.P.; supervision, Z.L. All authors have read and agreed to the published version of the manuscript.

Funding: The Project is supported by the European Union and co-financed by the European Social Fund (grant agreement no. EFOP-3.6.3-VEKOP-16-2017-00005).

Conflicts of Interest: The authors declare no conflict of interest.

References

1. Hawkes, C. Defining "healthy" and "unhealthy" foods. An international review. Prepared for the Office of Nutrition Policy and Promotion. *Health Can.* **2009**. Available online: https://www.canada.ca/en/health-canada/services/food-nutrition/healthy-eating/nutrition-policy-reports/defining-healthy-unhealthy-foods-international-review-2009-executive-summary.html (accessed on 23 June 2020).
2. Lobstein, T.; Davies, S. Defining and labelling 'healthy' and 'unhealthy' food. *Public Health Nutr.* **2009**, *12*, 331–340. [CrossRef]
3. Campbell, N.; Duhaney, T.; Ashley, L.; Arango, M.; Berg, A.; Flowitt, F.; Gelfer, M.; Kaczorowski, J.; Mang, E.; Morris, D.; et al. A National Model for Defining Healthy and Unhealthy Foods and Beverages—Canadian Health and Scientific Organization. Consensus Statement. 2016. Available online: www.hypertensiontalk.com/position-statements/ (accessed on 23 June 2020).
4. Dickson-Spillmann, M.; Siegrist, M. Consumers' knowledge of healthy diets and its correlation with dietary behaviour. *J. Hum. Nutr. Diet.* **2011**, *24*, 54–60. [CrossRef] [PubMed]
5. Rodman, S.O.; Palmer, A.M.; Zachary, D.A.; Hopkins, L.C.; Surkan, P.J. "They Just Say Organic Food Is Healthier": Perceptions of Healthy Food among Supermarket Shoppers in Southwest Baltimore. *Cult. Agric. Food Environ.* **2014**, *36*, 83–92. [CrossRef]
6. Gogus, U. *A Fundamental Guide for a Healthy Lifestyle and Nutrition*; AuthorHouse: Bloomington, IN, USA, 2011.
7. Zaheer, I.S.; Bach, C. Consumers Demand Response Patterns. University of Bridgeport. Available online: https://www.researchgate.net/publication/261993663_consumers_Demand_article_journal_Bach_Finalx (accessed on 1 March 2019).
8. University of Washington Center for Public Health Nutrition (CPHN) Defining "Healthy Foods". Available online: https://nutr.uw.edu/resource/opportunities-for-increasing-access-to-healthy-foods-washington/ (accessed on 26 June 2013).
9. Mai, R.; Hoffmann, S. How to combat the unhealthy= tasty intuition: The influencing role of health consciousness. *J. Public Policy Mark.* **2015**, *34*, 63–83. [CrossRef]
10. Howlett, E.A.; Burton, S.; Bates, K.; Huggins, K. Coming to a restaurant near you? Potential consumer responses to nutrition information disclosure on menus. *J. Consum. Res.* **2009**, *36*, 494–503. [CrossRef]
11. Steinhauser, J.; Janssen, M.; Hamm, U. Who Buys Products with Nutrition and Health Claims? A Purchase Simulation with Eye Tracking on the Influence of Consumers' Nutrition Knowledge and Health Motivation. *Nutrients* **2019**, *11*, 2199. [CrossRef]
12. Plasek, B.; Temesi, Á. The credibility of the effects of functional food products and consumers' willingness to purchase/willingness to pay–review. *Appetite* **2019**, *143*, 104398. [CrossRef]
13. Niebylski, M.L.; Redburn, K.A.; Duhaney, T.; Campbell, N.R. Healthy food subsidies and unhealthy food taxation: A systematic review of the evidence. *Nutrition* **2015**, *31*, 787–795. [CrossRef] [PubMed]
14. Provencher, V.; Jacob, R. Impact of perceived healthiness of food on food choices and intake. *Curr. Obes. Rep.* **2016**, *5*, 65–71. [CrossRef]
15. Alba, J.W.; Williams, E.F. Pleasure principles: A review of research on hedonic consumption. *J. Consum. Psychol.* **2013**, *23*, 2–18. [CrossRef]
16. Krishna, A. An integrative review of sensory marketing: Engaging the senses to affect perception, judgment and behavior. *J. Consum. Psychol.* **2012**, *22*, 332–351. [CrossRef]
17. Raghunathan, R.; Naylor, R.W.; Hoyer, W.D. The unhealthy= tasty intuition and its effects on taste inferences, enjoyment, and choice of food products. *J. Mark.* **2006**, *70*, 170–184. [CrossRef]
18. Jo, J.; Lusk, J.L. If it's healthy, it's tasty and expensive: Effects of nutritional labels on price and taste expectations. *Food Qual. Prefer.* **2018**, *68*, 332–341. [CrossRef]
19. Lusk, J.L. Consumer beliefs about healthy foods and diets. *PLoS ONE* **2019**, *14*, e0223098. [CrossRef] [PubMed]
20. Petrescu, D.C.; Vermeir, I.; Petrescu-Mag, R.M. Consumer Understanding of Food Quality, Healthiness, and Environmental Impact: A Cross-National Perspective. *Int. J. Environ. Res. Public Health* **2020**, *17*, 169. [CrossRef]
21. Riebl, S.K.; Estabrooks, P.A.; Dunsmore, J.C.; Savla, J.; Frisard, M.I.; Dietrich, A.M.; Peng, Y.; Zhang, X.; Davy, B.M. A systematic literature review and meta-analysis: The Theory of Planned Behavior's application to understand and predict nutrition-related behaviors in youth. *Eat. Behav.* **2015**, *18*, 160–178. [CrossRef]

22. Dorota Rudawska, E. Customer loyalty towards traditional products–Polish market experience. *Br. Food J.* **2014**, *116*, 1710–1725. [CrossRef]
23. Marques da Rosa, V.; Spence, C.; Miletto Tonetto, L. Influences of visual attributes of food packaging on consumer preference and associations with taste and healthiness. *Int. J. Consum. Stud.* **2019**, *43*, 210–217. [CrossRef]
24. Pires, M.A.; de Noronha, R.L.F.; Trindade, M.A. Understanding consumer's perception and acceptance of bologna sausages with reduced sodium content and/or omega-3 addition through conjoint analysis and focus group. *J. Sens. Stud.* **2019**, e12495. [CrossRef]
25. Yarar, N.; Machiels, C.J.; Orth, U.R. Shaping up: How package shape and consumer body conspire to affect food healthiness evaluation. *Food Qual. Prefer.* **2019**. [CrossRef]
26. Machín, L.; Aschemann-Witzel, J.; Curutchet, M.R.; Giménez, A.; Ares, G. Does front-of-pack nutrition information improve consumer ability to make healthful choices? Performance of warnings and the traffic light system in a simulated shopping experiment. *Appetite* **2018**, *121*, 55–62. [CrossRef] [PubMed]
27. Hartmann, C.; Hieke, S.; Taper, C.; Siegrist, M. European consumer healthiness evaluation of 'Free-from'labelled food products. *Food Qual. Prefer.* **2018**, *68*, 377–388. [CrossRef]
28. Festila, A.; Chrysochou, P. Implicit communication of food product healthfulness through package design: A content analysis. *J. Consum. Behav.* **2018**, *17*, 461–476. [CrossRef]
29. Polizer Rocha, Y.J.; Lapa-Guimarães, J.; de Noronha, R.L.F.; Trindade, M.A. Evaluation of consumers' perception regarding frankfurter sausages with different healthiness attributes. *J. Sens. Stud.* **2018**, *33*, e12468. [CrossRef]
30. Wijayaratne, S.P.; Reid, M.; Westberg, K.; Worsley, A.; Mavondo, F. Food literacy, healthy eating barriers and household diet. *Eur. J. Mark.* **2018**, *52*, 2449–2477. [CrossRef]
31. Lee, H.C.; Chang, C.T.; Cheng, Z.H.; Chen, Y.T. Will an organic label always increase food consumption? It depends on food type and consumer differences in health locus of control. *Food Qual. Prefer.* **2018**, *63*, 88–96. [CrossRef]
32. Vila-López, N.; Küster-Boluda, I. Commercial versus technical cues to position a new product: Do hedonic and functional/healthy packages differ? *Soc. Sci. Med.* **2018**, *198*, 85–94. [CrossRef]
33. Lidón, I.; Rebollar, R.; Gil-Pérez, I.; Martín, J.; Vicente-Villardón, J.L. The influence the image of the product shown on food packaging labels has on product perception during tasting: Effects and gender differences. *Packag. Technol. Sci.* **2018**, *31*, 689–697. [CrossRef]
34. Acton, R.B.; Hammond, D. Do Consumers Think Front-of-Package "High in" Warnings are Harsh or Reduce their Control? A Test of Food Industry Concerns. *Obesity* **2018**, *26*, 1687–1691. [CrossRef]
35. Carabante, K.M.; Ardoin, R.; Scaglia, G.; Malekian, F.; Khachaturyan, M.; Janes, M.E.; Prinyawiwatkul, W. Consumer Acceptance, Emotional Response, and Purchase Intent of Rib-Eye Steaks from Grass-Fed Steers, and Effects of Health Benefit Information on Consumer Perception. *J. Food Sci.* **2018**, *83*, 2560–2570. [CrossRef] [PubMed]
36. Miraballes, M.; Gámbaro, A. Influence of Images on the Evaluation of Jams using Conjoint Analysis Combined with Check-All-That-Apply (CATA) Questions. *J. Food Sci.* **2018**, *83*, 167–174. [CrossRef]
37. Wardy, W.; Jack, A.R.; Chonpracha, P.; Alonso, J.R.; King, J.M.; Prinyawiwatkul, W. Gluten-free muffins: Effects of sugar reduction and health benefit information on consumer liking, emotion, and purchase intent. *Int. J. Food Sci. Technol.* **2018**, *53*, 262–269. [CrossRef]
38. Benson, T.; Lavelle, F.; Bucher, T.; McCloat, A.; Mooney, E.; Egan, B.; Collins, C.E.; Dean, M. The impact of nutrition and health claims on consumer perceptions and portion size selection: Results from a nationally representative survey. *Nutrients* **2018**, *10*, 656. [CrossRef]
39. Shan, L.C.; Regan, Á.; Monahan, F.J.; Li, C.; Lalor, F.; Murrin, C.; Wall, P.G.; McConnon, Á. Consumer preferences towards healthier reformulation of a range of processed meat products: A qualitative exploratory study. *Br. Food J.* **2017**, *119*, 2013–2026. [CrossRef]
40. Shan, L.C.; De Brún, A.; Henchion, M.; Li, C.; Murrin, C.; Wall, P.G.; Monahan, F.J. Consumer evaluations of processed meat products reformulated to be healthier–A conjoint analysis study. *Meat Sci.* **2017**, *131*, 82–89. [CrossRef] [PubMed]
41. Labbe, D.; Rytz, A.; Godinot, N.; Ferrage, A.; Martin, N. Is portion size selection associated with expected satiation, perceived healthfulness or expected tastiness? A case study on pizza using a photograph-based computer task. *Appetite* **2017**, *108*, 311–316. [CrossRef]

42. Prada, M.; Garrido, M.V.; Rodrigues, D. Lost in processing? Perceived healthfulness, taste and caloric content of whole and processed organic food. *Appetite* **2017**, *114*, 175–186. [CrossRef]
43. Tijssen, I.; Zandstra, E.H.; de Graaf, C.; Jager, G. Why a 'light'product package should not be light blue: Effects of package colour on perceived healthiness and attractiveness of sugar-and fat-reduced products. *Food Qual. Prefer.* **2017**, *59*, 46–58. [CrossRef]
44. Marino, R.; Della Malva, A.; Seccia, A.; Caroprese, M.; Sevi, A.; Albenzio, M. Consumers' expectations and acceptability for low saturated fat 'salami': Healthiness or taste? *J. Sci. Food Agric.* **2017**, *97*, 3515–3521. [CrossRef]
45. Cavallo, C.; Piqueras-Fiszman, B. Visual elements of packaging shaping healthiness evaluations of consumers: The case of olive oil. *J. Sens. Stud.* **2017**, *32*, e12246. [CrossRef]
46. Gineikiene, J.; Kiudyte, J.; Degutis, M. Functional, organic or conventional? Food choices of health conscious and skeptical consumers. *Balt. J. Manag.* **2017**, *12*, 139–152. [CrossRef]
47. Rebouças, M.C.; Rodrigues, M.D.C.P.; Freitas, S.M.D.; Ferreira, B.B.A.; Costa, V.D.S. Effect of nutritional information and health claims related to cashew nut and soya milk beverages on consumers' acceptance and perception. *Nutr. Food Sci.* **2017**, *47*, 721–730. [CrossRef]
48. Tleis, M.; Callieris, R.; Roma, R. Segmenting the organic food market in Lebanon: An application of k-means cluster analysis. *Br. Food J.* **2017**, *119*, 1423–1441. [CrossRef]
49. Brečić, R.; Mesić, Ž.; Cerjak, M. Importance of intrinsic and extrinsic quality food characteristics by different consumer segments. *Br. Food J.* **2017**, *119*, 845–862. [CrossRef]
50. Thomson, N.; Worsley, A.; Wang, W.; Sarmugam, R.; Pham, Q.; Februhartanty, J. Country context, personal values and nutrition trust: Associations with perceptions of beverage healthiness in five countries in the Asia Pacific region. *Food Qual. Prefer.* **2017**, *60*, 123–131. [CrossRef]
51. Apaolaza, V.; Hartmann, P.; Echebarria, C.; Barrutia, J.M. Organic label's halo effect on sensory and hedonic experience of wine: A pilot study. *J. Sens. Stud.* **2017**, *32*, e12243. [CrossRef]
52. Anders, S.; Schroeter, C. Estimating the effects of nutrition label use on Canadian consumer diet-health concerns using propensity score matching. *Int. J. Consum. Stud.* **2017**, *41*, 534–544. [CrossRef]
53. Talati, Z.; Pettigrew, S.; Dixon, H.; Neal, B.; Ball, K.; Hughes, C. Do health claims and front-of-pack labels lead to a positivity bias in unhealthy foods? *Nutrients* **2016**, *8*, 787. [CrossRef]
54. Samoggia, A. Wine and health: Faraway concepts? *Br. Food J.* **2016**, *118*, 946–960. [CrossRef]
55. Seegebarth, B.; Behrens, S.H.; Klarmann, C.; Hennigs, N.; Scribner, L.L. Customer value perception of organic food: Cultural differences and cross-national segments. *Br. Food J.* **2016**, *118*, 396–411. [CrossRef]
56. Puska, P.; Luomala, H.T. Capturing qualitatively different healthfulness images of food products. *Mark. Intell. Plan.* **2016**, *34*, 605–622. [CrossRef]
57. Larkin, D.; Martin, C.R. Caloric estimation of healthy and unhealthy foods in normal-weight, overweight and obese participants. *Eat. Behav.* **2016**, *23*, 91–96. [CrossRef] [PubMed]
58. Szocs, C.; Lefebvre, S. The blender effect: Physical state of food influences healthiness perceptions and consumption decisions. *Food Qual. Prefer.* **2016**, *54*, 152–159. [CrossRef]
59. Lazzarini, G.A.; Zimmermann, J.; Visschers, V.H.; Siegrist, M. Does environmental friendliness equal healthiness? Swiss consumers' perception of protein products. *Appetite* **2016**, *105*, 663–673. [CrossRef]
60. Jo, J.; Lusk, J.L.; Muller, L.; Ruffieux, B. Value of parsimonious nutritional information in a framed field experiment. *Food Policy* **2016**, *63*, 124–133. [CrossRef]
61. Fenko, A.; Lotterman, H.; Galetzka, M. What's in a name? The effects of sound symbolism and package shape on consumer responses to food products. *Food Qual. Prefer.* **2016**, *51*, 100–108. [CrossRef]
62. Hipp, J.A.; Becker, H.V.; Marx, C.M.; Tabak, R.G.; Brownson, R.C.; Yang, L. Worksite nutrition supports and sugar-sweetened beverage consumption. *Obes. Sci. Pract.* **2016**, *2*, 144–153. [CrossRef]
63. Rizk, M.T.; Treat, T.A. Sensitivity to portion size of unhealthy foods. *Food Qual. Prefer.* **2015**, *45*, 121–131. [CrossRef]
64. Rizk, M.T.; Treat, T.A. Perceptions of food healthiness among free-living women. *Appetite* **2015**, *95*, 390–398. [CrossRef]
65. Sütterlin, B.; Siegrist, M. Simply adding the word "fruit" makes sugar healthier: The misleading effect of symbolic information on the perceived healthiness of food. *Appetite* **2015**, *95*, 252–261. [CrossRef] [PubMed]

66. Wąsowicz, G.; Styśko-Kunkowska, M.; Grunert, K.G. The meaning of colours in nutrition labelling in the context of expert and consumer criteria of evaluating food product healthfulness. *J. Health Psychol.* **2015**, *20*, 907–920. [CrossRef] [PubMed]
67. Luomala, H.; Jokitalo, M.; Karhu, H.; Hietaranta-Luoma, H.L.; Hopia, A.; Hietamäki, S. Perceived health and taste ambivalence in food consumption. *J. Consum. Mark.* **2015**, *32*, 290–301. [CrossRef]
68. Xie, B.; Wang, L.; Yang, H.; Wang, Y.; Zhang, M. Consumer perceptions and attitudes of organic food products in Eastern China. *Br. Food J.* **2015**, *117*, 1105–1121. [CrossRef]
69. Grubor, A.; Djokic, N.; Djokic, I.; Kovac-Znidersic, R. Application of health and taste attitude scales in Serbia. *Br. Food J.* **2015**, *117*, 840–860. [CrossRef]
70. Vasiljevic, M.; Pechey, R.; Marteau, T.M. Making food labels social: The impact of colour of nutritional labels and injunctive norms on perceptions and choice of snack foods. *Appetite* **2015**, *91*, 56–63. [CrossRef]
71. Reutner, L.; Genschow, O.; Wänke, M. The adaptive eater: Perceived healthiness moderates the effect of the color red on consumption. *Food Qual. Prefer.* **2015**, *44*, 172–178. [CrossRef]
72. Thomsen, T.U.; Hansen, T. Perceptions that matter: Perceptual antecedents and moderators of healthy food consumption. *Int. J. Consum. Stud.* **2015**, *39*, 109–116. [CrossRef]
73. Dharni, K.; Gupta, K. Exploring antecedents of healthy food choices: An Indian experience. *Int. J. Consum. Stud.* **2015**, *39*, 101–108. [CrossRef]
74. Annunziata, A.; Vecchio, R.; Kraus, A. Awareness and preference for functional foods: The perspective of older Italian consumers. *Int. J. Consum. Stud.* **2015**, *39*, 352–361. [CrossRef]
75. Maehle, N.; Iversen, N.; Hem, L.; Otnes, C. Exploring consumer preferences for hedonic and utilitarian food attributes. *Br. Food J.* **2015**, *117*, 3039–3063. [CrossRef]
76. Bucher, T.; Müller, B.; Siegrist, M. What is healthy food? Objective nutrient profile scores and subjective lay evaluations in comparison. *Appetite* **2015**, *95*, 408–414. [CrossRef]
77. Kraus, A. Development of functional food with the participation of the consumer. Motivators for consumption of functional products. *Int. J. Consum. Stud.* **2015**, *39*, 2–11. [CrossRef]
78. Orquin, J.L. A Brunswik lens model of consumer health judgments of packaged foods. *J. Consum. Behav.* **2014**, *13*, 270–281. [CrossRef]
79. Carrete, L.; Arroyo, P. Social marketing to improve healthy dietary decisions: Insights from a qualitative study in Mexico. *Qual. Mark. Res. Int. J.* **2014**, *17*, 239–263. [CrossRef]
80. Lin, H.C. The effects of food product types and affective states on consumers' decision making. *Br. Food J.* **2014**, *116*, 1550–1560. [CrossRef]
81. Available online: http://eisz.mtak.hu/index.php/en/open-access-english/338-access-to-sciencedirect-scopus-and-scival-open-for-the-hungarian-research-community-as-eisz-and-elsevier-work-towards-an-open-access-pilot-agreement.html (accessed on 15 June 2020).

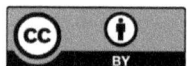

© 2020 by the authors. Licensee MDPI, Basel, Switzerland. This article is an open access article distributed under the terms and conditions of the Creative Commons Attribution (CC BY) license (http://creativecommons.org/licenses/by/4.0/).

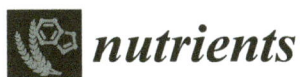 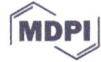

Article

The Effect of an Online Sugar Fact Intervention: Change of Mothers with Young Children

Yi-Chun Chen [1,2,*], Ya-Li Huang [2,3,4], Yi-Wen Chien [1,5] and Mei Chun Chen [1]

[1] School of Nutrition and Health Sciences, Taipei Medical University, Xinyi District, Taipei City 110, Taiwan; ychien@tmu.edu.tw (Y.-W.C.); gshejenny@gmail.com (M.C.C.)
[2] Research Center of Health Equity, College of Public Health, Taipei Medical University, Xinyi District, Taipei City 110, Taiwan; ylhuang@tmu.edu.tw
[3] Department of Public Health, School of Medicine, College of Medicine, Taipei Medical University, Xinyi District, Taipei City 110, Taiwan
[4] School of Public Health, College of Public Health, Taipei Medical University, Xinyi District, Taipei City 110, Taiwan
[5] Graduate Institute of Metabolism and Obesity Sciences, College of Nutrition, Taipei Medical University, Xinyi District, Taipei City 110, Taiwan
* Correspondence: yichun@tmu.edu.tw

Received: 21 April 2020; Accepted: 19 June 2020; Published: 22 June 2020

Abstract: Research indicates that high sugar intake in early childhood may increase risks of tooth decay, obesity and chronic disease later in life. In this sugar fact study, we explored whether an online intervention which focused on comprehensive and useful information about nutrition labels impacted mother's choice of low sugar food. The intervention was developed on the basis of the theory of planned behavior. In total, 122 mothers were recruited. Mothers were divided into an online-only group and a plus group. Knowledge of sugar and nutrition labels, behavioral attitudes, perceived behavioral control, behavioral intentions and behavior towards purchasing low-sugar products with nutrition labels were collected. After the intervention, both groups exhibited significantly enhanced sugar and nutrition label knowledge, perceived behavioral control, behavioral intentions and behavior. Compared to the online-only group, knowledge, perceived behavioral control and behavior of the plus group significantly improved. After the intervention, about 40% of the plus group and 80% of the online-only group still did not know the World Health Organization (WHO) sugar recommendations. Understanding sugar recommendations and using nutrition labels are crucial to help people control calorie and sugar intake. Further research with a larger sample is warranted to evaluate the effects of the intervention on long-term changes in shopping behavior. More efficient and convenient nutrition education is required to increase public awareness of sugar recommendations and help people control calorie and sugar intake.

Keywords: online nutrition intervention; theory of planned behavior; nutrition labels; sugar; consumer behavior; consumer attitude; consumer perception

1. Background

Being overweight and obese increases the risks of many health problems, including diabetes, heart disease and certain cancers [1–3]. An examination of the 2015 data of the World Obesity Federation reveals that overweight rates of children in Taiwan were the highest in Asia [4]. A long-term follow-up study in Taiwan found that approximately 90% of young children consume sugary drinks and snacks once per day, and one-third of 5 year-old children more than 10% of their caloric intake from refined sugar [5]. Studies have confirmed that sugar promotes a high energy balance and children who consume more sugar have higher obesity rates than those who consume less sugar [6–8]. Thus, the World Health Organization (WHO) strongly recommends that it is good to reduce the sugar intake to <10% of total energy intake for both adults and children [9].

Products with low- or no-sugar-related claims, such as "sugar free", "no added sugar" and "reduced sugar", may be particularly appealing to parents who want to manage their child's sugar intake [10,11]. However, a Canadian study found that half of 3048 prepackaged foods with sugar-related claims contained excessive sugar, and a greater proportion contained sweeteners than did products without such claims [12]. A survey in Taiwan also found that more than 90% of popular snacks and drinks with no-added-sugar claims consumed by children were high in sugar [13]. A study in Australia and New Zealand found that 28% of consumers misunderstood the meaning of the claim of "no added sugar", believing that products with such a claim contained no sugar [14]. In addition, 95.7% of mothers know that excessive sugar intake increases future health risks in children, but only 21.9% know the WHO sugar recommendations [15].

Nutrition labeling is an important tool to help people choose healthy foods. A previous study has discovered that although most consumers trust nutrition labels, they perceive that the information on them is difficult to understand and confusing, including information on recommended daily allowances, percent daily values and servings [16]. Because of limited time, consumers normally only read one or two of the facts on nutrition labels, such as calories and fats [17]. The Health Information National Trends Survey in the US suggested that although most people have difficulty interpreting nutrition labels, they cannot effectively utilize such facts to make informed dietary choices they possess insufficient reading comprehension and calculation skills [18]. Education can help the public improve those skills required to understand nutrition labels, thereby allowing consumers to effectively purchase suitable foods according to nutrition labels [19]. A study in the US applied a multimedia intervention to participants in an experimental group and significantly improved their comprehension of nutrition labels [20]. Another study in the US demonstrated that online courses helped the public improve skills required to effectively use nutrition labels to buy healthy foods [21]. In brief, effective education can improve people's comprehension of nutrition labels, thereby enabling the public to select healthy foods.

Despite the desire of parents to maintain their children's optimal health, they may not provide healthy foods to their children if they lack nutrition knowledge. A survey of Taiwanese mothers with young children demonstrated that the less sugar-related knowledge they had, the more positive their attitude was toward no-added-sugar infant cereal and the higher their purchase intention was for these infant cereals [15]. Moreover, some parents who lack this knowledge consider providing healthy diets to their children a challenge [22]. Under such circumstances, desirable nutrition education can improve parents' beliefs and behaviors concerning their children's diets, allowing them to provide a healthy diet for their children. The theory of planned behavior (TPB) has been widely adopted in studies that explore or predict various health behaviors as well as those that explore health promotion. This theory posits that behavioral intentions are a pivotal antecedent that affects actual behaviors; furthermore, attitudes toward a behavior, subjective norms and perceived behavioral control are possible controlling factors that affect behavioral intentions [23]. Increasing one's relevant knowledge and developing relevant skills help to change attitudes toward a specific behavior and in turn enhance individuals' intentions to perform such a behavior, thereby encouraging individuals to improve that behavior. A study of Australian mothers with preschool-aged children demonstrated that perceived behavioral control and intention were positively associated with mothers' healthy feeding behavior perceived behavioral control was the only variable positively associated with the mothers' perceptions of their children's fruit and vegetable consumption [22]. A study in South Australia indicated that a parent-focused nutrition intervention can affect maternal feeding practices, which reduced growth-related indicators of future obesity risk in young children [24]. Similarly, an Australian study regarding breakfast consumption indicated that people's attitudes and perceived behavioral control significantly affected their intention to eat breakfast; such an intention affected an individual's breakfast consumption [25]. A podcast-based research study in the US determined that listening to a podcast about omega-3 fatty acids in the grocery store enhanced customers' attitudes and perceived behavioral control toward purchasing foods rich in omega-3 fatty acids [26]. According to the aforementioned studies, it was assumed that nutrition educational interventions based on the TPB can promote the public's health behaviors.

In Taiwan, nutrition labeling regulations regarding sugar content apply to the products manufactured after July 2015 [27] and sugar recommendation was available on 2018 [28]. Encouraging people to use nutrition labels is crucial. Traditionally, interventions targeting parents with young children which required face-to-face classes had low attendance and high dropout rates [29,30]. Online interventions are an efficient and cost-effective way to provide nutrition education. Previous studies confirmed that online nutrition educational programs should be considered to expand outreach and decrease barriers to attending traditional face-to-face classes [31,32]. According a 2017 Taiwanese Internet usage survey, there was an 80% Internet usage rate across the nation [33]. Therefore, online education is feasible in Taiwan. In the present study, the TPB was used to develop an online intervention program to enhance mothers' use of nutrition labels to buy low-sugar foods for their children.

2. Methods

2.1. Design and Participants

This Sugar Fact intervention was a quasi-experimental trial, which was conducted from December 2017 to August 2018 in Taiwan. Online videos and a small-group discussion were used to encourage mothers to use nutrition labeling to buy low-sugar foods for their children. The intervention was designed for the senior high school level because 95% of Taiwanese women aged 25–44 years have at least a senior high school education [34]. Mothers who live in Taiwan, communicate in Chinese, had a child aged 1–6 years, and were their child's primary caregiver and the family's food purchaser were eligible for the study. Various parenting social networks (e.g.; BabyHome, a mothers' groups on Facebook and BabyMother on a bulletin board system) were approached and those who agreed to distribute or advertise the study posted a link to the online recruitment questionnaire on their network. Participants were classified into an online-only group or a plus group according to their intentions. An official Line account (a social networking app popular in Taiwan) was used to contact and follow-up participants. A notification message by Line was sent once per week to remind participants to continue the intervention. The intervention for the online-only group consisted of watching two online videos. The intervention of the plus group included watching two online video and participating in one small-group discussion.

In total, 236 mothers were recruited, and 185 mothers were enrolled in the intervention. Finally, 90 mothers in the online-only group and 32 mothers in the plus group completed the intervention and posttest questionnaire (Figure 1). The completion rate was 62.1% for the online-only group and 80% for the plus group. Participants who completed the intervention received a commercial voucher as an incentive (NT$100 for the online-only group and NT $300 for the plus group; about US $3 and $9, respectively).

2.2. Ethical Considerations

The study was approved by the Taipei Medical University—Joint Institutional Review Board (N201711059) and written informed consent was obtained from all mothers.

2.3. Developed Educational Intervention

The educational intervention was developed based on results of a previous study [15]. Considering the difficulty of attending classes by mothers with young children [35], online video courses were used. The purpose of the online video session for mothers was to increase their positive attitudes and perceived behavioral control of using nutrition labels to buy low-sugar foods for their child (Figure 2). The purpose of the first video was to increase the mother's perceptions of "sugar and health" and "sugar and nutrition". The purpose of the second video was to improve the mothers' understanding of "sugar recommendations", "sugar-related claims" and "nutrition labeling on food packages". All of the contents of the videos were reviewed by three public health nutrition professionals. Five mothers eligible for recruitment were included in a pilot intervention. They were asked to watch the first version of the two videos and give comments. The two videos were uploaded on YouTube after being revised.

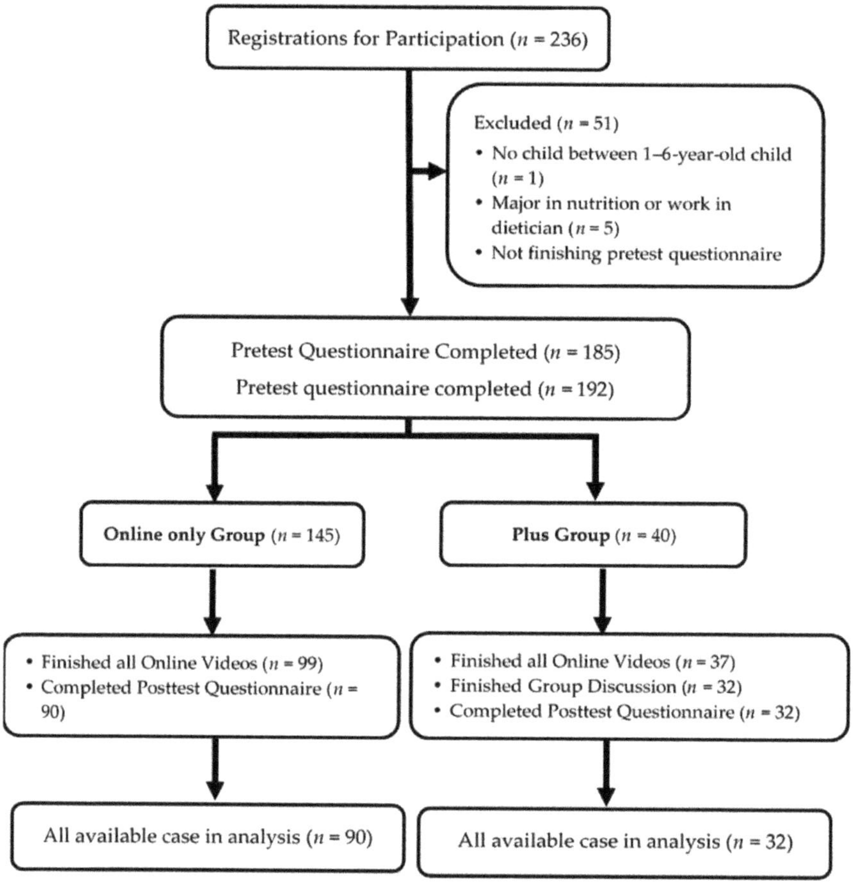

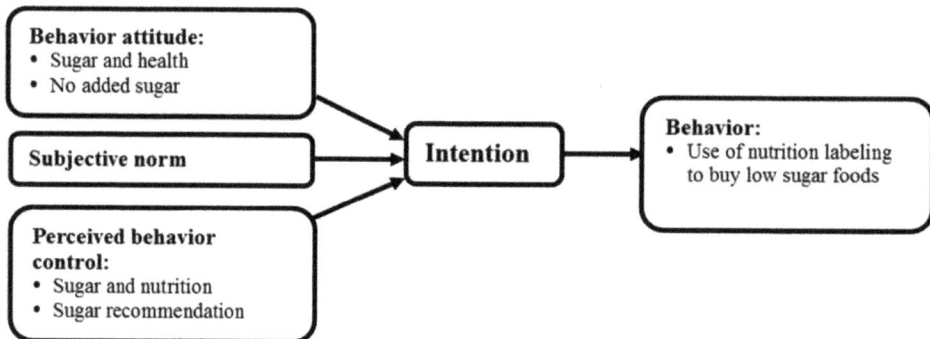

Figure 1. Recruitment of participants.

Figure 2. Intervention concept.

For the online-only group, the nutrition intervention included two 15 min online video sessions. For the plus group, the nutrition intervention included two 15 min online video sessions and one small-group discussion led by the researchers (for 2–3 h). Additional educational materials included a booklet for the online videos and a pamphlet for the small-group discussion. The aims of the small-group discussion were to help mothers clarify the content of the online videos and improve their perceived behavioral control structure. The small-group discussion session focused on barriers that mothers encounter when selecting low-sugar foods and controlling their children's sugar intake. From January to May 2018, the small-group discussion sessions were held 10 times. There were three to five mothers in each small-group discussion. In total, 32 mothers participated in small-group discussions, and all group discussions were recorded. Several topics on a list were discussed to gain an in-depth understanding of participants' reactions to the online video courses and barriers when the mothers practiced their skills of choosing low-sugar foods for their children. The mothers were also allowed to practice using nutrition labels to choose low-sugar foods.

2.4. Questionnaire

A theory-based questionnaire containing the mother's demographic characteristics was used to collect data. All participants completed the questionnaire before the intervention, and they also completed a posttest questionnaire within 2 weeks of finishing the intervention.

The theory-based questionnaire was prepared by reviewing other questionnaires applied in similar studies [15,26,36,37]. Three nutrition and statistical professionals reviewed and revised the questionnaire. The questionnaire was also tested by 15 mothers who had a child aged 1–6 years. Questionnaire items were tested for consistency and comprehensibility. The questionnaire included the following sections; demographic characteristics of the mothers, including age, education (≤high school, undergraduate or ≥graduate), medical background (mother were health professional, such as medical doctors, dietitians or nurses: yes or no), parity (child was firstborn or non-firstborn), household income (≤NT $50,000 or >NT $50,000) and the child's age. Second, data on the mother's behaviors and intentions were collected. Behaviors: I used nutrition labels to buy low-sugar foods for my child/children during the past week? (always, usually, sometimes or seldom); Behavioral intentions: I am going to use nutrition labels to buy low-sugar foods for my child/children in the coming week. The third part was about the mothers' sugar-related knowledge. It included "sugar and health", "sugar and carbohydrates", "daily sugar recommendation", "no-added-sugar claims" and "nutrition labels". The last part included mother's attitudes, subjective norms and perceived behavioral control. There were four questions about attitudes (e.g., I believe that using nutrition labels to buy low-sugar foods for my child/children is very important), three question about subjective norms e.g., My family members expect me to use nutrition labels to buy low-sugar foods for my child/children) and four questions about perceived behavioral control (e.g., It is difficult for me to use nutrition labels to buy low-sugar foods for my child/children). A Likert scale was used to score the data collection instruments. In order to avoid neutral feedback, this section used a Likert 6-point scale divided into "very disagree", "disagree", "disagree a little", "consent a little", "agree" and "very agree". These were scored 1–6 points, respectively [38].

2.5. Data Analysis

A statistical software package (SPSS, Chicago, IL, USA) was utilized. The Kolmogorov-Smirnov test was used to examine the normal distribution of all continuous variables (the test of normality was present at Supplementary Table S1). Nonparametric statistics were used due to most variables did not match normal distribution. Baseline data for demographic characteristics and TPB variables of the two groups were analyzed using a chi-squared and Mann-Whitney U test. A Wilcoxon signed-rank test was used to study changes before and after the educational intervention and a Mann–Whitney U test was used to evaluate the mean of changes and compare the mean of study variables in the two groups. Spearman's rank correlation was used to examine the correlation among the difference of TPB variables. Statistical significance was set as $p < 0.05$.

3. Results

Table 1 shows the demographic characteristics of participants. There was no significant difference in demographic characteristics between the two groups ($p > 0.05$). The mothers' average ages were 35.3 ± 4.5 years in the online-only group and 34.9 ± 4.5 years in the plus group. The children's average ages were 2.7 ± 1.6 years in the online-only group and 2.9 ± 1.6 years in the plus group. Most mothers of the two groups had more than one child, had a university/college degree, worked full-time. The average family monthly income was NT $30,000–50,000 and more than 80% of the mothers had no medical background, such as medical doctors, dietitians or nurses.

Table 1. Demographic characteristics of participants by the intervention condition [1].

Characteristics	Total ($n = 122$)	Online Only Group ($n = 90$)	Plus Group [2] ($n = 32$)	p Value
Mother's Age (years)	35.3 ± 4.5	35.3 ± 4.5	34.9 ± 4.5	0.456
Child's Age (years)	2.8 ± 1.6	2.7 ± 1.6	2.9 ± 1.6	0.573
Number of Children				0.270
One	52 (42.6)	41 (45.6)	11 (34.4)	
More than One	70 (57.4)	49 (54.4)	21 (65.6)	
Education				0.241
Senior High School	13 (10.7)	9 (10.0)	4 (12.5)	
University/College	84 (68.8)	65 (72.2)	19 (59.4)	
≥Master's	25 (20.5)	16 (17.8)	9 (28.1)	
Working status				0.605
Housewife	47 (38.5)	36 (40.0)	11 (34.4)	
Full-time	61 (50.0)	44 (48.9)	17 (53.1)	
Part-time	14 (11.5)	10 (11.1)	4 (12.5)	
Medical Background				0.398
No	107 (87.7)	79 (87.8)	28 (87.5)	
Yes	15 (12.3)	11 (12.2)	4 (12.5)	
Family Income, NT$/month [3]				0.718
<30,000	16 (13.1)	11 (12.2)	5 (15.6)	
30,001–50,000	33 (27.0)	25 (27.8)	8 (25.0)	
50,001–70,000	28 (23.0)	22 (24.4)	6 (18.8)	
70,001–100,000	26 (21.3)	20 (22.2)	6 (18.8)	
≥100,001	19 (15.6)	12 (13.3)	7 (21.9)	

[1] Data are presented as the number (percentage) or mean ± standard deviation; [2] participants of the plus group finished online videos and a group discussion; [3] the average exchange rate in 2018 was US1.00 ≈ New Taiwan (NT) $30.

Table 2 presents the results after the educational intervention, including changes in nutrition knowledge and TPB variables in the two groups and differences between the online-only and plus groups. After the educational intervention, sugar and nutrition label knowledge in both groups significantly improved ($p < 0.001$). The change in the plus group was greater than that in the online-only group (4.3 ± 2.4 vs. 2.0 ± 2.3, $p < 0.001$). No significant difference was observed between the groups regarding the mean scores for behavioral attitudes, perceived behavioral control or subjective norms before the intervention. Mean changes in scores for behavioral attitudes, perceived behavioral control, and subjective norms were significant in the plus group ($p < 0.05$), but the change in behavioral attitudes in the online-only group was not. The mean change in perceived behavioral control in the plus group was greater than that in the online-only group (0.3 ± 0.7 vs. 0.7 ± 0.9, $p = 0.026$). After the intervention, the mean changes in intentions and behavior significantly improved in both groups. The improvement in behavior for the plus group was significantly greater than that of the online-only group (1.8 ± 1.7 vs. 0.8 ± 1.7, $p = 0.005$).

Table 2. Changes in knowledge and theory of planned behavior (TPB) before and after the intervention in both groups. [1]

Variable	Online-Only Group Mean ± SD	Plus Group [2] Mean ± SD	p Value [3]
Knowledge of Sugar and Labels (0–16 score)			
Before	9.4 ± 2.0	8.3 ± 2.2	0.039 *
After	11.4 ± 2.1	12.6 ± 1.6	0.006 *
Difference	2.0 ± 2.3	4.3 ± 2.4	<0.001 **
p value [4]	<0.001 **	<0.001 **	
Behavioral Attitudes (1–6 score)			
Before	5.0 ± 0.8	4.9 ± 0.7	0.351
After	5.1 ± 0.7	5.3 ± 0.7	0.294
Difference	0.2 ± 0.7	0.3 ± 0.9	0.071
p value [4]	0.166	0.030 *	
Perceived Behavioral Control (1–6 score)			
Before	4.6 ± 0.8	4.6 ± 0.7	0.713
After	5.0 ± 0.7	5.3 ± 0.6	0.056
Difference	0.3 ± 0.7	0.7 ± 0.9	0.026 *
p value [4]	<0.001 **	<0.001 **	
Subjective Norms (1–6 score)			
Before	4.5 ± 1.0	4.4 ± 0.9	0.375
After	4.8 ± 1.0	4.7 ± 0.8	0.197
Difference	0.3 ± 0.9	0.3 ± 0.8	0.965
p value [4]	0.001 *	0.035 *	
Behavioral Intentions (1–6 score)			
Before	5.1 ± 1.0	4.9 ± 0.9	0.122
After	5.4 ± 0.7	5.4 ± 0.6	0.636
Difference	0.3 ± 0.8	0.5 ± 0.8	0.054
p value [4]	0.001 *	0.002 *	
Behaviors (1–5 score)			
Before	2.8 ± 1.7	2.1 ± 1.6	0.040 *
After	3.5 ± 1.5	3.9 ± 1.3	0.356
Difference	0.8 ± 1.7	1.8 ± 1.7	0.005 *
p value [4]	<0.001 **	<0.001 **	

[1] Data are presented as mean and standard deviation (SD); [2] participants of the plus group finished online videos and a group discussion; [3] difference between the online-only group and plus group; [4] difference between the before and after scores; * $p < 0.05$; ** $p < 0.001$ by Mann-Whitney U test and Wilcoxon signed-rank test.

Figure 3 presents the correlation among changes in TPB constructs. The figure indicates significant predictive associations with mothers' intentions to use nutrition labeling to buy low-sugar food and the positive associations between mothers' intentions and behaviors.

Table 3 presents changes in the mothers' sugar-related knowledge in both groups after the intervention. The correct rate of all questions had increased in the plus group, but not in the online-only group. Both before and after the intervention, more than 90% of mothers in both groups knew of the association of sugar with health. After the intervention, the change in the correct rate of "No-added-sugar claim" had increased 25% in the online-only group and more than 50% in the plus group. In particular, the correct rate of "comparing sugar contents of foods with 'no added sugar' and those without 'no added sugar' on the label" had increased 68.7% in the plus group. In the small discussion group session, most mothers expressed that they really cared about the sugar content of foods and they would buy the food with "no added sugar" claim, since they did not realize the difference between "sugar-free" claim and "no added sugar" claim. During the small-group discussion session, they practiced reading several child food packages to understand the difference and found it was important to read the sugar content on nutrition labels.

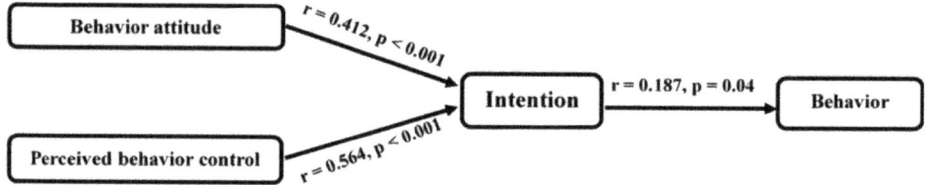

Figure 3. Constructs of the theory of planned behavior in this study ($n = 122$).

Table 3. Correct knowledge rates about sugar and nutrition labels in both groups [1].

Section Question	Answer	Online-Only Group ($n = 90$)			Plus Group ($n = 32$)		
		Before	After	Change (%)	Before	After	Change (%)
A. Sugar and Health Average Rate		96.3	97.1	0.8	96.9	99.0	2.1
High sugar intake increases the risk of obesity.	T	89 (98.9)	88 (97.8)	1.0	31 (96.9)	32 (100.0)	1.0
High sugar intake increases the risk of tooth decay.	T	88 (97.8)	87 (96.7)	−1.1	32 (100.0)	32 (100.0)	0.0
High sugar intake increases the preference for sweets.	T	83 (92.2)	87 (96.7)	4.5	30 (93.8)	31 (96.9)	3.1
B. No-added-sugar Claims		48.9	73.9	25.0	29.7	86.0	56.3
"No added sugar" signifies "sugar free".	F	61 (67.8)	77 (85.6)	17.8	16 (50.0)	30 (93.8)	43.8
The sugar content of food with "No added sugar" is lower than food without "no added sugar".	F	27 (30.0)	56 (62.2)	32.2	3 (9.4)	25 (78.1)	68.7
C. Sugar and nutrition		55.9	77.0	21.1	46.9	82.0	35.1
Whole-grain foods and sugar are carbohydrates.	T	63 (70.0)	78 (86.7)	16.7	20 (62.5)	29 (90.6)	28.1
Honey is one type of sugar.	T	61 (67.8)	78 (86.7)	18.9	23 (71.9)	32 (100.0)	28.1
Sugar contains 4 calories per gram.	T	51 (56.7)	86 (95.6)	38.9	15 (46.9)	32 (100.0)	53.1
Brown sugar is healthier than white sugar.	F	26 (28.9)	35 (38.9)	10.0	2 (6.3)	12 (37.5)	31.2
D. Sugar recommendations		3.3	13.7	10.4	2.1	39.6	37.5
Calories from daily sugar intake should be greater than 20% of total calories.	F	3 (3.3)	17 (18.9)	15.6	1 (3.1)	20 (62.5)	59.4
The sugar content of one Yakult [2] is higher than the daily sugar recommendation for 1–3-year-old children.	F	1 (1.1)	3 (3.3)	2.2	0 (0.0)	6 (18.8)	18.8
Fifty grams of sugar of intake/per day is acceptable for 4–6-year-old children.	F	5 (5.6)	22 (24.4)	18.8	1 (3.1)	12 (37.5)	34.4
E. Nutrition labels		79.6	87.5	7.9	71.9	86.0	14.1
Product A contains 26 g of sugar.	F	65 (72.2)	72 (80.0)	7.8	26 (81.3)	28 (87.5)	6.2
Product B contains 65 g of carbohydrates.	T	74 (82.8)	90 (100.0)	17.2	23 (71.9)	31 (96.9)	25.0
Product A contains fewer calories than product B.	T	75 (83.3)	77 (85.6)	2.3	20 (62.5)	24 (75.0)	12.5
Product B contains a lower sugar content than product A.	T	72 (80.0)	76 (84.4)	4.4	23 (71.9)	27 (84.4)	12.5

[1] Data are presented as the number (percentage); [2] a popular yogurt drink; T: True; F: False.

After the intervention, the correct rates of "sugar and nutrition" exceeded 80% in both groups, and the correct rates of "brown sugar is healthier than white sugar" were still lower than 40% in both groups. The "sugar recommendation" had the lowest correct rates in both groups. After the intervention, changes in the correct rate of "calories from daily sugar intake" was 59.4% in the plus group and only 15.6% in the online-only group. Even after the intervention, correct rates of the other two questions about "sugar recommendations" was still <40% in both groups. During the small-group discussion, most mothers expressed that they knew that the recommended sugar intake differed by age, but it was difficult to memorize different sugar recommended gram for different ages.

After the intervention, the correct rates of "nutrition labeling" were >80% for the online-only group and >75% for the plus group. During the small-group discussion, some mothers expressed confusion about the information presented by nutrition labels. Mothers were confused why some products contained only one serving while other products contained two servings (Figure 4) and they had trouble calculating sugar contents or calories for all products and comparing or choosing products.

Nutrition Facts (Product A)			Nutrition Facts (Product B)		
Amount per serving 250 mL			Amount per serving 500 mL		
2 serving per container			1 serving per container		
	Serving	100mL		Serving	100mL
Calories	128kcal	51.2kcal	Calories	299kcal	74.8kcal
Protein	2.0g	0.8g	Protein	3.0g	0.6g
Fat	0g	0g	Fat	3.0g	0.6g
Saturated	0g	0g	Saturated	0g	0g
Trans Fat	0g	0g	Trans Fat	0g	0g
Carbohydrate	30g	12g	Carbohydrate	65g	13g
Sugar	26g	10.4g	Sugar	42g	8.4g
Sodium	47mg	18mg	Sodium	50mg	10mg

Figure 4. Nutrient labeling information for knowledge part E. nutrition labeling.

4. Discussion

4.1. Application of the TPB in a Low-Sugar Educational Intervention

This study employed the behavior attitude and perceived behavior control elements of the TPB to design an online educational intervention program. The study results revealed that at one week after participation in the intervention program, both the plus group and online-only group showed increases in intentions and behavioral frequencies toward using nutrition labels to buy food products with lower sugar content for their children. Moreover, changes in behavioral attitudes and perceived behavioral control were positively associated with mothers' intentions. According to the TPB, behavioral attitudes and perceived behavioral control are crucial factors influencing the behavioral intentions and actual behaviors of people [23]. By applying this theory in the context of this study, it was possible to use an educational intervention to increase the health-related behavioral intentions of participants, which in turn promoted positive behavioral attitudes and ultimately increased actual positive health behaviors. The results of this study supported that educational interventions could influence a person's behavioral intentions; the stronger the personal behavioral intention is, the greater is the frequency of health behavior execution. Approximately 10% of Taiwanese women aged 25–44 years have at least a master's-level education [34]. Compared with women's education level in Taiwan, more participants in this study, particularly in the plus group, had a master's-level education. Future interventions should be modified to enable more mothers to benefit from the online class.

4.2. Advantages of the Online Nutritional Education Intervention

In considering both the pervasiveness of Internet services and mothers with young children may have difficulties attending face-to-face learning sessions, this study used online videos to deliver the intervention program; some mothers who were interested could participate in the small-group discussion sessions. The online learning program seemed to be a suitable educational intervention tool for the mothers who participated in this study were highly educated (90% had greater than a college educational level). A study conducted in the US revealed that online teaching media (e.g., emails and websites) are low-cost intervention tools for nutrition education, and more important, these online teaching media can enhance the willingness of learners to participate [39]. The completion rate of this study was 62.1% for the online-only group and 80.0% for the plus group. This finding indicated that although online videos could increase the mothers' convenience to participate in the intervention program, some mothers still had insufficient time available to finish watching two 15-minute online videos. As for the plus group, the participants may have had stronger intentions and motivation to learn and were therefore willing to overcome obstacles to complete the intervention program. The online videos used in the present study should be modified to increase mothers' participation rates; for instance, the videos should be split into shorter, more-manageable videos, and also the content could be modified according to results of the group discussions in the present study.

This study revealed that compared to the online-only group, the plus group consciously enhanced their perceived behavioral control and frequency of using nutrition labels to buy low-sugar food products after participating in the intervention program. This indicated that the small-group discussions can improve the ability of mothers to read and use nutrition labels. A study conducted in the UK revealed that group interventions are useful for teaching mothers about child feeding techniques and helping them achieve desired dietary targets for their children [40]. In another study analyzing parents as nutritional education participants, group discussions had a positive role in remedying parents' difficulties with feeding their children and improving their feeding techniques [41]. Although the small-group discussions are a useful intervention tool, it was difficult to identify a group meeting time that suited three or more participants in this study, because more than half of the participants were working mothers. Therefore, eight participants (20%) of the plus group could not even complete one required face-to-face discussion session. Because an increasing number of web conferencing software programs, such as Skype business, are becoming popular, future studies may use this kind of software to conduct the small-group discussions and increase the participation rate of mothers.

4.3. Improvement of Mothers' Knowledge of Nutrition Labels

Results of the current study revealed that after the intervention, the knowledge, behavioral attitudes, perceived behavioral control, intentions and behaviors of the plus group participants had significantly improved. Specifically, their knowledge, perceived behavioral control, and behaviors significantly improved compared to those of the online-only group. Regarding the plus group, in addition to watching the online educational videos, they participated in a small-group discussion to clarify doubts regarding the videos and engage in nutritional-label-use practices. Both their behavioral attitudes and perceived behavioral control in terms of using nutrition labels to shop for low-sugar foods improved after the intervention. A previous study found that nutrition knowledge can improve the ability of participants to shop for healthy food items [42], while another study demonstrated that knowledge influences purchasing behaviors through its influence on attitudes [43]. Berg et al. [44] asserted that behavioral attitudes and perceived behavioral control are crucial factors that influence personal food choice intentions. A study in Iran that employed the TPB to increase participants' fruit and vegetable intake revealed that compared to pre-intervention levels, participants' post-intervention behavioral attitudes, perceived behavioral control, and behavioral intentions significantly improved [45]. However, the researchers asserted that even if a person had positive behavior attitudes toward such food items, if he or she did not possess the ability to implement autonomous control, then they would still be unable to modify their behavior [45]. Results of a study about fruit and vegetable intake also confirmed that perceived behavioral control is a fundamental factor in predicting food choice intentions and behaviors [46]. Results of the present study revealed that after the educational intervention was administered, mothers in both groups had a significantly improved ability to consciously shop for low-sugar foods using nutrition labels. This indicates that enhancing perceived behavioral control is an important factor in increasing participants' positive nutrition-label-use behaviors.

Although the present study did not incorporate subjective norms into the design of the educational program, the subjective norm scores of both groups significantly increased from the pre- to post-intervention stages. It is possible that during the study period, participants may have engaged in additional discussions related to sugar, health, and/or nutrition labels with their family and friends, which subsequently led to an increase in support from friends and family with regard to controlling the sugar intake of their children. This would ultimately have led to an increase in subjective norm scores. To further increase the support of family and friends towards participants, in future studies, intervention sessions could be designed in which the participants could engage in discussions with their friends and family.

4.4. Understanding No-Added-Sugar Claims and Changing Behavioral Attitudes

In terms of behavioral attitudes, this study demonstrated that before the educational intervention was implemented, fewer than 50% of the online-only group participants and fewer than 40% of the plus group had correct perceptions about the "no-added-sugar" claim, whereas more than 50% of the total participants believed that food items with the "no-added-sugar" label contained less sugar than food items without it. During the group discussions, several participants reported that they would buy the "no-added-sugar" food items for their children, but they did not know considered the actual sugar content. A survey conducted in Taiwan reported that more than half of mothers believed that infant cereals with "no-added-sugar" claims contained less sugar than products without such claims [15]. After the educational intervention was implemented, the mean percentage of correct responses improved by 25.0% for the online-only group and 56.3% for the plus group. A study conducted in the UK revealed that approximately 40% of responding parents took the initiative to search for food items with the "no-added-sugar" label when shopping for food for their children [47]. Furthermore, a snack and beverage marketing survey conducted in Taiwan also revealed that more than 90% of children's popular snacks and beverages with "no-added-sugar" or "no-artificial-sweeteners" claims actually had high sugar contents [13]. If parents do not possess sufficient knowledge about sugar claims, they may be easily misled by the "no-added-sugar" claims and end up choosing food items that actually have high sugar contents. In the future, stricter sugar claims regulations should be implemented to prevent the public from being misled. Additionally, the present study revealed that mothers' incorrect perceptions could be effectively modified using online videos and/or group discussions. Furthermore, group discussions can enhance mothers' positive attitudes toward paying attention to nutrition labels. To promote the effects of online videos, future interventions could include explanations (with relevant examples) about "no-added-sugar" claims and sugar contents of common foods.

4.5. Awareness of Sugar Recommendations

In this study, although 90% of mothers in this study had a college education, after the intervention, about 40% of the plus group and 80% of the online-only group did not know the WHO sugar recommendations. These findings are consistent with the previous study that even highly educated people are rarely aware of sugar recommendations [48]. An online survey in Northern Ireland found that even about 90% of participants were college level, there were still 65% of them were unaware of the WHO guidelines for sugar intake, only 4% of respondents correctly classified sugar and artificial sweeteners [48]. Another online survey among Canadian young people also found that only 4.8% of participants correctly identified Canadian recommendations for sugar intake [49]. The present study also found that during the small-group discussion, mothers mentioned the difficulty of remembering WHO recommendations or were confused about the different acceptable daily sugar intake for different age groups. Understanding sugar recommendations and using nutrition labels to choose foods are important to help people control their sugar intake. Therefore, more nutrition education or campaign are needed to raise people's awareness of the sugar recommendations and control their sugar intake.

4.6. Difficulties with Nutrition Labels

The study found that after the intervention, about 15% of both groups still had difficulty interpreting nutrition labels. During the group discussion, the mothers expressed difficulties in using nutrition labels to calculate sugar contents and selecting foods with low-sugar contents. Mothers were confused why some products contain only one serving, but other products contain more than two servings thus they had trouble using nutrition labels to compare or determine sugar contents of products. An experiment about the efficacy of nutrition label formats found that the percent daily value information could help consumers correctly identify the relative amount of total sugar, and the added sugar information could help people correctly identify the relative amount of added sugar in a food [49]. A previous web-based label-reading training intervention also found that web-based practice led to improvements in nutrition label-reading skills; however, consumers may not bother using nutrition labels if reading them is too difficult or time-consuming [21]. Previous studies showed that graphic symbols, such as a traffic light, were easily understood by people with different education or income levels [50–52]. In Taiwan, the percent daily value of sugar or graphic symbols are not available. Further studies are needed to develop the simple label to help parents to choose the low sugar food.

4.7. Limitations and Further Developments

First, although the online video course made it convenient for mothers with young children to participate, it is not possible to confirm whether all the mothers watched and understood all of the online videos. Second, the importance of knowledge on sugar and intention to use food labels for mothers' food purchasing decisions remains unclear. Third, because the groups were assigned by participant preference, the motivation of those in the plus group may have been higher than that in the online-only group. This may have been a factor causing differing results between the two groups.

The results suggest that an online intervention increases mothers' intentions to use nutrition labeling to buy low-sugar foods for their children. Online video s should be improved using the feedback from small-group discussions; therefore, more mothers can benefit from online classes. Furthermore, more research with a larger sample size is warranted to evaluate the effects of the intervention on long-term changes in mothers' real shopping behaviors. Purchases over one week after the intervention may be an inadequate reflection of change. Therefore, an examination of purchases over time, such as one or two months later, is required.

5. Conclusions

This study demonstrated that after the online sugar educational intervention, mothers in both the online-only and plus groups exhibited increased intentions and behavioral frequencies of using nutrition labels when selecting low-sugar food products for their children. In addition, after the intervention, approximately 40.0% of the plus group and 80% of the online-only group still did not know the WHO sugar recommendations. Awareness of the WHO sugar recommendations and using nutrition labels to select foods are instrumental in helping people control their calorie and sugar intake. Therefore, more efficient and convenient nutrition education is required to increase public awareness of sugar recommendations and help people control their calorie and sugar intake.

Supplementary Materials: The following are available online at http://www.mdpi.com/2072-6643/12/6/1859/s1, Table S1: Test of normality for knowledge and constructs of TPB.

Author Contributions: Y.-C.C. conceived and designed the intervention; Y.-C.C. and M.C.C. performed the intervention; Y.-L.H. and Y.-W.C. analyzed the data; Y.-C.C. was responsible for data interpretation writing original draft preparation. The datasets generated and/or analyzed during the current study are not publicly available because new manuscripts are in preparation. They can be available from the corresponding author on reasonable request. All authors have read and agree to the published version of the manuscript.

Funding: This work was supported by the Ministry of Science and Technology [Grant Number MOST 107-2511-H-038 -001 -MY2].

Acknowledgments: The author wishes to acknowledge the help of Shwu-Chen Kuo and Shwu-Huey Yang in commenting on an early draft of the manuscript.

Conflicts of Interest: The authors declare no conflict of interest.

References

1. Bhaskaran, K.; Douglas, I.; Forbes, H.; Dos-Santos-Silva, I.; Leon, D.A.; Smeeth, L. Body-mass index and risk of 22 specific cancers: A population-based cohort study of 5·24 million UK adults. *Lancet* **2014**, *384*, 755–765. [CrossRef]
2. Malik, V.S.; Popkin, B.M.; Bray, G.A.; Després, J.-P.; Hu, F.B. Sugar-sweetened beverages, obesity, type 2 diabetes mellitus, and cardiovascular disease risk. *Circulation* **2010**, *121*, 1356–1364. [CrossRef] [PubMed]
3. Akil, L.; Ahmad, H.A. Relationships between obesity and cardiovascular diseases in four southern states and Colorado. *J. Health Care Poor Underserved* **2011**, *22*, 61–72. [CrossRef] [PubMed]
4. Ministry of Health and Welfare Obesity prevention of white paper. Available online: https://www.hpa.gov.tw/Pages/Detail.aspx?nodeid=1405&pid=8920 (accessed on 20 April 2020).
5. Lyu, L.-C.; Yang, Y.-C.; Yu, H.-W. A long-term follow-up study of sugar sweetened beverages, snacks and desserts, and refined sugar consumption among preschoolers aged 2 to 5 in Taiwan. *Taiwan J. Public Health* **2013**, *32*, 346–357.
6. Pan, L.; Li, R.; Park, S.; Galuska, D.A.; Sherry, B.; Freedman, D.S. A longitudinal analysis of sugar-sweetened beverage intake in infancy and obesity at 6 years. *Pediatrics* **2014**, *134*, S29–S35. [CrossRef]
7. Cantoral, A.; Téllez-Rojo, M.M.; Ettinger, A.; Hu, H.; Hernández-Ávila, M.; Peterson, K. Early introduction and cumulative consumption of sugar-sweetened beverages during the pre-school period and risk of obesity at 8–14 years of age. *Pediatr. Obes.* **2016**, *11*, 68–74. [CrossRef]
8. He, B.; Long, W.; Li, X.; Yang, W.; Chen, Y.; Zhu, Y. Sugar-sweetened beverages consumption positively associated with the risks of obesity and hypertriglyceridemia among Children aged 7–18 years in South China. *J. Atheroscler. Thromb.* **2018**, *25*, 81–89. [CrossRef]
9. World Health Organization. *Guideline: Sugars Intake for Adults and Children*; World Health Organization: Geneva, Switzerland, 2015.
10. Seburg, E.M.; Kunin-Batson, A.; Senso, M.M.; Crain, A.L.; Langer, S.L.; Levy, R.L.; Sherwood, N.E. Concern about child weight among parents of children at-risk for obesity. *Health Behav. Policy Rev.* **2014**, *1*, 197–208. [CrossRef]
11. Young, B.M.; De Bruin, A.; Eagle, L. Attitudes of parents toward advertising to children in the UK, Sweden and New Zealand. *J. Mark. Manag.* **2003**, *19*, 475–490. [CrossRef]
12. Bernstein, J.T.; Franco-Arellano, B.; Schermel, A.; Labonté, M.; L'Abbé, M.R. Healthfulness and nutritional composition of Canadian prepackaged foods with and without sugar claims. *Appl. Physiol. Nutr. Metab.* **2017**, *42*, 1217–1224. [CrossRef]
13. Chen, M.C.; Chien, Y.W.; Yang, H.T.; Chen, Y.C. Marketing strategy, serving size, and nutrition information of popular children's food packages in Taiwan. *Nutrients* **2019**, *11*. [CrossRef] [PubMed]
14. Food Standards Australia New Zealand Food Standards Australia and New Zealand. Food labelling Issues: Quantitative Research with Consumers. Available online: http://foodstandards.gov.au/publications/documents/Part_1_with%20App_A.pdf (accessed on 20 April 2020).
15. Chien, T.-Y.; Chien, Y.-W.; Chang, J.-S.; Chen, Y.C. Influence of mothers' nutrition knowledge and attitudes on their purchase intention for infant cereal with no added sugar claim. *Nutrients* **2018**, *10*. [CrossRef] [PubMed]
16. Campos, S.; Doxey, J.; Hammond, D. Nutrition labels on pre-packaged foods: A systematic review. *Public Health Nutr.* **2011**, *14*, 1496–1506. [CrossRef]
17. Institute of Medicine. *Front-of-Package Nutrition Rating Systems and Symbols: Promoting Healthier Choices*; The National Academies Press: Washington, DC, USA, 2012; p. 180.
18. Persoskie, A.; Hennessy, E.; Nelson, W.L. US Consumers' understanding of nutrition labels in 2013: The importance of health literacy. *Prev. Chronic Dis.* **2017**, *14*, E86. [CrossRef]
19. Malloy-Weir, L.; Cooper, M. Health literacy, literacy, numeracy and nutrition label understanding and use: A scoping review of the literature. *J. Hum. Nutr. Diet.* **2017**, *30*, 309–325. [CrossRef] [PubMed]
20. Jay, M.; Adams, J.; Herring, S.J.; Gillespie, C.; Ark, T.; Feldman, H.; Jones, V.; Zabar, S.; Stevens, D.; Kalet, A. A randomized trial of a brief multimedia intervention to improve comprehension of food labels. *Pre. Med.* **2009**, *48*, 25–31. [CrossRef]
21. Miller, L.M.S.; Beckett, L.A.; Bergman, J.J.; Wilson, M.D.; Applegate, E.A.; Gibson, T.N. Developing nutrition label reading skills: A web-based practice approach. *J. Med. Internet Res.* **2017**, *19*. [CrossRef]

22. Duncanson, K.; Burrows, T.; Holman, B.; Collins, C. Parents' perceptions of child feeding: A qualitative study based on the theory of planned behavior. *J. Dev. Behav. Pediatr.* **2013**, *34*, 227–236. [CrossRef]
23. Ajzen, I. The theory of planned behavior. *Organ. Behav. Hum. Dec. Process.* **1991**, *50*, 179–211. [CrossRef]
24. Daniels, L.; Mallan, K.; Battistutta, D.; Nicholson, J.; Perry, R.; Magarey, A. Evaluation of an intervention to promote protective infant feeding practices to prevent childhood obesity: Outcomes of the NOURISH RCT at 14 months of age and 6 months post the first of two intervention modules. *Inter. J. Obesity* **2012**, *36*, 1292–1298. [CrossRef]
25. Kothe, E.J.; Mullan, B.A.; Amaratunga, R. Randomised controlled trial of a brief theory-based intervention promoting breakfast consumption. *Appetite* **2011**, *56*, 148–155. [CrossRef] [PubMed]
26. Bangia, D.; Palmer-Keenan, D.M. Grocery store podcast about omega-3 fatty acids influences shopping behaviors: A pilot study. *J. Nutr. Educa. Behav.* **2014**, *46*, 616–620. [CrossRef] [PubMed]
27. Ministry of Health and Welfare. Regulations on Nutrition Labeling for Prepackaged Food Products. Available online: http://www.fda.gov.tw/EN/law.aspx (accessed on 20 April 2020).
28. Ministry of Health and Welfare. Dietary Guidelines. Available online: https://www.hpa.gov.tw/Pages/EBook.aspx?nodeid=1217 (accessed on 20 April 2020).
29. Østbye, T.; Krause, K.M.; Stroo, M.; Lovelady, C.A.; Evenson, K.R.; Peterson, B.L.; Bastian, L.A.; Swamy, G.K.; West, D.G.; Brouwer, R.J. Parent-focused change to prevent obesity in preschoolers: Results from the KAN-DO study. *Prev. Med.* **2012**, *55*, 188–195. [CrossRef] [PubMed]
30. Fitzgibbon, M.L.; Stolley, M.R.; Schiffer, L.; Kong, A.; Braunschweig, C.L.; Gomez-Perez, S.L.; Odoms-Young, A.; Van Horn, L.; Christoffel, K.K.; Dyer, A.R. Family-based hip-hop to health: Outcome results. *Obesity* **2013**, *21*, 274–283. [CrossRef] [PubMed]
31. Swindle, T.M.; Ward, W.L.; Whiteside-Mansell, L.; Bokony, P.; Pettit, D. Technology use and interest among low-income parents of young children: Differences by age group and ethnicity. *J. Nutr. Educ. Beha.* **2014**, *46*, 484–490. [CrossRef] [PubMed]
32. Stotz, S.; Lee, J.S.; Rong, H.; Murray, D. The feasibility of an eLearning nutrition education program for low-income individuals. *Health Promot. Pract.* **2017**, *18*, 150–157. [CrossRef] [PubMed]
33. Taiwan Network Information Center 2017 TWNIC Annual Report. Available online: https://www.twnic.net.tw/nt/61.pdf (accessed on 20 April 2020).
34. Gender Equality Committee of the Executive Yuan, 2019 Important Gender Statistics Database. Available online: https://www.gender.ey.gov.tw/gecdb/Stat_Statistics_Query.aspx?sn=Mm4ACreYMwEr7cuT6no39g%3d%3d&statsn=MUwvQW33tN8mhRl94KFn2g%3d%3d&d=m9ww9odNZAz2Rc5Ooj%2fwIQ%3d%3d&Create=1 (accessed on 20 April 2020).
35. Griffiths, M.; Parke, A.; Wood, R.; Parke, J. Internet gambling: An overview of psychosocial impacts. *UNLV Gaming Res. Rev. J.* **2005**, *10*, 27–39.
36. Blanchard, C.M.; Fisher, J.; Sparling, P.B.; Shanks, T.H.; Nehl, E.; Rhodes, R.E.; Courneya, K.S.; Baker, F. Understanding adherence to 5 servings of fruits and vegetables per day: A theory of planned behavior perspective. *J. Nutr. Educ. Behav.* **2009**, *41*, 3–10. [CrossRef]
37. Menozzi, D.; Sogari, G.; Mora, C. Explaining vegetable consumption among young adults: An application of the theory of planned behaviour. *Nutrients* **2015**, *7*, 7633–7650. [CrossRef]
38. Kothe, E.; Mullan, B. Acceptability of a theory of planned behaviour email-based nutrition intervention. *Health Promot. Inter.* **2012**, *29*, 81–90. [CrossRef]
39. Kolasa, K.M.; Miller, M.G. New developments in nutrition education using computer technology. *J. Nutr. Educ.* **1996**, *28*, 7–14. [CrossRef]
40. Jones, C.; Bryant-Waugh, R. Development and pilot of a group skills-and-support intervention for mothers of children with feeding problems. *Appetite* **2012**, *58*, 450–456. [CrossRef]
41. Mitchell, G.L.; Farrow, C.; Haycraft, E.; Meyer, C. Parental influences on children's eating behaviour and characteristics of successful parent-focussed interventions. *Appetite* **2013**, *60*, 85–94. [CrossRef] [PubMed]
42. Howlett, E.; Burton, S.; Kozup, J. How modification of the nutrition facts panel influences consumers at risk for heart disease: The case of trans fat. *J. Public Policy Mark.* **2008**, *27*, 83–97. [CrossRef]
43. Aertsens, J.; Mondelaers, K.; Verbeke, W.; Buysse, J.; Van Huylenbroeck, G. The influence of subjective and objective knowledge on attitude, motivations and consumption of organic food. *Br. Food J.* **2011**, *113*, 1353–1378. [CrossRef]

44. Berg, C.; Jonsson, I.; Conner, M. Understanding choice of milk and bread for breakfast among Swedish children aged 11–15 years: An application of the theory of planned behaviour. *Appetite* **2000**, *34*, 5–19. [CrossRef]
45. Taghdisi, M.H.; Babazadeh, T.; Moradi, F.; Shariat, F. Effect of educational intervention on the fruit and vegetables consumption among the students: Applying theory of planned behavior. *J. Res. Health Sci.* **2016**, *16*, 195–199.
46. Bogers, R.; Brug, J.; Van Assema, P.; Dagnelie, P. Explaining fruit and vegetable consumption: The theory of planned behaviour and misconception of personal intake levels. *Appetite* **2004**, *42*, 157–166. [CrossRef] [PubMed]
47. Patterson, N.; Sadler, M.; Cooper, J. Consumer understanding of sugars claims on food and drink products. *Nutr. Bull.* **2012**, *37*, 121–130. [CrossRef]
48. Tierney, M.; Gallagher, A.M.; Giotis, E.S.; Pentieva, K. An online survey on consumer knowledge and understanding of added sugars. *Nutrients* **2017**, *9*, 37. [CrossRef]
49. Vanderlee, L.; White, C.M.; Bordes, I.; Hobin, E.P.; Hammond, D. The efficacy of sugar labeling formats: Implications for labeling policy. *Obesity* **2015**, *23*, 2406–2413. [CrossRef] [PubMed]
50. Borgmeier, I.; Westenhoefer, J. Impact of different food label formats on healthiness evaluation and food choice of consumers: A randomized-controlled study. *BMC Public Health* **2009**, *9*, 184. [CrossRef] [PubMed]
51. Hawley, K.L.; Roberto, C.A.; Bragg, M.A.; Liu, P.J.; Schwartz, M.B.; Brownell, K.D. The science on front-of-package food labels. *Public Health Nutr.* **2013**, *16*, 430–439. [CrossRef] [PubMed]
52. Siegrist, M.; Leins-Hess, R.; Keller, C. Which front-of-pack nutrition label is the most efficient one? The results of an eye-tracker study. *Food Qual. Prefer.* **2015**, *39*, 183–190. [CrossRef]

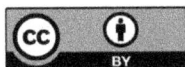

© 2020 by the authors. Licensee MDPI, Basel, Switzerland. This article is an open access article distributed under the terms and conditions of the Creative Commons Attribution (CC BY) license (http://creativecommons.org/licenses/by/4.0/).

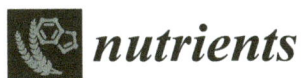 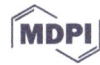

Article

The Impact of the Food Labeling and Other Factors on Consumer Preferences Using Discrete Choice Modeling—The Example of Traditional Pork Sausage

Péter Czine [1], Áron Török [2,*], Károly Pető [3], Péter Horváth [3] and Péter Balogh [1]

1 Department of Statistics and Methodology, Institute of Statistics and Methodology, Faculty of Economics and Business, University of Debrecen, 4032 Debrecen, Hungary; czine.peter@econ.unideb.hu (P.C.); balogh.peter@econ.unideb.hu (P.B.)
2 Department of Agricultural Economics and Rural Development, Institute for the Development of Enterprises, Corvinus University of Budapest, 1093 Budapest, Hungary
3 Department of Rural Development and Regional Economics, Institute of Rural Development, Regional Management and Tourism Management, Faculty of Economics and Business, University of Debrecen, 4032 Debrecen, Hungary; peto.karoly@econ.unideb.hu (K.P.); horvath.peter@econ.unideb.hu (P.H.)
* Correspondence: aron.torok@uni-corvinus.hu; Tel.: +36-1-4825397

Received: 8 May 2020; Accepted: 9 June 2020; Published: 12 June 2020

Abstract: In our study, we examined whether product characteristics indicated by food labels matter in purchasing decisions for sausage made from traditional Hungarian mangalica pork; and how much consumers are willing to pay for them. On the other hand, we also tried to measure whether any changes in consumers' preferences occurred in recent years. Two product characteristics (label of origin and different mangalica meat content) and two other factors (place of purchase and price) are examined in a discrete choice experiment based on stated preference data. According to our expectations, government-funded consumer campaigns in recent years have had an impact on consumers purchase of this traditional product, and they pay more attention to food labels, which can also be influenced by sociodemographic characteristics. Our results have been compared to a previous choice-model based research, investigating consumers' attitude towards similar mangalica pork products. Three different types of models (multinomial logit, random parameter logit, and latent class) are employed, from which two types of models account for the heterogeneity in preferences. Based on the results, it can be concluded that the advertisements promoting traditional meat consumption had only a partial effect on consumer attitudes. Consumers clearly prefer the label of origin indicating meat from registered animals and purchasing on the farmers' market, but according to the indication of the different mangalica meat content in the product, we have already reached conflicting results. Three consumer segments were identified: "price sensitive, loyal to label, label neutral" based on latent class model estimates.

Keywords: food labeling; latent class modeling; traditional meat product, mangalica sausage

1. Introduction

Research in consumer preferences has always been a central topic of economics, especially in microeconomics, which is highly related to the field of marketing. This relationship is mainly focused on answering questions on the preferences of members of groups with different characteristics and how they make their purchasing decisions [1]. Food labels may represent a marketing tool and may influence consumers' perception of food quality [2].

In Hungary, there is growing interest and increasing consumer demand for high-quality and healthy local products [3,4]. The intensification of local food products' production would contribute improving ecosystems and would help towards improving the economic situations of farmers, who form the basis of local development, and are directly related to the achievement of United Nations' second, 12th, and 15th sustainable development goals [5].

Habits and traditions linked to countries and territories have always played an important role in food choices; therefore, it is often investigated by agricultural marketing. In six European regions, Guerrero et al. [6] examined what the word "traditional" means for consumers in terms of food. They found that consumers from southern Europe mostly associate to heritage, culture, or history, while central and northern Europeans rather to convenience, health, or appropriateness. In contrast, Kühne et al. [7] tried to gauge how people perceive traditional product innovation. Consumers' reactions indicated openness towards innovations in this product category, however, with preserving the traditional character as a prerequisite for innovations. Pieniak et al. [8] analyzed the relationship between traditional food consumption and food choice motifs and found that the familiarity with the product and the natural contents are positively associated with the attitudes towards traditional foods. Chrysochou et al. [9] examined the role of quality labels as a driver of consumer loyalty in traditional foods. Based on French scanner data, results showed that standalone labels assuring the designation of origin are less important than brands accompanied with such origin labels.

Mangalica pig is considered a traditional Hungarian breed with Serbian origin, emerged in the Carpathian basin [10], widely used in Hungary from the middle of the 19th century, mainly due to its undemanding nature and excellent lard producing capacity [11]. However, due to changing consumer habits requiring a less fatty diet, the number of registered sows fell from 18,000 heads in 1955 to 243 in ten years, and in another five years, to a few dozens of animals [12]. The breed was rescued after the political change in Hungary, in the mid-1990s when the Hungarian National Association of Mangalica Breeders was established, which certifies the pigs and officially guarantees the origin of genuine mangalica products. In 2004, the Hungarian Parliament claimed mangalica a national treasure representing a high genetic value. Since then, several governmental initiatives took place to strengthen its position, among others marketing campaigns, to promote mangalica food products. Therefore, in recent years, the number of registered sows has increased from 7327 to 10,050 [13]. There has been a continuous growth in the economic importance of the breed due to the increase in demand both in the domestic and export market: Hungarian consumers mainly seek for sausage made from mangalica meat, while a Spanish serrano ham producer sources mangalica meat, producing top quality products [10,11].

Individuals make decisions daily, choose from alternatives; therefore, it is exciting how and based on what they do this [14,15]. The full explanation is probably impossible to find because decision-making is characterized by a high degree of variability and heterogeneity due to several uncertain factors that are mostly difficult or impossible to measure [16]. The purpose of examining the decision-making process is to identify as much information as possible to facilitate a fuller, more detailed understanding. Closer analysis of the chosen alternative (product or service) can provide significant help in this regard [17]. The term preference is rarely used in everyday life, but it is a regular part of life. These are mostly based on the attributes of the product/service (e.g., label, taste, price, etc.), which can be positive or negative (avoiding something). So it can also be said that choices are made within specific attributes of alternatives in the decision-making process. However, it is essential to know which characteristics (e.g., label, taste) are relevant and how important they are for decision-makers. If one aspect is considered important, this factor will be the basis for comparing alternatives. However, if several aspects are decisive, combinations thereof are compared [18]. By assigning a numerical value to them, we can find out the satisfaction or utility level of the consumers. An important consideration when examining preferences is to take proper account of the various limitations. These may include income limits (resulting from not necessarily having the amount of money at which the alternative could be obtained) and technological limitations (resulting from the fact that the product/service requested is no longer or not yet available under current market conditions) [19].

In the literature, there are two main methods identified to assess consumers' choices. The revealed methods observe the behavior of individuals in real-world market situations. In contrast, the stated methods confront consumers with a hypothetical situation to evaluate alternatives of labels that are not yet available in the real market environment [20–22]. The latter can be particularly useful when it is about whether certain products/services with different labels should be introduced to the market [23,24]. It is important to mention that there are many investigations with a combination of revealed and stated data together, with labels aimed at gaining more relevant information through the results [25,26]. This approach is often used in the process of evaluating consumer preferences, also known as discrete choice experiment [27–29].

The discrete choice experiment is based on the utility-maximizing behavior of individuals. It means that the element with the highest utility value is always selected from a deciding set. Furthermore, according to the theory of characteristics, the utility of products/services derives from their attributes. In addition, it assumes a discrete choice situation (only one element is selected from the choice set) [30]. Finally, the utility function is broken down into a systematic and a random part [31].

The method is increasingly appearing in the field of agricultural marketing, where the focus is on examining the expected attributes of different foods (e.g., label of origin, price, fat, or meat content) and the willingness to pay for product attributes (e.g., how much they are willing to pay for a label indicating 25% higher meat content) [31–35].

Therefore, in this paper, we would like to answer several questions. First, which kind of characteristics of the traditional Hungarian mangalica sausage matters for the consumers. Second, what is their willingness to pay for these attributes, third can we distinguish different traditional product consumer segments using the latent class (LC) model and fourth, can we observe any kind of change in consumers' preference for this traditional product in the recent years, mainly due to the government-funded promotions.

2. Literature Review

Among foods, the traditional and regional meat products have always played a prominent role, especially if they are certified (e.g., geographical indication, country of origin, etc.). In the regions related to production, usually, local consumers prefer traditional meat products, and it is often accompanied by a higher willingness to pay [36]. On average, meat products have the highest price premium among foods with geographical indication in the European Union [37]. In the case of raw meat, the literature is mainly focusing on beef (e.g., [38–41]) and lamb (e.g., [42–46]), indicating that consumers are positive and willing to pay more for local and traditional products or with origin with high reputation. In the case of pork meat, for hams, in particular, several studies indicated that consumers are particularly fond of these traditional products and are ready to pay more for them (e.g., [47–49]). However, certifications and trademarks are only relevant up to a certain level of quality and in the very premium segment, other product attributes matter more [29]. It is also important to point out that for meat products with a high reputation, consumers living near the place of production tend to be willing to pay a lower premium than those from remote areas [50].

Many research focused on consumers' attitudes toward pork meat. Among others, Balcombe et al. [51] examined consumer preferences for different meat products with special emphasis on country of origin, using a discrete choice experiment. Based on their results, the country of origin information is positively assessed for all food products. However, it was already considered less important compared to other food product attributes. Shan et al. [52] investigated consumer ratings for processed meat products. The study identified consumer purchase intentions and quality perceptions of basic meat products. These included the price, base meat product, and healthy ingredients. Di Vita et al. [53] emphasized that the price is one of the most important factors in determining the quality level of the salami investigated. Besides, the authors concluded that certain socio-economic segments of consumers show a significant willingness to pay extra for low salt content and nitrate-free salami. Ngapo [54] explored consumer preferences in the direction of pork ribs in five Canadian provinces. According to his findings, fat cover and slight color were among the factors most influencing consumer choices. Špička et al. [55] investigated consumer behavior in the Czech pork retail market. They identified that the Czech consumers preferred packaged meat or counter sales over sourcing from a butcher. Furthermore, the relatively high proportion of low education consumers and one-person households do not favor quality; people with lower education are more price-sensitive than those with higher education; older consumers prefer price to quality; in general, the majority of consumers prefer domestic pork by origin. Font-i-Furnols and Guerrero [56] examined consumer behavior and perception of meat and meat products. Based on their results, consumer behavior is influenced by several factors related to meat and meat products, so consumer preferences are heterogeneous. Effective information strategies (labels in particular) can help to promote a better understanding of the process. Xazela et al. [57] examined perceptions of rural consumers regarding meat consumption. They assessed that the main place of purchase was the supermarket, which was rated the most hygienic and with a fresh supply. They further conclude that consumers' perceptions of meat quality are also influenced by their income and cultural background. Merlino et al. [58] examined the behavior of households concerning meat consumption, with a particular focus on households with and without children. The results showed that weekly meat consumption was higher in households without children. Both groups preferred sourcing from the butcher, followed by supermarkets. Kallas et al. [59] attempted to assess consumer preferences for traditional and innovative pig products. Their results showed that preferences are heterogeneous among the countries included, moreover eating experiences have a significant effect on preferences. Kallas et al. [60] used a non-hypothetical discrete choice experiment with a hedonic evaluation to find out the importance of food neophobia in consumer purchases and to calculate willingness to pay before and after tasting the products. Their results showed that traditional pork products preventing cardiovascular disease achieved higher purchase intention and willingness to pay (WTP) than expected. However, after tasting, consumers showed a lower WTP for all innovative traditional pork products. Food neophobia was closely related to WTP prior to hedonic evaluation. Candek-Potokar et al. [61] examined the sustainability of local pig breeds by establishing a collaborative trademark. Among others, they suggested to have a label attracting end-users (farmers), breeders associations, and meat processors to sufficiently support conserving local pig breeds.

Balogh et al. [62] also focused on a traditional meat product: salami made of mangalica pork. The survey they employed was conducted between August and October 2012, in the Northern Great Plain region of Hungary, using a discrete choice experiment with 309 participants. The main findings of the research were that consumers prefer a salami product made entirely of mangalica meat and sourced from a butcher. During the years after the experiment (between 2012 and 2018), the Hungarian government placed great emphasis on encouraging the consumption of locally produced (labeled) traditional products, including mangalica meat, from reliable sources. In 2019, with the support of the Ministry of Agriculture, the incentive program of the Agricultural Marketing Center was launched (including so-called "Mangalica Festivals", tastings, chef competition, conference held in several cities), which was explicitly aimed at promoting mangalica meat and encouraging its consumption [63]. In the light of the above, our research tries to find out whether there has been a change in consumer preferences for labeled mangalica meat (represented by a sausage product in the present study) compared to the results of this previous research.

Against this background, we tried to investigate four different aspects of consumers' attitude towards mangalica sausage.

First, what are the product attributes that matter for the consumers?

Second, what are their willingness to pay for these attributes?

Third, can we distinguish different traditional product consumer segments using the LC model?

Finally, is there any change in consumer preference as a result of the marketing campaigns financed by the Hungarian government? Here, as a benchmark, we used the results of similar research conducted in 2012 [63].

3. Materials and Methods

Before the survey, two focus group interviews were conducted (with six regular consumers per group) in October 2019 to determine the product attributes to be included. We identified four attributes including price (representing four typical price levels for similar products available in the region of the research *and our price levels are the same as the previous research of Balogh et al. (2016) used, as the price of mangalica sausage and salami did not change significantly in the recent years and to get more comparable results*), mangalica meat content (the proportion of mangalica in the product), label of origin (official label of the breeding association certifying that the product was made from registered mangalica pigs raised in a registered barn), and the place of the purchase (the type of sales channel) were included, similar to the research of Balogh, Békési, Gorton, Popp, and Lengyel [62]. Subsequently, we determined their attribute levels, all referring to the real market conditions (Table 1).

Table 1. Attributes, their levels, and their coding.

Attribute	Attribute Level	Coding
Price (HUF/kg) [1,2]	1500 HUF 2000 HUF 2500 HUF 3000 HUF	Continuous variable
Mangalica meat content (from the total meat) (%)	50% 75% 100%	1 2 3
Label of origin (NAMB label of origin [3])	No Yes	0 1
Place of purchase	'Farmers' market Butcher Hyper-/supermarket	1 2 3

[1] 1 EUR is 332 HUF based on the exchange rate of on 9 December 2019. [2] The levels of price attribute are divided by 1000 in order to get fewer ranges. [3] The National Association of Mangalica Breeders (NAMB) certifies that registered mangalica pig meat has been used in the preparation of the product.

We used so-called "design" coding for categorical variables (here, there was a difference compared with Balogh et al. [62] because they used "effect" coding in their models run in STATA software). In all cases, the same levels were the base levels during the model estimations (50% meat content, No NAMB label of origin, Farmers' market). To select the experimental design, we first estimated how many decision situations the full factorial design would include in the experiment. Based on the selected attributes and their levels, this number became too high (72), so we used a partial D-efficient design (to reduce the number of product combinations while minimizing the number of D-errors), through the use of Ngene 1.2. software in the final questionnaire, with eight decision situations (with three alternatives per situation, each with a "no answer" option) [64]. See Table 2, for example.

Table 2. An example of a decision situation.

	Alternative 1	Alternative 2	Alternative 3
Price (HUF/kg)	3000	2000	
Meat content (%)	75%	75%	None of these products
Label of origin	Yes	No	
Place of purchase	'Farmers' market	Butcher	

In addition to the decision situations, the final questionnaire included additional questions on purchasing and consumption habits and the sociodemographic characteristics of the respondents. Before the survey, we did a pilot survey to get feedback on difficult-to-understand parts.

Our research was carried out in the three most populous cities of the Northern Great Plain region (Nyíregyháza, Debrecen, Szolnok), where 26% of the registered Hungarian mangalica sows are kept, and the headquarter of the National Association of Mangalica Breeders (NAMB) is also located. Moreover, the most substantial volume of mangalica products is purchased in this region. In the three selected cities, respondents were reached in front of the stores of the Tesco hypermarkets, between December 2019 and February 2020. The sample contains 477 persons (155–165–157 answers, respectively), detailed in Table 3. During the data collection, great emphasis was placed on ensuring representativeness for several sociodemographic variables through quota sampling. We have successfully achieved this by gender, age, and place of residence [65,66].

Table 3. Sociodemographic characteristics of respondents.

Sociodemographic Factors	Sample ($N = 477$)	Regional Distribution *
Gender (%)		
Female	56.0	51.7
Male	44.0	48.3
Age (category) (%)		
Age1 (<30)	22.0	21.8
Age2 (30–39)	26.5	27.1
Age3 (40–49)	22.0	21.0
Age4 (50<)	29.5	30.1
Age (mean)	41.54	41.7
Highest level of education (%)		
Elementary	8.2	-
Secondary	44.6	-
Higher education	47.2	-
Monthly gross income (%) **		
Substantially below average	33.3	-
Below average	17.6	-
Average	25.8	-
Above average	23.3	-
Residence (%)		
Urban	72.3	68.3
Rural	27.7	31.7

* [66]; ** Net average regional income in 2019: 187,366 HUF/month.

The dataset was processed via the R: Apollo 0.0.6 software extension [67,68]. In the following, we describe the characteristics of the model specifications used in estimates.

3.1. Multinomial Logit Model (MNL)

The widely used multinomial logit model is related to McFadden and Zarembka [69], which has the advantage that estimates can be easily interpreted. It is based on the theory of random utility; it assumes the utility-maximizing behavior of individuals. For the model, the systematic and random part of utility can be written according to Equation (1):

$$U_{n,i} = \beta X_{n,i} + \varepsilon_{n,i}, \tag{1}$$

where U denotes the total utility, βX the systematic part, ε the random part, n the respondent, and i denotes the alternative.

The probability of choosing alternative *i* is given by Equation (2):

$$Prob_{n,i} = \frac{\exp \sum_{k=1}^{K} \beta_k X_{n,i,k}}{\sum_{i=1}^{I} \exp \sum_{k=1}^{K} \beta_k X_{n,i,k}}, \qquad (2)$$

where *k* is the product/service attribute, *X* is the variable, β is the coefficient value for that variable.

One of the drawbacks of the model is that it is unable to capture the heterogeneity of individual tastes and assumes the independence of irrelevant alternatives. As a result, more complex models are often used to analyze discrete choice experiments [70].

3.2. Random Parameter Logit Model (RPL)

The major advantage of the random parameter logit model is its ability to capture preference heterogeneity. This is reached by allowing the coefficients of β to be randomized among the respondents, along with a particular pre-selected distribution by the researcher. At the same time, their parameters (mean, standard deviation) can also be set up [71]. The other great advantage is to allow a flexible variance-covariance structure for the random term, thus resolving the restrictive assumption known as the independence of irrelevant alternatives [72,73]. In the model, the systematic part of the utility can be decomposed by Equation (3):

$$V_{n,i} = \left(\overline{\beta}' + \eta_n'\right) X_{n,i}, \qquad (3)$$

where $\overline{\beta}$ is the mean value, and η_n a person-specific difference.

The probability of choice (for alternative *i* by person *n* in decision situation *t*) can be described by Equation (4):

$$Prob_{i,n,t} = \frac{\exp(\alpha' + \beta' X_{i,n,t} + \varphi' F_{i,n,t})}{\sum_{j=1}^{J} \exp(\alpha' + \beta' X_{j,n,t} + \varphi' F_{j,n,t})}, \qquad (4)$$

where α' is the alternative-specific constant value, β' is the random parameter, φ' is the fixed parameter, $X_{i,n,t}$ is the attribute variable for the alternative, and $F_{i,n,t}$ is the variable of personal characteristics [74].

3.3. Latent Class Model (LC)

An advantage of the latent class model is that it captures heterogeneity among individuals. This is reached by grouping individuals into distinct *Q* groups, which are distinct and have their own β parameter [75]. In the model, the probability of choosing alternative *i* by person *n* from class *q* can be described by Equation (5) [76,77]:

$$Prob_{i,nq} = \frac{\exp(\beta'_q X_{i,n})}{\sum_{i=1}^{I_n} \exp(\beta'_q X_{i,n})} \quad q = 1, \ldots, Q. \qquad (5)$$

One of the features of the latent class model is to estimate class probability values ($H_{n,q}$), which allows estimating the probability of individuals falling into different classes. Accordingly, the probability of choice changes to Equation (6):

$$Prob_{i,n} = \sum_{q=1}^{Q} Prob_{i,nq} H_{n,q}. \qquad (6)$$

The limitations of the model most often refer to the ideal definition of the number of classes. Most decisions are made based on information criteria (Akaike information criterion (AIC), consistent Akaike information criterion (CAIC), (Bayesian information criterion (BIC)) [78].

4. Results

In the following, we intend to present estimates of the three models. Firstly, we use multinomial logit, then the random parameter logit models, and finally, we estimate latent class model in order to find whether we can distinguish different consumer segments based on their preferences for a food product [79,80]. The utility functions used for the different models, and how the willingness to pay (in case of MNL model) was calculated, are explained in Appendix A.

4.1. Importance of Different Product Attributes and Willingness to Pay among Mangalica Sausage Consumers

The results of our estimates based on MNL and RPL (where we used a special form utility function to make direct estimates for the willingness to pay [73]) specifications are presented in Table 4.

Table 4. The results of multinomial logit (MNL) and random parameter logit (RPL) model estimates.

Attributes and Model Details	MNL Model		RPL Model (Direct WTP)	
	Coefficient	Standard Error	Coefficient	Standard Error
ASC (alternative 2)	0.652 ***	0.071	0.673 ***	0.061
ASC (opt-out)	−1.583 ***	0.138	−3.191 ***	0.156
Price/1000	−0.885 ***	0.058	−1.215 *** (2.909) ***	0.138
75% meat content	0.697 ***	0.078	0.895 ***	0.039
100% meat content	0.844 ***	0.065	0.862 ***	0.044
Label of origin	1.843 ***	0.089	1.682 *** (0.677) ***	0.073
Butcher	−0.759 ***	0.09	−0.657 ***	0.064
Hyper-/supermarket	−1.009 ***	0.101	−1.058 *** (0.585) ***	0.101
Observations		3816		
Pseudo R^2	0.1608		0.2634	
Adj R^2	0.1589		0.2607	
Log-likelihood	−3518.227		−3088.236	
AIC	7052.45		6198.47	

Note: ASC represents the alternative-specific constant value.; ASC (alternative 1), 50% meat content, no label of origin, and the 'farmers' market variables reported the base levels in the estimates.; The standard deviation values in the RPL model (for random variables) are shown in parentheses below the parameter estimates.; *** indicate statistical significance at the 1% level.; ASC (alternative 2), ASC (opt-out), and price coefficients in RPL model mean the coefficient of utility, while the others (75% meat content, 100% meat content, label of origin, butcher, hyper-/supermarket) mean the coefficients of willingness to pay (WTP).; Adj R^2 denotes the adjusted value of R^2; AIC denotes the Akaike information criterion.

In the RPL model, all parameters were first randomized; however, we got significant standard deviation values only for the price, label of origin, and hyper-/supermarket variables. As a result, only these were randomized in the final specification (as shown in Table 4) [19]. We chose log-uniform distribution for the price, while we used normal distribution for the label of origin and hyper-/supermarket [81]. For the estimates, we used 500 so-called halton draws.

Based on the results of the MNL model parameter estimates, it can be concluded that the opt-out alternative (no buying sausage) was preferred significantly less often than the alternative 1; as the price of the mangalica sausage increases, the level of consumer utility decreases; as the mangalica meat content increases, consumers sense of utility increases; the existence of label of origin has a positive impact on utility; they prefer purchasing on the 'farmers' market over butcher and much over the hyper-/supermarket. According to the significance values, all parameters in the model can be considered significant.

For the MNL model, calculations of willingness to pay were based on point estimate [19]. The results are shown in Table 5.

Table 5. Willingness to pay (WTP) estimates for the multinomial logit model.

Product Attributes	Willingness to Pay
75% meat content	0.787 ***
100% meat content	0.954 ***
Label of origin	2.082 ***
Butcher	−0.858 ***
Hyper-/supermarket	−1.139 ***

Note: *** indicate statistical significance at the 1% level.

According to the WTP estimates, consumers would pay more for higher meat content, ca. 787 HUF more for products with 75%, and 954 HUF more with 100% mangalica meat content, compared to 50% meat content. In addition, they would pay about 2082 HUF extra for a labeled product certifying the origin. Finally, they would pay less outside of 'farmers' market, while results estimated a discount of 858 HUF at a butcher and 1139 HUF in a hyper-/supermarket.

Comparing the results of MNL and RPL models, we can see that the RPL model specification shows a significantly better fit (Pseudo R^2 in MNL: 0.1608; Pseudo R^2 in RPL: 0.2634). Furthermore, significant standard deviation values are present for some attributes (price, label of origin, hyper-/supermarket), indicating that there is heterogeneity in preferences which the MNL model cannot handle. The significant ASC (opt-out) value of RPL model (−3.191) means that consumers preferred more alternative 1 over the no-choice alternative. According to the negative value of the price coefficient, consumer utility decreases when the price increases. There is a statistically significant standard deviation value for the price attribute, which means that there is heterogeneity in consumer preferences regarding price. There is a difference in mangalica meat content compared to the estimates of the MNL model. Consumers prefer more a 75% than a 100% mangalica meat content product compared to a 50% mangalica meat content product (they would pay about 895 HUF more for 75% and 862 HUF more for 100% mangalica meat content product, compared to 50%). Although the presence of the label of origin can be considered highly preferred in both cases (based on RPL model estimates, they are willing to pay about 1682 HUF for a product with the label of origin, compared to non-labeled product), the significant standard deviation value of the RPL model suggests that there is heterogeneity in willingness to pay for the attribute. In terms of place of purchase, we can draw similar conclusions in RPL as in the case of the MNL model (they prefer the farmers' market over butcher and hyper-/supermarket and are willing to pay about 657 HUF less at a butcher, 1058 HUF less at a hyper-/supermarket purchase, compared to buying at the farmers' market). However, it is important to note that we obtained a significant standard deviation value for the hyper-/supermarket, which suggests that there is heterogeneity in consumer willingness to pay for this level of attribute.

4.2. Consumer Segments of the Mangalica Sausage

Before presenting the results, it is important to note that several model configurations have been tested for the latent class model (Table 6). The best values came from the three-class specification shown in Table 7 (based on class probability values, Pseudo R^2, Log-likelihood, and AIC aspects).

Table 6. Comparison of information criteria.

	2 Segments Model		3 Segments Model			4 Segments Model		
Estimated parameters	22		36			50		
Log-likelihood (LL)	−3092.223		−2993.281			−2943.919		
AIC	6228.45		6058.56			5987.84		
BIC	6365.88		6283.45			6300.19		
Pseudo R^2	0.2624		0.286			0.2978		
Class probability values	0.40	0.60	0.28	0.57	0.15	0.13	0.54	0.04	0.29

Note: Log-likelihood evaluated at zero is: −4192.304.; AIC denotes the Akaike information criterion, while BIC denotes the Bayesian information criterion.

It should also be noted that several sociodemographic variables were tested to find the source of heterogeneity among groups (members of groups with different characteristics, what preferences they have for each product feature). Among these, we found significant effects in terms of gender, age groups, and income levels (Table 7).

Table 7. The results of the latent class (LC) model estimates.

Attributes and Model Details	Coefficient			Standard Error		
	Price Sensitive	Loyal to Label	Label Neutral	Price Sensitive	Loyal to Label	Label Neutral
ASC (alternative 2)		0.62 ***			0.088	
ASC (opt-out)		−2.845 ***			0.184	
Price/1000	−3.663 ***	−0.55 ***	−1.915 ***	0.247	0.099	0.129
75% meat content	3.457 ***	0.584 ***	1.53 ***	0.315	0.142	0.256
100% meat content	3.07 ***	0.73 ***	2.223 ***	0.341	0.112	0.265
Label of origin	6.98 ***	1.26 ***	0.722 ***	0.388	0.174	0.255
Butcher	−2.214 ***	−0.524 ***	−0.714 ***	0.25	0.167	0.228
Hyper-/supermarket	−2.478 ***	−0.711 ***	−2.783	0.257	0.145	0.00
Female	−0.859 ***		−0.029	0.24		0.35
Age2	0.00		0.153	0.357		0.494
Age3	1.141 ***		1.073 **	0.355		0.46
Age4	0.771 **		0.668	0.327		0.47
Income2	0.203		1.573 ***	0.35		0.45
Income3	−0.035		−0.025	0.285		0.481
Income4	−0.986 ***		−0.279	0.329		0.457
Delta	−0.558		−2.112 ***	0.313		0.539
Class probability values	0.28	0.57	0.15			
Observations	3816					
Pseudo R^2	0.286					
Adj R^2	0.2774					
Log-likelihood	−2993.281					
AIC	6058.56					

Note: ASC represents the alternative-specific constant value.; Female: type of gender, Age 2 (30–40 years), Age 3 (40–50 years), Age 4 (above 50 year) the age, Income 2 (below average), Income 3 (average), and Income 4 (above average) represent the monthly gross income classification for respondents.; ASC (alternative 1), 50% meat content, no label of origin, 'farmers' market, male, the lowest age group (below 30 years) and income level (substantially below average), and the delta variable for class "B" reported the base levels in the estimates.; Delta is a constant value for the classes of the latent class model.; **, and *** indicate statistical significance at the 5% and 1% levels.

The parameter estimates clearly show that the coefficients of product attributes differ in size from the multinomial logit model, but similar conclusions can be drawn. The only significant difference is in Class 1 ("price sensitive"), where members prefer 75% mangalica meat content product more than 50% and 100% meat content (with a similar conclusion like in the RPL model). Based on significance values, all product attributes can be considered significant, except hyper-/supermarket level for Class 3 ("label neutral").

It is important to note that for Class 1 ("price sensitive"), we found several significant sociodemographic variables, including gender, age 3, age 4, and income 4. Based on these, we can conclude that older (above 40 years) men with lower income level (average or below average) are most likely to be in Class 1 ("price sensitive"). They are significantly more price sensitive in case of the product investigated than the other two classes, preferring a product with a mangalica meat content of 75%, possessing the label of origin and obtaining the product from the 'farmers' market is very important to them.

The willingness to pay estimates for the model are shown in Table 8, where in addition to point estimates for each class, parameters for the entire model are indicated, corrected by class probability values.

Table 8. WTP estimates for the LC model.

Product Attributes	Willingness to Pay			
	Price Sensitive	Loyal to Label	Label Neutral	Full Model
75% mangalica meat content	0.944 ***	1.061 ***	0.799 ***	0.993 ***
100% mangalica meat content	0.838 ***	1.326 ***	1.161 ***	1.165 ***
Label of origin	1.906 ***	2.289 ***	0.377 **	1.897 ***
Butcher	−0.604 ***	−0.952 **	−0.373 **	−0.768 **
Hyper-/supermarket	−0.677 ***	−1.291 ***	−1.453 ***	−1.143 ***

Note: **, and *** indicate statistical significance at the 5% and 1% levels.

Based on the results of the WTP estimates (for the full model), we can conclude that consumers would pay about 993 HUF more for a 75% and 1165 HUF more for a 100% mangalica meat content product compared to 50% meat content product; pay a higher price of about 1897 HUF for a labeled product; and would give about 768 HUF less when purchasing at a butcher, while about 1143 HUF at a hyper-/supermarket shopping, compared to buying on 'farmers' market. Based on these results (shown in Tables 7 and 8), we named the classes, which we have used earlier (price sensitive, loyal to label, and label neutral).

4.3. Changes in Consumer Willingness to Pay for a Traditional Mangalica Product

To answer our last question, we compared the results of the 2012 and 2019 WTP estimates (shown in Table 9).

Table 9. Comparisons of WTP estimates for MNL and RPL models between 2012 and 2019.

Product Attributes	WTP for MNL (HUF)		WTP for RPL (HUF)	
	2012	2019	2012	2019
Label of origin	0.457	2.082	0.942	1.682
75% meat content	0.235	0.787	0.623	0.895
100% meat content	0.445	0.954	0.736	0.862
Butcher	0.349	−0.858	0.827	−0.657
Hyper-/supermarket	−0.715	−1.139	−1.347	−1.058

5. Discussion

In our paper, we tried to investigate the consumers' preferences toward mangalica sausages, in terms of utilities and willingness to pay, and we also tried to compare our results to previous research of 2012. Regarding the willingness to pay, it can be concluded that while in the case of the MNL model, consumers would pay more for the 100% meat content product than for the 75% product (considering the 50% product as a base). In contrast, in the case of the RPL model, they would pay the most for the 75% meat content product. The fit of the applied LC model (based on the Pseudo R^2 value) shows a better fit than the RPL model. Similar conclusions can be drawn for classes as for the MNL and RPL models. However, in terms of meat content, we can see contradictory results here as well (in the case of two classes, the product with 100% meat content is the most preferred, while in the case of one class, the product with 75% meat content).

Our results suggest that for this traditional Hungarian pork, there is heterogeneity in consumer preferences, in which the conclusion is similar to inferences of Font-i-Furnols and Guerrero [56] and Kallas, Čandek-Potokar, Tomažin, Pugliese, Aquilani, and Gil [59]. Our assumption that the changes in preferences are mainly related to the food labels and their information content can be confirmed, in line with other consumer studies focusing on traditional meat products (e.g., [82–84]). Comparing the willingness to pay for different product characteristics with the 2012 results, we can conclude that consumers would pay significantly more for both labeled and high-meat content products. They prefer to buy at the farmers' market, though, in the 2012 survey [62], sourcing at the butcher was the most preferred place of purchase (for a detailed comparison, see Table 9).

Moreover, the influence of consumers' sociodemographic characteristics was also confirmed and supported by the results as older men with lower income represented a distinct class. Previous research including Van Loo, Caputo, Nayga, Meullenet, and Ricke [34], Wang, Ge, and Ma [35], Kallas et al. [60], Lusk [85], Lusk et al. [86], Verbeke et al. [87] reached a similar consequence. Based on their conclusions, product labeling is a determining factor in decisions, and they also shed light on the impact of sociodemographic characteristics in decision-making.

Regarding price levels and willingness to pay, a remarkable premium was identified. Our survey was conducted in the region (Northern Great Plain) where mangalica production is traditionally the most important in Hungary; therefore these local consumers prefer traditional meat products, and also have a higher willingness to pay, just as found for local consumers by van Zyl, Vermeulen, and Kirsten [36]. On the contrary, unlike another central European investigation found (Špička, Náglová, and Mezera [55] for the Czech Republic), for Hungarian mangalica pork meat consumers, sourcing from the butcher was preferred over purchasing in large scale food retails. This difference could be explained by the fact that the subject of the Czech research was conventional pork meat. This also suggests that for traditional food products, traditional sales channels are preferred and in Hungary, the farmers' market is still considered as one of the most important channels [88], and with other types of short food supply chains are expected to have increasing importance in the case of quality food purchase [89].

For traditional pork products, Candek-Potokar, Giusto, Conti, Cosola, and Fontanesi [61] suggested—among others—a trademark which attracts both farmers, breeders' associations, and processors; therefore, it could contribute to the self-sustainability of comprised local pig breeds. Our results show, that in the case of mangalica, the label of the producers' associations testifying genuine origin has already filled this gap and consumers are attracted to this label, both in terms of utility and price premium.

This study has some limitations and further research opportunities. First, due to limited funding, it was conducted only in one region of Hungary. This study could be repeated in a national survey. Through this, we could examine the attitude of the entire Hungarian population to the purchase of mangalica sausage and could gain even more evidence. Second, the preference assessment procedures based on a hypothetical situation do not take into account many of the factors that arise in real choices [90]. Besides, the graphical representation of cards in decision situations were weak, sketchy, and less realistic, as opposed to other experiments [85,91,92]. Finally, the structure of the corresponding model specification also involves several limitations and issues (assigning random parameters, determining the number of latent classes).

6. Conclusions

In our research, we aimed to explore consumer preferences for a labeled traditional product, the mangalica sausage, using a discrete choice experiment and comparing our results with the previous investigation in the same topic with a very similar methodology and with the same attributes [62].

Our study was conducted on a sample of 477 persons. Product attributes featured in the experiment included label of origin, meat content, product price, and place of purchase. We made our estimates using multinomial logit, latent class, and random parameter logit models. Based on our results, we concluded that the existence of the label of origin positively influences the consumers' sense of utility; purchasing at the farmers' market is more preferred over the butcher and even more over hyper-/supermarket. However, the role of the level of mangalica meat content was contradictory.

The overall results of our research have clear messages for the stakeholders of the value chain of this traditional pork variety. On the one hand, the label of the Hungarian National Association of

Mangalica Breeders testifying genuine origin has an added value, as consumers acknowledge it. On the other hand, mangalica sausage producers should be encouraged to use direct sales channels to reach their target groups.

Regarding willingness to pay, higher mangalica meat content is accepted by the consumers with a remarkable price premium compared to sausages with a lower level of mangalica meat content. This indicates that the higher quality level of this traditional variety over the conventional pork meat is recognized. This could also stimulate the production of mangalica meat. In addition, the label of the producers' association is accompanied by a higher price level, indicating that it is worthy of investing by the producers and of maintaining the testifying system through their association. Last but not least, the negative price premium to be paid for non-direct sales (outside of farmers' market) also reveals the importance of short food supply chains for mangalica producers.

In our paper, as a reference point, we used the results of a similar survey conducted in 2012. Since then, a change in consumers' attitude can be recognized. Although the same product characteristics are still considered the most important, the governmental promotion campaigns and the initiatives of the Hungarian National Association of Mangalica Breeders have met their expectations. Mangalica products are consumed and preferred even more over mainstream alternative products, in terms of willingness to pay. The demand of this traditional product has moved to even more authentic channels and farmers' markets providing direct interactions between the producers and the final consumers seem to be the place where this traditional product can fulfil a real niche of the market and can attract a determinative number of consumers. According to our LC model results, three consumer segments were identified: "price sensitive, loyal to label, label neutral" due to the preference heterogeneity. Furthermore, we can conclude that older (above 40 years) men with lower income level (average or below average) are most likely to be in the "price sensitive" separate group according to habits of mangalica sausage. These characteristics of the mangalica meat consumers should be also bear in mind once targeting this traditional product.

However, further research might also be addressed on the preferences of other traditional food products to investigate whether consumers consider the existence of product labeling properties also important. Besides, it may be worthy of testing additional model specifications and of including additional sociodemographic variables to refine the estimates, using a nation-wide sample.

Author Contributions: Conceptualization, Á.T., P.C. and P.B.; methodology, P.C. and P.B.; software, P.C. and P.B.; validation, K.P. and P.H.; formal analysis, P.H.; investigation, K.P. and P.H.; resources, P.B.; data curation, P.C. and P.B.; writing–original draft preparation, Á.T., K.P., P.H., P.C. and P.B.; writing–review and editing, Á.T., K.P., P.H., P.C. and P.B.; supervision, Á.T., P.C. and P.B.; funding acquisition, P.B. All authors have read and agreed to the published version of the manuscript.

Funding: This research and the APC was funded by National Research, Development, and Innovation Fund of Hungary grant number Project no. 130443.

Conflicts of Interest: The authors declare no conflict of interest.

Appendix A

In the multinomial logit model, the systematic part of the utility for alternative i can be written according to Equation (A1):

$$V_i = ASC_{alt.i} + \beta_{Price} * Price_{alt.i} + \beta_{75\% \; Meat \; content} * 75\% \; Meat \; content_{alt.i} \\ + \beta_{100\% \; Meat \; content} * 100\% \; Meat \; content_{alt.i} + \beta_{Label \; of \; origin} \\ * Label \; of \; origin_{alt.i} + \beta_{Butcher} * Butcher_{alt.i} \\ + \beta_{Hyper-/supermarket} * Hyper_{alt.i}. \tag{A1}$$

The systematic part of the utility in the RPL model can be written according to Equation (A2):

$$V_i = ASC_{alt.i} + \beta_{Price} * (Price_{alt.i} + V_{75\% \text{ Meat content}} * 75\% \text{ Meat content}_{alt.i} \\ + V_{100\% \text{ Meat content}} * 100\% \text{ Meat content}_{alt.i} + V_{Label\ of\ origin} \\ * Label\ of\ origin_{alt.i} + V_{Butcher} * Butcher_{alt.i} \\ + V_{Hyper-/supermarket} * Hyper_{alt.i}), \quad (A2)$$

where the V parameters represent the willingness to pay for that attribute.

The willingness to pay calculation in the MNL model is based on Equation (A3):

$$WTP_{attribute\ k} = (-)\frac{\beta_{attribute\ k}}{\beta_{attribute\ Price}}, \quad (A3)$$

where β expresses the value of the coefficients for attributes.

For the latent class model, the systematic part of utility for alternative i and class q can be written according to Equation (A4):

$$V_i = ASC_{alt.i} + \beta_{Price}[q] * Price_{alt.i} + \beta_{75\% \text{ Meat content}}[q] \\ * 75\% \text{ Meat content}_{alt.i} + \beta_{100\% \text{ Meat content}}[q] \\ * 100\% \text{ Meat content}_{alt.i} + \beta_{Label\ of\ origin}[q] \\ * Label\ of\ origin_{alt.i} + \beta_{Butcher}[q] * Butcher_{alt.i} \\ + \beta_{Hyper-/supermarket}[q] * Hyper_{alt.i}. \quad (A4)$$

References

1. Novemsky, N.; Dhar, R.; Schwarz, N.; Simonson, I. Preference Fluency in Choice. *J. Mark. Res.* **2007**, *44*, 347–356. [CrossRef]
2. Kumar, N.; Kapoor, S. Do labels influence purchase decisions of food products? Study of young consumers of an emerging market. *Br. Food J.* **2017**, *119*, 218–229. [CrossRef]
3. Szakály, Z.; Horvát, A.; Soós, M.; Pető, K.; Szente, V. A minőségre és származásra utaló jelölések szerepe a fogyasztói döntéshozatalban. *Élelmiszertáplálkozás Mark.* **2014**, *10*, 3–10.
4. Szakály, Z.; Soós, M.; Szabó, S.; Szente, V. Role of labels referring to quality and country of origin in food consumers' decisions. *Acta Aliment.* **2016**, *45*, 323–330. [CrossRef]
5. The United Nations. The Division for Sustainable Development Goals (DSDG). Available online: https://sustainabledevelopment.un.org/ (accessed on 29 March 2020).
6. Guerrero, L.; Claret, A.; Verbeke, W.; Enderli, G.; Zakowska-Biemans, S.; Vanhonacker, F.; Issanchou, S.; Sajdakowska, M.; Granli, B.S.; Scalvedi, L.; et al. Perception of traditional food products in six European regions using free word association. *Food Qual. Prefer.* **2010**, *21*, 225–233. [CrossRef]
7. Kühne, B.; Vanhonacker, F.; Gellynck, X.; Verbeke, W. Innovation in traditional food products in Europe: Do sector innovation activities match consumers' acceptance? *Food Qual. Prefer.* **2010**, *21*, 629–638. [CrossRef]
8. Pieniak, Z.; Verbeke, W.; Vanhonacker, F.; Guerrero, L.; Hersleth, M. Association between traditional food consumption and motives for food choice in six European countries. *Appetite* **2009**, *53*, 101–108. [CrossRef]
9. Chrysochou, P.; Krystallis, A.; Giraud, G. Quality assurance labels as drivers of customer loyalty in the case of traditional food products. *Food Qual. Prefer.* **2012**, *25*, 156–162. [CrossRef]
10. Török, Á. Spanyolul tanul a magyar mangalica! *Gazdálkodás* **2011**, *55*, 412–420.
11. Balogh, P.; Szabó, P.; Pocsai, K. Introduction of different mangalica breeds's prolificacy and rearing performances. *Res. Pig Breed.* **2013**, *7*, 34–37.
12. National Association of Mangalica Breeders. Introduction. Available online: http://www.moe.org.hu/en/association/introduction/ (accessed on 5 May 2020).
13. National Association of Mangalica Breeders. Available online: https://magyarmezogazdasag.hu/cimkek/mangalicatenyesztok-orszagos-egyesulete-moe (accessed on 18 March 2020).
14. Simon, H.A. A Behavioral Model of Rational Choice. *Q. J. Econ.* **1955**, *69*, 99–118. [CrossRef]
15. Simon, H.A. Rationality in Psychology and Economics. *J. Bus.* **1986**, *59*, S209–S224. [CrossRef]

16. Kroneberg, C.; Kalter, F. Rational Choice Theory and Empirical Research: Methodological and Theoretical Contributions in Europe. *Annu. Rev. Sociol.* **2012**, *38*, 73–92. [CrossRef]
17. McFadden, D. Economic Choices. *Am. Econ. Rev.* **2001**, *91*, 351–378. [CrossRef]
18. Hess, S.; Daly, A. *Handbook of Choice Modelling*; Edward Elgar Publishing: Cheltenham, UK, 2014. [CrossRef]
19. Hensher, D.A.; Rose, J.M.; Greene, W.H. *Applied Choice Analysis*; Cambridge University Press: New York, NY, USA, 2005. [CrossRef]
20. Georgescu, I. Fuzzy choice functions. In *Fuzzy Choice Functions*; Springer: Berlin, Germany, 2007; pp. 75–106.
21. Kroes, E.P.; Sheldon, R.J. Stated preference methods: An introduction. *J. Transp. Econ. Policy* **1988**, *22*, 11–25.
22. Mark, T.L.; Swait, J. Using stated preference and revealed preference modeling to evaluate prescribing decisions. *Health Econ.* **2004**, *13*, 563–573. [CrossRef] [PubMed]
23. Hensher, D.A.; Barnard, P.O.; Truong, T.P. The role of stated preference methods in studies of travel choice. *J. Transp. Econ. Policy* **1988**, 45–58.
24. McCluskey, J.J.; Huffman, W.E. Using Stated Preference Techniques and Experimental Auction Methods: A Review of Advantages and Disadvantages for Each Method in Examining Consumer Preferences for New Technology. *Int. Rev. Environ. Resour. Econ.* **2017**, *10*, 269–297. [CrossRef]
25. Hensher, D.A.; Bradley, M. Using stated response choice data to enrich revealed preference discrete choice models. *Mark. Lett.* **1993**, *4*, 139–151. [CrossRef]
26. Train, K.; Wilson, W.W. Estimation on stated-preference experiments constructed from revealed-preference choices. *Transp. Res. Part B Methodol.* **2008**, *42*, 191–203. [CrossRef]
27. Costanigro, M.; Onozaka, Y. A Belief-Preference Model of Choice for Experience and Credence Goods. *J. Agric. Econ.* **2019**, *71*, 70–95. [CrossRef]
28. Louviere, J.J.; Hensher, D.A.; Swait, J.D. *Stated Choice Methods: Analysis and Applications*; Cambridge University Press: Cambridge, UK, 2000. [CrossRef]
29. Loureiro, M.L.; McCluskey, J.J. Assessing consumer response to protected geographical identification labeling. *Agribusiness* **2000**, *16*, 309–320. [CrossRef]
30. Lancaster, K.J. A New Approach to Consumer Theory. *J. Political Econ.* **1966**, *74*, 132–157. [CrossRef]
31. Ceschi, S.; Canavari, M.; Castellini, A. Consumer's Preference and Willingness to Pay for Apple Attributes: A Choice Experiment in Large Retail Outlets in Bologna (Italy). *J. Int. Food Agribus. Mark.* **2017**, *30*, 305–322. [CrossRef]
32. Denver, S.; Jensen, J.D. Consumer preferences for organically and locally produced apples. *Food Qual. Prefer.* **2014**, *31*, 129–134. [CrossRef]
33. Lockshin, L.; Jarvis, W.; d'Hauteville, F.; Perrouty, J.-P. Using simulations from discrete choice experiments to measure consumer sensitivity to brand, region, price, and awards in wine choice. *Food Qual. Prefer.* **2006**, *17*, 166–178. [CrossRef]
34. Van Loo, E.J.; Caputo, V.; Nayga, R.M.; Meullenet, J.-F.; Ricke, S.C. Consumers' willingness to pay for organic chicken breast: Evidence from choice experiment. *Food Qual. Prefer.* **2011**, *22*, 603–613. [CrossRef]
35. Wang, J.; Ge, J.; Ma, Y. Urban Chinese Consumers' Willingness to Pay for Pork with Certified Labels: A Discrete Choice Experiment. *Sustainability* **2018**, *10*, 603. [CrossRef]
36. van Zyl, K.; Vermeulen, H.; Kirsten, J.F. Determining South African consumers' willingness to pay for certified Karoo lamb: An application of an experimental auction. *Agrekon* **2013**, *52*, 1–20. [CrossRef]
37. AND International. *Value of Production of Agricultural Products and Foodstuffs, Wines, Aromatised Wines and Spirits Protected by a Geographical Indication (GI)*; AND International: Paris, France, 2012.
38. Ardeshiri, A.; Rose, J.M. How Australian consumers value intrinsic and extrinsic attributes of beef products. *Food Qual. Prefer.* **2018**, *65*, 146–163. [CrossRef]
39. Gao, Z.; Schroeder, T.C.; Yu, X. Consumer Willingness to Pay for Cue Attribute: The Value Beyond Its Own. *J. Int. Food Agribus. Mark.* **2010**, *22*, 108–124. [CrossRef]
40. Loureiro, M.L.; Umberger, W.J. Estimating consumer willingness to pay for country-of-origin labeling. *J. Agric. Resour. Econ.* **2003**, *28*, 287–301.
41. Revoredo-Giha, C.; Lamprinopoulou, C.; Leat, P.; Kupiec-Teahan, B.; Toma, L.; Cacciolatti, L. How Differentiated Is Scottish Beef? An Analysis of Supermarket Data. *J. Food Prod. Mark.* **2011**, *17*, 183–210. [CrossRef]
42. Arnoult, M.; Lobb, A.; Tiffin, R. Willingness to Pay for Imported and Seasonal Foods: A UK Survey. *J. Int. Food Agribus. Mark.* **2010**, *22*, 234–251. [CrossRef]

43. Bernabeu, R.; Rabadan, A.; El Orche, N.E.; Diaz, M. Influence of quality labels on the formation of preferences of lamb meat consumers. A Spanish case study. *Meat Sci* **2018**, *135*, 129–133. [CrossRef]
44. Gracia, A. Consumers' preferences for a local food product: A real choice experiment. *Empir. Econ.* **2013**, *47*, 111–128. [CrossRef]
45. Gracia, A.; de Magistris, T.; Nayga, R.M. Importance of Social Influence in Consumers' Willingness to Pay for Local Food: Are There Gender Differences? *Agribusiness* **2012**, *28*, 361–371. [CrossRef]
46. Imami, D.; Chan-Halbrendt, C.; Zhang, Q.; Zhllima, E. Conjoint analysis of consumer preferences for lamb meat in central and southwest urban Albania. *Int. Food Agribus. Manag. Rev.* **2011**, *14*, 111–126.
47. Arfini, F.; Mancini, M.C. The effect of information and co-branding strategies on consumers willingness to pay (WTP) for Protected Designation of Origin (PDO) products: The case of pre-sliced Parma Ham. *Prog. Nutr.* **2015**, *17*, 15–22.
48. Mesías, F.; Gaspar, P.; Escribano, M.; Pulido, F. The role of protected designation of origin in consumer preference for Iberian dry-cured ham in Spain. *Ital. J. Food Sci.* **2010**, *22*, 367.
49. Resano, H.; Sanjuán, A.I.; Albisu, L.M. Consumers' response to the EU Quality policy allowing for heterogeneous preferences. *Food Policy* **2012**, *37*, 355–365. [CrossRef]
50. Garavaglia, C.; Mariani, P. How Much Do Consumers Value Protected Designation of Origin Certifications? Estimates of willingness to Pay for PDO Dry-Cured Ham in Italy. *Agribusiness* **2017**, *33*, 403–423. [CrossRef]
51. Balcombe, K.; Bradley, D.; Fraser, I.; Hussein, M. Consumer preferences regarding country of origin for multiple meat products. *Food Policy* **2016**, *64*, 49–62. [CrossRef]
52. Shan, L.C.; De Brún, A.; Henchion, M.; Li, C.; Murrin, C.; Wall, P.G.; Monahan, F.J. Consumer evaluations of processed meat products reformulated to be healthier–A conjoint analysis study. *Meat Sci.* **2017**, *131*, 82–89. [CrossRef]
53. Di Vita, G.; Blanc, S.; Mancuso, T.; Massaglia, S.; La Via, G.; D'Amico, M. Harmful Compounds and Willingness to Buy for Reduced-Additives Salami. An Outlook on Italian Consumers. *Int. J. Environ. Res. Public Health* **2019**, *16*, 2605. [CrossRef]
54. Ngapo, T. Consumer preferences for pork chops in five Canadian provinces. *Meat Sci.* **2017**, *129*, 102–110. [CrossRef]
55. Špička, J.; Náglová, Z.; Mezera, J. Consumers Behaviour in the Czech Pork Meat Retail Market. In Proceedings of the INPROFORUM 2017, České Budějovice, Czech Republic, November 2017.
56. Font-i-Furnols, M.; Guerrero, L. Consumer preference, behavior and perception about meat and meat products: An overview. *Meat Sci.* **2014**, *98*, 361–371. [CrossRef]
57. Xazela, N.M.; Hugo, A.; Marume, U.; Muchenje, V. Perceptions of rural consumers on the aspects of meat quality and health implications associated with meat consumption. *Sustainability* **2017**, *9*, 830. [CrossRef]
58. Merlino, V.M.; Borra, D.; Verduna, T.; Massaglia, S. Household behavior with respect to meat consumption: Differences between households with and without children. *Vet. Sci.* **2017**, *4*, 53. [CrossRef]
59. Kallas, Z.; Čandek-Potokar, M.; Tomažin, U.; Pugliese, C.; Aquilani, C.; Gil, J.M. Measuring consumers' preferences for traditional and innovative pork products. *Agric. Conspec. Sci.* **2017**, *82*, 137–141.
60. Kallas, Z.; Varela, E.; Čandek-Potokar, M.; Pugliese, C.; Cerjak, M.; Tomažin, U.; Karolyi, D.; Aquilani, C.; Vitale, M.; Gil, J.M. Can innovations in traditional pork products help thriving EU untapped pig breeds? A non-hypothetical discrete choice experiment with hedonic evaluation. *Meat Sci.* **2019**, *154*, 75–85. [CrossRef]
61. Candek-Potokar, M.; Giusto, A.; Conti, C.; Cosola, C.; Fontanesi, L. Improving sustainability of local pig breeds using quality labels–case review and trademark development in project TREASURE. *Arch. Zootec.* **2018**, 235–238.
62. Balogh, P.; Békési, D.; Gorton, M.; Popp, J.; Lengyel, P. Consumer willingness to pay for traditional food products. *Food Policy* **2016**, *61*, 176–184. [CrossRef]
63. AMC. Kampány Indult a Mangalicahús Népszerűsítéséért. Available online: https://www.amc.hu/belpiaci-hirek/kampany-indult-a-mangalicahus-nepszerusiteseert/576/ (accessed on 17 March 2020).
64. Ngene, C. *1.2 User Manual & Reference Guide*; ChoiceMetrics Pty Ltd.: Sydney, Australia, 2018.
65. Hungarian Central Statistical Office. National Data—Summary Tables. Available online: http://www.ksh.hu/stadat (accessed on 24 May 2020).
66. Hungarian Central Statistical Office. National Data—Dissemination Database. Available online: http://statinfo.ksh.hu/Statinfo/themeSelector.jsp?lang=hu (accessed on 24 May 2020).

67. Hess, S.; Palma, D. Apollo: A flexible, powerful and customisable freeware package for choice model estimation and application. *J. Choice Model.* **2019**, *32*, 100170. [CrossRef]
68. Hess, S.; Palma, D. Apollo Version 0.0.6, User Manual. Available online: www.ApolloChoiceModelling.com (accessed on 20 February 2020).
69. McFadden, D.; Zarembka, P. Frontiers in econometrics. Cond. Logit Anal. Qual. Choice Behav. In *Frontiers in Econometrics*; Zarembka, P., Ed.; Academic Press: New York, NY, USA, 1973; pp. 105–142.
70. Fiebig, D.G.; Keane, M.P.; Louviere, J.; Wasi, N. The Generalized Multinomial Logit Model: Accounting for Scale and Coefficient Heterogeneity. *Mark. Sci.* **2010**, *29*, 393–421. [CrossRef]
71. Fosgerau, M.; Bierlaire, M. A practical test for the choice of mixing distribution in discrete choice models. *Transp. Res. Part B Methodol.* **2007**, *41*, 784–794. [CrossRef]
72. Train, K.E. *Discrete Choice Methods with Simulation*; Cambridge University Press: Cambridge, UK, 2003. [CrossRef]
73. Train, K.; Weeks, M. Discrete Choice Models in Preference Space and Willingness-to-Pay Space. In *Applications of Simulation Methods in Environmental and Resource Economics*; Scarpa, R., Alberini, A., Eds.; Springer: Dordrecht, The Netherlands, 2005; pp. 1–16. [CrossRef]
74. Hensher, D.A.; Rose, J.M.; Greene, W.H. Combining RP and SP data: Biases in using the nested logit '-contrasts with flexible mixed logit incorporating panel and scale effects. *J. Transp. Geogr.* **2008**, *16*, 126–133. [CrossRef]
75. Boxall, P.C.; Adamowicz, W.L. Understanding heterogeneous preferences in random utility models: A latent class approach. *Environ. Resour. Econ.* **2002**, *23*, 421–446. [CrossRef]
76. Greene, W.H.; Hensher, D.A. A latent class model for discrete choice analysis: Contrasts with mixed logit. *Transp. Res. Part B Methodol.* **2003**, *37*, 681–698. [CrossRef]
77. Morey, E.; Thacher, J.; Breffle, W. Using Angler Characteristics and Attitudinal Data to Identify Environmental Preference Classes: A Latent-Class Model. *Environ. Resour. Econ.* **2006**, *34*, 91–115. [CrossRef]
78. Cavanaugh, J.E.; Neath, A.A. The Akaike information criterion: Background, derivation, properties, application, interpretation, and refinements. *Wiley Interdiscip. Rev. Comput. Stat.* **2019**, *11*, e1460. [CrossRef]
79. Ballco, P.; De Magistris, T. Spanish Consumer Purchase Behaviour and Stated Preferences for Yoghurts with Nutritional and Health Claims. *Nutrients* **2019**, *11*, 2742. [CrossRef] [PubMed]
80. Jurado, F.; Gracia, A. Does the valuation of nutritional claims differ among consumers? Insights from Spain. *Nutrients* **2017**, *9*, 132. [CrossRef]
81. Hess, S.; Daly, A.; Dekker, T.; Cabral, M.O.; Batley, R. A framework for capturing heterogeneity, heteroskedasticity, non-linearity, reference dependence and design artefacts in value of time research. *Transp. Res. Part B Methodol.* **2017**, *96*, 126–149. [CrossRef]
82. Bernués, A.; Olaizola, A.; Corcoran, K. Labelling information demanded by European consumers and relationships with purchasing motives, quality and safety of meat. *Meat Sci.* **2003**, *65*, 1095–1106. [CrossRef]
83. Bernués, A.; Ripoll, G.; Panea, B. Consumer segmentation based on convenience orientation and attitudes towards quality attributes of lamb meat. *Food Qual. Prefer.* **2012**, *26*, 211–220. [CrossRef]
84. Cerjak, M.; Karolyi, D.; Kovačić, D. Effect of information about pig breed on consumers' acceptability of dry sausage. *J. Sens. Stud.* **2011**, *26*, 128–134. [CrossRef]
85. Lusk, J.L. Consumer preferences for and beliefs about slow growth chicken. *Poult. Sci.* **2018**, *97*, 4159–4166. [CrossRef]
86. Lusk, J.L.; Schroeder, T.C.; Tonsor, G.T. Distinguishing beliefs from preferences in food choice. *Eur. Rev. Agric. Econ.* **2013**, *41*, 627–655. [CrossRef]
87. Verbeke, W.; Guerrero, L.; Almli, V.L.; Vanhonacker, F.; Hersleth, M. European Consumers' Definition and Perception of Traditional Foods. In *Traditional Foods*; Springer: Boston, MA, USA, 2016. [CrossRef]
88. Vittersø, G.; Torjusen, H.; Laitala, K.; Tocco, B.; Biasini, B.; Csillag, P.; de Labarre, M.D.; Lecoeur, J.-L.; Maj, A.; Majewski, E.; et al. Short Food Supply Chains and Their Contributions to Sustainability: Participants' Views and Perceptions from 12 European Cases. *Sustainability* **2019**, *11*, 4800. [CrossRef]
89. Delicato, C.; Collison, M.; Myronyuk, I.; Symochko, T.; Boyko, N. Is Local Better? Consumer Value in Food Purchasing and the Role of Short Food Supply Chains. *Stud. Agric. Econ.* **2019**, *121*, 75–83. [CrossRef]
90. Lopéz-Galán, B.; de-Magistris, T. Personal and Psychological Traits Influencing the Willingness to Pay for Food with Nutritional Claims: A Comparison between Vice and Virtue Food Products. *Foods* **2020**, *9*, 733. [CrossRef] [PubMed]

91. Grashuis, J.; Magnier, A. Product differentiation by marketing and processing cooperatives: A choice experiment with cheese and cereal products. *Agribusiness* **2018**, *34*, 813–830. [CrossRef]
92. Profeta, A.; Hamm, U. Do consumers prefer local animal products produced with local feed? Results from a Discrete-Choice experiment. *Food Qual. Prefer.* **2019**, *71*, 217–227. [CrossRef]

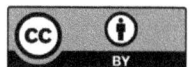

© 2020 by the authors. Licensee MDPI, Basel, Switzerland. This article is an open access article distributed under the terms and conditions of the Creative Commons Attribution (CC BY) license (http://creativecommons.org/licenses/by/4.0/).

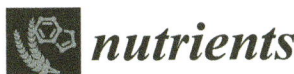

Review

Destigmatizing Carbohydrate with Food Labeling: The Use of Non-Mandatory Labelling to Highlight Quality Carbohydrate Foods

Christopher P.F. Marinangeli [1,*], Scott V. Harding [2], Andrea J. Glenn [3,4], Laura Chiavaroli [3,4], Andreea Zurbau [3,4], David J.A. Jenkins [3,4,5,6], Cyril W.C. Kendall [3,4,7], Kevin B. Miller [8] and John L. Sievenpiper [3,4,5,6]

1. Pulse Canada, 920-220 Portage Avenue, Winnipeg, MB R3C 0A5, Canada
2. Department of Biochemistry, Faculty of Science, Memorial University of Newfoundland, St. John's, NL A1C 5S7, Canada; sharding@mun.ca
3. Department of Nutritional Sciences, University of Toronto, Toronto, ON M5B 1W8, Canada; andrea.glenn@utoronto.ca (A.J.G.); laura.chiavaroli@alumni.utoronto.ca (L.C.); andreea.zurbau@mail.utoronto.ca (A.Z.); David.jenkins@utoronto.ca (D.J.A.J.); cyril.kendall@utoronto.ca (C.W.C.K.); john.sievenpiper@utoronto.ca (J.L.S)
4. Clinical Nutrition and Risk Factor Modification Centre, St. Michael's Hospital, Toronto, ON M5B 1W8, Canada
5. Li Ka Shing Knowledge Institute, St. Michael's Hospital, Toronto, ON M5B 1W8, Canada
6. Division of Endocrinology and Metabolism, St. Michael's Hospital, Toronto, ON M5B 1W8, Canada
7. College of Pharmacy and Nutrition, University of Saskatchewan, Saskatoon, SK S7N 5E5, Canada
8. General Mills Inc., Global Scientific & Regulatory Affairs, Golden Valley, MN 55427-3870, USA; kevin.miller2@genmills.com
* Correspondence: cmarinangeli@pulsecanada.com; Tel.: +1-905-330-0514

Received: 30 April 2020; Accepted: 4 June 2020; Published: 9 June 2020

Abstract: Dietary carbohydrates are components of healthy foods, but many carbohydrate foods have recently been stigmatized as primary causes of diet-related risk factors for chronic disease. There is an opportunity to enhance efforts within the food landscape to encourage the consumption of higher quality carbohydrate foods. The use of labelling is one strategy that permits consumers to identify healthy carbohydrate foods at the point-of-purchase. This review discusses the regulatory frameworks and examples of associated non-mandatory food labelling claims that are currently employed to highlight healthy carbohydrate foods to consumers. The existing labelling frameworks discussed here align with established measures of carbohydrate quality, such as 1. dietary fibre nutrient content claims and associated dietary fibre-based health claims; 2. the presence of whole carbohydrate foods and ingredients that are intact or reconstituted, such as whole grains; and 3. low glycemic index and glycemic response claims. Standards from Codex Alimentarius, and regulations from Australia and New Zealand, Canada, Europe, and the United States will be used to illustrate the means by which food labelling can be used by consumers to identify quality carbohydrate foods.

Keywords: quality carbohydrate; dietary fibre; whole grains; health claims; glycemic index

1. Introduction

"Quality carbohydrate" is a relatively new term that has been introduced as a means of discussing the contribution of carbohydrate foods to healthy diets. While not formally defined, individual and aggregated measures of carbohydrate quality have been discussed and applied within the literature, and have included one or more criteria, including total dietary fibre, whole versus refined grains, glycemic index (GI) or glycemic response, solid-to-liquid carbohydrate ratio, carbohydrate-to-fibre ratio, whole grain-to-total grain ratio, and sugar content [1–5].

Dietary carbohydrates are components of many healthy foods, including dairy, fruits and vegetables, legumes, seeds and nuts, and whole grains, yet carbohydrate foods are often stigmatized publicly as primary causes of diet-related risk factors for chronic disease. However, similar to dietary fat, the term carbohydrate encompasses various food components that, on their own and within foods, can have a spectrum of benefits on physiological function and health within dietary patterns. Fundamentally, the digestible carbohydrates obtained from foods are a source of energy for cells. Non-digestible carbohydrates, including dietary fibres and resistant starches promote stool regularity, lower circulating LDL-cholesterol, blunt postprandial glycemic responses, encourage mineral absorption in the large intestine, and impose positive effects on the human intestinal microbiome [6]. The fact that carbohydrate-rich foods are emphasized in national dietary guidelines and within dietary patterns shown to reduce cardiovascular and diabetes risk factors demonstrates their value in healthy diets [7–9].

Across jurisdictions, labelling tools exist to help consumers identify foods that align with healthy dietary patterns; this includes foods of higher carbohydrate quality. From a regulatory perspective, many jurisdictions permit the use of nutrient content claims to communicate the presence of nutrients or other healthy food components, including dietary fibre, in foods. Health claims that refer to a physiological function or a health benefit could be supported by the presence of a carbohydrate, such as specific types of dietary fibre. Other claims and labelling programs communicate the presence of intact or reconstituted foods and ingredients, such as whole grains, that contain carbohydrates and other nutrients, but also align with a jurisdiction's nutritional policies. While polarizing, low glycemic index (GI) or glycemic response claims have also been permitted where it has been acknowledged that a lower peak rise in postprandial glucose levels is a physiological benefit to consumers and a nutritional strategy for managing blood glucose levels amongst people with diabetes.

This review provides an overview of the existing regulatory frameworks and examples of associated non-mandatory food labelling claims that are currently employed to highlight high-quality carbohydrate foods to consumers. The labelling frameworks discussed align with established measures of carbohydrate quality, such as 1. dietary fibre content claims and associated dietary fibre-based health claims; 2. the presence of whole carbohydrate foods and ingredients that are intact or reconstituted, such as whole grains; and 3. low GI and glycemic response claims. Standards from Codex Alimentarius, and regulatory frameworks from Australia and New Zealand, Canada, Europe, and the United States (the US) will be used to illustrate the means by which food labelling is used to identify quality carbohydrate foods to consumers. The benefits of expanding labelling regulations to further encourage consumption of higher quality carbohydrate foods will also be discussed.

2. Defining Quality Carbohydrate and Considering Consumer Perception

The term "carbohydrate quality" can be controversial and is open to interpretation, not only from a scientific perspective, but also from the perspective of the consumer. One common feature is that quality carbohydrate foods refer to those foods that support healthy dietary patterns. Carbohydrates contribute significantly to diets around the world [10]. Indeed, carbohydrate foods are ubiquitous in the food supply, found in many forms (processed and unprocessed) with various physiological and health benefits. Therefore, it is reasonable that carbohydrate quality would not be defined by a single attribute. Often, dietary guidelines have focused on sugar, starch, and dietary fibre to inform the consumption of quality carbohydrate foods [11]. Some of these attributes are often quantified on the nutrition declaration labels of pre-packaged foods. However, in addition to these qualities, there are opportunities to use non-mandatory labelling to highlight attributes that permit the identification of quality carbohydrate foods, that resonate with consumers. For example, emphasizing the presence of whole grains, legumes, and fruits and vegetables within multi-component food products can capture the presence of dietary fibre and complex starch, but also promote vitamin and mineral intakes, along with other plant components (e.g., polyphenols, etc.) with health benefits.

With multiple domains of carbohydrate quality, the next challenge is leveraging labelling tools that encourage consumers to choose higher quality carbohydrate foods over lower quality carbohydrate foods. Increased consumption of refined and rapidly digestible carbohydrates, where dietary fibre, micronutrients, and in some cases, proteins have been removed, has been linked to the development of cardiometabolic diseases and some cancers [4]. Studies demonstrate that diets containing higher levels of dietary fibre and intact carbohydrate foods, such as whole grains, are associated with lower mortality and risk of chronic disease [12,13]. However, it seems that, in some cases, consumers have often extrapolated information referring to refined carbohydrate and negative effects on health to all types of carbohydrate and carbohydrate foods. In a recent study in Canada, when consumers from three major metropolitan cities were asked to use word associations to convey their feelings toward carbohydrates, negative descriptions revolved around overeating, weight gain, risk, and feelings of guilt [14]. In the same study however, participants distinguished between "good" and "bad" carbohydrate foods, where the former was associated with fruits and vegetables, dietary fibre, whole grains, and slowly digestible carbohydrates [14]. These findings mirror a recent consumer survey by the International Food Information Council Foundation, where 23% of US adults believed carbohydrates cause weight gain, which was second to sugar at 27% [15]. Conversely, only 13% of participants believed fats caused weight gain. While these perceptions stigmatize carbohydrates, in the same survey, over 80% of participates identified dietary fibre and whole grains as healthy foods [15].

From the consumer data, there is an opportunity to enhance efforts within the food landscape to encourage higher consumption of quality carbohydrates. As outlined previously, various measures of quality carbohydrates have been applied to foods and diets in a research setting to quantify their characterization as quality carbohydrate foods. While all measures of quality carbohydrates used academically may not be suitable for labelling initiatives, there are broad domains of carbohydrate quality that can and are already used in the marketplace. In 2017, a workshop hosted by the International Life Science Institute North America put forth vision statements that identified three domains of quality carbohydrate foods: 1. a source of dietary fibre; 2. whole food credentials; and 3. low GI or glycemic response. These three domains are closely related to those used in a systematic review and meta-analyses of carbohydrate quality on chronic disease by Reynolds et al. [16]. In addition to dietary fibre and the GI, rather than a broad evaluation of whole foods, whole grain foods were specifically reviewed. Across regions, regulatory frameworks and dietary guidelines already permit the use consumer-facing non-mandatory labelling tools that align with these domains of quality carbohydrates.

The use of labelling is one strategy that permits consumers to easily identify healthy foods at the point-of-purchase. The following sections of this review will discuss and summarize regulations and provide non-mandatory labelling examples that have been used across jurisdictions that have been leveraged to facilitate higher consumption of quality carbohydrates. While some labelling initiatives must follow specific compositional criteria for claims, other labelling initiatives communicate the presence or an attribute of the food. Fundamental to all labelling initiatives, it is imperative that the information communicated to the consumer is not misleading.

3. Labelling Foods for Carbohydrate Quality

3.1. Dietary Fibre

3.1.1. Direct Dietary Fibre Claims: Fibre Nutrient Content Claims

The presence of dietary fibre is a commonly identified measure of carbohydrate quality. Although dietary fibre is not a nutrient per se, it is considered to be a beneficial component of dietary patterns. Across regions, Australia and New Zealand, Canada, Europe, and the US have set specific regulatory targets for dietary fibre consumption as well as dietary fibre nutrient content claims (Table 1). In the US and Canada, although a recommended daily allowance (RDA) has not been established, an adequate intake of 14 g fibre/1000 kcal is recommended and is based on reduced risk for coronary heart disease [17–19]. In Australia and New Zealand, adequate intakes for dietary fibre of 14–30 g/day were derived from median intakes of fibre in populations where issues with laxation did not occur [20]. Similarly, dietary fibre recommendations in Europe are based on effects on laxation with 25 g fibre/day recommended for adults (2–3 g fibre/MJ), and 2 g fibre/MJ for children ≥1 year of age [21]. Given that daily dietary fibre recommendations are relative to energy intake, recommendations can differ between life stages. Note that Codex Alimentarius implements food standards that consider the input from membership countries with different food landscapes, and dietary recommendations for dietary fibre have been left to individual countries [22].

Despite different dietary fibre recommendations across regions, recommendations are based on the observation that dietary fibre can improve physiological function or prevent chronic disease and supports the value of identifying high fibre foods as nutrient content claims. While the criteria differ, nutrient content claims provide a fundamental platform for communicating that foods are a source of quality carbohydrates. However, confusion can arise because of differences in the definition of dietary fibre across regions. As outlined in Table 2, definitions of dietary fibre commonly include indigestible carbohydrates from plants. With the exception of Codex, a degree of polymerization of monomeric units of ≥3 is common among Australia and New Zealand, Canada, Europe, and the US. For extracted and/or novel dietary fibres (including synthetic fibre), a physiological benefit must be demonstrated before the carbohydrate can be considered a dietary fibre. Laxation, cholesterol-lowering, and decreased postprandial glucose and insulin responses are common physiological benefits between countries. However, the US has an expanded list that includes mineral absorption and effects on energy intake from food consumption. Canada and Europe have also included microbial fermentation in the large intestine. However, the directive from the European Commission that outlined the accepted physiological benefits for novel dietary fibres was repealed [28] and replaced by regulation 1169/2011 [29]. It is assumed that the physiological benefits outlined in the previous directive remain as acceptable. Canada explicitly indicates that other benefits not outlined in the dietary fibre policy could also be accepted for novel fibre sources [30].

The common ability to claim that foods are a source dietary fibre is a straightforward opportunity for consumers to identify food sources of quality carbohydrates. For industry, studies to substantiate accepted physiological benefits of extracted, novel, or synthetic dietary fibres can be challenging to demonstrate in healthy populations, but are minimally invasive. However, given that the requirements for dietary fibre claims can differ across jurisdictions, similar foods may not always have the ability to leverage "source of fibre" claims in different countries. Nevertheless, consumers and industry have access to many fibre-containing unprocessed and processed foods, and fibre ingredients, respectively, that can be leveraged as an attribute of quality carbohydrates.

3.1.2. Indirect Dietary Fibre Claims: Function and Disease Risk Claims

Health claims that communicate a functional or health benefit from the presence of a specific type of dietary fibre could also be used to increase the consumption of quality carbohydrates. Functional-type health claims (general level health claims in Australia and New Zealand) refer to a physiological benefit from the food. Therapeutic or disease risk reduction health claims (high-level health claims in Australia and New Zealand) refer to effects of a food or ingredient on chronic disease risk factors such as cholesterol and blood pressure lowering, or disease prevention. Recall that physiological and health benefits can be used to characterize novel carbohydrate ingredients as dietary fibres (see Section 3.1.1.). However, the criteria for leveraging physiological and health benefits as a standalone claim on foods from the inclusion of dietary fibre can require higher standards of evidence, and can differ between regions.

Table 1. Summary of dietary fibre recommendations and criteria for nutrient content claims for dietary fibre from Codex and in Australia and New Zealand, Canada, Europe, and the US.

	Codex Alimentarius Standards [22]	Australia and New Zealand [20,23]	Canada [17,19]	Europe [21,24]	United States [17,25]
Dietary fibre Recommendation	Recommendation to be determined at the national level	14–30 g/day (based on median intakes to prevent laxation)	14 g/1000 kcal	2–3 g/MJ (239 kcal)	14 g/1000 kcal
Basis for Dietary fibre Recommendation	N/A	↑ Laxation	↓ Coronary heart disease risk	↑ Laxation	↓ Coronary heart disease risk
Dietary fibre Nutrient Content Claims	**Source** ■ 3 g dietary fibre per 100 g; or ■ 1.5 g dietary fibre per 100 kcal; or ■ 10% of the DRV per serving **High Source** ■ 6 g dietary fibre per 100 g; or ■ 3 g dietary fibre per 100 kcal; or ■ 20% of the DRV per serving	**General Claim** ■ A serving of the food contains at least 2 g of dietary fibre. **Good Source** ■ A serving of the food contains at least 4 g of dietary fibre. **Excellent Source** ■ A serving of the food contains at least 7 g of dietary fibre.	**Source** ■ 2 g or more of dietary fibre per reference amount[†] and serving size. **High Source** ■ 4 g or more of dietary fibre per reference amount[†] and serving size. **Very High Source** ■ 6 g or more of dietary fibre per reference amount[†] and serving size.	**Source** ■ 3 g of dietary fibre per 100 g or at least 1.5 g of fibre per 100 kcal **High Source** ■ 6 g dietary of fibre per 100 g or at least 3 g of fibre per 100 kcal	**Good Source** ■ ≥10% to ≤19.9% of the DRV [*] for dietary fibre per RACC[§] of food **High Source** ■ ≥20% of the DRV [*] for dietary fibre per RACC[§] of food

Abbreviations: DRV: daily reference value; RACC, reference amount customarily consumed. [†] Canada: A reference amount is a regulated serving size that is typically consumed in a single meal event [26]. [*] US DRV for dietary fiber: Adults and children ≥4 years, 28 g/day; children 1–3 years, 14 g/day; pregnant and lactating women, 28 g/day [§] US: An RACC is a regulated serving size consumed in a single meal event [27].

Table 2. Definitions of fibre from Codex and regulatory agencies in Australia and New Zealand, Canada, Europe, and the US.

Jurisdiction	Definition of Dietary Fibre
Codex Alimentarius [31]	■ Carbohydrate polymers with ≥10 or more monomeric units (DP * ≥ 10), which are not hydrolyzed by the endogenous enzymes in the small intestine of humans and belong to the following categories: • Edible carbohydrate polymers naturally occurring in the food as consumed; • Carbohydrate polymers, which have been obtained from food raw material by physical, enzymatic, or chemical means and which have been shown to have a physiological effect of benefit to health as demonstrated by generally accepted scientific evidence to competent authorities; • Synthetic carbohydrate polymers which have been shown to have a physiological effect of benefit to health as demonstrated by generally accepted scientific evidence to competent authorities.
Australia and New Zealand [20]	■ Dietary fibre means the fraction of the edible parts of plants or their extracts, or synthetic analogues, that are resistant to digestion and absorption in the small intestine, usually with complete or partial fermentation in the large intestine. ■ Dietary fibre includes polysaccharides, oligosaccharides (DP * > 2), and lignins, and promotes one or more of the following beneficial physiological effects: • Laxation; • Reduction in blood cholesterol; • Modulation of blood glucose.

Canada [30]	■ Carbohydrates with a DP * ≥3 that naturally occur in foods of plant origin and that are not digested and absorbed by the small intestine; and
	■ Accepted novel dietary fibres:
	• Novel dietary fibres are ingredients manufactured to be sources of dietary fibre and consist of carbohydrates with a DP * of 3 or more that are not digested and absorbed by the small intestine.
	• They are synthetically produced or are obtained from natural sources which have no history of safe use as dietary fibre or which have been processed so as to modify the properties of the fibre contained therein.
	• Accepted novel dietary fibres have at least one physiological effect demonstrated by generally accepted scientific evidence:
	  ■ Improves laxation or regularity by increasing stool bulk;
	  ■ Reduces blood total and/or LDL-cholesterol levels;
	  ■ Reduces postprandial blood glucose and/or insulin levels, or increases sensitivity to insulin;
	  ■ Provides energy-yielding metabolites through colonic fermentation.
	• Other physiological benefits of novel dietary fibres could be accepted.

Table 2. Cont.

Jurisdiction	Definition of Dietary Fibre
Europe [28,29]	■ "Fibre" means carbohydrate polymers with 3 or more monomeric units, which are neither digested nor absorbed in the human small intestine and belong to the following categories: • Edible carbohydrate polymers naturally occurring in the food as consumed; • Edible carbohydrate polymers which have been obtained from food raw material by physical, enzymatic, or chemical means and which have a beneficial physiological effect demonstrated by generally accepted scientific evidence; • Edible synthetic carbohydrate polymers which have a beneficial physiological effect demonstrated by generally accepted scientific evidence. ■ Accepted physiological benefits are not defined in Regulation 1169/2011. However, repealed Directive 90/496/EEC (replaced by regulation 1169/2011) indicated that that physiological benefits of dietary fibre include: • Decrease intestinal transit time; • Increase stool bulk; • Fermentable by colonic microflora; • Reduce blood total cholesterol, reduce blood LDL-cholesterol levels; • Reduce postprandial blood glucose, or reduce blood insulin levels.
United States [32]	■ Dietary fibre is defined as non-digestible soluble and insoluble carbohydrates (DP * of ≥3 monomeric units), and lignin that are intrinsic and intact in plants; ■ Isolated or synthetic non-digestible carbohydrates (DP * of ≥3 monomeric units) determined by the FDA to have physiological effects that are beneficial to human health. Examples include: • Attenuation of blood glucose and/or insulin levels; • Reductions in fasting blood total and LDL-cholesterol levels; • Improved laxation; • Increased intestinal absorption of minerals; • Reduced energy intake from food consumption.

Abbreviations: DP, degree of polymerization; FDA, US Food and Drug Administration; LDL, low-density lipoprotein; * DP refers to the number of monomeric units of the carbohydrate molecule.

Table 3 provides examples of physiological function claims that have been identified by regulatory agencies across regions that are based on the presence of dietary fibres. Laxation claims are common. In Australia and New Zealand, all dietary fibres can claim an effect on laxation if the levels of fibre within a food meet the general conditions for a fibre nutrient content claim (Table 1: 2 g/serving). This is reasonable given that dietary fibre recommendations are based on laxation. This is similar to Europe where claims related to increasing fecal bulk, decreased transit time, or normal bowel function can be used if the level of fibre in the food qualifies for a "high in fibre" claim. In Canada, the Canadian Food Inspection Agency (CFIA) has indicated that function claims referring to the effect of wheat bran and psyllium on laxation are permitted. Claims referring to a reduced postprandial glycemic response, maintenance of normal cholesterol levels, and contribution to weight loss in the context of a calorie-restricted diet are also considered to be function-type health claims in Europe and have been approved for a variety of dietary fibres.

Table 3. Summary of function-type health claims supported by dietary fibre in Australia and New Zealand, Canada, and Europe [§].

Region	Fibre Type	Claim	Claim Type	Criteria
Australia and New Zealand	Dietary Fibre [23]	Contributes to regular laxation	General level health claim *	■ Food meets the general conditions for making a nutrient content claim.
	Beta-glucan [23]	Reduces dietary and biliary cholesterol absorption	General level health claim *	■ One or more of the following oat or barley foods: Oat bran; or ■ Whole grain oats; or ■ Whole grain barley; and ■ At least 1 g per serving beta-glucan from the abovementioned foods; and ■ Indicate that 3 g/day beta glucan is required; and ■ The food meets the nutritional criteria of the NPSC [23,33].
	Psyllium fibre [34]	Increased laxation	Function claim	■ Food contains ≥3.5 g/serving psyllium fibre; or ■ If the food contains <3.5 g/serving psyllium fibre, the claim must indicate 3.5 g/day psyllium fibre promotes laxation or regularity.
Canada	Wheat bran fibre [34]	Increased laxation	Function claim	■ Food contains ≥7 g/serving course wheat bran fibre; or ■ If the food contains <7 g/serving course wheat bran fibre, the claim must indicate 7 g/day course wheat bran fibre promotes laxation or regularity
	Polysaccharide complex (glucomannan, xanthan gum, sodium alginate) [35]	Lowers postprandial glycemic response	Function claim	■ Food contains ≥5 g per serving of stated size and reference amount [†] of polysaccharide complex; and ■ Food contains <15 g total sugars per serving of stated size and reference amount [†]; or ■ Food contains <15 g total sugars per serving of stated size, if the food is a prepackaged meal, supplement, or meal replacement.

Table 3. Cont.

Region	Fibre Type	Claim	Claim Type	Criteria
	Barley grain fibre [36]	Increased laxation (increased fecal bulk)	Function health claim	■ Food contains sufficient barley grain fibre to qualify for a "high in fibre claim" (see Table 1)
	Rye fibre [36]	Normal bowel function	Function health claim	■ Food contains sufficient rye fibre to qualify for a "high in fibre claim" (see Table 1)
	Sugar beet fibre [37]	Increased laxation (increased fecal bulk)	Function health claim	■ Food contains sufficient sugar beet fibre to qualify for a "high in fibre claim" (see Table 1)
	Wheat bran fibre [36]	Increased laxation (increased fecal bulk)	Function health claim	■ Food contains sufficient wheat bran fibre to qualify for a "high in fibre claim" (see Table 1)
	Wheat bran fibre [36]	Laxation (decreased transit time)	Function health claim	■ Food contains sufficient wheat bran fibre to qualify for a "high in fibre claim" (see Table 1) ■ Information provided to the consumer that 10 g/day wheat bran fibre is required.
Europe	Arabinoxylan produced from wheat endosperm [36]	Lowers postprandial glycemic response	Function health claim	■ Food contains at least 8 g of arabinoxylan fibre produced from wheat endosperm per 100 g of available carbohydrates in a quantified portion as part of the meal; and ■ Arabinoxylan fibre from wheat endosperm represents 60% arabinoxylan by weight; and ■ Information is provided to the consumer that the beneficial effect is obtained by consuming arabinoxylan-rich fibre as part of the meal.
	Beta-glucans from oats and barley [36]	Lowers postprandial glycemic response	Function health claim	■ Food which contains at least 4 g of beta-glucans from oats or barley for each 30 g of available carbohydrates in a quantified portion as part of the meal; and ■ Information is provided to the consumer that the beneficial effect is obtained by consuming the beta-glucans from oats or barley as part of the meal.
	Hydroxypropyl methylcellulose (HPMC) [36]	Lowers postprandial glycemic response	Function health claim	■ Food which contains at least 4 g of HPMC per quantified portion as part of the meal; and ■ Information is provided to the consumer that the beneficial effect is obtained by consuming HPMC as part of the meal; and ■ Warning of choking for people with swallowing difficulties; and ■ Advice on consuming with water to ensure HPMC reaches the stomach.

Table 3. Cont.

Region	Fibre Type	Claim	Claim Type	Criteria
Europe	Pectins [36]	Lowers postprandial glycemic response	Function health claim	<ul><li>10 g of pectins per quantified portion; and</li><li>Information is provided to the consumer that the beneficial effect is obtained by consuming 10 g of pectins as part of the meal; and</li><li>Warning of choking for people with swallowing difficulties; and</li><li>Advice on consuming with water to ensure pectins reach the stomach.</li></ul>
	Resistant starch [36]	Lowers postprandial glycemic response	Function health claim	<ul><li>Food in which digestible starch has been replaced by resistant starch so that the final content of resistant starch is at least 14% of total starch.</li></ul>
	Beta-glucans [36]	Maintains normal blood cholesterol levels	Function health claim	<ul><li>The claim may be used only for food which contains at least 1 g of beta-glucans from oats, oat bran, barley, barley bran, or from mixtures of these sources per quantified portion; and</li><li>Information is provided to the consumer that the beneficial effect is obtained with a daily intake of 3 g of beta-glucans from oats, oat bran, barley, barley bran, or from mixtures of these beta-glucans.</li></ul>
	Glucomannan (Konjac mannan) [36]	Maintains normal blood cholesterol levels	Function health claim	<ul><li>Food provides at least 4 g/day of glucomannan; and</li><li>The claim indicates that the benefit is obtained with 4 g/day of glucomannan;</li><li>Warning of choking for people with swallowing difficulties; and</li><li>Advice on consuming with water to ensure glucomannan reaches the stomach.</li></ul>
	Guar Gum [36]	Maintains normal cholesterol levels	Function health claim	<ul><li>Food provides at least 10 g/day of guar gum; and</li><li>The claim indicates that the benefit is obtained with 10 g/day of guar gum; and</li><li>Warning of choking for people with swallowing difficulties; and</li><li>Advice on consuming with water to ensure guar gum reaches the stomach.</li></ul>

Table 3. *Cont.*

Region	Fibre Type	Claim	Claim Type	Criteria
	Hydroxypropyl methylcellulose (HPMC) [36]	Maintains normal blood cholesterol levels	Function health claim	■ Food provides at least 5 g/day of HPMC; and ■ The claim indicates that the benefit is obtained with 5 g/day of HPMC; and ■ Warning of choking for people with swallowing difficulties; and ■ Advice on consuming with water to ensure HPMC reaches the stomach.
Europe	Pectins [36]	Maintains normal blood cholesterol levels	Function health claim	■ Food provides at least 6 g/day of pectins; and ■ The claim indicates that the benefit is obtained with 6 g/day of pectins; and ■ Warning of choking for people with swallowing difficulties; and ■ Advice on consuming with water to ensure that pectins reach the stomach.
	Glucomannan (Konjac mannan) [36]	Contributes to weight loss in the context of an energy restricted diet	Function health claim	■ Food provides 1 g glucomannan per quantified portion; and ■ Information is provided to the consumer that the beneficial effect is obtained with 3 g/day glucomannan in 3 doses of 1 g each that is consumed with 1–2 glasses of water before meals in the context of an energy restricted diet.

Abbreviations: HPMC, hydroxypropyl methylcellulose; NPSC, Nutrient Profiling Scoring Criterion; RACC, reference amount customarily consumed. * Australia and New Zealand: A general level health claim refers to a claim that is not considered a high-level health claim. A high-level health claim refers to a serious disease or biomarker for a serious disease. A serious disease is a disease, disorder, or condition that is generally diagnosed, treated, or managed in consultation with or with supervision by a health care professional [38]. † Canada: A reference amount is a regulated serving size that is typically consumed in a single meal event [26]. § Structure/function health claims in the US for conventional foods do not require pre-approval and the US code of the federal registrar does not provide a list of corresponding claims [39].

In Europe, all claims regardless of their scope must be reviewed by the European Food Safety Authority and subsequently added to EU regulation 432/2012 [36]. In the US, structure/function-type health claims do not undergo pre-approval, and thus a list of function claims is not provided within the US Code of Federal Regulations but does not preclude their use on food labels [39]. In some regards, the US is similar to Australia and New Zealand, and Canada, where function-type claims do not require regulatory approval. However, regulatory agencies in these regions will review function-type claims if requested, and subsequently publish their assessment and approval. An example of this has been demonstrated in Canada, where a proprietary combination of viscous fibres characterized as a "polysaccharide complex (glucomannan, xanthan gum, sodium alginate)" was reviewed by Health Canada and accepted as an ingredient that can lower the postprandial glycemic response [35]. In Australia and New Zealand, if a review is not requested prior to utilization, the Chief Executive Officer of Food Standards Australia New Zealand must be notified of the claim [33]. In all three regions, function-type claims used by industry that have not undergone review are required to have adequately substantiated the claim internally and could be asked by regulators to present a claim dossier.

In addition to fibre claims that disseminate an effect on physiological function, various fibres have been reviewed and approved for claims that communicate their ability to decrease cardiometabolic disease risk factors (Table 4). Across the regions included in this review, claims that promote the cholesterol-lowering efficacy of beta-glucan from oats and barely are permitted. For Australia and New Zealand, and Europe, a minimum of 1 g/serving beta-glucan is required to make a cholesterol-lowering claim [23,40,41]. In Canada, at least 0.75 g beta-glucan from oat and 1.0 g beta-glucan from barley per reference amount and serving of the stated size of a food are required [42,43]. In the US, the minimum level of beta-glucan for a lower risk of coronary heart disease claim is 0.75 g per reference amount customarily consumed (RACC) [44]. For all regions summarized, labelling must also communicate a contextual statement that 3 g/day beta-glucan is required. In Europe, it is important to highlight the distinction between the effect of fibres on maintaining cholesterol levels as a function claim (Table 3) and cholesterol-lowering as a risk reduction claim (Table 4). Canada has approved cholesterol-lowering claims for soluble psyllium fibre at 1.75 g/reference amount (and serving of stated size) and 7 g/day [45]. A similar claim referring to a lower risk of coronary heart disease risk is permitted in the US for soluble psyllium fibre at 1.7 g/RACC (US) (and 7 g psyllium fibre/day) [44]. The cholesterol-lowering efficacy of a proprietary polysaccharide complex has also been approved as a cholesterol-lowering ingredient in Canada [46]. The US has authorized health claims for high-fibre grains, fruits, and vegetables for their effects on decreasing the risk of coronary heart disease and cancer, and is based on those grains, fruits, and vegetables that contain at least 0.6 g soluble fibre per RACC [47] and is at least a "good source of fibre" [48] (Table 2), respectively. Regulations indicate that numerous fibre ingredients have been approved for claims relating to physiological benefits and reduced risk for cardiometabolic disease, which are based on the presence of fibre as a quality carbohydrate source.

Table 4. Summary of therapeutic and disease reduction claims supported by dietary fibre in Australia and New Zealand, Canada, Europe, and the US.

Region	Fibre Type	Claim	Claim Type	Criteria
Australia and New Zealand	Beta-glucan [23]	Reduces blood cholesterol	High-level health claim *	■ One or more of the following oat or barley foods: Oat bran; or Whole grain oats; or Whole grain barley; and ■ At least 1 g per serving beta-glucan from the abovementioned foods; and ■ Claim is in the context of a diet low in saturated fatty acids; and ■ Indication that 3 g/day beta glucan is required; and ■ The food meets the nutritional criteria of the NPSC [23,33].
Canada	Barley beta-glucan [43]	Reduces cholesterol levels	Therapeutic claim	■ Food contains at least 1.0 g barley beta-glucan per reference amount [†] and per serving of stated size; and ■ Claim must indicate that 3 g/day beta-glucan from barley fibre lowers cholesterol levels; and ■ Food must meet specific nutritional requirements.
	Oat beta-glucan [42]	Reduces cholesterol levels	Therapeutic claim	■ Food contains at least 0.75 g oat beta-glucan per reference amount [†] and per serving of stated size; and ■ Claim must indicate 3 g/day beta-glucan from oat fibre lowers cholesterol levels; and ■ Food must meet specific nutritional requirements.
	Polysaccharide complex (glucomannan, xanthan gum, sodium alginate) [46]	Reduces cholesterol levels	Therapeutic claim	■ Food contains at least 3.3 g/of polysaccharide complex per reference amount [†] and per serving of stated size; and ■ Claim must indicate 10 g/day polysaccharide complex lowers cholesterol levels; and ■ Food must meet specific nutritional requirements.
	Psyllium [45]	Reduces cholesterol levels	Therapeutic claim	■ Food contains at least 1.75 g psyllium soluble fibre per reference amount [†] and per serving of stated size; and ■ Claim must indicate 7 g/day psyllium fibre lowers cholesterol levels; and ■ Food must meet specific nutritional requirements.

Table 4. Cont.

Region	Fibre Type	Claim	Claim Type	Criteria
Europe	Barley beta-glucans [41]	Reduces cholesterol levels	Reduced disease risk factor health claim	■ The claim can be used for foods which provide at least 1 g of barley beta-glucan per quantified portion; and ■ Information is provided to the consumer that the beneficial effect is obtained with 3 g/day of barley beta-glucan.
	Oat beta-glucan [40]	Reduces cholesterol levels	Reduced disease risk factor health claim	■ The claim can be used for foods which provide at least 1 g of oat beta-glucan per quantified portion; and ■ Information is provided to the consumer that the beneficial effect is obtained with 3 g/day of oat beta-glucan.
United States	Barley beta-glucan [44]	May reduce risk of coronary heart disease	Authorized health claim	■ Food contains at least 0.75 g beta glucan soluble fibre from barley per RACC §; and ■ Claim must indicate 3 g/day beta-glucan from barley fibre lowers cholesterol levels; and ■ Food must meet specific nutritional requirements.
	Oat beta-glucan [44]	May reduce risk of coronary heart disease	Authorized health claim	■ Food contains at least 0.75 g beta-glucan soluble fibre from oat per RACC §; and ■ Claim must indicate 3 g/day beta-glucan from oat fibre lowers cholesterol levels; ■ Food must meet specific nutritional requirements.
	Psyllium husk [44]	May reduce risk of coronary heart disease	Authorized health claim	■ Food contains at least 1.7 g psyllium soluble fibre per RACC §; and ■ Claim must indicate 7 g/day soluble psyllium fibre lowers cholesterol levels; and ■ Food must meet specific nutritional requirements.
	Fruit, vegetables, and grain products that contain soluble fibre [47]	May reduce risk of coronary heart disease	Authorized health claim	■ Food contains at least 0.6 g soluble fibre (without fortification) per RACC §; and ■ Content of soluble fibre is listed in the nutrition information panel; and ■ Food must meet specific nutritional requirements.
	Fiber-containing grain products, fruits, and vegetables and cancer [48]	May reduce the risk of some types of cancers	Authorized health claim	■ Food meets the nutrient content requirements to be considered a "good source of fibre" (without fortification) (Table 1); and ■ Food must meet specific nutritional requirements.

Abbreviations: NPSC, nutrient profiling scoring criterion; RACC, reference amount customarily consumed. * Australia and New Zealand: A high-level health claim refers to a serious disease or biomarker for a serious disease. A serious disease is a disease, disorder, or condition that is generally diagnosed, treated, or managed in consultation with or with supervision by a health care professional [38]. † Canada: A reference amount is a regulated serving size that is typically consumed in a single meal event [21]. § US: RACC is a regulated serving size consumed at a single meal event [27].

3.2. Emphasis on Whole Foods

Whole foods, such as whole grains, or their presence in multicomponent and manufactured foods, can resonate with consumers as healthier food options. When intact foods or all of their components are consumed, it can facilitate the consumption of quality carbohydrates, as well as vitamins, minerals, and other possible bioactives that are often removed when ingredients are refined.

Randomized clinical trials and prospective cohorts studies have demonstrated that higher consumption of whole carbohydrate foods, such as low-fat dairy, legumes, whole grains, nuts, fruits, and vegetables, have been shown to decrease disease risk factors and/or are associated with reduced disease incidence [13,49–64]. Options for labelling that a multicomponent food contains whole food ingredients that are intact or reconstituted to the proportions of their native form are often permitted. This has been demonstrated with labelling programs that highlight whole grains.

The use of food labelling to identify the presence of a broad category of quality carbohydrates within foods, like whole grains, that align with consumer perceptions of a healthy dietary pattern and dietary guidelines could be an effective labelling tool for the consumer. Whole grain cereals and pseudocereals can be consumed as intact cereals, as in the case of brown rice and whole oats (groats), or used as ingredients in multi-component foods. The Cereals & Grains Association (formally the American Association of Cereal Chemists) has defined whole grains as cereals and pseudocereals that "consist of the intact, ground, cracked or flaked caryopsis, whose principal anatomical components—the starchy endosperm, germ and bran—are present in the same relative proportions as they exist in the intact caryopsis [65]." Australia and New Zealand have formally adopted a similar definition of whole grains in the Food Standards Code [66]. Similar definitions of whole grains have been provided by Health Canada and the US as statements or proposed guidance, respectively [67,68]. In Europe, a legal definition of whole grains for use in human food has not been established with different definitions of whole grains being used across countries [69]. The European Food Safety Authority has referenced Cereals & Grains Association's definition in an opinion for health claims related to whole grains [70]. Despite established definitions, without some level of dietary knowledge, it could be difficult for some consumers to identify foods that are indeed whole grains or contribute a meaningful amount of whole grains expected to convey some health benefit. Whole grains are emphasized in most dietary guidelines in Europe, as well as Canada, the US [71], Australia [9], and New Zealand [72], with evidence demonstrating dose-dependent relationships between higher whole grain consumption and reduced risk of all-cause mortality, coronary heart disease incidence, type 2 diabetes, and colorectal cancer [12,13,16].

Messaging that identifies wholes grains within the marketplace, such as oats, could help increase consumption, regardless of whether the consumer is knowledgeable about quality carbohydrate foods. Labelling statements or symbols that indicate that these foods contain a significant level of whole grains can also facilitate increased consumption. As an example, The Oldways Whole Grains Council has developed and implemented a Whole Grain Stamp labelling program that communicates the presence of whole grains in food products in 62 countries, including Canada and the US (Figure 1) [73]. Utilization of the front-of-pack labelling symbol is contingent on a minimum of 8 g/serving of whole grains, which is one-half of the US Department of Agriculture's defined serving of whole grains (16 g) [8]. Similarly, Australia's Grains & Legumes Nutrition Council implemented a voluntary code of practice for claiming that foods are a source of whole grains. The code permits the use of whole grain claims on foods to indicate they contain ≥8 g/serving ("contains whole grain"), ≥16 g/serving ("high level in whole grain"), or ≥24 g/serving ("very high in whole grain") [74]. Additionally, all general and health claims in Australia and New Zealand must comply with the Nutrient Profiling Scoring Criterion (NPSC) [33] outlined in Schedule 4 of the Food Standards Code [23]. A systematic audit of foods in major retail outlets in Sydney showed that utilization of whole grain content claims increased by 71% across food categories evaluated between 2013 and 2019 [75]. Although whole grain labelling has been discussed in detail, similar programs that emphasize the nutritional contribution of other whole quality carbohydrate foods could also be developed. It is also worth noting that front-of-pack labelling symbols cannot be used in a manner that interferes or detracts from mandatory nutrition labelling [29,76–78].

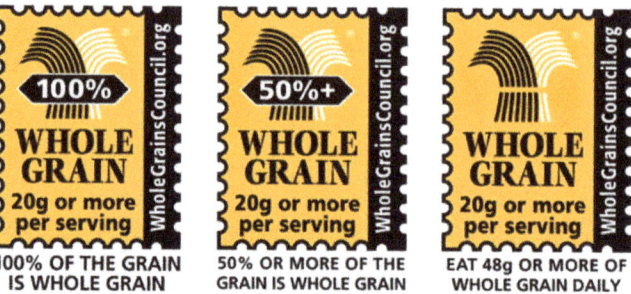

Figure 1. Examples of the Oldways Whole Grains Council's Whole Grains Stamp that assists consumers to identify foods that contain significant levels of whole grains [73]. Reproduced with permission from the Oldways Whole Grains Council.

Although similar, claims that emphasize the presence of a whole food by using "made with" or "contains" claims do not necessarily have the same utility as front-of-pack symbols or claims that are supported by nutritional and dietary guidance. Consumers may not understand that the former is often solely based on the presence of the ingredient and is not necessarily founded on the ingredient's contribution to a healthy dietary pattern, and, in the context of this review, quality carbohydrates. For example, Canada's "Safe Food for Canadians" regulations do not permit the use of words or symbols that falsely communicate the presence of an ingredient [79]. The CFIA's corresponding policy on highlighted ingredients indicates that "it is misleading to over-emphasize the importance, presence or absence of an ingredient or substance in a food because of its desirable or undesirable qualities, or for any other reason [80]." While one could extrapolate this to the presence of an ingredient, such as a quality carbohydrate food or ingredient, ambiguous claims or symbols may not provide sufficient information to the consumer that the claim is referring to nutritional or dietary criteria. For example, an ambiguous claim highlighting the presence of the ingredient could refer to attributes other than nutrition, such as flavour, texture, or the absence of artificial ingredients.

The US and Australia and New Zealand do not have regulations and policies that qualify the use of claims that communicate the presence of particular ingredients. An analysis of fruit and vegetable "presence," "proportion," or "serving" claims in Australia demonstrated that 31%, 52%, and 8% did not meet the cut off from the NPSC, respectively [81]. In some cases, without a reference level, whole food claims could be challenging and, if not implemented correctly, could trigger enforcement from regulatory agencies.

3.3. The Glycemic Index and Glycemic Response

The GI is a measure of the postprandial glycemic response of a carbohydrate food relative to an equal carbohydrate portion of a reference food as liquid glucose or white bread. Postprandial glycemic responses are measured directly on a glucose scale or converted to the glucose scale when bread is used as the reference food [82]. The test food and reference food are consumed in servings that contain 50 g of available carbohydrates. When levels of carbohydrates are low in the test food, 25 g available carbohydrates is used for both the test and reference food [82]. Given that the GI is determined by using a standardized reference (glucose or bread), foods can be characterized as having a low (<55), medium (56–69), or high (≥70) GI (based on a glucose scale) [82,83]. The GI is only applicable to foods with physiologically relevant levels of available carbohydrates per serving [84]. Many foods with significant levels of carbohydrates that also have a low GI are acknowledged in dietary guidelines across regions and include specific whole grains, legumes, nuts, dairy, temperate climate fruits, and a variety of vegetables [85].

From a scientific perspective, the GI has been successfully used as part of a diet-based approach to manage blood glucose levels in individuals with diabetes [86–91]. Guidelines for the management of diabetes in Canada, Australia, Europe, the UK, and the US acknowledge that low GI dietary patterns can be used to assist with blood glucose management [92–95]. In Canada, low glycemic index diets have also been acknowledged as a strategy for the prevention and management for cardiovascular disease [96].

From a regulatory perspective, the GI is the most contentious labelling strategy for identifying quality carbohydrate foods. In a recent systemic review and meta-analysis of prospective cohorts, Reynolds et al. [16] concluded that, compared with dietary fibre and whole grains, the GI might not be as useful a measure of carbohydrate quality for the prevention of chronic disease. Conversely, subsequent dose–response meta-analyses of prospective cohorts showed that the risk of coronary heart disease and type 2 diabetes increased by 24% and 27% per 10 unit increase in GI, respectively [97,98]. Food Standards Australia New Zealand permits "low," "medium," and "high" GI claims. However, historically, GI claims have not been permitted in Canada and Europe [99,100]. To our knowledge, there is no regulation in the US that would discourage GI labelling on food.

The rationale for not permitting the use of GI labelling are multifaceted and include the following: perceived challenges with the precision and accuracy of the methods used to measure the GI [101], risk of low-GI foods misaligning with regional healthy eating policies [99], and poor characterization of low-GI foods [100]. Uncertainties around the precision and accuracy of GI values have largely been addressed in the scientific literature [101]. The International Organization for Standardization (ISO) has published an official method for determining the GI of a food [84]. A recent study demonstrated that the ISO method generated accurate GI values with an interlaboratory standard deviation of 5.1% and a coefficient of variation of 8.1% [102]. Results also showed that the ISO GI method was sufficiently precise to distinguish between low- and high-GI foods with 97–99% probability [103]. From a labelling perspective, it is valid that published tables on GI values can demonstrate variability between similar products [85]. However, as with any labelling framework, it is the responsibility of the industry stakeholder using the claim to ensure that the GI of a specific product is assessed using a validated method and confirmed to have a low GI, and not extrapolated from other data sources.

The GI is an attribute of the food. Thus, it is fair that some low-GI foods may or may not align with national dietary policies. Health Canada has outlined concerns that snack-type foods, such as ice cream, and naturally or artificially sweetened beverages could be classified as low-GI foods and mislead consumers to perceiving these foods as healthy and encourage consumption [99]. However, mechanisms can be implemented to mitigate this risk. For example, in Australia and New Zealand, health claims, including GI claims, can only be made if food products meet specific nutritional criteria quantified by the NPSC [23]. The Glycemic Index Foundation (GIF) is an Australia-based non-profit organization supported by the University of Sydney, and Diabetes New South Wales and the Australian Capital Territory, that provides the food industry with a front-of-pack GI symbol program to permit consumers to quickly identify low-GI foods in the marketplace (Figure 2). In addition to regulatory requirements, the GIF has additional nutritional and testing requirements before the symbol program can be used on food products [103]:

1. The food must contain ≥7.5 g carbohydrate/serving, or be ≥80% carbohydrate (served in multiple units of small servings sizes as part of one meal or snack) [104];
2. The GI of the food is measured using the ISO method [104];
3. The nutritional profile of foods meet category-specific criteria for energy, saturated fat, sodium, and dietary fibre, specified by the GIF [104];
4. Adhere to the GIF's glycemic index testing policy [105].

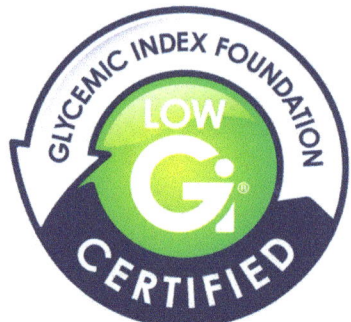

Figure 2. The Glycemic Index Foundation's low glycemic symbol used by consumers to identify that foods have a low GI [104]. Reproduced with permission from the Glycemic Index Foundation.

The GIF symbol program focuses on the identification of "low-GI" foods (GI ≤ 55) and negates the need to linking the symbol to a GI number, which could cause confusion amongst consumers. It is generally accepted that "low-GI" foods have a GI value ≤ 55, which has been used as the cut-off for demonstrating beneficial effects on blood sugar management and reduced cardiometabolic risk. Data from the Australian National Nutrition Survey demonstrated that the GI and glycemic load of diets had decreased by 5% and 12% respectively, from 1995 to 2012 [106]. Combining the GI with nutrition profiling ensures that potential benefits of decreasing postprandial glycemic responses from carbohydrate foods are not counteracted by dietary factors associated with unhealthy dietary patterns.

Regulations in Australia and New Zealand also permit "medium GI" and "high GI" claims on food. However, the latter two claims have little, if any utility for the consumer for identifying quality carbohydrate foods. Again, the benefits of the GI as a tool to facilitate healthy carbohydrate choices are supported by patterns that incorporate foods with a "low GI" designation. Thus, adopting GI as a labeling strategy is only supported by foods with a GI ≤ 55. It is also reasonable that when a food is reformulated, it is retested to ensure that it qualifies for a low GI designation.

Although Canada and Europe do not permit labelling to identify low-GI foods, both jurisdictions have been receptive to the use of postprandial glycemic response claims, which itself is also considered a function-type health claim (Table 3). Similar to the GI, the postprandial glycemic response is determined by measuring the incremental area under the blood glucose curve of the test food. However, rather than indexing against a standardized control, in theory, any food can be used as the reference food. Considered to be a function-type health claim, in 2013, Health Canada published a draft guidance document for postprandial glycemic response claims, where reference foods were suggested to be similar to the test foods [107]. It was also indicated that the postprandial glycemic response should be at least 20% lower than the reference food without a disproportionate rise in insulin levels to make the claim [107]. Few stakeholders in Canada have applied glycemic response labelling to foods as the approach can be limiting to stakeholders. Furthermore, given that the proposed claim is relative to a specific food, the incorporation of "low glycemic response claims" and its efficacy for blood glucose management through the adoption of dietary patterns is arbitrary. While a review for function-type health claims is not required, Health Canada has reviewed and approved a low glycemic response claim for a proprietary polysaccharide complex that contains various viscous dietary fibres (glucomannan, xanthan gum, and sodium alginate) [35]. Reference to the control food has not been identified in the claim statement [35] and is a departure from Health Canada's draft guidance [107]. In Europe, similar to the GI, The European Food Safety Authority (EFSA) has published the opinion that carbohydrate foods that induce a low glycemic response are insufficiently characterized [21]. Nevertheless, since 2010, numerous dietary fibres in Europe that have been appropriately characterized have been authorized to facilitate "a reduction in blood glucose rise after a meal" (Table 2).

An overarching challenge with glycemic response claims is that they are indiscriminate. Labelling and advertising that a food reduces the postprandial glycemic response is only relative to the reference food used. While a significant decrease in the glycemic response might be observed with test food compared with the reference food, the response may not be particularly useful for individuals with diabetes or impaired glucose tolerance. Thus, the utilization of the postprandial glycemic response in the context of a dietary pattern, which would be required to demonstrate meaningful benefits of blood glucose management and decreased cardiometabolic risk over time, can be difficult for the consumer to implement and quantify. On the other hand, low-GI foods, with values ≤55, are characterized by comparing a test food to a standardized reference of glucose (or bread). This enables foods to be definitively labelled as "low-GI foods" and incorporated into dietary patterns that can be adopted and, over time, result in a predictable outcome, which corresponds with the purpose of a claim and quality carbohydrates.

4. Discussion

There are multiple opportunities to use labelling to promote the consumption of quality carbohydrates. Given that carbohydrate is a macronutrient, high-quality carbohydrate foods can encompass various characteristics. For the most part, source of dietary fibre, dietary fibre-related health claims, whole carbohydrate foods, including whole grains, and low GI and response claims have been implemented internationally into non-mandatory labelling strategies to assist consumers with choosing carbohydrate foods that align with nutrient-dense dietary patterns and/or prevent non-communicable diseases. However, as demonstrated in this review, although the parameters of carbohydrate quality are similar, regulatory frameworks corresponding to quality carbohydrate criteria can differ between regions.

Just as there is no "one-size-fits-all" healthy dietary pattern, this review demonstrates that there are multiple attributes that can be used to highlight carbohydrate quality in foods to the consumer. The laws that underpin regulations and policies that permit the characteristics of foods to be communicated to the consumer are predicated on the fact that food labels and claims cannot be misleading [29,108–112]. Labelling for "source of fibre," fibre-derived health claims, and programs that highlight the presence of whole food credentials are straightforward with similar claims made across jurisdictions, whereas labelling with regard to the GI and glycemic response continues to be debated and varies across regions.

The effects of carbohydrate foods on postprandial glycemia are the most contentious measure of carbohydrate quality. The ongoing polarized debate around "low GI" labelling frameworks is an example of the disconnect between developments in nutrition science and labelling regulations. Jurisdictions have acknowledged the value of managing postprandial glycemia, which, over time, can assist with decreasing the risk of vascular complications linked to diabetes [113]. Australia and New Zealand permit claims that identify foods as "low GI," which has been successfully leveraged and implemented by the GIF. Canada and Europe have been transparent by presenting their rationale for refuting labelling claims that identify low-GI foods or permitting foods that facilitate a lower glycemic response. Although the GI is an attribute of the food that is not presented in the same manner as glycemic response, scientific validity has been presented regarding its benefits when used to help facilitate blood glucose management. This review has highlighted that various metrics of quality carbohydrates exist, and will resonate differently for consumers depending on their food values and needs. Canada's position on GI labelling contradicts Canadian expert opinions for the management of diabetes and cardiovascular disease risk since guidelines recommend low-GI dietary patterns [92,96]. A recent study demonstrated that Canadians would be receptive to GI labelling as a tool to destigmatize carbohydrates and assist with choosing healthy carbohydrate foods [14]. Similar to Australia and New Zealand, when used alongside nutrient profiling, GI labelling can be an efficacious strategy for implementing dietary patterns with higher carbohydrate quality.

Sugar content in foods has not been included as a domain used to identify quality carbohydrate foods. Given that the levels of sugar in specific foods have been raised as a nutritional concern for its effects on cardiometabolic risk, characterizing foods with a high level of sugar as foods of lower quality carbohydrate could be considered. Across regions, policies, including mandatory front-of-pack labelling initiatives, have been used to help consumers choose foods with lower levels of sugar [114]. However, while sugar is a carbohydrate, the absence of sugar is not necessarily a proxy for the carbohydrate quality of foods. Although foods with higher levels of added sugars are linked to cardiometabolic risk, risk is not ubiquitous across all food types. High consumption of added sugars in sugar-sweetened beverages (SSBs) have been consistently shown to be associated with increased risk for diabetes and cardiovascular disease [12,13,115,116]. Conversely, total sugar consumption or intrinsic sugars in solid and liquid foods have not demonstrated the same associations [117–119]. A global review on the effects of dietary factors on the global burden of disease identified higher consumption of SSBs as a significant contributor to disability-adjusted life years (DALYs) and deaths from cardiovascular disease (DALYs: 2.8 million; deaths: 117 thousand) and type 2 diabetes (DALYs: 1.6 million; deaths: 21 thousand) [120]. Other sugar-containing foods were not identified. Comparatively, low consumption of other quality carbohydrate foods, such as fruit (DALYs: 65 million; deaths: 2.4 million), vegetables (DALY: 34 million; deaths: 1.5 million), whole grains (DALYs: 82 million; deaths, 3.1 million), nuts and seeds (DALYs: 50 million; deaths: 2.1 million), legumes (DALYs: 11 million; deaths: 535 thousand), milk (DALYs: 2.7 million; deaths: 126 thousand), and dietary fibre (DALYs: 20 million; deaths: 873 thousand), was ranked higher than increased SSBs consumption as dietary factors that prevent non-communicable diseases [120]. The purpose of mandatory front-of-pack labelling for added sugars in foods, is in part, to prevent high intakes of added sugars that could displace healthy food options from the diet and increase the risk of cardiometabolic disease [121]. However, in the context of labelling for quality carbohydrate foods, sugar on its own, may not be as useful as other domains outlined in this review [122].

It is important to acknowledge that, from an academic perspective, measurements of carbohydrate quality in dietary patterns can be more comprehensive than parameters used to inform consumer food choices. The SUN cohort used a comprehensive approach that combined attributes of carbohydrate quality outlined in this review (dietary fibre and the GI), as well as other indicators (whole grains-to-total grains ratios, solid-to-total carbohydrate ratio) to determine associations with obesity, cardiovascular disease incidence, and micronutrient intake adequacy [1,123,124]. It is undetermined if these approaches are useful as a labelling strategy. Mozaffarian et al. [5] compared various strategies for identifying whole grain foods in grocery stores, which included the Whole Grain Stamp cited in this review. Results demonstrated that using a ≤10:1 ratio of carbohydrate-to-fibre was the most effective at identifying foods with higher levels of dietary fibre, and lower levels of sodium, and sugar. While promising, this approach could require a regulatory assessment. The successful implementation of any labelling strategy by industry would require consumer education and industry support. Labelling concepts that are overly complex may hinder their adoption and usefulness in the marketplace.

Labelling that highlights the quality carbohydrates of a food is not mandatory. It is ultimately up to industry stakeholders to decide on the labelling messages that best align with the foods provided to their consumers, and then for consumers to choose attributes of carbohydrate quality that align with their dietary needs and values. The attributes of a food and corresponding labelling strategy will differ depending on the targeted consumer, and their preferences. Having multiple labelling tools at the industry's disposal across multiple domains of carbohydrate quality can assist with the widespread consumption of quality carbohydrate foods. The scientific community ensures that parameters used to characterize quality carbohydrates, or other attributes, are scientifically valid and applied within a regulatory framework that is not misleading to the consumer. The food environment must enable scientifically valid labelling tools to be accessible to industry to facilitate innovation across multiple parameters of carbohydrate quality.

In the regions discussed in this review, mandatory nutritional information is required on most prepackaged food products. Fresh foods or some single ingredient foods are exempt from nutrition labelling [18,29,125,126]. In Canada and the US, the dietary fibre content of a food per serving is a mandatory component of nutrient declaration panels [18,125], while it is optional in Australia and New Zealand, and Europe, unless a food presents a dietary fibre nutrient content claim [29,126]. While claims and front-of-pack labelling can be useful for quickly identifying the carbohydrate quality of foods, fundamental nutritional literacy and habitual use of mandatory nutrition information on products could help consumers better evaluate foods for their nutrition value, including quality carbohydrates, and make better selections, and thus enhance the nutritional quality of their diets. Buyuktuncer et al. [127] demonstrated that students that had consistently used nutrition facts tables on food products had higher composite Healthy Eating Index-2005 scores, and higher intakes of total fruit, whole fruit, total vegetables, whole grains, and milk. Consistent users also had higher scores associated with lower intakes of added sugars [127].

5. Conclusions

Over the last decade, carbohydrate foods have been increasingly stigmatized by consumers. While some types of carbohydrate (i.e., sugar) may not confer a nutritional or health benefit, regulatory agencies and dietary guidelines recognize carbohydrate-rich foods and specific carbohydrate fractions, such as dietary fibre, to be part of healthy dietary patterns. High-quality carbohydrate foods can be identified as those that are high in dietary fibre, contain meaningful levels of whole carbohydrate foods and ingredients that are intact or reconstituted, such as whole grains, or have a low GI or glycemic response. Regulatory agencies around the world permit the use of non-mandatory labelling tools to promote quality carbohydrate foods to consumers across these domains of carbohydrate quality. While not exhaustive, this review provided examples of quality carbohydrate labelling that has been leveraged across Australia, New Zealand, Canada, Europe, and the US. This review does not promote one labelling strategy over another and acknowledges that different facets of carbohydrate quality will resonate differently between consumers. However, as nutrition science continues to evolve, it is crucial that government agencies are equipped to adapt to developments in nutrition science to ensure regulatory frameworks enable the use of labelling to relay messages that destigmatize carbohydrates and steer consumers to healthy quality carbohydrate choices.

Author Contributions: Conceptualization: C.P.F.M. and J.L.S.; Investigation: C.P.F.M., S.V.H., A.J.G., L.C., A.Z., D.J.A.J., C.W.C.K., K.B.M., and J.L.S.; Writing—Original draft: C.P.F.M.; Writing—Review and editing: S.V.H., A.J.G., L.C., A.Z., D.J.A.J., C.W.C.K., K.B.M., and J.L.S. All authors have read and agreed to the published version of the manuscript.

Funding: This research received no external funding.

Acknowledgments: The authors would like to thank Oldways Whole Grains Council for providing pictures of their Whole Grains Stamp (Figure 1) and the Glycemic Index Foundation for providing a picture of their Glycemic Index Symbol (Figure 2).

Conflicts of Interest: C.P.F.M. is an employee of Pulse Canada and former employee of Kellogg Canada. S.V.H. has received research funding from Natural Sciences and Engineering Council of Canada, Canada Foundation for Innovation, Ocean Frontier Institute and Memorial University. S.V.H. has consulted, and/or received honoraria, and/or travel support from Apotex Canada, Dairy UK, Merck/Seven Seas UK, Unilever R&D Vlaardingen, and MSPrebiotics (Manitoba, Canada). A.J.G. has received funding from the Banting & Best Diabetes Centre Tamarack Graduate Award in Diabetes Research and is a consultant for Solo GI Nutrition. L.C. is a Mitacs-Elevate post-doctoral fellow jointly funded by the Government of Canada and the Canadian Sugar Institute. A.Z. is a part-time research associate at Inquis Clinical Research Ltd., a contract research organization. D.J.A.J. has received research grants from Saskatchewan & Alberta Pulse Growers Associations, the Agricultural Bioproducts Innovation Program through the Pulse Research Network, the Advanced Foods and Material Network, Loblaw Companies Ltd., Unilever Canada and Netherlands, Barilla, the Almond Board of California, Agriculture and Agri-food Canada, Pulse Canada, Kellogg's Company, Canada, Quaker Oats, Canada, Procter & Gamble Technical Centre Ltd., Bayer Consumer Care, Springfield, NJ, Pepsi/Quaker, International Nut & Dried Fruit (INC), Soy Foods Association of North America, the Coca-Cola Company (investigator initiated, unrestricted grant), Solae, Haine Celestial, the Sanitarium Company, Orafti, the International Tree Nut Council Nutrition Research and Education Foundation, the Peanut Institute, Soy Nutrition Institute (SNI), the Canola and Flax Councils of Canada, the Calorie Control Council, the Canadian Institutes of Health Research (CIHR), the Canada Foundation for Innovation (CFI)and the Ontario Research Fund (ORF). He has received in-kind supplies for trials as a research support from the Almond board of California, Walnut Council of California, American Peanut Council, Barilla, Unilever, Unico, Primo, Loblaw Companies, Quaker (Pepsico), Pristine Gourmet, Bunge Limited, Kellogg Canada, WhiteWave

Foods. He has been on the speaker's panel, served on the scientific advisory board and/or received travel support and/or honoraria from the Almond Board of California, Canadian Agriculture Policy Institute, Loblaw Companies Ltd., the Griffin Hospital (for the development of the NuVal scoring system), the Coca-Cola Company, EPICURE, Danone, Diet Quality Photo Navigation (DQPN), Better Therapeutics (FareWell), Verywell, True Health Initiative (THI), Institute of Food Technologists (IFT), Soy Nutrition Institute (SNI), Herbalife Nutrition Institute (HNI), Saskatchewan & Alberta Pulse Growers Associations, Sanitarium Company, Orafti, the American Peanut Council, the International Tree Nut Council Nutrition Research and Education Foundation, the Peanut Institute, Herbalife International, Pacific Health Laboratories, Nutritional Fundamentals for Health (NFH), Barilla, Metagenics, Bayer Consumer Care, Unilever Canada and Netherlands, Solae, Kellogg, Quaker Oats, Procter & Gamble, Abbott Laboratories, Dean Foods, the California Strawberry Commission, Haine Celestial, PepsiCo, the Alpro Foundation, Pioneer Hi-Bred International, DuPont Nutrition and Health, Spherix Consulting and WhiteWave Foods, the Advanced Foods and Material Network, the Canola and Flax Councils of Canada, Agri-Culture and Agri-Food Canada, the Canadian Agri-Food Policy Institute, Pulse Canada, the Soy Foods Association of North America, the Nutrition Foundation of Italy (NFI), Nutra-Source Diagnostics, the McDougall Program, the Toronto Knowledge Translation Group (St. Michael's Hospital), the Canadian College of Naturopathic Medicine, The Hospital for Sick Children, the Canadian Nutrition Society (CNS), the American Society of Nutrition (ASN), Arizona State University, Paolo Sorbini Foundation and the Institute of Nutrition, Metabolism and Diabetes. He received an honorarium from the United States Department of Agriculture to present the 2013 W.O. Atwater Memorial Lecture. He received the 2013 Award for Excellence in Research from the International Nut and Dried Fruit Council. He received funding and travel support from the Canadian Society of Endocrinology and Metabolism to produce mini cases for the Canadian Diabetes Association (CDA). He is a member of the International Carbohydrate Quality Consortium (ICQC). His wife, Alexandra L Jenkins, is a director and partner of Glycemic Index Laboratories, Inc., and his sister, Caroline Brydson, received funding through a grant from the St. Michael's Hospital Foundation to develop a cookbook for one of his studies. C.W.C.K. has received grants or research support from the Advanced Food Materials Network, Agriculture and Agri-Foods Canada (AAFC), Almond Board of California, American Peanut Council, Barilla, Canadian Institutes of Health Research (CIHR), Canola Council of Canada, International Nut and Dried Fruit Council, International Tree Nut Council Research and Education Foundation, Loblaw Brands Ltd., Pulse Canada and Unilever. He has received in-kind research support from the Almond Board of California, American Peanut Council, Barilla, California Walnut Commission, Kellogg Canada, Loblaw Companies, Quaker (PepsiCo), Primo, Unico, Unilever, WhiteWave Foods/Danone. He has received travel support and/or honoraria from the American Peanut Council, Barilla, California Walnut Commission, Canola Council of Canada, General Mills, International Nut and Dried Fruit Council, International Pasta Organization, Loblaw Brands Ltd., Nutrition Foundation of Italy, Oldways Preservation Trust, Paramount Farms, Peanut Institute, Pulse Canada, Sun-Maid, Tate & Lyle, Unilever and White Wave Foods/Danone. He has served on the scientific advisory board for the International Tree Nut Council, International Pasta Organization, McCormick Science Institute and Oldways Preservation Trust. He is a member of the International Carbohydrate Quality Consortium (ICQC), Executive Board Member of the Diabetes and Nutrition Study Group (DNSG) of the European Association for the Study of Diabetes (EASD), is on the Clinical Practice Guidelines Expert Committee for Nutrition Therapy of the EASD and is a Director of the Toronto 3D Knowledge Synthesis and Clinical Trials foundation. K.B.M. is a former employee of Novartis, Nestle, and The Kellogg Company. He is a current employee of General Mills Inc. J.L.S. has received research support from the Canadian Foundation for Innovation, Ontario Research Fund, Province of Ontario Ministry of Research and Innovation and Science, Canadian Institutes of health Research (CIHR), Diabetes Canada, PSI Foundation, Banting and Best Diabetes Centre (BBDC), American Society for Nutrition (ASN), INC International Nut and Dried Fruit Council Foundation, National Dried Fruit Trade Association, The Tate and Lyle Nutritional Research Fund at the University of Toronto, The Glycemic Control and Cardiovascular Disease in Type 2 Diabetes Fund at the University of Toronto (a fund established by the Alberta Pulse Growers), and the Nutrition Trialists Fund at the University of Toronto (a fund established by an inaugural donation from the Calorie Control Council). He has received in-kind food donations to support a randomized controlled trial from the Almond Board of California, California Walnut Commission, American Peanut Council, Barilla, Unilever, Unico/Primo, Loblaw Companies, Quaker, Kellogg Canada, and WhiteWave Foods. He has received travel support, speaker fees and/or honoraria from Diabetes Canada, Dairy Farmers of Canada, FoodMinds LLC, International Sweeteners Association, Nestlé, Pulse Canada, Canadian Society for Endocrinology and Metabolism (CSEM), GI Foundation, Abbott, Biofortis, ASN, Northern Ontario School of Medicine, INC Nutrition Research & Education Foundation, European Food Safety Authority (EFSA), Comité Européen des Fabricants de Sucre (CEFS), and Physicians Committee for Responsible Medicine. He has or has had ad hoc consulting arrangements with Perkins Coie LLP, Tate & Lyle, and Wirtschaftliche Vereinigung Zucker e.V. He is a member of the European Fruit Juice Association Scientific Expert Panel and Soy Nutrition Institute (SNI) Scientific Advisory Committee. He is on the Clinical Practice Guidelines Expert Committees of Diabetes Canada, European Association for the study of Diabetes (EASD), Canadian Cardiovascular Society (CCS), and Obesity Canada. He serves or has served as an unpaid scientific advisor for the Food, Nutrition, and Safety Program (FNSP) and the Technical Committee on Carbohydrates of the International Life Science Institute (ILSI) North America. He is a member of the International Carbohydrate Quality Consortium (ICQC), Executive Board Member of the Diabetes and Nutrition Study Group (DNSG) of the EASD, and Director of the Toronto 3D Knowledge Synthesis and Clinical Trials foundation. His wife is an employee of AB InBev.

References

1. Santiago, S.; Zazpe, I.; Bes-Rastrollo, M.; Sanchez-Tainta, A.; Sayon-Orea, C.; de la Fuente-Arrillaga, C.; Benito, S.; Martinez, J.A.; Martinez-Gonzalez, M.A. Carbohydrate quality, weight change and incident obesity in a Mediterranean cohort: The SUN Project. *Eur. J. Clin. Nutr.* **2015**, *69*, 297–302. [CrossRef]
2. Blaak, E.E. Carbohydrate quantity and quality and cardio-metabolic risk. *Curr. Opin. Clin. Nutr. Metab. Care* **2016**, *19*, 289–293. [CrossRef]
3. Brand-Miller, J.; McMillan-Price, J.; Steinbeck, K.; Caterson, I. Carbohydrates—the good, the bad and the whole grain. *Asia Pac. J. Clin. Nutr.* **2008**, *17* (Suppl. 1), 16–19.
4. Ludwig, D.S.; Hu, F.B.; Tappy, L.; Brand-Miller, J. Dietary carbohydrates: Role of quality and quantity in chronic disease. *BMJ* **2018**, *361*, k2340. [CrossRef]
5. Mozaffarian, R.S.; Lee, R.M.; Kennedy, M.A.; Ludwig, D.S.; Mozaffarian, D.; Gortmaker, S.L. Identifying whole grain foods: A comparison of different approaches for selecting more healthful whole grain products. *Public Health Nutr.* **2013**, *16*, 2255–2264. [CrossRef] [PubMed]
6. Anderson, J.W.; Baird, P.; Davis, R.H., Jr.; Ferreri, S.; Knudtson, M.; Koraym, A.; Waters, V.; Williams, C.L. Health benefits of dietary fiber. *Nutr. Rev.* **2009**, *67*, 188–205. [CrossRef]
7. Government of Canada. *Canada's Dietary Guidelines for Health Professionals and Policy Makers*; Health Canada: Ottawa, ON, Canadian, 2019.
8. Department of Health and Human Services; U.S. Department of Agriculture. *2015–2020 Dietary Guidelines for Americans*, 8th ed. Available online: http://health.gov/dietaryguidelines/2015/guidelines (accessed on 18 March 2020).
9. *Australian Dietary Guidelines*; National Health and Medical Research Council: Canberra, Australia, 2013.
10. Schmidhuber, J.; Sur, P.; Fay, K.; Huntley, B.; Salama, J.; Lee, A.; Cornaby, L.; Horino, M.; Murray, C.; Afshin, A. The Global Nutrient Database: Availability of macronutrients and micronutrients in 195 countries from 1980 to 2013. *Lancet Planet. Health* **2018**, *2*, e353–e368. [CrossRef]
11. Slavin, J.L. Carbohydrate Quality: Who Gets to Decide? *Cereal Foods World* **2018**, *63*, 96–98.
12. Schlesinger, S.; Neuenschwander, M.; Schwedhelm, C.; Hoffmann, G.; Bechthold, A.; Boeing, H.; Schwingshackl, L. Food Groups and Risk of Overweight, Obesity, and Weight Gain: A Systematic Review and Dose-Response Meta-Analysis of Prospective Studies. *Adv. Nutr.* **2019**, *10*, 205–218. [CrossRef] [PubMed]
13. Schwingshackl, L.; Hoffmann, G.; Lampousi, A.M.; Knuppel, S.; Iqbal, K.; Schwedhelm, C.; Bechthold, A.; Schlesinger, S.; Boeing, H. Food groups and risk of type 2 diabetes mellitus: A systematic review and meta-analysis of prospective studies. *Eur. J. Epidemiol.* **2017**, *32*, 363–375. [CrossRef] [PubMed]
14. Marinangeli, C.P.F.; Castellano, J.; Torrance, P.; Lewis, J.; Gall Casey, C.; Tanuta, J.; Curran, J.; Harding, S.V.; Jenkins, D.J.A.; Sievenpiper, J.L. Positioning the Value of Dietary Carbohydrate, Carbohydrate Quality, Glycemic Index, and GI Labelling to the Canadian Consumer for Improving Dietary Patterns. *Nutrients* **2019**, *11*, 457. [CrossRef] [PubMed]
15. International Food Information Council Foundation. 2019 Food and Health Survey. Available online: https://foodinsight.org/2019-food-and-health-survey/ (accessed on 5 March 2020).
16. Reynolds, A.; Mann, J.; Cummings, J.; Winter, N.; Mete, E.; Te Morenga, L. Carbohydrate quality and human health: A series of systematic reviews and meta-analyses. *Lancet* **2019**, *393*, 434–445. [CrossRef]
17. Institute of Medicine. Chapter 7: Dietary, Functional, and Total Fiber. In *Dietary Reference Intakes for Energy, Carbohydrate, Fiber, Fat, Fatty Acids, Cholesterol, Protein, and Amino Acids*; The National Academies Press: Washington, DC, USA, 2005; p. 1358. [CrossRef]
18. Food and Drug Administration. Electronic Code of Federal Regulations. Title 21. Part 101 Food Labelling. Subpart A: 101.9 Nutrition Labeling of Food. Available online: https://www.ecfr.gov/cgi-bin/text-idx?SID=204cb193309beffa421b1d0df1fcf8a0&mc=true&node=pt21.2.101&rgn=div5#se21.2.101_19 (accessed on 8 April 2020).
19. Government of Canada. Dietary Reference Intakes. Available online: https://www.canada.ca/en/health-canada/services/food-nutrition/healthy-eating/dietary-reference-intakes/tables/reference-values-macronutrients-dietary-reference-intakes-tables-2005.html (accessed on 8 April 2020).
20. Australian Government Department of Health and Ageing; New Zealand Ministry of Health. Nutrient Reference Values for Australia and New Zealand. In *Nutrient Reference Values for Australia and New Zealand Including Recommended Dietary Intakes*; National Health and Medical Research Council: Canberra, Australia, 2006.

21. EFSA Panel on Dietetic Products, Nutrition, and Allergies (NDA). Scientific Opinion on Dietary Reference Values for carbohydrates and dietary fibre. *EFSA J.* **2010**, *8*, 1462. [CrossRef]
22. Food and Agriculture Organization of the United Nation. *Codex Alimentarius. Guidelines on Nutrition Labelling: CAC/GL2-1985*; World Health Organization: Rome, Italy, 2017.
23. *Schedule 4—Nutrition, Health and Related Claims (F2017C00711)*; Food Standards Australia New Zealand: Canberra, Australia, 2017.
24. *Regulation (EU) No 1924/2006 of the European Parliament and of the the Council of of 20 December 2006 on Nutrition and Health Claims Made on Foods*; European Commission: Brussels, Belgium, 2006.
25. The Food and Drug Administration. *Electronic Code of Federal Regulations. Title 21: Food and Drugs*; Part 101—Food labelling; Subpart A—General provisions. 101.9 Nutrition Labeling of Food; Office of the Federal Register: Washington, DC, USA, 2020.
26. Government of Canada. Table of Reference Amounts for Food. Available online: https://www.canada.ca/en/health-canada/services/technical-documents-labelling-requirements/table-reference-amounts-food.html (accessed on 13 April 2020).
27. Food and Drug Administration. Electronic Code of Federal Regulations. Title 21. Part 101 Food Labelling. Subpart A: 101.12 Reference Amounts Customarily Consumed Per Eating Occasion. Available online: https://www.ecfr.gov/cgi-bin/textidx?SID=81de530b0bca2d6c4dea96523cdefbd7&\T1\textquotedblrightmc=true&node=pt21.2.101&rgn=div5#se21.2.101_112 (accessed on 13 April 2020).
28. *Comission Directive 2008/100/EC of 28 October 2008: Amending Council Directive 90/496/EEC on Nutrition Labelling for Foodstuffs as Regards Recommended Daily Allowances, Energy Conversion Factors and Definitions*; European Commission: Brussels, Belgium, 2008.
29. *Regulation (EC) No 1169/2011 of the Euopean Parlimant and of the Council of 25 October 201 on the Provision of Food Information to Consumers, Amending Regulations (EC) No 1924/2006 and (EC) No 1925/2006 of the European Parliament and of the Council, and Repealing Commission Directive 87/250/EEC, Council Directive 90/496/EEC, Commission Directive 1999/10/EC, Directive 2000/13/EC of the European Parliament and of the Council, Commission Directives 2002/67/EC and 2008/5/EC and Commission Regulation (EC) No 608/2004*; European Commission: Brussels, Belgium, 2011.
30. Government of Canada. Policy for Labelling and Advertising of Dietary Fibre-Containing Food Products. Available online: https://www.canada.ca/en/health-canada/services/publications/food-nutrition/labelling-advertising-dietary-fibre-food-products.html (accessed on 8 April 2020).
31. Codex Alimentarius. Guidelines on Nturition Labelling CAC/GL 2-1985. In *Section 2—Definitions: Fibre*; FAO: Rome, Italy; WHO: Geneva, Switzerland, 2017.
32. U.S. Department of Health and Human Services; Food and Drug Administration; Center for Food Safety and Applied Nutrition. *Scientific Evaluation of the Evidence on the Beneficial Physiological Effects of Isolated or Synthetic Non-Digestible Carbohydrates Submitted as a Citizen Petition (21 CFR 10.30): Guidance for Industry*; Office of Nutrition and Food Labeling: Boston, MA, USA, 2018.
33. *Standard 1.2.7—Nutrition, Health and Related Claims (F2018C00942)*; Food Standards Australia New Zealand: Canberra, Australia, 2018.
34. Government of Canada. Food Labelling Tool: Function Claims—Acceptable Function Claims Table. Available online: https://www.inspection.gc.ca/food-label-requirements/labelling/industry/health-claims-on-food-labels/eng/1392834838383/1392834887794?chap=8#s13c8 (accessed on 13 April 2020).
35. Health Canada. Summary of Health Canada's Assessment of a Health Claim about a Polysaccharide Complex (Glucomannan, Xanthan Gum, Sodium Alginate) and a Reduction of the Post-Prandial Blood Glucose Response. Available online: https://www.canada.ca/en/health-canada/services/food-nutrition/food-labelling/health-claims/assessments/summary-assessment-health-claim-about-polysaccharide-complex-glucomannan-xanthan-sodium-alginate-reduction-post-prandial-blood-glucose.html (accessed on 9 April 2020).
36. *Commission Regulation (EU) No 432/2012 of 16 May 2012: Establishing a List of Permitted Health Claims Made on Foods, Other than Those Referring to the Reduction of Disease Risk and to Children's Development and Health*; European Commission: Brussels, MA, USA, 2012.
37. *Comission Regulation (EU) No 40/2014 of 17 January 2014: Authorising a Health Claim Made on Foods, Other than Those Referring to the Reduction of Disease Risk and to Children's Development and Health and Amending Regulation (EU) No 432/2012*; European Commission: Brussels, MA, USA, 2014.

38. *Standard 1.1.2—Definitions Used throughout the Code (F2018C00912)*; Food Standards Australia New Zealand: Canberra, Australia, 2018.
39. Food and Drug Administration. Structure/Function Claims. Available online: https://www.fda.gov/food/food-labeling-nutrition/structurefunction-claims (accessed on 28 April 2020).
40. *Commission Regulation (EU) No 1160/2011 of 14 November 2011 on the Authorisation and Refusal of Authorisation of Certain Health Claims Made on Foods and Referring to the Reduction of Disease Risk*; European Commission: Brussels, MA, USA, 2011.
41. *Commission Regulation (EU) No 1048/2012 of 8 November 2012 on the Authorisation of a Health Claim Made on Foods and Referring to the Reduction of Disease Risk*; European Commission: Brussels, MA, USA, 2012.
42. Health Canada. Summary of Assessment of a Health Claim about Oat Products and Blood Cholesterol Lowering. Available online: https://www.canada.ca/en/health-canada/services/food-nutrition/food-labelling/health-claims/assessments/products-blood-cholesterol-lowering-summary-assessment-health-claim-about-products-blood-cholesterol-lowering.html (accessed on 9 April 2020).
43. Health Canada. Summary of Health Canada's Assessment of a Health Claim about Barley Products and Blood Cholesterol Lowering. Available online: https://www.canada.ca/en/health-canada/services/food-nutrition/food-labelling/health-claims/assessments/assessment-health-claim-about-barley-products-blood-cholesterol-lowering.html (accessed on 9 April 2020).
44. Food and Drug Administration. Electronic Code of Federal Regulations. Title 21. Part 101 Food Labelling. Subpart E: 101.81 Health Claims: Soluble Fiber from Certain Foods and Risk of Coronary Heart Disease (CHD). Available online: https://www.ecfr.gov/cgi-bin/text-idx?SID=46c4b638cff1090093f7997b0d293de9&mc=true&node=pt21.2.101&rgn=div5 (accessed on 8 April 2020).
45. Health Canada. Summary of Health Canada's Assessment of a Health Claim about Food Products Containing Psyllium and Blood Cholesterol Lowering. Available online: https://www.canada.ca/en/health-canada/services/food-nutrition/food-labelling/health-claims/assessments/psyllium-products-blood-cholesterol-lowering-nutrition-health-claims-food-labelling.html (accessed on 9 April 2020).
46. Health Canada. Summary of Health Canada's Assessment of a Health Claim about a Polysaccharide Complex (Glucomannan, Xanthan Gum, Sodium Alginate) and Cholesterol Lowering. Available online: https://www.canada.ca/en/health-canada/services/food-nutrition/food-labelling/health-claims/assessments/polysaccharide-complex-glucomannan-xanthan-sodium-alginate-cholesterol-lowering-nutrition-health-claims-food-labelling.html (accessed on 13 April 2020).
47. Food and Drug Administration. Electronic Code of Federal Regulations. Title 21. Part 101 Food Labelling. Subpart E: 101.77 Health Claims: Fruits, Vegetables, and Grain Products that Contain Fiber, Particularly Soluble Fiber, and Risk of Coronary Heart Disease. Available online: https://www.ecfr.gov/cgi-bin/text-idx?SID=46c4b638cff1090093f7997b0d293de9&mc=true&node=pt21.2.101&rgn=div5 (accessed on 8 April 2020).
48. Food and Drug Administration. Electronic Code of Federal Regulations. Title 21. Part 101 Food Labelling. Subpart E: 101.76 Health Claims: Fiber-Containing Grain Products, Fruits, and Vegetables and Cancer. Available online: https://www.ecfr.gov/cgi-bin/text-idx?SID=46c4b638cff1090093f7997b0d293de9&mc=true&node=pt21.2.101&rgn=div5 (accessed on 8 April 2020).
49. Fabiani, R.; Naldini, G.; Chiavarini, M. Dietary Patterns in Relation to Low Bone Mineral Density and Fracture Risk: A Systematic Review and Meta-Analysis. *Adv. Nutr.* **2019**, *10*, 219–236. [CrossRef]
50. Viguiliouk, E.; Glenn, A.J.; Nishi, S.K.; Chiavaroli, L.; Seider, M.; Khan, T.; Bonaccio, M.; Iacoviello, L.; Mejia, S.B.; Jenkins, D.J.A.; et al. Associations between Dietary Pulses Alone or with Other Legumes and Cardiometabolic Disease Outcomes: An Umbrella Review and Updated Systematic Review and Meta-analysis of Prospective Cohort Studies. *Adv. Nutr.* **2019**, *10*, S308–S319. [CrossRef]
51. Kim, Y.; Keogh, J.B.; Clifton, P.M. Does Nut Consumption Reduce Mortality and/or Risk of Cardiometabolic Disease? An Updated Review Based on Meta-Analyses. *Int. J. Environ. Res. Public Health* **2019**, *16*, 4957. [CrossRef]
52. Sochol, K.M.; Johns, T.S.; Buttar, R.S.; Randhawa, L.; Sanchez, E.; Gal, M.; Lestrade, K.; Merzkani, M.; Abramowitz, M.K.; Mossavar-Rahmani, Y.; et al. The Effects of Dairy Intake on Insulin Resistance: A Systematic Review and Meta-Analysis of Randomized Clinical Trials. *Nutrients* **2019**, *11*, 2237. [CrossRef]
53. Abargouei, A.S.; Janghorbani, M.; Salehi-Marzijarani, M.; Esmaillzadeh, A. Effect of dairy consumption on weight and body composition in adults: A systematic review and meta-analysis of randomized controlled clinical trials. *Int. J. Obes.* **2012**, *36*, 1485–1493. [CrossRef]

54. Aune, D.; Keum, N.; Giovannucci, E.; Fadnes, L.T.; Boffetta, P.; Greenwood, D.C.; Tonstad, S.; Vatten, L.J.; Riboli, E.; Norat, T. Nut consumption and risk of cardiovascular disease, total cancer, all-cause and cause-specific mortality: A systematic review and dose-response meta-analysis of prospective studies. *BMC Med.* **2016**, *14*, 207. [CrossRef]
55. Becerra-Tomas, N.; Paz-Graniel, I.; Cyril, W.C.K.; Kahleova, H.; Rahelic, D.; Sievenpiper, J.L.; Salas-Salvado, J. Nut consumption and incidence of cardiovascular diseases and cardiovascular disease mortality: A meta-analysis of prospective cohort studies. *Nutr. Rev.* **2019**, *77*, 691–709. [CrossRef]
56. Liu, G.; Guasch-Ferre, M.; Hu, Y.; Li, Y.; Hu, F.B.; Rimm, E.B.; Manson, J.E.; Rexrode, K.M.; Sun, Q. Nut Consumption in Relation to Cardiovascular Disease Incidence and Mortality Among Patients With Diabetes Mellitus. *Circ. Res.* **2019**, *124*, 920–929. [CrossRef] [PubMed]
57. Tieri, M.; Ghelfi, F.; Vitale, M.; Vetrani, C.; Marventano, S.; Lafranconi, A.; Godos, J.; Titta, L.; Gambera, A.; Alonzo, E.; et al. Whole grain consumption and human health: An umbrella review of observational studies. *Int. J. Food Sci. Nutr.* **2020**, 1–10. [CrossRef] [PubMed]
58. Aune, D.; Keum, N.; Giovannucci, E.; Fadnes, L.T.; Boffetta, P.; Greenwood, D.C.; Tonstad, S.; Vatten, L.J.; Riboli, E.; Norat, T. Whole grain consumption and risk of cardiovascular disease, cancer, and all cause and cause specific mortality: Systematic review and dose-response meta-analysis of prospective studies. *BMJ* **2016**, *353*, i2716. [CrossRef] [PubMed]
59. Hebden, L.; O'Leary, F.; Rangan, A.; Singgih Lie, E.; Hirani, V.; Allman-Farinelli, M. Fruit consumption and adiposity status in adults: A systematic review of current evidence. *Crit. Rev. Food Sci. Nutr.* **2017**, *57*, 2526–2540. [CrossRef]
60. Hernaez, A.; Sanllorente, A.; Castaner, O.; Martinez-Gonzalez, M.A.; Ros, E.; Pinto, X.; Estruch, R.; Salas-Salvado, J.; Corella, D.; Alonso-Gomez, A.M.; et al. Increased Consumption of Virgin Olive Oil, Nuts, Legumes, Whole Grains, and Fish Promotes HDL Functions in Humans. *Mol. Nutr. Food Res.* **2019**, *63*, e1800847. [CrossRef]
61. Toh, D.W.K.; Koh, E.S.; Kim, J.E. Incorporating healthy dietary changes in addition to an increase in fruit and vegetable intake further improves the status of cardiovascular disease risk factors: A systematic review, meta-regression, and meta-analysis of randomized controlled trials. *Nutr. Rev.* **2019**, nuz104. [CrossRef]
62. Zhan, J.; Liu, Y.J.; Cai, L.B.; Xu, F.R.; Xie, T.; He, Q.Q. Fruit and vegetable consumption and risk of cardiovascular disease: A meta-analysis of prospective cohort studies. *Crit. Rev. Food Sci. Nutr.* **2017**, *57*, 1650–1663. [CrossRef]
63. Juan, J.; Liu, G.; Willett, W.C.; Hu, F.B.; Rexrode, K.M.; Sun, Q. Whole Grain Consumption and Risk of Ischemic Stroke: Results From 2 Prospective Cohort Studies. *Stroke* **2017**, *48*, 3203–3209. [CrossRef]
64. Dehghan, M.; Mente, A.; Rangarajan, S.; Sheridan, P.; Mohan, V.; Iqbal, R.; Gupta, R.; Lear, S.; Wentzel-Viljoen, E.; Avezum, A.; et al. Association of dairy intake with cardiovascular disease and mortality in 21 countries from five continents (PURE): A prospective cohort study. *Lancet* **2018**, *392*, 2288–2297. [CrossRef]
65. American Association of Cereal Chemists International. Whole Grain Definition. *Cereal Foods World* **1999**, *45*, 79.
66. *Standard 2.1.1—Cereal and Cereal Products (F2015L00420)*; Food Standards Australia New Zealand: Canberra, Australia, 2015.
67. Government of Canada. Whole Grains—Get the Facts. Available online: https://www.canada.ca/en/health-canada/services/canada-food-guide/resources/healthy-eating-recommendations/eat-a-variety/whole-grain/get-facts.html (accessed on 29 April 2020).
68. The Food and Drug Administration. Draft Guidance for Industry and FDA Staff: Whole Grain Label Statements (Docket Number: FDA-2006-D-0298). Available online: https://www.fda.gov/regulatory-information/search-fda-guidance-documents/draft-guidance-industry-and-fda-staff-whole-grain-label-statements (accessed on 29 April 2020).
69. European Commission. Health Promotion & Disease Prevention: Whole Grain. Available online: https://ec.europa.eu/jrc/en/health-knowledge-gateway/promotion-prevention/nutrition/whole-grain (accessed on 28 April 2020).
70. EFSA Panel on Dietetic Products, Nutrition and Allergies (NDA). Scientific Opinion on the substantiation of health claims related to whole grain (ID 831, 832, 833, 1126, *1268*, 1269, 1270, *1271*, 1431) pursuant to Article 13(1) of Regulation (EC) No 1924/2006. *EFSA J.* **2010**, *8*, 1766. [CrossRef]

71. Herforth, A.; Arimond, M.; Alvarez-Sanchez, C.; Coates, J.; Christianson, K.; Muehlhoff, E. A Global Review of Food-Based Dietary Guidelines. *Adv. Nutr.* **2019**, *10*, 590–605. [CrossRef] [PubMed]
72. *Eating and Activity Guidelines for New Zealand Adults*; Ministry of Health: Wellington, New Zealand, 2015.
73. Oldways Whole Grains Councel. Whole Grain Stamp. Available online: https://wholegrainscouncil.org/whole-grain-stamp (accessed on 18 March 2020).
74. Whole Grain and Legumes Council. *Code of Practice for Whole Grain Ingredient Content Claims*; GLNC: North Sydney, Australia, 2017.
75. Curtain, F.; Locke, A.; Grafenauer, S. Growing the Business of Whole Grain in the Australian Market: A 6-Year Impact Assessment. *Nutrients* **2020**, *12*, 313. [CrossRef] [PubMed]
76. Food and Drug Administration. Electronic Code of Federal Regulations. Title 21. Part 101 Food Labelling. Subpart A: 101.1. Principal Display Panel of Packaged Form Food. Available online: https://www.ecfr.gov/cgi-bin/text-idx?SID=204cb193309beffa421b1d0df1fcf8a0&mc=true&node=pt21.2.101&rgn=div5#se21.2.101_19 (accessed on 8 April 2020).
77. *Standard 1.2.1—Requirements to Have Labels or Otherwise Provide Information (F2018C00464)*; Food Standards Australia New Zealand: Canberra, Australia, 2018.
78. *Food and Drug Regulations. Part A Administration—Interpretation: A.01.016*; Government of Canada: Ottawa, ON, Canada, 2020.
79. *Safe Food for Canadians Regulations: Fasle, Misleding or Deceptive Labelling 199 (1) and (2)*; Government of Canada: Ottawa, ON, Canada, 2020; Volume 2020.
80. Government of Canada. Food Composition and Quality Claims: Highlighted Ingredients. Available online: https://www.inspection.gc.ca/food-label-requirements/labelling/industry/composition-and-quality-claims/eng/1391025998183/1391026062752?chap=2#s6c2 (accessed on 19 March 2020).
81. Wellard, L.; Hughes, C.; Tsang, Y.W.; Watson, W.; Chapman, K. Investigating fruit and vegetable claims on Australian food packages. *Public Health Nutr.* **2014**, *18*, 2729–2735. [CrossRef]
82. Brouns, F.; Bjorck, I.; Frayn, K.N.; Gibbs, A.L.; Lang, V.; Slama, G.; Wolever, T.M. Glycaemic index methodology. *Nutr. Res. Rev.* **2005**, *18*, 145–171. [CrossRef]
83. Augustin, L.S.; Kendall, C.W.; Jenkins, D.J.; Willett, W.C.; Astrup, A.; Barclay, A.W.; Bjorck, I.; Brand-Miller, J.C.; Brighenti, F.; Buyken, A.E.; et al. Glycemic index, glycemic load and glycemic response: An International Scientific Consensus Summit from the International Carbohydrate Quality Consortium (ICQC). *Nutr. Metab. Cardiovasc. Dis.* **2015**, *25*, 795–815. [CrossRef]
84. *ISO 26642:2010: Food Products—Determination of the Glycaemic Index (GI) and Recommendation for Food Classification*; International Organization for Standardization: Geneva, Switzerland, 2010.
85. Atkinson, F.S.; Foster-Powell, K.; Brand-Miller, J.C. International tables of glycemic index and glycemic load values: 2008. *Diabetes Care* **2008**, *31*, 2281–2283. [CrossRef]
86. Jenkins, D.J.; Kendall, C.W.; McKeown-Eyssen, G.; Josse, R.G.; Silverberg, J.; Booth, G.L.; Vidgen, E.; Josse, A.R.; Nguyen, T.H.; Corrigan, S.; et al. Effect of a low-glycemic index or a high-cereal fiber diet on type 2 diabetes: A randomized trial. *JAMA* **2008**, *300*, 2742–2753. [CrossRef]
87. Rizkalla, S.W.; Taghrid, L.; Laromiguiere, M.; Huet, D.; Boillot, J.; Rigoir, A.; Elgrably, F.; Slama, G. Improved plasma glucose control, whole-body glucose utilization, and lipid profile on a low-glycemic index diet in type 2 diabetic men: A randomized controlled trial. *Diabetes Care* **2004**, *27*, 1866–1872. [CrossRef]
88. Jenkins, D.J.; Kendall, C.W.; Augustin, L.S.; Mitchell, S.; Sahye-Pudaruth, S.; Blanco Mejia, S.; Chiavaroli, L.; Mirrahimi, A.; Ireland, C.; Bashyam, B.; et al. Effect of legumes as part of a low glycemic index diet on glycemic control and cardiovascular risk factors in type 2 diabetes mellitus: A randomized controlled trial. *Arch. Intern. Med.* **2012**, *172*, 1653–1660. [CrossRef]
89. Pavithran, N.; Kumar, H.; Menon, A.S.; Pillai, G.K.; Sundaram, K.R.; Ojo, O. The Effect of a Low GI Diet on Truncal Fat Mass and Glycated Hemoglobin in South Indians with Type 2 Diabetes-A Single Centre Randomized Prospective Study. *Nutrients* **2020**, *12*, 179. [CrossRef] [PubMed]
90. Zafar, M.I.; Mills, K.E.; Zheng, J.; Regmi, A.; Hu, S.Q.; Gou, L.; Chen, L.L. Low-glycemic index diets as an intervention for diabetes: A systematic review and meta-analysis. *Am. J. Clin. Nutr.* **2019**, *110*, 891–902. [CrossRef] [PubMed]
91. Thomas, D.E.; Elliott, E.J. The use of low-glycaemic index diets in diabetes control. *Br. J. Nutr.* **2010**, *104*, 797–802. [CrossRef] [PubMed]

92. Sievenpiper, J.L.; Chan, C.B.; Dworatzek, P.D.; Freeze, C.; Williams, S.L. Nutrition Therapy. *Can. J. Diabetes* **2018**, *42*, S64–S79. [CrossRef] [PubMed]
93. The Royal Australian College of General Practitioners. *General Practice Management of Type 2 Diabetes: 2016–18*; RACGP: East Melbourne, Australia, 2016.
94. *Evidence-Based Nutrition Guidelines for the Prevention and Management of Diabetes*; Diabetes UK 2018 Nutrition Working Group: London, UK, 2018.
95. Davies, M.J.; D'Alessio, D.A.; Fradkin, J.; Kernan, W.N.; Mathieu, C.; Mingrone, G.; Rossing, P.; Tsapas, A.; Wexler, D.J.; Buse, J.B. Management of hyperglycaemia in type 2 diabetes, 2018. A consensus report by the American Diabetes Association (ADA) and the European Association for the Study of Diabetes (EASD). *Diabetologia* **2018**, *61*, 2461–2498. [CrossRef]
96. Tobe, S.W.; Stone, J.A.; Anderson, T.; Bacon, S.; Cheng, A.Y.Y.; Daskalopoulou, S.S.; Ezekowitz, J.A.; Gregoire, J.C.; Gubitz, G.; Jain, R.; et al. Canadian Cardiovascular Harmonized National Guidelines Endeavour (C-CHANGE) guideline for the prevention and management of cardiovascular disease in primary care: 2018 update. *CMAJ* **2018**, *190*, E1192–E1206. [CrossRef]
97. Livesey, G.; Taylor, R.; Livesey, H.F.; Buyken, A.E.; Jenkins, D.J.A.; Augustin, L.S.A.; Sievenpiper, J.L.; Barclay, A.W.; Liu, S.; Wolever, T.M.S.; et al. Dietary Glycemic Index and Load and the Risk of Type 2 Diabetes: A Systematic Review and Updated Meta-Analyses of Prospective Cohort Studies. *Nutrients* **2019**, *11*, 1280. [CrossRef]
98. Livesey, G.; Livesey, H. Coronary Heart Disease and Dietary Carbohydrate, Glycemic Index, and Glycemic Load: Dose-Response Meta-analyses of Prospective Cohort Studies. *Mayo Clin. Proc. Innov. Qual. Outcomes* **2019**, *3*, 52–69. [CrossRef]
99. Aziz, A.; Dumais, L.; Barber, J. Health Canada's evaluation of the use of glycemic index claims on food labels. *Am. J. Clin. Nutr.* **2013**, *98*, 269–274. [CrossRef]
100. EFSA Panel on Dietetic Products, Nutrition and Allergies (NDA). Scientific Opinion on the substantiation of health claims related to carbohydrates that induce low/reduced glycaemic responses (ID 474, 475, 483, 484) and carbohydrates with a low glycaemic index (ID 480, 481, 482, 1300) pursuant to Article 13(1) of Regulation (EC) No 1924/2006. *EFSA J.* **2010**, *8*, 1491. [CrossRef]
101. Wolever, T.M. Is glycaemic index (GI) a valid measure of carbohydrate quality? *Eur. J. Clin. Nutr.* **2013**, *67*, 522–531. [CrossRef] [PubMed]
102. Wolever, T.M.S.; Meynier, A.; Jenkins, A.L.; Brand-Miller, J.C.; Atkinson, F.S.; Gendre, D.; Leuillet, S.; Cazaubiel, M.; Housez, B.; Vinoy, S. Glycemic Index and Insulinemic Index of Foods: An Interlaboratory Study Using the ISO 2010 Method. *Nutrients* **2019**, *11*, 2218. [CrossRef] [PubMed]
103. Gycemic Index Foundation. Glycemic Index Foundation: About the Program. Available online: https://www.gisymbol.com/gi-symbol-program/ (accessed on 30 March 2020).
104. Gycemic Index Foundation. Product Eligibility and Nutrition Criteria. Available online: https://www.gisymbol.com/wp-content/uploads/2017/08/GI-Foundation-Product-Eligibility-and-Nutrient-Criteria-November-2015-2.pdf (accessed on 30 March 2020).
105. Gycemic Index Foundation. Policy: Glycemic Index Testing: Low GI Declaration on Foods and Beverages. Available online: https://www.gisymbol.com/wp-content/uploads/2017/08/GI-Foundation-GI-testing-policy-October-2015.pdf (accessed on 30 March 2020).
106. Kusnadi, D.T.L.; Barclay, A.W.; Brand-Miller, J.C.; Louie, J.C.Y. Changes in dietary glycemic index and glycemic load in Australian adults from 1995 to 2012. *Am. J. Clin. Nutr.* **2017**, *106*, 189–198. [CrossRef] [PubMed]
107. Health Canada. *Draft Guidance Document on Food Health Claims Related to the Reduction in Post-Prandial Glycaemic Response*; Health Canada: Ottawa, ON, Canada, 2013.
108. Competition and Consumer Act 2010. Schedule 2 (Version C2019C00149). In *Chapter 2 General Protections. Part 2-1 Section 18: Misleading or Deceptive Conduct*; Government of Australia: Canberra, Australia, 2019.
109. Competition and Consumer Act 2010. Schedule 2 (Version C2019C00149). In *Chapter 3 Specific protections. Part 3-1 Unfair Practices. Divison 1 False or Misleading Representations etc. Section 29: False or Misleading Representations about Goods or Services*; Government of Australia: Canberra, Australia, 2019.
110. Food and Drugs Act. *Deception, etc., Regarding Food: Subsection 5(1)*; Government of Canada: Ottawa, ON, Canada, 2020.
111. *Fair Trading Act 1986*; Government of New Zealand: Wellington, New Zealand, 2020.

112. Chapter 9—Federal Food, Drug, and Cosmetic Act (sections 301–399d). In *Section 343 Misbranded Food*; United States Government: Washington, DC, USA, 2018.
113. Aryangat, A.V.; Gerich, J.E. Type 2 diabetes: Postprandial hyperglycemia and increased cardiovascular risk. *Vasc. Health Risk Manag.* **2010**, *6*, 145–155. [CrossRef] [PubMed]
114. Popkin, B.M.; Hawkes, C. Sweetening of the global diet, particularly beverages: Patterns, trends, and policy responses. *Lancet Diabetes Endocrinol.* **2016**, *4*, 174–186. [CrossRef]
115. Imamura, F.; O'Connor, L.; Ye, Z.; Mursu, J.; Hayashino, Y.; Bhupathiraju, S.N.; Forouhi, N.G. Consumption of sugar sweetened beverages, artificially sweetened beverages, and fruit juice and incidence of type 2 diabetes: Systematic review, meta-analysis, and estimation of population attributable fraction. *BMJ* **2015**, *351*, h3576. [CrossRef] [PubMed]
116. Xi, B.; Huang, Y.; Reilly, K.H.; Li, S.; Zheng, R.; Barrio-Lopez, M.T.; Martinez-Gonzalez, M.A.; Zhou, D. Sugar-sweetened beverages and risk of hypertension and CVD: A dose-response meta-analysis. *Br. J. Nutr.* **2015**, *113*, 709–717. [CrossRef]
117. Welsh, J.A.; Wang, Y.; Figueroa, J.; Brumme, C. Sugar intake by type (added vs. naturally occurring) and physical form (liquid vs. solid) and its varying association with children's body weight, NHANES 2009–2014. *Pediatr. Obes.* **2018**, *13*, 213–221. [CrossRef]
118. Tsilas, C.S.; de Souza, R.J.; Mejia, S.B.; Mirrahimi, A.; Cozma, A.I.; Jayalath, V.H.; Ha, V.; Tawfik, R.; Di Buono, M.; Jenkins, A.L.; et al. Relation of total sugars, fructose and sucrose with incident type 2 diabetes: A systematic review and meta-analysis of prospective cohort studies. *CMAJ* **2017**, *189*, E711–E720. [CrossRef]
119. Khan, T.A.; Chiavaroli, L.; Zurbau, A.; Sievenpiper, J.L. A lack of consideration of a dose-response relationship can lead to erroneous conclusions regarding 100% fruit juice and the risk of cardiometabolic disease. *Eur. J. Clin. Nutr.* **2019**, *73*, 1556–1560. [CrossRef]
120. Afshin, A.; Sur, P.J.; Fay, K.A.; Cornaby, L.; Ferrara, G.; Salama, J.S.; Mullany, E.C.; Abate, K.H.; Abbafati, C.; Abebe, Z.; et al. Health effects of dietary risks in 195 countries, 1990–2017: A systematic analysis for the Global Burden of Disease Study 2017. *Lancet* **2019**, *393*, 1958–1972. [CrossRef]
121. Billich, N.; Blake, M.R.; Backholer, K.; Cobcroft, M.; Li, V.; Peeters, A. The effect of sugar-sweetened beverage front-of-pack labels on drink selection, health knowledge and awareness: An online randomised controlled trial. *Appetite* **2018**, *128*, 233–241. [CrossRef] [PubMed]
122. Wang, Y.F.; Chiavaroli, L.; Roke, K.; DiAngelo, C.; Marsden, S.; Sievenpiper, J. Canadian Adults with Moderate Intakes of Total Sugars have Greater Intakes of Fibre and Key Micronutrients: Results from the Canadian Community Health Survey 2015 Public Use Microdata File. *Nutrients* **2020**, *12*, 1124. [CrossRef]
123. Zazpe, I.; Sanchez-Tainta, A.; Santiago, S.; de la Fuente-Arrillaga, C.; Bes-Rastrollo, M.; Martinez, J.A.; Martinez-Gonzalez, M.A. Association between dietary carbohydrate intake quality and micronutrient intake adequacy in a Mediterranean cohort: The SUN (Seguimiento Universidad de Navarra) Project. *Br. J. Nutr.* **2014**, *111*, 2000–2009. [CrossRef] [PubMed]
124. Zazpe, I.; Santiago, S.; Gea, A.; Ruiz-Canela, M.; Carlos, S.; Bes-Rastrollo, M.; Martinez-Gonzalez, M.A. Association between a dietary carbohydrate index and cardiovascular disease in the SUN (Seguimiento Universidad de Navarra) Project. *Nutr. Metab. Cardiovasc. Dis.* **2016**, *26*, 1048–1056. [CrossRef]
125. Food and Drug Regulations. *Division 1—Nutrition Labelling Core Information: B.01.401*; Government of Canada: Ottawa, ON, Canada, 2020.
126. *Standard 1.2.8—Nutrition Information Requirements (F2018C00944)*; Food Standards Australia New Zealand: Canberra, Australia, 2018.
127. Buyuktuncer, Z.; Ayaz, A.; Dedebayraktar, D.; Inan-Eroglu, E.; Ellahi, B.; Besler, H.T. Promoting a Healthy Diet in Young Adults: The Role of Nutrition Labelling. *Nutrients* **2018**, *10*, 1335. [CrossRef]

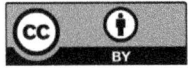

© 2020 by the authors. Licensee MDPI, Basel, Switzerland. This article is an open access article distributed under the terms and conditions of the Creative Commons Attribution (CC BY) license (http://creativecommons.org/licenses/by/4.0/).

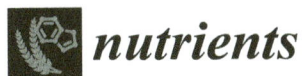

Review

Effects of Menu Labeling Policies on Transnational Restaurant Chains to Promote a Healthy Diet: A Scoping Review to Inform Policy and Research

Sofía Rincón-Gallardo Patiño [1,*], Mi Zhou [1], Fabio Da Silva Gomes [2], Robin Lemaire [3], Valisa Hedrick [1], Elena Serrano [1] and Vivica I. Kraak [1]

1. Department of Human Nutrition, Foods, and Exercise, College of Agriculture and Life Sciences, Virginia Polytechnic Institute and State University, Blacksburg, VA 24061, USA; mi14@vt.edu (M.Z.); vhedrick@vt.edu (V.H.); serrano@vt.edu (E.S.); vivica51@vt.edu (V.I.K.)
2. Department of Non-Communicable Diseases and Mental Health, Pan American Health Organization, World Health Organization, Washington, DC 20037, USA; gomesfabio@paho.org
3. Center for Public Administration and Policy, School of Public and International Affairs, Virginia Polytechnic Institute and State University, Blacksburg, VA 24061, USA; rlemaire@vt.edu
* Correspondence: sofiargp@vt.edu

Received: 30 April 2020; Accepted: 20 May 2020; Published: 26 May 2020

Abstract: There is insufficient evidence that restaurant menu labeling policies are cost-effective strategies to reduce obesity and diet-related non-communicable diseases (NCDs). Evidence suggests that menu labeling has a modest effect on calories purchased and consumed. No review has been published on the effect of menu labeling policies on transnational restaurant chains globally. This study conducted a two-step scoping review to map and describe the effect of restaurant menu labeling policies on menu reformulation. First, we identified national, state, and municipal menu labeling policies in countries from global databases. Second, we searched four databases (i.e., PubMed, CINHAL/EBSCO, Web of Science, and Google Scholar) for peer-reviewed studies and gray-literature sources in English and Spanish (2000–2020). Step 1 identified three voluntary and eight mandatory menu labeling policies primarily for energy disclosures for 11 upper-middle and high-income countries, but none for low- or middle-income countries. Step 2 identified 15 of 577 studies that met the inclusion criteria. The analysis showed reductions in energy for newly introduced menu items only in the United States. We suggest actions for governments, civil society organizations, and the restaurant businesses to develop, implement, and evaluate comprehensive menu labeling policies to determine whether these may reduce obesity and NCD risks worldwide.

Keywords: food labeling; menu labeling; nutrition declaration; food and nutrition policy; restaurant chains; reformulation; serving size; energy; obesity

1. Introduction

Unhealthy dietary patterns characterized by the rapid nutrition transition are associated with obesity and diet-related non-communicable diseases (NCDs) [1]. Over the past several decades, dietary patterns have shifted from eating home-cooked meals to eating out more frequently [2,3]. Eating away from home is linked to an increased consumption of ultra-processed food and beverage products with excessive calories, fat, and added sugars and sodium [4–7]. Cafeterias, fast-food restaurant chains, independent take-out-restaurants, and food retailers contribute substantially to the daily energy intake [8,9]. A global survey conducted with 30,000 online respondents across 61 countries found that 48% of participants reported eating away from home weekly or more often with quick-service restaurants (QSRs) and fast-casual restaurants (FCRs) being the most preferred [10].

Evidence suggests that food labeling at point-of-purchase may inform shoppers to choose healthier options [11–13]. The World Health Organization (WHO) has recommended nutrition labeling and reducing portion sizes as strategies to reduce energy intake; however, there is insufficient evidence to show that menu labeling legislation for chain restaurants and food retailers is a cost-effective "best buy" policy to improve diet quality and reduce NCD-related disability and mortality in low- and middle-income countries [14].

The aim of menu labeling policies is to reduce energy intake and improve diet quality by helping consumers make better-informed decisions and to encourage food retailers and restaurant businesses to reformulate menu items and reduce and standardize serving sizes to meet recommended nutrient targets [15,16]. This dual goal has the potential to improve the nutrition and diet quality of individuals who eat away from home frequently because it may impact entire populations and does not require conscious individual behavior changes [17,18].

The restaurant business sector, which includes QSRs, FCRs, and full-service restaurant (FSR) chains and independent restaurants, has the resources and capacity to reformulate menu items or introduce new items [19–21]. United States (US) chain restaurant establishments have demonstrated progress to improve the nutrition composition of items and reduce meal size or portions served to meet recommended nutrient targets of public health experts, namely, the United States Department of Agriculture and the Dietary Guidelines for Americans [20]. A systematic review conducted in 2019 identified trends for restaurant chains to reformulate food and beverage products and reduce or standardize portions in 30 countries across six regions worldwide between 2000 and 2018 [21]. Recommendations by public health practitioners have been issued to downsize and standardize portions to 600–700 calories or 2510–2930 kilojoules/meal as an important strategy for restaurants to help costumers reduce obesity and NCD risks. However, this research found a lack of clear, universal, and internationally accepted standards for transnational restaurant chains to adopt portion or serving sizes for meals, beverages, side dishes, and desserts served to children, adolescents and adults [21]. The studies reviewed ($n = 50$) also revealed wide variation within and across countries, regions, firms, and restaurant chains to reduce energy, saturated fats, trans fats, sodium, and standardized portions. In addition, menu labeling may influence some of the documented progress [21].

The implementation of menu labeling policies in countries has led to 12 published systematic reviews and/or meta-analyses that examined the influence of restaurant menu labeling on consumer dietary behaviors between 2008 and 2018. These studies documented a modest yet statistical reduction in calories purchased and/or consumed at chain restaurants and other food-service settings [15,22–32]. However, only one published literature review examined the restaurant industry's reformulation of menu items [15]. No review has been published on whether menu labeling policies have an effect on reformulation, introduction of new or existing products, or reduction of serving sizes on menus from transnational restaurant chains globally.

Given the lack of published evidence on this topic, a better understanding is needed of the effects of mandatory and voluntary menu labeling on the restaurant sector's businesses. The results may be used to inform governments, civil society organizations, researchers, and the restaurant sector across countries on whether and how to develop comprehensive and robust policies that encourage industry changes to promote healthy dietary choices that will help to reduce obesity and NCD risks worldwide.

Study Purpose

The purpose of this study is two-fold: (1) to conduct a scoping review to map and describe the menu labeling policies enacted across countries and regions from 2000 to 2020; and (2) and to examine evaluations for any measurable effects (i.e., positive, no, or mixed) that restaurant menu labeling policies have on businesses to reformulate products or introduce new products and reduce the serving size of menus items served and sold to customers. The results are discussed within the context of government actions needed to strengthen policies and invest in external monitoring and evaluations of menu labeling legislation. We also discuss the need to make a compelling business case to encourage restaurant businesses to reformulate menu items to meet recommended healthy nutrient targets. This objective is part of a broader marketing-mix choice-architecture approach to improve their corporate image and attract new customers interested in health and wellness. Finally, we examine the implications for actions for diverse stakeholders, including governments, the WHO, restaurant businesses, private foundations, researchers, and civil society organizations to develop comprehensive menu labeling policies to determine whether these may reduce obesity and NCD risks worldwide.

2. Materials and Methods

This study was a two-step scoping review, conducted between 1 January and 29 February 2020 to examine the influence of restaurant menu labeling policies on product reformulation and reducing the serving sizes of menu items across countries and regions globally. This study utilized a scoping review, defined by Sucharew as a "research method and strategy to map, describe, and provide an overview of the published literature to identify relevant data and gaps to inform policymaking and research" [33]. The approach differs from a systematic evidence review that gathers, analyzes, and formally assesses the data to draw robust conclusions from the existing evidence for a well-defined issue.

2.1. Scoping Review Step 1: Identify Restaurant Menu Labeling Policies

Step 1 of the scoping review was guided by the following research question: "What restaurant menu labeling policies have been implemented by countries across regions worldwide between January 2000 and February 2020?". The lead investigator (S.R.G.P.) searched the WHO Global database on the Implementation of Nutrition Action (GINA) [34] and the World Cancer Research Fund International's NOURISHING framework [35,36] for national, state, or municipal policies. Then, the data were screened, extracted, compiled and triangulated. The lead investigator used a cross-checked consultation process by reviewing the evidence with other relevant sources (i.e., governmental or health ministry websites and databases, international organizations, and governmental and nongovernmental agency reports) in English and Spanish.

2.2. Scoping Review—Step 2: Identify Evidence for Restaurant Menu Labeling Effects

Step 2 of the scoping review step was conducted using the five steps described by Arksey and O'Malley's 2015 framework [37]. To enhance this methodology, we integrated scoping review recommendations by Levac et al. 2010 and Daudt et al. 2012 [38]. The process included identifying the research question, identifying relevant studies that met the inclusion criteria, study selection, charting the data, and summarizing the results. This research followed an iterative approach and used evidence and investigator triangulation to select and analyze the studies.

2.2.1. Identifying the Research Question

The development of the research question was guided by the Population, Exposure, Outcome (PEO) framework that is widely used in qualitative social science or policy research rather than the PICO framework (i.e., population, intervention, comparison, and outcome) framework that is used to assess quantitative research outcomes [39–41]. This review defined population as transnational restaurants, including fast-food or QSR, FCR, and FSR chains; exposure was defined as voluntary and/or mandatory menu labeling policies, and the outcomes as food and beverage product reformulation and serving size reduction of restaurant menu items. Step 2 of the scoping review was guided by the following research question was: "What were the effects of voluntary and mandatory restaurant menu labeling policies on food reformulation and serving size available to restaurant consumers between January 2000 and February 2020?"

2.2.2. Identifying Relevant Studies

The initial search was conducted using four electronic databases, including PubMed, CINAHL, Web of Science, and Google Scholar for peer-reviewed literature and gray literature. Only the first 100 hits sorted by relevance were considered for the Google Scholar database search. The databases were selected to be comprehensive and cover a broad range of disciplines, with guidance from a university research librarian. The PEO framework guided the identification of appropriate Medical Subject Headings (MeSH) terms and a combination of synonyms (Table 1; Table S1 provides MeSH terms definitions, and Table S2 provides the search details on each database). The reference sections of relevant articles were handsearched to identify further evidence not captured in the electronic database search.

Table 1. Systematic search strategy for the scoping review.

PEO Framework	MeSH Terms and Synonyms
Population	"Restaurants"[MeSH] OR "Food Services"[MeSH] OR "Food Supply"[MeSH] OR "Fast Foods"[MeSH] OR "Food Industry"[MeSH] OR "Food-Processing Industry"[MeSH] "Chain restaurant*" OR restaurant or "food retail" OR "food services*" OR "food supply" OR "food supplies" OR "fast food*" NOT Schools [MeSH] AND
Exposure	"Policy"[MeSH] OR "Nutrition Policy"[MeSH] OR "Public Policy"[MeSH] OR "Health Policy"[MeSH] OR "Government Regulation"[MeSH] OR "Legislation" [Publication Type] OR "Legislation, Food"[MeSH] OR "Voluntary Programs"[MeSH] OR "Mandatory Programs"[MeSH] OR "Patient Protection and Affordable Care Act"[MeSH] OR "Mandatory Policy" OR "Voluntary Policy" OR "Self-regulation" OR "Nutrition policies" OR Guideline OR "Food Policy" AND "Food Labeling"[MeSH] OR "Product Labeling"[MeSH] OR "Food product label*" OR "Menu label*" OR "Restaurant label*" OR "Restaurant label" OR "Restaurant menu label*" OR "Food calories" OR "Nutrient label*" OR "Food content" NOT "Food Packaging"
Outcome	"Food"[MeSH] OR "Beverages"[MeSH] OR "Food and Beverages"[MeSH] OR "Food Ingredients"[MeSH] OR "food product*" OR "Fast food" AND "Food Quality"[MeSH] OR "Food, Formulated"[MeSH] OR "Serving Size"[MeSH] OR "Portion Size"[MeSH] OR "Food reformulation" OR "Reduce* Portion*" OR "Reduce* size*" OR "Product reformulation"

PEO framework: (P) Population—transnational restaurants; (E) Exposure—voluntary and mandatory policies; (O) Outcome—food reformulation and serving size reductions.

2.2.3. Study Selection

The evidence selection was based on a priori inclusion and exclusion criteria. This scoping review was limited to peer-reviewed and gray literature published between 1 January 2000 and 29 February 2020 for English and Spanish-language studies and publications that explored the effect of menu labeling for restaurant chains that measured or evaluated the effects of menu labeling on product reformulation and serving size reductions. Studies were excluded for non-restaurant settings including cafeterias, laboratory settings, vending machines, schools, supermarkets, or independent food-retail establishments. Other evidence excluded was based on other outcomes related to consumers, purchase or consumption of nutrients, sales, pricing data, or described prevalence of business compliance. Literature reviews and studies based on packaged food labeling or other marketing strategies were considered to be different interventions and not included. Exclusion criteria also included literature reviews (i.e., scoping reviews, systematic reviews, and meta-analysis), which were removed and classified as the wrong type of study. All citations were imported into an EndNote X9 citation manager system and uploaded to the Covidence software, Cochrane's primary screening and data extraction tool to support scoping and systematic reviews [42]. The screening process used the Preferred Reporting Items for Systematic Reviews and Meta-Analyses (PRISMA; Figure 1) guidelines that enabled the systematic searching, selection, and synthesis of the identified evidence [43]. The primary investigator (S.R.G.P.) removed duplicates, and a co-investigator (M.Z.) independently reviewed the title, abstract, and the full text of studies for inclusion against the eligibility criteria. A third co-investigator (V.I.K.) resolved any disagreements related to study inclusion.

2.2.4. Charting the Data

From each selected study, two investigators (S.R.G.P. and M.Z.) extracted data on the author, year, country, study design, study purpose, sample, setting, data source, main outcomes, and disclosure of conflicts of interest. The data extraction was compiled in a single Microsoft Excel sheet. To assess the study quality, two investigators (S.R.G.P. and M.Z.) used the Johanna Briggs Institute's critical appraisal eight-item checklist for analytical observational studies [44] and assigned a quality score ranging from poor, fair, or good. A third co-investigator (V.I.K.) was consulted to resolve any discrepancies to reach consensus through investigator triangulation.

2.2.5. Collating, Summarizing and Reporting Results

We used a narrative synthesis [45] to report and summarize the evidence compiled for restaurant menu labeling policies related to the reformulation and serving size reductions of restaurant menu items, and to compare similarities, differences, and patterns among the evidence. A thematic analysis was also completed during the examination of the studies to identify topics and categorize the main results [46]. We disassembled the evidence to identify relevant themes based on the main outcomes. Thereafter, we reassembled the data across studies and organized it by positive effect if results showed a statistically significant p-value, no effect if results showed no statistically significant p-value or negative effects, and mixed-effects if results showed both findings for the effects of menu labeling.

3. Results

The search identified 3 voluntary and 8 mandatory menu labeling policies in 11 upper–middle and high-income countries defined by The World Bank classification. No policies were identified for low- or middle-income countries. Out of 577 screened studies, 15 studies met the inclusion criteria. Eleven studies were conducted in the Americas region (i.e., Canada and the US), two studies were conducted in the European region (i.e., the UK and Ireland), and two studies were conducted in the Western Pacific region (i.e., Australia) (Table 2).

Table 2. Two-step scoping review results across countries by world region*.

* World Region	Scoping Review—Step 1	Scoping Review—Step 2
	Identify Policies (Policies = 11)	Identify Evidence (Studies n = 15)
Africa	None identified (n = 0)	None identified
Americas (n = 2)	Canada and US (n = 2)	Canada (n = 1): Scourboutakos et al. (2019) [47]. US (n = 11): Bleich et al. (2015) [48], Bleich et al. (2016) [49], Bleich et al. (2017) [50], Bleich et al. (2018) [19], Bleich et al. (2020) [51], Bruemmer et al. (2012) [16], Namba et al. (2013) [52], Petimar et al. (2019) [53], Saelens et al. (2012) [54], Tran et al. (2019) [55], Wu et al. (2014) [56]
South-East Asia	None identified (n = 0)	None identified
Europe	Ireland and the UK (n = 2)	UK (n = 1): Theis et al. (2019) [57]
Eastern Mediterranean	Bahrain, Saudi Arabia, United Arab Emirates (n = 3)	None identified
Western Pacific	Australia, Malaysia, South Korea, Taiwan (n = 4)	Australia (n = 2): Wellard-Cole et al. (2018) [58], Wellard-Cole et al. (2019) [59].

US: United States; UK: United Kingdom. * World Health Organization regional groups [60].

3.1. Scoping Review Results for Step 1: Identify Restaurant Menu Labeling Policies

The implementation of voluntary or mandatory menu labeling policies has become popular throughout upper–middle and high-income countries of the world by region including the Americas n = 2, Europe n = 2, Eastern Mediterranean n = 3, Western Pacific n = 4; including Australia, Bahrain,

Canada, Ireland, Malaysia, Saudi Arabia, South Korea, Taiwan, United Arab Emirates, the UK and the US (Table 3). No policies were found in the Africa and South-East Asian regions.

We identified eight mandatory menu labeling policies across 11 countries. The US was the first country that enacted a mandatory national menu labeling law in 2010 that became effective on 1 May 2018 [61]. The Food and Drug Administration (FDA) has oversight for implementing the law and provided compliance guidance for industry. Section 4205 of the 2010 Affordable Care Act, Public Law 111-148 (HR 3590) mandated that restaurant chains and other retail establishments (i.e., convenience stores, coffee shops, grocery stores, cafeterias) with 20 or more US locations disclose calories on menus and menu boards and make other nutrition information available to customers upon request [61].

Several countries implemented a mandatory policy at national, state/provincial/territorial levels, including Australia [62], Canada [63], and the United Arab Emirates [64]. Between 2011 and 2018, the Australian government and Obesity Policy Coalition implemented various menu labeling schemes throughout four states and one territory. The current legislative schemes provide detailed requirements for chain food outlets, which include displaying the energy content in kilojoules for items on the menus, drive-through boards, tags, and other materials that display the name or price of products [62].

While mandatory policies have emerged, other countries have launched voluntary recommendations and guidelines to encourage restaurant chains and food industry businesses to display menu labeling for food and beverage items, which include Malaysia in 2008, followed by Bahrain in 2010, and the UK in 2011 [36]. These three countries are moving towards mandatory policies, and initiatives are being debated or incorporated into national plans. In 2016, the Malaysian government included the menu labeling strategy into its National Plan of Action for Nutrition 2016–2025, and plans to have a mandatory menu labeling policy by 2025 [65]. In 2018, Bahrain submitted a proposal to the Ministerial Cabinet that is currently under review for restaurants and cafes to voluntarily display calories [66]. Since 2015, mandatory menu labeling in Ireland has been under consideration and is now included in the National Obesity Policy and Action Plan 2016–2020 [67]. In 2011, the UK government released the voluntary policy for the Out of Home Calorie Labeling pledge as part of The Public Health Responsibility Deal, where businesses voluntarily committed to display the calorie content on menus [68]. The UK government is currently undertaking a consultation to implement menu labeling as a mandatory national policy [69–71].

All the policies across countries require the disclosure of energy content as calories or kilojoules. The US, Australia, and Dubai have mandatory policies that also require the display of daily energy intake statements so a customer can compare specific menu items to 2000 calories/day or 8700 kilojoules/day. Malaysia, Bahrain, and Korea expanded the nutrients that restaurants are required to report to include fat, protein, sodium, and added sugars. Taiwan is the only country that has a mandatory policy that requires the disclosure of caffeine and added sugars for beverages.

Table 3. Implemented menu labeling policies across countries worldwide, 2008–2020 *.

Country, Year	Policy Type	Action
Australia, 2011–2018	Mandatory, four states and one territory	Restaurant chains with ≥20 outlets in the state, or 50 or more across the country, are required to present the energy content (kilojoules) and include a daily intake statement on menus and menu boards. Similar food businesses are invited to voluntarily implement menu labeling. States of New South Wales, 2011: Food regulation 2011 Australia Capital Territory, 2012: Amendments to Food Regulation 2002 Australia, South Australia, 2012: Amendments to Food Regulation 2002 Australia, Queensland, 2017: Amendments to Food Act 2006 Australia, Victoria, 2018: Amendment to Food Act 1984
Bahrain, 2010	Voluntary, national	The Nutrition Section of the Ministry of Health recommends that fast-food chain restaurants display nutrients per serving, including calories, fat, protein, carbohydrates, salt/sodium, and sugar.
Canada, Ontario, 2017	Mandatory, province	In 2015, Ontario's Healthy Menu Choices Act, part of the Making Healthier Choices Act (Bill 45) in the Ontario Regulation 50/16, requires food service establishments with 20 or more businesses to depict calories for menu items on paper and electronic menus, menu boards, drive-through menus, menu applications, and advertisements or promotional flyers.
Ireland, 2015	Mandatory, national	In 2015, the Health Service Executive approved the implementation of Calorie Posting Policy across health services in all food and beverage facilities (i.e., restaurants, coffee shops, catering services, and vending machines).
Malaysia, 2008	Voluntary, national	In 2008, the Malaysian government released voluntary guidelines for the advertising and nutrition labeling of restaurant chains to display nutrient information on the menu items (i.e., calories, carbohydrates, protein, fat, and sodium for food and total sugar for beverages).
Saudi Arabia, 2018	Mandatory, national	In 2018, the Saudi Food and Drug Authority launched mandatory measures that require calorie labeling on menu items for all food facilities, including cashier desks, menu boards, table menus, drive-through menus, phone, and web applications.
South Korea, 2010	Mandatory, national	In 2010, the South Korean government enforced through the Special Act on Safety Control of Children's Dietary Life that restaurants with more than 100 outlets are required to report energy, total sugars, protein, saturated fat and sodium on the menus
Taiwan, 2015	Mandatory, national	From 2015, the Taiwanese Act Governing Food Safety and Sanitation that regulates business chains (i.e., convenience stores, drink vendors, and fast-food restaurants) requires the labeling of the sugar and caffeine content of prepared-when-ordered drinks.
United Arab Emirates, 2020	Mandatory, state/emirate	The 2017–2020 National Nutrition Agenda for Dubai requires food retailers to display the calorie content of menu items and a daily intake statement, effective 1 January 2020.
United Kingdom, 2011	Voluntary, national	From 2011–2015, the Out of Home Calorie Labelling pledge, part of the government's Responsibility Deal (2010 to 2015), established for businesses with 45 or more food establishments the need to provide calorie information on menus in England, Scotland, and Wales. In 2012, the Food Standards Agency worked with Northern Ireland and the local food industry to encourage calorie labeling on menus
United States, 2010-2018	Mandatory, national	In 2010, Section 4205 of the Affordable Care Act, Public Law 111-148 (HR 3590), mandated that restaurant chains and other food retail establishments (i.e., convenience stores, coffee shops, grocery stores, cafeterias) with 20 or more locations would be required to disclose calories and daily intake statements on menus and menu boards and make other nutrition information available to customers upon request. The law became effective on 1 May 2018.

* Policy is defined as a law, procedure, regulation, rule, or standard that guides how government, businesses, and organizations operate and how citizens live their lives [72].

3.2. Scoping Review Results for Step 2: Identify Evidence for Restaurant Menu Labeling Effects

The search yielded 560 articles across four electronic databases, and 17 additional records identified manually were included. After removing 58 duplicates, 519 records were screened. Of these, 369 records were excluded by title. Thereafter, 150 records were screened by abstract, 19 selected for full-text assessment, and 15 studies were included in the final scoping review (Figure 1).

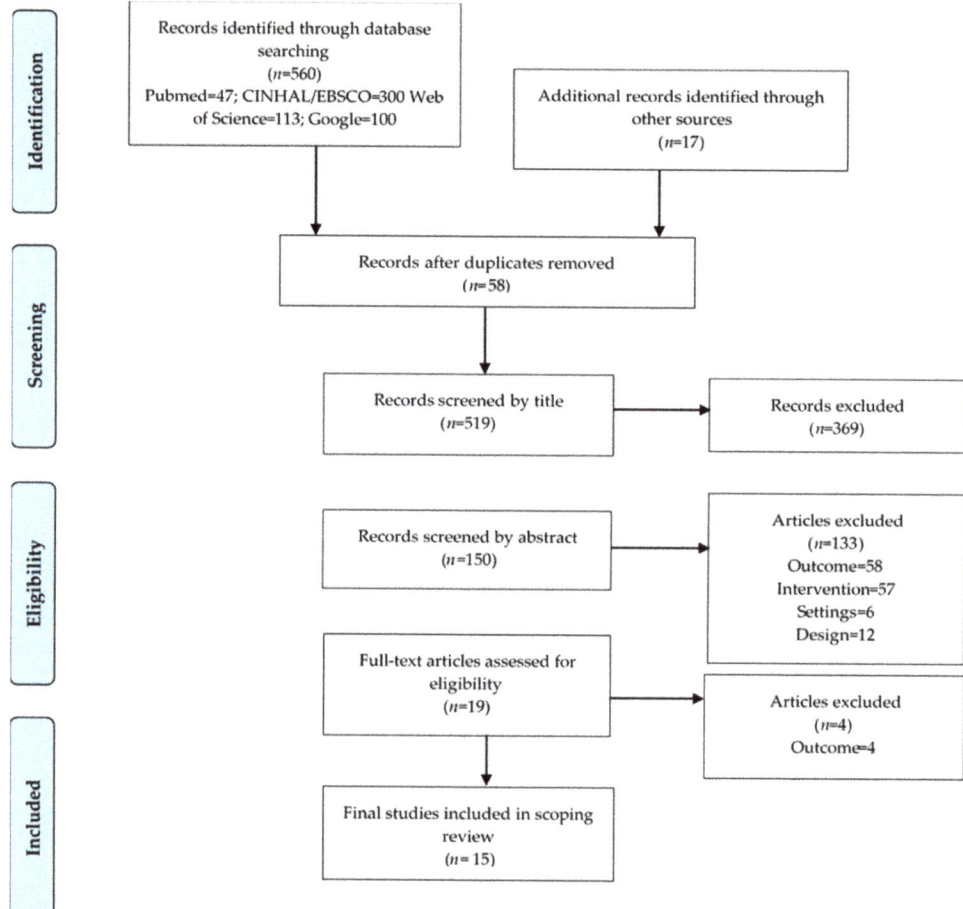

Figure 1. PRISMA flow diagram of the systematic study identification, screening, and selection of the studies for the scoping review.

Table 4 summarizes the studies that met all the inclusion criteria for the scoping review. Despite the search strategy including a wide range of years (from 2000 to 2020), all the included studies were published between 2012 and 2020, and more than half of the studies were published from 2018 to 2020. Eleven studies were conducted in the US, two in Australia, one in Canada, and one in the UK. A majority of studies ($n = 14$) were observational (i.e., longitudinal, case-control, and cross-sectional); and one study was a quasi-experimental design. The analyzed studies ($n = 14$) were conducted in diverse QSR, FCR and FSR chain settings, and a single study included convenience stores [55]. Diverse evidence sources were used across studies to assess the potential effects of menu labeling on food reformulation of food and beverage menu items and the serving reductions. Most of the studies used either the MenuStat Database (i.e., a free nutritional database provided by the New York City Department of Health and Mental Hygiene that provides nutritional information on menu items offered by the largest US chain restaurants; $n = 7$) or consulted business websites, visited establishments, or requested information via email and telephone ($n = 7$) to obtain nutrition content and serving size on menu items offered by restaurants chains. A single study for Canada used the Menu-FLIP database developed by the University of Toronto that provides nutrition data for chain restaurants [73]. The thematic analysis identified three main outcomes: (1) menu items, (2) the nutrition composition of menu items, and (3) newly introduced versus common or regular menu items. No conflicts of interest were found between the studies that could potentially influence the results. Table S3 shows the results of the study quality assessment. No studies were judged as being poor quality, four studies scored fair quality, and 11 studies were considered good quality.

3.2.1. Changes to Menu Items by Food and Beverage Category

The classification of menu items across studies varied. Most of the studies included appetizers and side dishes, main courses or entrees, and desserts. Six studies included children's meals [49,50,52,56,59,74] and six studies examined beverages [19,48–50,53,57]. The evidence suggests that most of the changes made by restaurants were for appetizers and side dishes. Four studies showed statistically significant positive effects for calorie reduction [16,49,50,55], and two studies from the UK and the US reported mixed results [52,57].

Positive effects: Tran et al. (2019) conducted a study in the US during the period leading up to the federal menu labeling implementation date of May 2018 and found a reduction on calories mainly in entrees and dropping higher-calorie appetizers, sides, entrees, and desserts from the menus of pizzeria chains [55]. Bleich et al. (2017) described trends in calories from 19,391 US restaurant chain items that found differences in toppings: 93 kcal in 2008 to 84 kcal in 2015 (p-value for trend = 0.001) [50]. Bleich et al. (2016) found that calories declined between 2012 and 2014 for the main course items and children's menu items at QSR, FCR, and FSR chains that suggested restaurants had voluntarily reduced calories in advance of the national menu labeling law [49]. Bruemmer et al. (2012) examined the calorie content of menu items in King County, Washington, and demonstrated statistically significant differences for the calorie content of entrees between 6 and 18 months of the menu labeling county law enactment. These results were presumably due to the reformulation of menu items for selected QSR and independent restaurant chains [16].

Mixed effects: A UK study assessed the effects of a national voluntary menu labeling guidelines for the top 100 UK chain restaurants ranked by sales [57]. Theis and Adams (2019) showed that while there was a reduction of calories and sodium for pizza, sandwiches, and toppings, baked goods items were higher in nutrients of concern (i.e., calories, fat, sugar, and sodium) in restaurants that provided menu labeling for customers [57]. Namba et al. (2013) found evidence that despite the increase in healthier entrees sold by US chain restaurants, a limited improvement was observed for the nutritional content of children's entrees [52].

Table 4. Summary of articles included in the scoping review.

Author Year	Country	Study Design	Purpose	Sample	Setting	Data Sources	Menu Items	Nutrition Composition	New vs. Common Menu Items	Effect *
Bleich et al. 2015 [48]	USA	Observational, longitudinal	Compare differences in calorie counts from menu labeling, 2012–2014	23,066 menu items from 66	Restaurant chains	MenuStat	Food and beverages	Calories. Average per item calories restaurants with voluntary labeling was significantly lower than those without the labeling (−286 kcal: 232 vs. 519)	Lower calorie content for new menu items introduced in 2013 (−182 kcal: 263 vs. 445; and in 2014 (−110 kcal: 309 vs. 419)	Positive
Bleich et al. 2016 [49]	USA	Observational, longitudinal	Describe trends in calories available in US chain restaurants from 2012 to 2014 to better understand restaurant-driven changes	23,066 menu items over 3 years in 66 large chain restaurants	QSR, FCR and FSR chains	MenuStat	Appetizers and sides, main courses, desserts, toppings, beverages, and children's menu items. New food, beverages, and children's menu items all had fewer mean calories relative to old menu items (66, 47, 43, and 35 fewer calories, respectively)	Calories. Predicted mean per-item calories in new main course items in 2013 had 85 fewer calories relative to old main course items in 2012. Calories declined in pizza (−120 calories), sandwiches (−82 calories), and salads (−68 calories)	Menu items newly introduced in 2013 and 2014 had significantly fewer calories relative to items on the menu in 2012 (2012 vs. 2013: −71 calories; 2012 vs. 2014, −69 calories)	Positive
Bleich et al. 2017 [50]	USA	Observational, longitudinal	Understand trends in calories in chain restaurants before and after the passage of the menu labeling rule	19,391 menu items from chain restaurants	QSR, FCR and FSR chains	MenuStat	Appetizers and sides, fried potatoes, main courses, toppings, beverages, and children's menu items. Largest differences were found for toppings that reduced from 93 kcal in 2008 to 84 kcal in 2015	Calories. Overall calories declined from 327 kcal in 2008 to 318 kcal in 2015	-	Positive
Bleich et al. 2018 [19]	USA	Observational, longitudinal	Compare mean calories for items that remained on restaurant menus with items dropped from the menu	27,238 menu items from restaurant chains	Restaurant chains	MenuStat	Appetizers and sides, main courses, desserts, and beverages	Calories. Items that were dropped had 71 more calories	Items that stayed on the menu in all years had fewer calories than those items that were dropped (448 calories vs. 733 calories)	Positive

Table 4. *Cont.*

Author Year	Country	Study Design	Purpose	Sample	Setting	Data Sources	Menu Items	Nutrition Composition	New vs. Common Menu Items	Effect *
Bleich et al. 2020 [51]	USA	Observational, longitudinal	Update calorie and nutrient trends 2012–2018 of menu items across restaurants	28,238 menu items from chain restaurants	Fast-food, fast-casual, and full-service restaurant chains	MenuStat	Appetizers and sides, main courses, fried potatoes, desserts and baked goods	Calories, saturated fat, sodium, sugar and protein. Significant changes in food (sugar −0.67 g) and beverages (unsaturated fat −1.8 g, protein −2.7 g). Trend in years: calories −120 kcals (−25%), saturated fat (−25%), saturated fat −3.4 g (−41%), unsaturated fat −4.5 g (−37%), non-sugar carbohydrates −10.3 g (−40%), and protein −4.3 g (−25%)	Significant changes were found among all newly introduced items. It is possible that the declines in calories and nutrients in this study are related to local or national nutrition policies	Positive
Bruemmer et al. 2012 [16]	USA	Observational, longitudinal	Evaluated changes in energy, saturated fat, and sodium content of entrées 6 and 18 months that occurred following the implementation of menu labeling regulation	37 chains	QSR and FSR chains	Personnel visited and recorded energy content from menu labels, and websites	Entrée items. Calorie content decline in overall average entrée calories post labeling (41 fewer calories at full-service restaurants and 19 fewer calories at QSR) when comparing 6 and 18 months post menu labeling	Calories and sodium. Decrease in energy, saturated fat, and sodium content between the two study periods following implementation of menu regulation for menu items that were present at both time periods. Saturated fat and sodium levels decreased significantly across all chains and SD chains	-	Positive

Table 4. Cont.

Author Year	Country	Study Design	Purpose	Sample	Setting	Data Sources	Menu Items	Nutrition Composition	New vs. Common Menu Items	Effect *
Namba et al. 2013 [52]	USA	Observational, case-control	Evaluate the effect of menu labeling on menu offerings over 7 years, from 2005 through 2011	3887 menu items from chain restaurants	Top 50 QSR chains	Restaurant websites	Entrées, sides, and children's entrées. Case restaurants increased the proportion of healthier entrées after labeling regulations: from 13% during years 2005 through 2008, up to 20% by 2011 with a mean difference of 5% pre-post 2008 in cases relative to controls. The prevalence of healthier side dishes was higher among case restaurants than controls (23% vs. 15%, respectively). Healthier children's entrées at case restaurants were higher	Calories. Regression models found no statistically significant changes over time in nutrient averages and no statistically significant differences between the nutritional averages of case and control restaurants	3 of 5 labeled restaurants improved their offerings. Control restaurants had a lower proportion of healthier items than cases. 2 of 5 showed no improvement and even launched new options, that increased average calories by over 20% and cholesterol by almost 140%	Mixed
Petimar et al. 2019 [53]	USA	Observational, longitudinal	Evaluate calorie labeling in mean calories purchased, pre-2015–2017 and post menu labeling implementation period 2017–2018	59 restaurants	Restaurants	Menustat	Entrées, sides, sugar-sweetened beverages	Calories. The top 50 menu offerings purchased in 2017–18 had a median of 350 calories (interquartile range 440–760) pre-implementation and a median of 340 calories (440–760) post-implementation.	-	Positive

Table 4. *Cont.*

Author Year	Country	Study Design	Purpose	Sample	Setting	Data Sources	Menu Items	Nutrition Composition	New vs. Common Menu Items	Effect *
Saelens et al. 2012 [54]	USA	Experimental, quasi-experimental	Examine changes in restaurants from before to after nutrition-labeling regulation in a regulated county versus a nonregulated county of Washington state	Top 10 QSR chains	QSR and independent restaurant chains	Nutrition Environment Measures Survey Restaurant (NEMS-R)	Healthy vs. Unhealthy based on 10 items examined by the Nutrition Environment Measures Surveys—Restaurant version (NEMS-R)	The healthfulness of children's menus improved modestly over time, but not differentially by county. Availability of reduced portions decreased in the regulated county	-	No effect
Scourboutakos et al. 2019 [47]	Canada	Observational, longitudinal	Investigate the early impact of Canada's mandatory menu labeling legislation on calorie levels in foods offered on chain restaurant menus before, leading up to, and at the point-of-implementation, 2010 - 2017	2988 foods sold by 28 restaurant chains	QSR and FSR chains	Menu-FLIP database	Entrées, pizza, breakfast foods, side dishes, baked goods/desserts, kids' foods	Calories. The average calories per serving on restaurant menus increased from 306 (SD = 6) kcal to 346 (SD = 6) kcal, between 2010 and 2017. An increase in serving size, from 155 (SD = 3) to 172 (SD = 3) grams, between 2010 and 2017. Calorie density (kcal per 100 g) did not significantly differ between 2010 and 2017. Significant increase in serving sizes among sit-down restaurants of 12 g per serving between 2010 and 2017	Overall, new foods introduced in 2017 were significantly higher in calories per serving compared with those introduced in 2016. New foods introduced in 2017 had significantly higher serving sizes compared with new foods in 2013 and 2016	No effect

Table 4. *Cont.*

Author Year	Country	Study Design	Purpose	Sample	Setting	Data Sources	Menu Items	Nutrition Composition	New vs. Common Menu Items	Effect *
Theis et al. 2019 [57]	UK	Observational, cross-sectional	Determine whether there are differences in the energy and nutritional content of menu items served by UK restaurants vs. without voluntary menu labeling	100 UK chain restaurants	QSR and FSR chains ranked by sales	Restaurant websites	Appetizers and sides, baked goods, beverages, burgers, desserts, fried potatoes, mains, pizza, salads, sandwiches, soup, toppings, and ingredients. Main dishes (i.e., pizza and sandwich) had less sugar and salt. Toppings and ingredients had less fat and protein than items from restaurants without menu labeling. Baked goods items from restaurants with menu labeling had, more energy, fat, saturated fat, sugar but protein and more salt	Calories, saturated fat, sodium, sugar, carbohydrates, and protein. Restaurants with menu labeling had 45% less fat (beta coefficient 0.55; 95% CI 0.32 to 0.96) and 60% less salt (beta coefficient 0.40; 95% CI 0.18 to 0.92)	-	Mixed
Tran et al. 2019 [55]	USA	Observational, longitudinal	Describe trends in calories among food items sold in US convenience stores and pizza restaurant chains from 2013 to 2017	1522 food items from convenience stores and 2085 items from pizza restaurant chains	Pizza restaurant chains	MenuStat	Appetizers and sides, main courses, and desserts. Lower calories among items that stayed on the menu compared to items dropped (overall: −60 kcal; appetizers and sides: −200 kcal *p* < 0.001; main courses: −50 kcal *p* = 0.03; desserts −60 kcal)	Calories. Reduced calories in menu items (−56 kcal: 390 kcal in 2013 vs. 334 kcal in 2017), appetizers (−230 kcal: 367 kcal in 2013 vs. 137 kcal in 2017)	Calories were lower among items that stayed on the menu compared to items dropped. Lower-calorie pizza options were introduced, but no significant changes	Positive

Table 4. Cont.

Author Year	Country	Study Design	Purpose	Sample	Setting	Data Sources	Menu Items	Nutrition Composition	New vs. Common Menu Items	Effect *
Wellard-Cole et al. 2018 [58]	Australia	Observational, longitudinal	Examine the energy content of Australian fast-food menu items before and after menu board labeling	522 menu items from fast-food chains	5 of the largest Australian QSR chains	Fast-food websites	Breakfast, burgers, desserts, chicken and seafood, salads, sides, sandwiches and wraps	Calories. No differences in energy per serving items, content per 100 g for burgers was higher after implementation (1040 vs. 999 kJ/100 g before implementation.)		No effect
Wellard-Cole et al. 2019 [59]	Australia	Observational, longitudinal	Investigate the nutrient composition of children's meals offers at fast-food chains, compare with children's daily requirements and recommendations and determine if results have changed prior to the implementation of menu labeling	289 children's meals	Australian QSR and FCR chains	Fast-food websites, email and telephone requests, and personnel visits	Children's meals per restaurant chain	Calories, saturated fat, sodium and sugar. Minimal changes were found. Meals from Chicken Treat reduced mean energy (−600 kJ/serving), saturated fat (−9.4 g/serving) and Na (−121 mg/serving), and from Red Rooster (−410 kJ/serving) and sugars (−11.8 g/serving), KFC reduced saturated fat (−10.5 g/serving). However, meals from Hungry Jack's increased in energy (345 kJ/serving), sugars (8.6 g/serving), and Na (187 mg/serving)	-	Mixed

Table 4. *Cont.*

Author Year	Country	Study Design	Purpose	Sample	Setting	Data Sources	Menu Items	Nutrition Composition	New vs. Common Menu Items	Effect *
Wu et al. 2014 [56]	USA	Observational, longitudinal	Track changes in the energy and sodium content of US chain restaurant main entrées between spring 2010 (when the Affordable Care Act was passed) and spring 2011	25,256 regular menu entrées from 213 restaurant brands	Top US chain restaurants based on 2008 sales	Restaurant websites, and email request	Regular menu entrées and children's menu entrées	Calories and sodium. 26 restaurants reduced sodium in newly added items by 707 mg on average. Significant decrease in mean energy (−40 kcal. Two upscale restaurants with children's menu entrées had a significant increase in mean energy (46 kcal). Items removed from children's menus were 36 kcal lower	Higher-sodium items decreased by 70 mg ($p = 0.027$) in added vs. removed items on regular menus. Calories decreased by 57 kcal ($p = 0.047$) for added vs. removed children's entrées	Mixed

* Effect: positive (if results showed a statistically significant *p*-value), no effect (if results showed no statistically significant *p*-value or negative effects), and mixed-effects (if results showed both) on menu labeling. QSR: quick-service restaurants; FCR: fast-casual restaurants; FSR: full-service restaurant. kJ: kilojoules.

3.2.2. Changes in the Nutritional Composition by Nutrients of Concern

The effects of menu labeling were measured by changes in the nutrition composition of menu items for four nutrients of concern, including calories ($n = 14$), sodium ($n = 5$), saturated fat ($n = 3$), and sugar ($n = 3$). A single US study from Washington state did not use these nutrients; rather the authors classified healthy versus unhealthy items based on 10 items examined by the Nutrition Environment Measures Surveys—Restaurant version (NEMSR) [54]. Two studies from the US and one from Canada assessed serving size reductions of menu items [16,47,54].

Positive effects: Bleich et al. (2020) reported the results of a longitudinal study (2012–2018) that examined nutrient trends for 28,238 food and beverage menu items from 28,238 US chain restaurants. The results found less calories in food items, and less calories and saturated fat in beverages, with results attributed to the US national menu labeling law [51]. Similar results were noted for six US studies that documented a significant decline in calories of certain items [19,48–50,53,55]. Besides energy, positive changes were reported for reducing the saturated fat and sodium content of menu items after the menu labeling implementation period in King County, Washington, that had more stringent menu labeling requirements before the national menu labeling law was passed in 2010 [16].

No effects: Two studies in Canada and Australia did not show significant results [47,58]. Saelens et al. (2012) reported that the availability of reduced portions actually decreased in King County, Washington, where menu labeling was implemented [54].

Mixed effects: Wu and Sturm (2014) assessed the energy and sodium changes from items offered by US chain restaurants after the national menu labeling law was passed in 2010 and in 2011. Results showed that QSR chains reduced the mean energy content of children's menu entrees by 40 calories; however, upscale restaurants had increased the mean energy content of children's menu entrees by 46 calories [56]. Similarly, Namba et al. (2013) examined the nutrient content of menu items after the national menu labeling law was passed in 2010 and in 2011, and found that the proportion of healthier menu items was higher in locations implementing restaurant labeling despite the mean calories of items that did not change [52]. Wellard-Cole et al. (2019) conducted a study in New South Wales, Australia, and found minimal decreases in energy, saturated fat, and sodium by specific QSR chains but and an increase in energy, sugars, and sodium from the QSR franchise called Hungry Jack's (Burger King) [59].

3.2.3. Newly Introduced Menu Items Versus Common or Regular Menu Items

Seven studies conducted in the US and Canada [47–49,51,52,55,56] compared the differences between newly introduced menu items after the baseline year of the implementation of a menu labeling policy in 2018 with those that were dropped and/or stayed the same over the years. Five studies found positive effects [48,49,51,55,56], one study mixed effects [47], and one study found no effects [52].

Positive effects: Five US studies found significant changes made for newly introduced menu items that had fewer calories (from −57 kcal to −285 kcal) relative to popular menu items that were offered regularly and consistently at the chain restaurants [48,49,51,55,56].

No effects: Scourbutakos et al. (2019) investigated the early impact of the mandatory menu labeling law in the province of Ontario, Canada, that documented opposite results from the US studies that measured similar outcomes. The study found that newly introduced food items in 2017 contained more energy per serving compared with the newly introduced food items in 2016. The newly introduced menu items in 2017 also had significantly higher serving sizes compared with the newly introduced items from 2013 and 2016 [47].

Mixed effects: Namba et al. (2013) reported the results of a case-control study that examined five QSR chains that had voluntarily implemented menu labeling before the US national menu labeling law was passed in 2010. Three of the chains had improved the nutritional quality of items with healthier profiles of side dishes and children's meals. However, two chains showed no reduction in calories of any menu items [52].

4. Discussion

This is the first comprehensive review published to document the number of countries that have enacted menu labeling policies, to compare the features of these policies, and to examine evaluations about the effect of menu labeling policies on the business practices of transnational restaurant chains globally. Step 1 of the scoping review identified 11 menu labeling policies or laws enacted by national, state or provincial, and/or municipal authorities in upper–middle and high-income countries between 2010 and 2020. The governments in eight countries had enacted mandatory policies (i.e., Australia, Canada, Ireland, Saudi Arabia, South Korea, Taiwan, United Arab Emirates, and the US). The governments in three countries had enacted voluntary policies (i.e., Bahrain, Malaysia, and the UK). Step 2 of the scoping review summarizes the results and evidence gaps from 15 published studies (2012 to 2020) on existing menu labeling policies across four countries (i.e., Australia, Canada, the UK, and the US). Overall, the studies found mixed results, and only the US studies showed positive effects of restaurant menu labeling policies to reformulate items or introduce new healthier items ranging from 57calories to 285 fewer calories/item. Studies conducted in Australia, Canada, and the UK found either no effect or mixed effects of menu labeling policies on businesses to reformulate or introduce new menu offerings.

Step 2 of the scoping review revealed a major lack of published evidence for the effects of menu labeling on restaurant business for other regions of the world that have policies in place identified in step 1 (Table 2). No studies were found on the effects of menu labeling policies on restaurant food reformulation and serving sizes in the Asian region (i.e., Malaysia, South Korea, and Taiwan); Middle East region (i.e., Bahrain, Dubai, Saudi Arabia, and the United Arab Emirates); and European region (i.e., Ireland). This may have been due to no evaluations conducted, evaluations that were not available in the public domain, or published in languages other than English or Spanish.

The mandatory restaurant menu labeling policy compliance rate for disclosing energy (calories or kilojoules) was high in the US (94% after May 2018) [75] and in New South Wales, Australia (95%) [76]. However, subsequent evaluations in New South Wales showed that this compliance had not translated into restaurants making significant reductions in energy for menu items by 2016 [59]. A 2018 evaluation of restaurant menu labeling compliance across four Australian states (including New South Wales) and one territory showed high menu labeling compliance reported by 11 chain restaurants [77]. However, independent evaluations are needed to verify industry-reported results.

The menu labeling policies reviewed were found across upper–middle and high-income countries. However, the existing evidence highlights that eating away from home is increasing among populations creating room for menu labeling policies. The 2015 Nielsen Global Out-of-Home Dining Survey conducted among more than 30,000 adults in 61 countries found that about half of respondents (48%) reported eating out one or more times weekly (REF). Consumers (22%–26%) in the Asia-Pacific region (i.e., Hong Kong, Taiwan, Malaysia and Thailand) reported eating out daily, and other countries with menu labeling legislation (i.e., Saudi Arabia and the US) reported rates of eating away from home daily (12%–15%) that exceeded the global average of 9 percent [10]. The survey found that three out of the top five countries with the highest percentage of respondents that eat lunch away from home are in Latin America: Chile, Brazil, and Colombia [10]. Popkin and Reardon (2018) confirmed that since 1995, people are increasingly spending more of their income on eating out of home, with higher significant increases in Brazil, Chile, and Colombia [78]. A Nielsen Global Survey of food labeling trends among 25,000 consumers in 56 countries found that 80 percent of respondents expressed that fast-food restaurants should include calorie labeling and other nutrition information either sometimes or always, and, support was strongest in Latin America, North America and Europe [79]. Given these trends, there is a need to evaluate menu labeling policies of countries in these regions.

The small number of studies that assessed other nutrients of concern (i.e., saturated fats, trans fats, sodium, and added sugars) [16,51,56,57,59] rather than just energy might be the consequence of policies limiting the regulation to reporting the energy content. All 11 countries that have implemented restaurant menu labeling policies require the disclosure of energy (i.e., calories or kilojoules). Only three countries (i.e., Australia, United Arab Emirates, and the US) require contextual information to display the daily energy intake recommended for the average adult (i.e., 2000 calories/day or 8700 kilojoules/day). Of these three countries, no evaluation was available for Dubai, and only two published evaluations were available for New South Wales, Australia, that found no significant effects. Results showed that two voluntary policies (Malaysia and Bahrain) and one mandatory policy (South Korea) included disclosure of fat, protein, sodium, and sugar besides calories. However, no evaluations were available to assess industry changes to reduce the availability of nutrients of concern (i.e., sodium, saturated fat, trans fat, and added sugar) linked to obesity, and diet-related NCDs have not been assessed yet.

It is important to note that the US studies showed a positive effect of menu labeling on restaurants to reduce calories for newly introduced items, especially appetizers and side dishes, may have been related to a longer time frame between the legislation enactment in 2010 and the published studies with positive effects (2015–2020) [16,19,48–51,53,55]. It is possible that the US restaurant sector had a longer period of time to implement changes that complied with the national law. Two US studies showed mixed results where the time factor could have influenced. Namba et al. (2013) evaluated the effect of menu labeling on QSR chain menus from 2005 through 2011, and most of the assessed years were before the national menu labeling law was passed [52]. In contrast, the menu labeling legislation passed in 2015 in Ontario, Canada, was implemented in January 2017. The Canadian study showed baseline data (2010–2016) no effects of menu labeling on the chain restaurants reformulating to offer healthier items [47]. Australia initiated mandatory menu labeling legislation in New South Wales in 2011, which was expanded to the Australian Canberra Territory and three states, including Victoria, which enacted mandatory menu labeling in 2018. The studies conducted in Australia showed both mixed [59] and no effect [58] of food reformulation or serving size reductions.

The type of policy might have influenced the study outcomes besides the time factor. The UK implemented a voluntary menu labeling policy that could have played a role in the mixed-effects found by Theis and Adams 2019 [57]. Several challenges are associated with mandatory policies enacted at the state or territorial levels (Australia) or the provincial level (Canada) that may lead to inconsistencies in legislation between jurisdictions and across the outlet threshold (chain versus non-chain), variations in the provision of voluntary, readable and standardized nutritional information to customers, and inability to customize menu ordering [77].

The study design may also explain the results from this review since the studies showing positive effects in the US were observational and longitudinal. The availability of longitudinal data from the MenuStat database could justify why the US studies showed positive effects for national menu labeling over eight years (2010–2018) compared to other countries that had a shorter time frame from the enactment of legislation. Experimental, quasi-experimental, and observational, case-control studies that compared non-regulated periods or jurisdiction versus regulated ones found no or mixed effects, respectively. This may indicate that industry changes may have happened for other reasons and/or policies independently from the menu labeling policy. In addition, studies that found positive effects have analyzed changes among items, and those that assessed effects among menus instead, have found no or mixed effects. These findings suggest that industry may have introduced positive changes to some items but kept the overall nutritional quality of the menu as a whole unchanged. The majority of study designs from the reviewed articles were observational, which cannot determine causation, and reverse causality needs to be explored. Restaurants could have changed their products before implementing menu labeling, or food businesses and non-restaurant businesses could have adopted pledges and commitments on items that are often offered in restaurants. Some recent US voluntary initiatives to improve the nutritional content of food and beverage products are the Healthy Weight Commitment [80] and the Children's Food and Beverage Advertising Initiative [81] in the US.

A robust body of evidence has shown that food reformulation may reduce or eliminate sodium and trans fats, both of which are identified by the WHO as a cost-effective strategy used across different countries to improve diet quality and reduce obesity and diet-related NCD risks [82–90]. Food and beverage product reformulation may have a greater impact on the entire population than strategies that encourage healthy choices that may or may not influence consumer behavior change because the decline in energy (calories or kilojoules) is distributed across populations that frequently consume the modified products [88,91,92].

Our scoping review results identified several challenges. First, evaluations were published for only four of 11 countries that had passed legislation between 2010 and 2020. This suggests that policymakers are not investing adequate resources to monitor and evaluate the effects of menu labeling policies. Second, only the US studies that evaluated the effects of a mandatory national policy showed that restaurants had reduced calories for some newly introduced menu item categories, but did not reduce calories or the serving sizes of popular items frequently consumed. This is a challenge because expert bodies have recommended nutrient targets for menu item categories that are not being used as reference points to evaluate industry progress [21]. Third, while the WHO has recommended nutrition labeling and reducing portion sizes as strategies to reduce energy intake, our study found no evidence to support menu labeling legislation as a cost-effectiveness "best buy" strategy to reduce NCD-related disability and mortality in low- and middle-income countries [14].

4.1. Implications for Policy, Practice, and Research

Our results suggest that menu labeling legislation in the absence of other supportive strategies is unlikely to produce a meaningful change among restaurant practices to expand healthy menu items for all customers. Menu labeling is one of eight marketing-mix and choice architecture strategies that restaurant businesses can use to nudge customers toward healthy food environments 20 [93,94]. A compelling business case must be made to persuade chain restaurants to adopt these strategies to improve their corporate image and attract new customers who want healthy meals [95].

Table 5 suggests several actions for stakeholders, including governments, the WHO, restaurant businesses, private foundations, researchers, and civil society organizations to develop, implement, and evaluate comprehensive restaurant menu labeling policies.

Table 5. Recommended actions for stakeholders to develop, implement, and evaluate comprehensive restaurant menu labeling policies.

Food System Actors	Recommended Actions
Governments	Provide enough support for food service restaurant businesses to facilitate a low-cost, sustainable, and accountable policy. Policies could be improved to incentivize more holistic menu changes by requiring the display of energy and other nutrients of concern, including fats, sodium, and added sugars for each item offered by restaurants.
World Health Organization	Issue recommendations for governments and transnational restaurants and their franchise businesses, and food service providers to harmonize, standardize, and apply a universal set of healthy dietary standards across countries and regions.
Restaurant businesses	Make commitments and increase transparency to meet product profile targets based on WHO- or expert-recommended guidelines
Private foundations	Provide technical assistance and incentivize transnational restaurant chains to implement, monitor, and evaluate menu labeling policies across countries and regions.
Researchers	Expand external monitoring and evaluation efforts of transnational restaurant chains to assess their compliance with WHO- or expert-recommended guidelines across countries and regions. Examine how digital technology could be used to leverage the effects of restaurant menu labeling policies.
Civil society organizations	Use social media advocacy, public awareness campaigns, and shareholder resolutions to encourage governments to implement comprehensive restaurant menu labeling policies for healthy product reformulation and portion size reduction for products sold to customers across countries and regions.

Government action is needed to implement national comprehensive menu labeling policies to have a significant effect on food reformulation and serving size reduction. Evidence still needs to be stronger to confirm these positive effects, and it is clear that voluntary efforts by industry are not enough. Only one study [57], based on the UK voluntary policy, discussed that food business initiatives and goodwill are insufficient for restaurant menu labeling to become a cost-effective strategy to address obesity and diet-related NCDs. Littlewood et al. (2016) have suggested that restaurants are more likely to improve their performance to offer healthier options with mandatory government requirements [25].

Digital technologies (i.e., online ordering through apps and digital menu boards) are being used more frequently to reach more customers that may either support or undermine the positive effect of menu labeling. The coronavirus or COVID-19 pandemic has created a new trend where restaurant businesses have moved to digital online and delivery, in response to the economic crisis that the pandemic has caused worldwide. Future policies and research should examine how restaurants change menu items based on customers' online ordering experience, use of onsite digital technology computerized touch screens and smartphones, use of algorithmic nudging to influence customers' choices, and how customers use digital technologies available through third-party delivery apps and businesses such as UberEats and DoorDash. Research could also examine how to leverage digital technology to encourage menu item reformulation and serving size reductions while encouraging customers to purchase the healthiest menu items [96].

Effective policy actions require regulatory oversight to ensure accountability [97]. The engagement of diverse sectors will help to strengthen the accountability process. Civil society organizations should mobilize efforts to support restaurant menu labeling initiatives and can perform independent evaluations that are shared with industry actors and government regulatory bodies. It is common for the industry sector to oppose these initiatives based on evidence from Ireland [67] and in the UK [69], where national menu labeling has been under consideration by Congress since 2015.

This research adds to the literature by identifying the knowledge gaps about the effects of restaurant and fast-food chain menu labeling on food reformulation and serving size reductions. Further research is needed to assess ongoing restaurant menu labeling policies from the Americas region (especially Latin and Central American countries), European, Eastern Mediterranean, African and Western Pacific regions for the short-term, mid-term, and long-term effects. More research is needed to explore whether restaurant menu labeling can reduce serving sizes of menu items in middle-and low-income countries. Experimental studies are needed to explore reverse causation and whether restaurant menu labeling policies will be effective in different countries by context. Finally, the WHO has clearly stated that obesity and NCDs are risk factors for COVID-19 [98]. Governments are implementing "new guidelines" for re-opening business and reset the economy and should prioritize in their political agenda policies that encourage healthier food environments to ensure that nutritious food is available for all populations as an integral strategy.

4.2. Study Strengths and Limitations

This scoping review has several limitations common to the nature of the study (i.e., map, describe, and provide an overview of the published literature to identify relevant data to inform policymaking and research). The exploratory scope of this review does not enable conclusions about the topic. However, these results may provide valuable insights for research and policy actions, especially regarding the monitoring and evaluation of implemented policies within and across countries to rigorously understand whether and under what conditions menu labeling could have an effect on restaurant businesses. It is possible that the use of additional literature databases would have yielded further articles. Given the involvement of an expert librarian, it was anticipated that the selected databases were appropriate to capture the breadth of research on this topic. In addition, this review also assessed the quality of the selected studies. We limited the search date to 2000. No studies that met the inclusion criteria were found between 2000 and 2011; therefore, we believe that our search captured the majority of relevant articles for the topic. Literature in other languages than English and

Spanish were excluded, so research for countries that had legislation and evaluations published in other languages may have been missed. Lastly, all the selected studies were conducted in high-income countries; therefore, these results cannot be generalized to middle- or low-income country settings.

5. Conclusions

The trend of increased eating away from home across countries is a call for mandatory menu labeling policies to improve healthy offerings to support a healthy diet worldwide. The overall evidence from this review is mixed on the effect of menu labeling policies for transnational restaurants and fast-food chains on food reformulation. The positive effects were from observational and longitudinal studies conducted within the period the legislation was enacted in the US and mainly for food reformulation of the energy content of menu items, and the introduction of new healthier menu items, not for overall changes among the menus. Case-control and quasi-experimental studies found no or mixed effects. Considerable gaps in the evidence remain, particularly regarding the effects of the implemented policies across regions at mid- and long-term, research in middle- and low-income countries, and reverse causation of restaurant menu labeling policies. Moreover, while all the enacted policies across countries request to display energy content, additional nutrients of concern could be included to have a greater impact. These results may inform governments, civil society, academics, and the restaurant industry to develop comprehensive and robust restaurant menu labeling policies that promote healthy dietary choices to reduce obesity and NCD risks worldwide.

Supplementary Materials: The following are available online at http://www.mdpi.com/2072-6643/12/6/1544/s1. Table S1: MeSH terms definitions. Table S2: Search details on each database. Table S3: Quality assessment results based on the Johanna Briggs Institute critical appraisal checklist.

Author Contributions: S.R.-G.P. led the study conception, methodology, data collection, formal analysis, and original draft manuscripts. The co-authors contributed as follows: Conceptualization, V.I.K., V.H., and E.S.; methodology, M.Z.; validation, M.Z. and V.I.K.; writing—review and editing, M.Z., V.H., E.S., R.L., F.D.S.G., and V.I.K. F.D.S.G. is a staff member of the Pan American Health Organization. The authors alone are responsible for the views expressed in this publication, and they do not necessarily represent the decisions or policies of the Pan American Health Organization. All authors have read and agreed to the published version of the manuscript.

Funding: We are grateful for the financial support provided by Virginia Tech Library's Open Access Subvention Fund to cover the publication and open access costs for this manuscript. In any use of this publication, there should be no suggestion that PAHO endorses specific organizations, products, or services.

Acknowledgments: The authors greatly appreciate Erin Smith for her guidance and input on developing the research question, finding the appropriate MeSH terms for the scoping review, and selecting the appropriate databases. We thank Sara Hendery and Jessica Agnew for their help in proofreading the manuscript.

Conflicts of Interest: The authors declare no conflict of interest.

References

1. Popkin, B.M. Relationship between shifts in food system dynamics and acceleration of the global nutrition transition. *Nutr. Rev.* **2017**, *75*, 73–82. [CrossRef] [PubMed]
2. Smith, L.P.; Ng, S.W.; Popkin, B.M. Resistant to the recession: Low-income adults' maintenance of cooking and away-from-home eating behaviors during times of economic turbulence. *Am. J. Public Health* **2014**, *104*, 840–846. [CrossRef] [PubMed]
3. Vandevijvere, S.; Jaacks, L.M.; Monteiro, C.A.; Moubarac, J.C.; Girling-Butcher, M.; Lee, A.C.; Pan, A.; Bentham, J.; Swinburn, B. Global trends in ultraprocessed food and drink product sales and their association with adult body mass index trajectories. *Obes. Rev.* **2019**, *20* (Suppl. 2), 10–19. [CrossRef] [PubMed]
4. Kant, A.K.; Graubard, B.I. A prospective study of frequency of eating restaurant prepared meals and subsequent 9-year risk of all-cause and cardiometabolic mortality in US adults. *PLoS ONE* **2018**, *13*, e0191584. [CrossRef] [PubMed]
5. Seguin, R.A.; Aggarwal, A.; Vermeylen, F.; Drewnowski, A. Consumption Frequency of Foods Away from Home Linked with Higher Body Mass Index and Lower Fruit and Vegetable Intake among Adults: A Cross-Sectional Study. *J. Environ. Public Health* **2016**, *2016*, 3074241. [CrossRef]

6. Alturki, H.A.; Brookes, D.S.; Davies, P.S. Comparative evidence of the consumption from fast-food restaurants between normal-weight and obese Saudi schoolchildren. *Public Health Nutr.* **2018**, *21*, 2280–2290. [CrossRef]
7. Tambalis, K.D.; Panagiotakos, D.B.; Psarra, G.; Sidossis, L.S. Association between fast-food consumption and lifestyle characteristics in Greek children and adolescents; results from the EYZHN (National Action for Children's Health) programme. *Public Health Nutr.* **2018**, *21*, 3386–3394. [CrossRef] [PubMed]
8. Llanaj, E.; Ádány, R.; Lachat, C.; D'Haese, M. Examining food intake and eating out of home patterns among university students. *PLoS ONE* **2018**, *13*, e0197874. [CrossRef]
9. Goffe, L.; Rushton, S.; White, M.; Adamson, A.; Adams, J. Relationship between mean daily energy intake and frequency of consumption of out-of-home meals in the UK National Diet and Nutrition Survey. *Int. J. Behav. Nutr. Phys. Act.* **2017**, *14*, 131. [CrossRef]
10. Nielsen. *Nielsen Global Out-of-Home Dining Survey*; The Nielsen Company: New York, NY, USA, 2015.
11. Kuo, T.; Jarosz, C.J.; Simon, P.; Fielding, J.E. Menu labeling as a potential strategy for combating the obesity epidemic: A health impact assessment. *Am. J. Public Health* **2009**, *99*, 1680–1686. [CrossRef]
12. Cawley, J.; Wen, K. Policies to Prevent Obesity and Promote Healthier Diets: A Critical Selective Review. *Clin. Chem.* **2018**, *64*, 163–172. [CrossRef] [PubMed]
13. World health Organization. *Follow-up to the Political Declaration of the High-Level Meeting of the General Assembly WHA66.10. Annex: Global Action Plan for Prevention and Control of Non-Communicable Diseases 2013–2020*; World Health Organization: Geneva, Switzerland, 2013.
14. World Health Organization. *Tackling NCDs: 'Best Buys' and other Recommended Interventions for the Prevention and Control of Noncommunicable Diseases*; World Health Organization: Geneva, Switzerland, 2017.
15. Bleich, S.N.; Economos, C.D.; Spiker, M.L.; Vercammen, K.A.; VanEpps, E.M.; Block, J.P.; Elbel, B.; Story, M.; Roberto, C.A. A Systematic Review of Calorie Labeling and Modified Calorie Labeling Interventions: Impact on Consumer and Restaurant Behavior. *Obesity* **2017**, *25*, 2018–2044. [CrossRef] [PubMed]
16. Bruemmer, B.; Krieger, J.; Saelens, B.E.; Chan, N. Energy, saturated fat, and sodium were lower in entrees at chain restaurants at 18 months compared with 6 months following the implementation of mandatory menu labeling regulation in King County, Washington. *J. Acad. Nutr. Diet.* **2012**, *112*, 1169–1176. [CrossRef] [PubMed]
17. Muth, M.K.; Karns, S.A.; Mancino, L.; Todd, J.E. How Much Can Product Reformulation Improve Diet Quality in Households with Children and Adolescents? *Nutrients* **2019**, *11*, 618. [CrossRef]
18. Federici, C.; Detzel, P.; Petracca, F.; Dainelli, L.; Fattore, G. The impact of food reformulation on nutrient intakes and health, a systematic review of modelling studies. *BMC Nutr.* **2019**, *5*, 2. [CrossRef]
19. Bleich, S.N.; Moran, A.J.; Jarlenski, M.P.; Wolfson, J.A. Higher-Calorie Menu Items Eliminated in Large Chain Restaurants. *Am. J. Prev. Med.* **2018**, *54*, 214–220. [CrossRef]
20. Kraak, V.; Englund, T.; Misyak, S.; Serrano, E. Progress Evaluation for the Restaurant Industry Assessed by a Voluntary Marketing-Mix and Choice-Architecture Framework that Offers Strategies to Nudge American Customers toward Healthy Food Environments, 2006–2017. *Int. J. Environ. Res. Public Health* **2017**, 760. [CrossRef]
21. Kraak, V.; Rincon-Gallardo Patino, S.; Renukuntla, D.; Kim, E. Progress Evaluation for Transnational Restaurant Chains to Reformulate Products and Standardize Portions to Meet Healthy Dietary Guidelines and Reduce Obesity and Non-Communicable Disease Risks, 2000-2018: A Scoping and Systematic Review to Inform Policy. *Int. J. Environ. Res. Public Health* **2019**, 2732. [CrossRef]
22. Fernandes, A.C.; Oliveira, R.C.; Proenca, R.P.; Curioni, C.C.; Rodrigues, V.M.; Fiates, G.M. Influence of menu labeling on food choices in real-life settings: A systematic review. *Nutr. Rev.* **2016**, *74*, 534–548. [CrossRef]
23. Harnack, L.J.; French, S.A. Effect of point-of-purchase calorie labeling on restaurant and cafeteria food choices: A review of the literature. *Int. J. Behav. Nutr. Phys. Act.* **2008**, *5*, 51. [CrossRef]
24. Kiszko, K.M.; Martinez, O.D.; Abrams, C.; Elbel, B. The influence of calorie labeling on food orders and consumption: A review of the literature. *J. Community Health* **2014**, *39*, 1248–1269. [CrossRef] [PubMed]
25. Littlewood, J.A.; Lourenco, S.; Iversen, C.L.; Hansen, G.L. Menu labelling is effective in reducing energy ordered and consumed: A systematic review and meta-analysis of recent studies. *Public Health Nutr.* **2016**, *19*, 2106–2121. [CrossRef] [PubMed]
26. Long, M.W.; Tobias, D.K.; Cradock, A.L.; Batchelder, H.; Gortmaker, S.L. Systematic review and meta-analysis of the impact of restaurant menu calorie labeling. *Am. J. Public Health* **2015**, *105*, e11–e24. [CrossRef] [PubMed]

27. Sinclair, S.E.; Cooper, M.; Mansfield, E.D. The influence of menu labeling on calories selected or consumed: A systematic review and meta-analysis. *J. Acad. Nutr. Diet.* **2014**, *114*, 1375–1388.e15. [CrossRef] [PubMed]
28. Swartz, J.J.; Braxton, D.; Viera, A.J. Calorie menu labeling on quick-service restaurant menus: An updated systematic review of the literature. *Int. J. Behav. Nutr. Phys. Act.* **2011**, *8*, 135. [CrossRef] [PubMed]
29. VanEpps, E.M.; Roberto, C.A.; Park, S.; Economos, C.D.; Bleich, S.N. Restaurant Menu Labeling Policy: Review of Evidence and Controversies. *Curr. Obes. Rep.* **2016**, *5*, 72–80. [CrossRef]
30. Sarink, D.; Peeters, A.; Freak-Poli, R.; Beauchamp, A.; Woods, J.; Ball, K.; Backholer, K. The impact of menu energy labelling across socioeconomic groups: A systematic review. *Appetite* **2016**, *99*, 59–75. [CrossRef] [PubMed]
31. Cantu-Jungles, T.M.; McCormack, L.A.; Slaven, J.E.; Slebodnik, M.; Eicher-Miller, H.A. A Meta-Analysis to Determine the Impact of Restaurant Menu Labeling on Calories and Nutrients (Ordered or Consumed) in U.S. Adults. *Nutrients* **2017**, 1088. [CrossRef]
32. Crockett, R.A.; King, S.E.; Marteau, T.M.; Prevost, A.T.; Bignardi, G.; Roberts, N.W.; Stubbs, B.; Hollands, G.J.; Jebb, S.A. Nutritional labelling for healthier food or non-alcoholic drink purchasing and consumption. *Cochrane Database Syst. Rev.* **2018**. [CrossRef]
33. Sucharew, H.; Macaluso, M. Progress Notes: Methods for Research Evidence Synthesis: The Scoping Review Approach. *J. Hosp. Med.* **2019**, *14*, 416–418. [CrossRef]
34. World Health Organization. *Global Database on the Implementation of Nutrition Action (GINA)*; World Health Organization: Geneva, Switzerland, 2012.
35. Hawkes, C.; Jewell, J.; Allen, K. A food policy package for healthy diets and the prevention of obesity and diet-related non-communicable diseases: The NOURISHING framework. *Obes. Rev.* **2013**, *14*, 159–168. [CrossRef] [PubMed]
36. World Cancer Research Fund International. *NOURISHING Framework*; World Cancer Research Fund International: London, UK, 2017.
37. Arksey, H.; O'Malley, L. Scoping studies: Towards a methodological framework. *Int. J. Soc. Res. Methodol.* **2005**, *8*, 19–32. [CrossRef]
38. Daudt, H.M.L.; van Mossel, C.; Scott, S.J. Enhancing the scoping study methodology: A large, inter-professional team's experience with Arksey and O'Malley's framework. *BMC Med Res. Methodol.* **2013**, *13*, 48. [CrossRef] [PubMed]
39. Doody, O.; Bailey, M.E. Setting a research question, aim and objective. *Nurse Res.* **2016**, *23*, 19–23. [CrossRef] [PubMed]
40. Moola, S.; Munn, Z.; Sears, K.; Sfetcu, R.; Currie, M.; Lisy, K.; Tufanaru, C.; Qureshi, R.; Mattis, P.; Mu, P. Conducting systematic reviews of association (etiology): The Joanna Briggs Institute's approach. *Int. J. Evid. -Based Healthc.* **2015**, *13*, 163–169. [CrossRef]
41. Richardson, W.S.; Wilson, M.C.; Nishikawa, J.; Hayward, R.S. The well-built clinical question: A key to evidence-based decisions. *ACP J. Club* **1995**, *123*, A12–A13.
42. Veritas Health. Covidence Systematic Review Software; Melbourne, Australia. 2019. Available online: https://www.medianet.com.au/releases/162025 (accessed on 15 February 2020).
43. Tricco, A.C.; Lillie, E.; Zarin, W.; O'Brien, K.K.; Colquhoun, H.; Levac, D.; Moher, D.; Peters, M.D.J.; Horsley, T.; Weeks, L.; et al. PRISMA Extension for Scoping Reviews (PRISMA-ScR): Checklist and Explanation. *Ann. Intern. Med.* **2018**, *169*, 467–473. [CrossRef]
44. The Johana Briggs Institute. *Checklist for Analytical Obesravtional Studies*; The University of Adelaide: Adelaide, Australia, 2017.
45. Ryan, R. Cochrane Consumer and Communication Review Group: Data Synthesis and Analysis. 2013. Available online: https://cccrg.cochrane.org/sites/cccrg.cochrane.org/files/public/uploads/Analysis.pdf (accessed on 15 January 2020).
46. Castleberry, A.; Nolen, A. Thematic analysis of qualitative research data: Is it as easy as it sounds? *Curr. Pharm. Teach. Learn.* **2018**, *10*, 807–815. [CrossRef]
47. Scourboutakos, M.J.; Orr, S.; Hobin, E.; Murphy, S.A.; Manson, H.; L'Abbé, M.R. Assessing the Early Impact of Menu-Labeling on Calories in Chain Restaurants in Ontario, Canada. *Am. J. Prev. Med.* **2019**, *56*, e195–e203. [CrossRef]

48. Bleich, S.N.; Wolfson, J.A.; Jarlenski, M.P.; Block, J.P. Restaurants With Calories Displayed On Menus Had Lower Calorie Counts Compared To Restaurants Without Such Labels. *Health Aff.* **2015**, *34*, 1877–1884. [CrossRef]
49. Bleich, S.N.; Wolfson, J.A.; Jarlenski, M.P. Calorie Changes in Large Chain Restaurants: Declines in New Menu Items but Room for Improvement. *Am. J. Prev. Med.* **2016**, *50*, e1–e8. [CrossRef] [PubMed]
50. Bleich, S.N.; Wolfson, J.A.; Jarlenski, M.P. Calorie changes in large chain restaurants from 2008 to 2015. *Prev. Med.* **2017**, *100*, 112–116. [CrossRef] [PubMed]
51. Bleich, S.N.; Soto, M.J.; Dunn, C.G.; Moran, A.J.; Block, J.P. Calorie and nutrient trends in large U.S. chain restaurants, 2012–2018. *PLoS ONE* **2020**, *15*, e0228891. [CrossRef] [PubMed]
52. Namba, A.; Auchincloss, A.; Leonberg, B.L.; Wootan, M.G. Exploratory analysis of fast-food chain restaurant menus before and after implementation of local calorie-labeling policies, 2005–2011. *Prev. Chronic Dis.* **2013**, *10*, E101. [CrossRef] [PubMed]
53. Petimar, J.; Zhang, F.; Cleveland, L.P.; Simon, D.; Gortmaker, S.L.; Polacsek, M.; Bleich, S.N.; Rimm, E.B.; Roberto, C.A.; Block, J.P. Estimating the effect of calorie menu labeling on calories purchased in a large restaurant franchise in the southern United States: Quasi-experimental study. *BMJ* **2019**, *367*, l5837. [CrossRef] [PubMed]
54. Saelens, B.E.; Chan, N.L.; Krieger, J.; Nelson, Y.; Boles, M.; Colburn, T.A.; Glanz, K.; Ta, M.L.; Bruemmer, B. Nutrition-labeling regulation impacts on restaurant environments. *Am. J. Prev. Med.* **2012**, *43*, 505–511. [CrossRef]
55. Tran, A.; Moran, A.; Bleich, S.N. Calorie changes among food items sold in U.S. convenience stores and pizza restaurant chains from 2013 to 2017. *Prev. Med. Rep.* **2019**, *15*, 100932. [CrossRef]
56. Wu, H.W.; Sturm, R. Changes in the energy and sodium content of main entrees in US chain restaurants from 2010 to 2011. *J. Acad. Nutr. Diet.* **2014**, *114*, 209–219. [CrossRef]
57. Theis, D.R.Z.; Adams, J. Differences in energy and nutritional content of menu items served by popular UK chain restaurants with versus without voluntary menu labelling: A cross-sectional study. *PLoS ONE* **2019**, *14*, e0222773. [CrossRef]
58. Wellard-Cole, L.; Goldsbury, D.; Havill, M.; Hughes, C.; Watson, W.L.; Dunford, E.K.; Chapman, K. Monitoring the changes to the nutrient composition of fast foods following the introduction of menu labelling in New South Wales, Australia: An observational study. *Public Health Nutr.* **2018**, *21*, 1194–1199. [CrossRef]
59. Wellard-Cole, L.; Hooper, A.; Watson, W.L.; Hughes, C. Nutrient composition of Australian fast-food and fast-casual children's meals available in 2016 and changes in fast-food meals between 2010 and 2016. *Public Health Nutr.* **2019**, *22*, 2981–2988. [CrossRef] [PubMed]
60. World Health Organization. *Health Statistics and Information Systems. Definition of Regional Grouping*; Global Health Estimates: Geneva, Switzerland, 2020.
61. Food and Drug Administration. Food Labeling: Revision of the Nutrition and Supplement Facts Labels. In *Final Rule. Fed. Regist*; 2016; 81, pp. 33741–33999. Available online: https://pubmed.ncbi.nlm.nih.gov/27236870/ (accessed on 15 January 2020).
62. Obesity Policy Coalition. Policy Brief: Menu Kilojoule Labelling in Chain Food Outlets in Australia; 2018. Available online: https://www.opc.org.au/downloads/policy-briefs/menu-kj-labelling-in-chain-food-outlets-in-australia.pdf (accessed on 15 January 2020).
63. Legislative Assembly of the Province of Ontario, Canada. Healthy Menu Choices Act, 2015 (Bill 45, Making Healthier Choices Act) O.Reg.50/16; Canada, G.o., Ed.; Ontario, Canada. 2017. Available online: https://labbelab.utoronto.ca/wp-content/uploads/2017/12/Evidence-Document-ON-reformat-Nov-8.pdf (accessed on 15 January 2020).
64. Food Safety Awareness and Applied Nutrition Unit; Department, F.S. Calorie Labeling in Food Service Establishments. In *Requirements and Guidelines*; Dubai Municipality: Dubai, United Arab Emirates, 2019. Available online: http://www.foodsafe.ae/pic/requirements/Calorie_Labeling_in_Food_Service_Establishments_Requirements_and_Guidelines_1907.pdf (accessed on 15 January 2020).
65. Ministry of Health Malaysia. National Plan of Action for Nutrition of Malaysia (2016–2025); Nutrition Division, M.o.H.M., Ed.; Putrajaya, Malaysia. 2016. Available online: http://nutrition.moh.gov.my/wp-content/uploads/2016/12/NPANM_III.pdf (accessed on 15 January 2020).

66. A'Ali, M. Bahrain News: Proposal for Restaurants and Cafés to Display Calories in Meals. GDNonline, 22 September. 2018. Available online: http://www.gdnonline.com/Details/402212/Proposal-for-restaurants-and-caf%E9s-to-display-calories-in-meals (accessed on 15 February 2020).
67. Department of Health. Consultation with Food Businesses on the Introduction of Mandatory Calorie Posting on Menus; Health, G.o.i.D.o., Ed.; 2020. Available online: https://www.gov.ie/en/consultation/d9bfcc-consultation-with-food-businesses-on-the-introduction-of-mandatory-c/ (accessed on 15 January 2020).
68. British Nutrition Foundation. The Public Health Responsibility Deal; Scotland. 2018. Available online: https://www.nutrition.org.uk (accessed on 15 January 2020).
69. Department of health and Social Care. Mandating Energy Labelling of Food and Drink in Out-of-Home Settings; IA No:13009; Department of health and Social Care: UK. 2018. Available online: https://assets.publishing.service.gov.uk/government/uploads/system/uploads/attachment_data/file/751532/impact-assessment-for-consultation-on-calorie-labelling-outside-of-the-home.pdf (accessed on 15 January 2020).
70. Secretary of State for Health and Social Care. Government Response to the House of Commons Health and Social Care Select Committee Report on Childhood Obesity: Time for Action, Eight Report of Session 2017-19; London, UK. 2019. Available online: https://www.parliament.uk/documents/commons-committees/Health/Correspondence/2017-19/Childhood-obesity-Government-Response-to-eighth-report-17-19.pdf (accessed on 15 January 2020).
71. Dame Sally Davies. Time to Solve Childhood Obesity. An Independent Report by the Chief Medical Officer. Annex A—Recommendations for Action. 2019. Available online: https://assets.publishing.service.gov.uk/government/uploads/system/uploads/attachment_data/file/837907/cmo-special-report-childhood-obesity-october-2019.pdf (accessed on 15 January 2020).
72. Center for Disease Control and Prevention. CDC Policy Process: Definition of Policy. In Office of the Associate Director for Policy; 2015. Available online: https://www.cdc.gov/policy/analysis/process/index.html (accessed on 15 January 2020).
73. Scourboutakos, M.J.; Semnani-Azad, Z.; L'Abbe, M.R. Added sugars in kids' meals from chain restaurants. *Prev. Med. Rep.* **2016**, *3*, 391–393. [CrossRef] [PubMed]
74. Scourboutakos, M.J.; L'Abbe, M.R. Restaurant menus: Calories, caloric density, and serving size. *Am. J. Prev. Med.* **2012**, *43*, 249–255. [CrossRef] [PubMed]
75. Cleveland, L.P.; Simon, D.; Block, J.P. Federal calorie labelling compliance at US chain restaurants. *Obes. Sci. Pract.* **2019**. [CrossRef]
76. Wellard, L.; Havill, M.; Hughes, C.; Watson, W.L.; Chapman, K. The availability and accessibility of nutrition information in fast food outlets in five states post-menu labelling legislation in New South Wales. *Aust. N. Z. J. Public Health* **2015**, *39*, 546–549. [CrossRef]
77. Sacks, G.; Robinson, E. *Inside Our Quick Service Restaurants: Assessment of Company Policies and Commitments Related to Obesity Prevention and Nutrition*; Deakin University: Melbourne, Australia, 2018.
78. Popkin, B.; Reardon, T. Obesity and the food system transformation in Latin America. *Obes. Rev.* **2018**, *19*, 1028–1064. [CrossRef]
79. Nielsen. *Battle of the Bulge & Nutrition Labels. Healthy Eating Trends Around the World*; The Nielsen Company: New York, NY, USA, 2012.
80. Healthy Weight Commitment Foundation. *Food and Beverage Manufacterers Pledging to Reduce Annual Calories By 1.5 Trillion By 2015*; CISION PR Newswire: London, UK, 2010.
81. Children's Food & Beverage Advertising Initiative. *Advertising Initiative Category-Specific Uniform Nutrition Criteria*; Council of Better Business Bureaus, Inc.: Arlington, VA, USA, 2018.
82. Mantilla Herrera, A.M.; Crino, M.; Erskine, H.E.; Sacks, G.; Ananthapavan, J.; Mhurchu, C.N.; Lee, Y.Y. Cost-Effectiveness of Product Reformulation in Response to the Health Star Rating Food Labelling System in Australia. *Nutrients* **2018**, *10*, 614. [CrossRef]
83. Pearson-Stuttard, J.; Hooton, W.; Critchley, J.; Capewell, S.; Collins, M.; Mason, H.; Guzman-Castillo, M.; O'Flaherty, M. Cost-effectiveness analysis of eliminating industrial and all trans fats in England and Wales: Modelling study. *J. Public Health* **2017**, *39*, 574–582. [CrossRef]
84. Shangguan, S.; Afshin, A.; Shulkin, M.; Ma, W.; Marsden, D.; Smith, J.; Saheb-Kashaf, M.; Shi, P.; Micha, R.; Imamura, F.; et al. A Meta-Analysis of Food Labeling Effects on Consumer Diet Behaviors and Industry Practices. *Am. J. Prev. Med.* **2019**, *56*, 300–314. [CrossRef]

85. Wilcox, M.L.; Mason, H.; Fouad, F.M.; Rastam, S.; al Ali, R.; Page, T.F.; Capewell, S.; O'Flaherty, M.; Maziak, W. Cost-effectiveness analysis of salt reduction policies to reduce coronary heart disease in Syria, 2010–2020. *Int. J. Public Health* **2015**, *60* (Suppl. 1), S23–S30. [CrossRef]
86. Watkins, D.A.; Olson, Z.D.; Verguet, S.; Nugent, R.A.; Jamison, D.T. Cardiovascular disease and impoverishment averted due to a salt reduction policy in South Africa: An extended cost-effectiveness analysis. *Health Policy Plan* **2016**, *31*, 75–82. [CrossRef] [PubMed]
87. Mason, H.; Shoaibi, A.; Ghandour, R.; O'Flaherty, M.; Capewell, S.; Khatib, R.; Jabr, S.; Unal, B.; Sozmen, K.; Arfa, C.; et al. A cost effectiveness analysis of salt reduction policies to reduce coronary heart disease in four Eastern Mediterranean countries. *PLoS ONE* **2014**, *9*, e84445. [CrossRef] [PubMed]
88. Spiteri, M.; Soler, L.G. Food reformulation and nutritional quality of food consumption: An analysis based on households panel data in France. *Eur. J. Clin. Nutr.* **2018**, *72*, 228–235. [CrossRef] [PubMed]
89. Downs, S.M.; Bloem, M.Z.; Zheng, M.; Catterall, E.; Thomas, B.; Veerman, L.; Wu, J.H. The Impact of Policies to Reduce trans Fat Consumption: A Systematic Review of the Evidence. *Curr. Dev. Nutr.* **2017**, *1*. [CrossRef] [PubMed]
90. Hendry, V.L.; Almiron-Roig, E.; Monsivais, P.; Jebb, S.A.; Neelon, S.E.; Griffin, S.J.; Ogilvie, D.B. Impact of regulatory interventions to reduce intake of artificial trans-fatty acids: A systematic review. *Am. J. Public Health* **2015**, *105*, e32–e42. [CrossRef] [PubMed]
91. Griffith, R.; O'Connell, M.; Smith, K. The Importance of Product Reformulation Versus Consumer Choice in Improving Diet Quality. *Economica* **2017**, *84*, 34–53. [CrossRef]
92. Leroy, P.; Requillart, V.; Soler, L.G.; Enderli, G. An assessment of the potential health impacts of food reformulation. *Eur. J. Clin. Nutr.* **2016**, *70*, 694–699. [CrossRef]
93. Kraak, V.I.; Englund, T.; Misyak, S.; Serrano, E.L. A novel marketing mix and choice architecture framework to nudge restaurant customers toward healthy food environments to reduce obesity in the United States. *Obes. Rev.* **2017**, *18*, 852–868. [CrossRef]
94. Roberto, C.A.; Khandpur, N. Improving the design of nutrition labels to promote healthier food choices and reasonable portion sizes. *Int. J. Obes.* **2014**, *38* (Suppl. 1), S25–S33. [CrossRef]
95. Kerins, C.; McHugh, S.; McSharry, J.; Reardon, C.M.; Hayes, C.; Perry, I.J.; Geaney, F.; Seery, S.; Kelly, C. Barriers and facilitators to implementation of menu labelling interventions from a food service industry perspective: A mixed methods systematic review. *Int. J. Behav. Nutr. Phys. Act.* **2020**, *17*, 48. [CrossRef]
96. Burke-Garcia, A.; Scally, G. Trending now: Future directions in digital media for the public health sector. *J. Public Health* **2014**, *36*, 527–534. [CrossRef] [PubMed]
97. World Health Organization. *Health Laws and Universal Health Coverage*; World Health Organization: Geneva, Switzerland, 2020.
98. World Health Organization. *Information Note on COVID-19 and NCDs*; World Health Organization: Geneva, Switzerland, 2020.

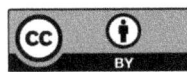

© 2020 by the authors. Licensee MDPI, Basel, Switzerland. This article is an open access article distributed under the terms and conditions of the Creative Commons Attribution (CC BY) license (http://creativecommons.org/licenses/by/4.0/).

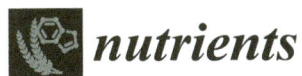

Article

Prevalence of Product Claims and Marketing Buzzwords Found on Health Food Snack Products Does Not Relate to Nutrient Profile

Maddison Breen [†], Hollie James [†], Anna Rangan and Luke Gemming *

Nutrition & Dietetics Department, Charles Perkins Centre, School of Life and Environmental Sciences, The University of Sydney, Sydney, NSW 2006, Australia; mbre6607@uni.sydney.edu.au (M.B.); holliejamesdietitian@gmail.com (H.J.); anna.rangan@sydney.edu.au (A.R.)
* Correspondence: luke.gemming@sydney.edu.au; Tel.: +61-286-275-209
† Maddison Breen and Hollie James should be considered joint first author.

Received: 18 April 2020; Accepted: 20 May 2020; Published: 22 May 2020

Abstract: Growth in the consumer health and wellness industry has led to an increase of packaged foods marketed as health food (HF) products. In consequence, a 'health halo' around packaged HF has arisen that influences consumers at point-of-purchase. This study compared product claims (nutrient content claims (NCC), health claims and marketing 'buzzwords') displayed on packaged HF snack products sold in HF stores and HF aisles in supermarkets to equivalent products sold in regular aisles (RA) of supermarkets. Product Health Star Rating (HSR), nutrient profile and price were also compared. Data were collected for 2361 products from three supermarket chains, two HF chains and one independent HF store in Sydney, Australia. Mann-Whitney U tests compared the product claims, HSR, nutrient composition and unit ($) price. HF snacks displayed significantly more product claims per product compared to RA foods (HSR ≤ 2.5), median (IQR) 5.0(4.0) versus 1.0(2) and (HSR > 2.5) 4.0(4.0) versus 3.0(4), respectively ($p < 0.001$). A significantly different HSR was evident between HF and RA snack products, median 2.5(0) versus 2.0(1.5), respectively ($p < 0.001$). HF snacks cost significantly more than RA snack foods, irrespective of product HSR ($p < 0.001$). These findings support the recommendation for revised labelling regulations and increased education regarding consumers food label interpretation.

Keywords: health food; nutrient content claims; health claims; food labelling; nutrient profile; health star rating

1. Introduction

Since 2004, the sales of packaged foods in Australia have nearly doubled and are predicted to continue to climb at a steady rate [1]. Likewise, in the past decade, ready-to-eat snack foods have increased in popularity amongst the Australian population [2]. Packaged, ready-to-eat snack foods can be defined as foods that have undergone a degree of processing and are designed to be consumed in the original state purchased [3,4]. Most fall within the discretionary food category (junk food) characterised by their high energy, saturated fat, added sugar and sodium content [2,5–7]. Thus, daily consumption should be limited due to their link with overweight and obesity, cardiovascular disease, diabetes and other co-morbidities [2,5,8].

Contrary to the rise in non-communicable diseases, such as obesity [9], consumer awareness of diet related health consequences has advanced [10]. It is evident that consumers are making a deliberate effort to modify certain dietary behaviours with the aim of improving their overall health and wellbeing [11–14]. According to a Nielsen report, sales of packaged health food (HF) products increased by 82% in supermarkets from 2012–2014, and most HF consumers report they shop in specialty retail stores that stock HF products [15]. In response, food manufacturers are constantly developing new HF products to capitalise on consumer demand [1]. These products are predominantly sold in HF aisles of supermarkets and specialty HF stores, which typically market themselves as food retailers in the health and wellness sector. In both locations, HF products are marketed and labelled as being nutritionally beneficial and often natural, organic or environmentally sustainable. Between 2012–2014, the sales of products with 'natural' or 'organic' claims grew by 24% and 28%, respectively [15]. Correspondingly, the value of 'natural' products has been influenced by consumer choice, with natural non-sugar sweetened product sales increasing by 186%, due to perceived health benefits, while artificially sweetened product sales decreased by 12% [15].

While the term healthy is defined as "beneficial to one's physical, mental, or emotional state: conducive to or associated with good health or reduced risk of disease" [16], the measured healthfulness of a product is difficult, given the differing attributes associated with health by consumers. Research indicates that consumers choose products that advertise 'healthy' qualities to attempt a more nutritionally balanced lifestyle [13]. Research also shows that consumers believe organic, gluten free and/or more expensive products to be healthier than the alternative [11–13,17,18]. Thus, a 'health halo' can exist [19,20], where consumers assume foods that are perceived to be 'healthy' have greater health benefits, more nutrients and fewer health risks than may actually be true [21–24].

With the aim to assist consumers in interpreting food labels more appropriately, the Health Star Rating (HSR) was implemented in Australia as a voluntary front of pack labelling (FoPL) scheme in 2014 [25]. Consumers prefer FoPL, including HSR and nutrition content claims (NCCs) over nutrition information panels (NIPs), because of their simplicity [24,26,27]. NCCs and health claims are images or words on product packaging that highlight particular properties and/or their health impact. Although the FoPL labels are strictly controlled by Food Standards Australia New Zealand (FSANZ), they may also contribute to the health halo effect when placed on products with other marketing messages with little to no restrictions, otherwise known as 'buzzwords', or when placed on products that are not necessarily healthier [21,23,26,28–32]. As such, questions have been raised regarding the use of NCCs and the HSR on packaged foods [33–37].

Due to the consumer confusion and vagueness of the term 'health' or 'healthy', products in the UK are not permitted to be labelled as such [38], while FSANZ does not mention this term specifically in nutrient and health claim regulations, neither permitting nor preventing its use [28]. Thus, a climate exists in food labelling where people who want to make healthier choices, by seeking healthy food products, may find it difficult to appropriately determine their value [39–42]. Concurrently, there has been significant growth in HF snack products sold in supermarket HF aisles and specialty HF stores. However, as there are no governing criteria of what can be stocked in these locations, the true health benefits of these products are largely unknown.

Accordingly, the primary aim of this study was to examine and compare the use of NCC, health claims and marketing 'buzzwords' on packaged HF snack products sold in supermarkets and specialty HF stores to equivalent products sold in RA of supermarkets. A secondary aim was to compare the nutrition profile and cost of these products.

2. Materials and Methods

2.1. Data Collection

Ethics approval was not required for the completion of this study. Data were collected from March 2018 to August 2019 as part of an audit of commercially available packaged snack foods in Australia [43]. Data were collected from the four major Australian supermarkets in the Sydney metropolitan area: Woolworths, Coles, Aldi and IGA. To capture additional HF snack products not sold in the major supermarkets, data were also collected from two national HF store chains, Go Vita and Healthy Life. To ensure data collection had reached saturation of the market, one large independent HF store was chosen at convenience for data collection. Several other HF stores across Sydney were subsequently visited to verify completeness of data collection. Assessment of the HF store's products indicated saturation was reached and therefore not used in the study. Not all supermarkets had entire dedicated HF aisles. Thus, HF aisle was defined as the aisle (complete or partly) that contained 'health foods', 'gluten free products' or 'sports nutrition products' as per aisle signage. Products located in all other aisles of supermarkets that contained a gluten free label were classified as RA foods.

Researchers captured images of the front and back packaging, ingredient list, Nutrition Information Panel (NIP) and barcode of all products using smartphones in-store. The products were classified into seven main categories and thirteen sub-categories (detailed in supplementary material Table S1). Once the data for HF snack foods was recorded, equivalent or 'like' products were sourced from the regular aisles (RA) of the supermarkets.

Product claims were divided into three categories; nutrient content claims (NCC), health claims and 'buzzwords'. Nutrient content and health claims were defined using the FSANZ definitions [28]. All other claims were categorised as 'buzzwords' (claim descriptions in supplementary material Table S2). Nutrition information from the NIP and full unit price values ($AUD) of all products were recorded and standardised per 100 g. Where the same products were available across multiple supermarkets or stores, price was taken from Coles or Woolworths, the first location where the product was recorded. All data were manually entered into an online database. Ready-to-eat packaged snack foods that were still wholefoods and/or were only minimally processed were excluded from collection, e.g., dried fruit and nut snack packs.

Data cleaning was carried out and duplicates of the same product within the same store type and duplicate products with different package sizes were removed from the database. The smallest package size was kept in the database and the unit cost was calculated from this. All outliers were checked against the original images. Any NIP values that stated nutrient content as <X, values were input as X - 1 for analysis, e.g., < 10 g was input as 9 g.

For those products that did not specify an HSR, the HSR was calculated using the Australian Government's HSR calculator (HSRC) [44]. Negative nutrients include energy (kJ), saturated fat, sugar and sodium, which accrue points, while positive nutrients such as protein, fibre and fruit, vegetable, nut and legume (FVNL) content deduct points; the higher the product score, the lower the HSR. Although, as many products did not declare ingredient percentage of product weight, the FVNL scores were estimated using a previously tested method [8]. As per other systematic analyses of the Australian food supply [37], for those products that did not specify fibre content in the NIP, a value was estimated from the nearest matched product from the AUSNUT 2011–2013 Food Nutrient database [45]. A sensitivity analysis was performed to determine whether these methods affected the derived fibre values and the derived HSR outcome.

2.2. Data Analysis

Data analysis was conducted using IBM SPSS Statistics Version 24 (2016), Armonk, NY, USA. The proportion (%) of products displaying NNC claims, health claims and buzzwords on HF snack products and equivalent RA foods was calculated and presented using descriptive statistics. The HSR was used to broadly classify product 'healthfulness'; products were classified as having an HSR ≤ 2.5 or >2.5 for NCC, health claim and buzzword comparisons. The data were checked for normality and found to be non-normal distribution; therefore, the median and interquartile range were used. The product claims, nutrient composition and unit price ($) per 100 g were compared between HF snack products and equivalent RA foods using Mann-Whitney U tests. A p-value of <0.001 was considered statistically significant due to the large number of tests undertaken. The HSR was used to group products for unit price comparisons using descriptive statistics.

3. Results

A total of 2361 snack products were collected; 1251 sold in RA and 1110 HF products sold in "health food" aisles of supermarkets and specialty "health food" stores; 621 products from HF aisles and 489 products from HF stores. The HSR was derived for 80% of RA products and 82% HF products. The fibre content was derived for 53% of RA and 11% of HF snack products. The sensitivity analysis revealed no apparent differences between original and derived fibre and HSR values; therefore, derived HSR values were used in the analysis. The largest category for HF snacks was snack bars (35%) and for RA products was confectionary (19%).

3.1. Nutrient Content Claims, Health Claims and 'Buzzwords'

A total of 8155 product claims were recorded, 5626 for HF snack products (2726 from HF aisles and 2900 from HF stores) and 2529 for RA snack products. Overall, 94% of the HF snack products and 73% of RA snack products reported/displayed NCC, health claims or 'buzzwords'.

Table 1 shows the proportion that different NCC, health claims or 'buzzwords', directly or indirectly related to health, were displayed on HF and RA snacks products (number of NCC, health claims and buzzwords/total HF or RA snack products).

Table 1. The proportion (%) of snack products that display nutrient content claims, health claims or 'buzzwords' on health food (HF) snack products sold in supermarkets and specialty HF stores, and equivalent products sold in regular aisles (RA) of supermarkets. FSANZ: Food Standards Australia New Zealand.

	Health Foods (%)	Regular Aisle Foods (%)
Nutrient content claims		
Gluten free	66.8	12.5
Sugar (e.g., no added sugar, low sugar etc.)	24.2	7.6
Fibre (e.g., source of fibre)	16.5	6.3
Protein (e.g., source of protein)	10.2	4.1
Fat (e.g., low fat, fat free etc.)	5.2	2.8
Sodium (e.g., low sodium/salt, salt reduced etc.)	2.7	0.5
Health claims		
All "health claims" (as per FSANZ)	2.5	2.4
Buzzwords		
"No Artificial" (e.g., no artificial colours, Flavours and/or preservatives)	27.6	34.5
Vegan	36.6	1.8
Natural	30.1	6.6
Organic	26.9	2.7
Dairy Free	27.0	28.9
Non-GMO	17.8	1.4
Wholegrain (e.g., Source of wholegrain)	5.0	6.6
Allergen free	26.6	1.4
Raw	7.8	0.1
Paleo	3.7	-
Keto	1.3	-
Environmental (e.g., green energy, Sustainable)	15.6	3.9
Superfood (e.g., 'supergrain', antioxidant, activated)	8.1	0.9
Nutritious (e.g., healthy, wholefood)	10.5	2.9
Good fats (e.g., good natural fats, omega 3)	5.3	4.6
Good sugars (e.g., natural sugars, fructose free, no refined sugar)	6.3	3.0
Made in Australia	4.2	29.7
All "other claims" directly and indirectly related to health and wellbeing (e.g., boost your inner health, burn fat, clean, FODMAP * friendly, low GI, made from real fruit, minimally processed, supports immune function, tone body ...)	100	35.6

* Fermentable Oligosaccharides, Disaccharides, Monosaccharides and Polyols.

'Gluten free' was the most common NCC displayed on both HF and RA snack products. 'Vegan' was the most common buzzword used on HF snack products and 'no artificial' was the most common for RA snack products. Other buzzwords, including 'no artificial', 'natural', 'dairy free', 'organic' and 'allergen free', were also frequently displayed (>25%) on HF snack products. 'Dairy free' was the only other buzzword displayed frequently (>25%) on RA snack products. Due to small individual numbers, a wide range of "other claims" were grouped together. At least one of these "other claims" were present on 100% of HF snack products and 39.6% of RA snack products.

Table 2 compares the proportion of HF and RA snack products with an HSR ≤ 2.5 or > 2.5, with 50% of HF and 25% RA snack products scoring an HSR > 2.5. Overall (all categories), HF snack products displayed significantly more NCC, health claims and buzzwords per product compared to RA products, median 5.0 versus 1.0 (HSR ≤ 2.5) and 4.0 versus 3.0 (HSR > 2.5), respectively ($p < 0.001$). For those products with an HSR ≤ 2.5, HF snacks displayed significantly more product claims per product for all categories. Similarly, for those products with an HSR > 2.5, HF snacks displayed significantly more product claims per product for all categories excluding chips and sweet biscuits was significantly lower. Small sample sizes ($n < 10$) for these two categories, chocolate and confectionary, were evident.

Table 2. Comparison of the median (IQR) product claims displayed on health food (HF) snack products sold in supermarkets and specialty HF stores to equivalent products sold in regular aisles (RA) of supermarkets, by product category for products with an HSR ≤ 2.5 and products with an HSR >2.5. Differences in median (IQR) claims displayed were assessed via Mann-Whitney U tests.

	Median Number of Product Claims Per Product with HSR ≤ 2.5			Median Number of Product Claims Per Product with HSR > 2.5		
	(N)	RA	HF	(N)	RA	HF
All categories	RA (n = 933) HF (n = 555)	1.0 (2.0)	5.0 (4.0) *	RA (n = 318) HF (n = 555)	3.0 (4.0)	4.0 (4.0) *
Beverages	RA (n = 54) HF (n = 49)	2.5 (3.0)	4.0 (4.0) *	RA (n = 89) HF (n = 46)	4.0 (3.5)	4.0 (2.0) *
Chips	RA (n = 97) HF (n = 61)	3.0 (2.0)	4.0 (5.0) *	RA (n = 11) HF (n = 133)	3.0 (2.0)	5.0 (2.0)
Chocolate	RA (n = 222) HF (n = 176)	1.0 (1.0)	6.0 (4.0) *	RA (n = 0) HF (n = 5)	-	4.0 (3.0)
Confectionary	RA (n = 193) HF (n = 34)	1.0 (1.0)	4.0 (4.0) *	RA (n = 49) HF (n = 6)	1.0 (1.0)	2.0 (2.5) *
Savoury biscuits	RA (n=108) HF (n=37)	2.0 (3.0)	2.0 (3.5) *	RA (n = 59) HF (n = 82)	3.0 (2.0)	6.0 (5.0) *
Snack bars	RA (n = 70) HF (n = 114)	3.0 (3.0)	5.0 (4.0) *	RA (n = 104) HF (n = 271)	3.0 (3.0)	4.0 (4.0) *
Sweet biscuits	RA (n = 189) HF (n = 84)	1.0 (2.0)	5.0 (3.5) *	RA (n = 6) HF (n = 12)	6.0 (4.0)	1.5 (2.5) *

Product claims include all nutrient content claims, health claims and 'buzzwords'. Health Star Rating abbreviated to HSR. Regular aisles abbreviated to RA. Health foods Abbreviated to HF. * Denotes p-value < 0.001.

3.2. Nutrient Composition and HSR

Table 3 shows the median HSR and nutrient composition of HF and RA snack products. Overall ('all categories'), the median HSR for HF snack products was significantly higher than RA products, 2.5 versus 2.0, respectively ($p < 0.001$). Compared to RA snacks, the median HSR for HF snack products was significantly higher for all categories, except beverages and confectionary. Overall ('all categories'), HF snack products were significantly higher in protein, total fat and fibre and RA snack products were significantly higher in carbohydrates and sugar ($p < 0.001$). No difference in energy, saturated fat or sodium was evident. For HF snack products, all categories, except beverages and confectionary, were significantly higher in fibre than RA products ($p < 0.001$).

Table 3. Comparative analysis of the differences in median (IQR) for HSR and nutrient content between health food (HF) snack products sold in supermarkets and specialty HF stores compared to equivalent products sold in regular aisles (RA) of supermarkets. Differences in median (IQR) nutrient values were assessed via Mann-Whitney U tests.

	HSR	Energy (kJ/100 g)	Protein (g/100 g)	Total Fat (g/100 g)	Saturated Fat (g/100 g)	CHO (g/100 g)	Sugar (g/100 g)	Sodium (mg/100 g)	Fibre (g/100 g)
All categories									
RA (n = 1251)	2.0(0.0)	1850(560)	5.6(4.3)	14.9(24.2)	4.3(11.7)	62.1(26.3)	25.9(41.5)	105(300)	2.3(2.8)
HF (n = 1110)	2.5(1.5)*	1805(553)	8.0(9.8)*	18.9(20.6)*	4.3(11.7)	44.8(41.5)*	11.1(27.4)*	153(327)	7.2(7.1)*
Beverages									
RA (n = 143)	3.5(2.5)	181(242)	0.9(2.6)	0.9(1.7)	0.9(1.0)	7.8(7.6)	6.3(7.1)	10(40)	0.2(0.9)
HF (n = 95)	2.5(3.0)	112(165)	0.7(3.9)	0.2(1.1)	0.2(0.9)	2.4(4.8)*	2.1(5.0)*	5.0(58.6)	0.4(0.9)
Chips									
RA (n = 108)	2.0(1.5)	2100(160)	6.7(1.8)	27.8(8.7)	4.3(10.5)	56.5(8.5)	2.3(2.4)	576(249)	3.5(1.7)
HF (n = 194)	3.5(2.0)*	1960(300)*	8.6(11.1)*	21.3(11.8)*	2.1(1.9)*	57.1(17.7)	2.8(5.9)	465(382)*	7.2(6.8)*
Chocolate									
RA (n = 222)	0.5(0.0)	2200(253)	6.0(2.3)	29.8(11.1)	17.6(6.1)	57.8(14.3)	50.9(13.2)	69(52)	2.3(1.1)
HF (n = 181)	1.0(1.5)*	2320(410)*	7.0(3.1)*	41.9(11.3)*	24.0(10.2)*	37.6(19.7)*	26.7(20.4)*	50(75)*	9.3(7.5)*
Confectionary									
RA (n = 242)	1.5(1.5)	1460(253)	1.0(2.7)	1.0(1.1)	1.0(0.9)	81.4(17.8)	51.2(33.3)	23(59)	0.0(1.0)
HF (n = 40)	2.0(1.0)	1462(224)	0.35(4.4)	0.1(0.9)*	0.0(0.9)*	80.5(15.7)	49.4(28.2)	61(65)	0.0(1.9)
Savoury biscuits									
RA (n = 167)	2.5(1.0)	1790(250)	8.9(3.2)	10.5(11.5)	2.0(3.3)	70.1(12.9)	2.7(3.7)	628(360)	3.6(1.1)
HF (n = 119)	3.0(1.5)*	1750(347)	9.0(5.5)	9.9(16.8)	1.6(3.9)	67.9(28.4)	1.8(3.5)	570(345)	4.4(9.1)*
Snack bars									
RA (n = 174)	3.0(1.5)	1795(370)	9.5(9.1)	17.2(17.5)	5.5(4.2)	51.5(25.0)	23.6(11.7)	126(186)	7.0(3.6)
HF (n = 385)	3.5(2.0)*	1670(422)*	15.0(21.7)*	16.2(14.5)	4.8(5.0)	37.3(40.6)*	19.8(27.4)	110(232)	9.1(4.9)*
Sweet biscuits									
RA (n = 195)	1.0(1.0)	2040(240)	5.4(1.8)	21.4(9.7)	11.9(7.2)	66.6(6.2)	34.6(12.6)	240(187)	1.9(1.2)
HF (n = 96)	1.5(1.0)*	1920(288)*	5.0(2.4)	22.3(8.7)	11.3(8.1)	62.1(13.8)*	26.1(14.9)*	221(220)	3.9(3.6)*

* Denotes p-value < 0.001. Regular aisles abbreviated to RA. Health foods abbreviated to HF.

3.3. Price

Figure 1 shows HF snack products in all food categories were substantially more expensive than RA foods. The largest overall price difference was between HF snack products and RA products was confectionary (253%). Median unit price ($) of HF snack products was significantly higher than RA products for all product categories (supplementary material Table S3).

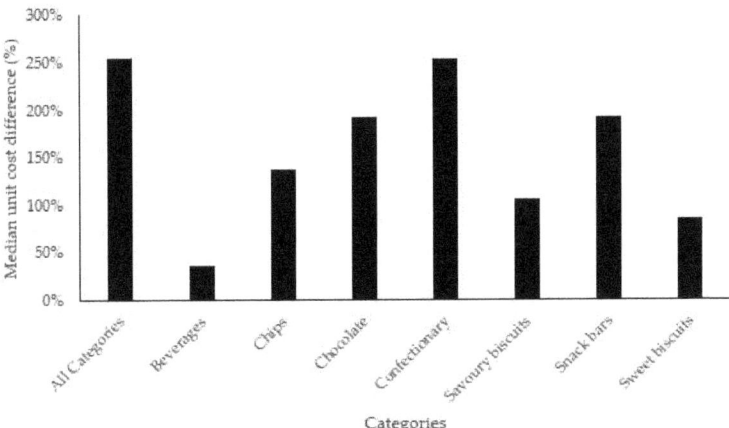

Figure 1. Median unit cost ($) per 100 g percent difference (%), per product category, between health food (HF) snack products sold in supermarkets and specialty HF stores compared to equivalent products sold in regular aisles (RA) of supermarkets.

Figure 2 shows unit cost ($) differences between product types, per HSR category. Health foods were substantially more expensive for all HSR categories. No clear trend between unit price ($) and HSR was evident. The greatest price difference was between HF and RA snack products scoring highest HSR of 5.0 (579%), followed by products scoring the lowest three HSR of 1.5, 1.0 and 0.5.

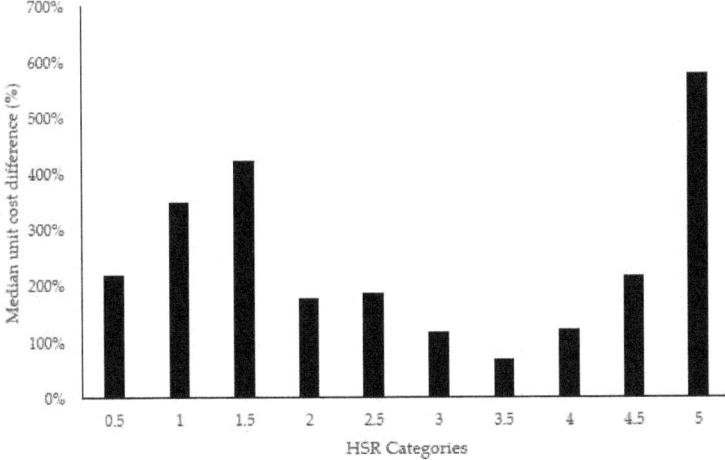

Figure 2. Median unit cost per 100 g percent difference (%), per HSR category, between health food (HF) snack products sold in supermarkets and specialty HF stores compared to equivalent products sold in regular aisles (RA) of supermarkets.

4. Discussion

This study sought to examine and compare NCC, health claims and 'buzzwords' displayed on pre-packaged snack HF products sold in supermarkets and specialty health food stores to equivalent products sold in RA of supermarkets. Secondary aims were to compare the nutrition profile and cost. The main findings of this study revealed manufactures of HF snack products use significantly more NCC, health claims and buzzwords to market their products compared to equivalent products sold in RA of supermarkets irrespective of their overall 'healthfulness'. Surprisingly, the greatest use of NCC, health claims and buzzwords was found on HF snack products with HSR ≤2.5 (median five claims per product). In contrast, equivalent products sold in RA only displayed one NCC, health claim or buzzword per product, revealing the presence and quantity of claims often does not relate to product healthfulness, and particularly for HF snack products, may instead encourage consumption of foods associated with increased health risks misleading consumers [8,21,23,26,33,46,47]. Furthermore, it must also be noted that the health halos that NCC may help create, also applies to the absence of misunderstood constituents, such as gluten. In the current study, a substantially higher proportion of HF snack products were labelled gluten free, despite 50% of products displaying an HSR ≤ 2.5. This is not surprising considering consumers often consider gluten free foods to be more beneficial to health [11,48].

The HSRC algorithm was used as a proxy to estimate a foods 'healthfulness' [44]. Overall, HF snack products were marginally superior to equivalent products sold in RA with a small but significant difference evident, median 2.5 versus 2.0, respectively. The slightly higher HSR achieved by HF snack products is likely attributed to greater fibre and lower sugar found across several categories, but no differences were evident for energy, saturated fat or sodium, all noted to be of concern by the World Health Organisation as detrimental to human health [9]. The significantly higher total fat and lower carbohydrate content in HF snack products was also notable and likely attributed to increased use of plant-based fats, nuts and seeds evident from the product ingredient lists. While our research used the mid-point of HSR system 2.5/5 to broadly classify foods into two distinct groups when examining differences in product labelling, a higher HSR cut-off ≥ 3.5 has been used by others to more clearly distinguish 'healthier' food choices and reduce the likelihood of discretionary foods being classified as healthy foods [7,37,49]. Accordingly, neither HF snacks nor equivalent RA products would meet this cut-off. This may be expected for products in RA, which are not always manufactured or viewed as the healthier options, but emphasises the concern surrounding HF snack products. Thus, the median HF score of 2.5/5 should be considered a minimum passing grade at best, a marked difference from the health halo surrounding products marketed as health foods [34].

Despite the limited research in this area, overall, these results were consistent with previous findings. Studies that have examined a range of products with and without NCC and health claims, or claimed to be 'organic', found that most products showed no difference in overall nutrient profile [8,21,23,26,33,46,47,50]. Pertinent to our own findings, Hughes et al. [33] found that a large number of NCC and health claims used on Australian products did not meet FSANZ nutrient profiling criteria [51] and this is likely true for a proportion of products examined in this study.

Previous literature has sought to determine appropriate FoPL to improve consumer perception of a products nutrition, without the strong influence of NCC, health claims and buzzwords, though not specifically for HF products [21,52–59]. Research shows that consumers have a poor understanding of food labels and cannot appropriately interpret the NIP [39,40], especially when a product claim is present [41,42]. In addition, qualitative literature has consistently found that consumers believe labels such as 'organic' [12,17,60], 'natural' and 'not artificial' [13] indicate that products are more nutritious [17] and are lower in sugar, fat and sodium [13]. Likewise, the placement of snack products within HF aisles and specialty HF stores marketed as 'health foods' (for which there is limited regulation) may act as a buzzword itself influencing consumer purchases. Evidence suggests the "reductive style" [55] of the HSR reduces consumer inclination to buy unhealthy products and guide more accurate interpretations [21,47,59,61]. However, our data show most products did not display

HSRs. Due to the voluntary nature of HSR, manufacturers may preferentially display HSRs on healthier products, therefore increasing consumer reliance on other product labels and claims [62]. Additionally, in agreement with other research, our data show that discretionary foods can obtain HSR scores >2.5, potentially distracting from the consumption of foods from the five food groups and showing poor alignment with the Australian Dietary Guidelines [34–37,49]. Together, these findings provide strong evidence for revised labelling regulations, and increased education initiatives for consumers on how to interpret nutrition labels, to make informed purchasing decisions [14,54].

Though the number of NCC, health claims and buzzwords that HF snack products displayed did not correlate to a higher HSR, they may partly explain the higher price of HF products. The majority of HF snack products in some categories claimed to be vegan, organic, environmentally conscious or made 'good sugar' claims. Thus, in conjunction with (likely) smaller production, the cost of organic and alternative ingredients such as coconut oil, increased use of nuts, wheat and cane sugar alternatives are likely more expensive. However, the large price differences observed are not likely due to production costs alone. In addition, the price premium for purchasing HF products was not related to the HSR. Other research has reported similar findings, with foods labelled 'organic' found to have a similar nutrition profile but cost significantly more than those that are not [50,63,64]. This is of significance as the use of 'buzzwords', along with higher price points, have been found to strongly influence consumers and generate a misleading health halo effect [13,15,17,29,31,32,65]. Consumers should have the right to seek and pay a premium for ethical, organic and sustainable food options, though this should not be confused with purchasing healthier choices.

When interpreting these data, limitations must be considered. The study was limited to snack foods, and therefore did not assess all products found in HF stores and aisles, such as cereal products. However, the remaining products (excluding whole foods e.g., nuts) do represent most other products found in HF stores and HF aisles. Over 80% of the HSR for all products from all store types were derived using the HSRC [44]. Furthermore, some fibre values also had to be derived for HSR calculation. Despite the sensitivity analysis conducted, and a validated approach used by others [8,62], the derived values are only estimates and might differ from the true values. Additionally, several researchers have raised concerns regarding the HSRC to appropriately assess foods 'healthfulness' [34–37]; thus, the system is not without limitations. 'Buzzwords' regarding environmentally conscious claims were grouped within the overall results for interpretation but do not directly imply a product is healthier. Some values may also be skewed due to the placement of supermarket products. For example, gluten free sections are often contained within HF aisles; thus, our HF data contains both formulated gluten free product alternatives such as gluten free biscuits and other HF products simply marketed as gluten free along with other buzzwords. Thus, the marketing intent of the gluten free label may be different between products. Due to nutrition labelling regulations in Australia, added sugars were not distinguished from natural sugars. Future research could analyse the difference between added and natural sugars between these store types using other datasets. Finally, these data are a snapshot of products from the Sydney metropolitan area, across a certain time. Due to constant fluctuation in product availability and pricing, the packaged food supply may have changed at time of publication. However, with over 2000 products analysed, the study has provided a reliable sample, and thus comparison, of packaged snack foods in HF stores, HF aisles and regular aisles in 2019.

5. Conclusions

The main findings of this study revealed manufactures of HF snack products use substantially more NCC, health claims and 'buzzwords' to market their products compared to equivalent products sold in RA of supermarkets irrespective of their overall 'healthfulness', and may actually encourage the consumption of foods associated with increased health risks, misleading consumers. Although the nutrition profiles of HF snack products were marginally better than equivalent products found in RA, overall, the HF snack products examined in the study often received low HSR ≤ 2.5, with most being discretionary choices, a marked difference from the consumer perception and health halo surrounding

HF products. Health food snack products were also found to be substantially more expensive, but this was not consistent with the 'healthfulness' of a product. If consumers pay a premium for ethical, organic and sustainable foods, they should not be confused with purchasing foods that are healthier. Thus, the findings of this research provide strong evidence to support recommendations for revised labelling regulations, particularly surrounding HF snack products. Increased efforts to educate consumers on label reading are required to help consumers make informed and healthy choices.

Supplementary Materials: The following are available online at http://www.mdpi.com/2072-6643/12/5/1513/s1, Table S1. Product category and subcategory descriptions. Table S2. Product claim categories. Table S3. Comparative analysis of median unit cost ($/100g) between health food (HF) snack products sold in supermarkets and specialty HF stores compared to equivalent products sold in regular aisles (RA) of supermarkets.

Author Contributions: Conceptualization, M.B., H.J., A.R. and L.G.; Formal analysis, M.B. and H.J.; Investigation, M.B. and H.J.; Methodology, M.B., H.J., A.R. and L.G.; Supervision, A.R. and L.G.; Writing—original draft, M.B., H.J. and L.G.; Writing—review and editing, M.B., H.J., A.R. and L.G. All authors have read and agreed to the published version of the manuscript.

Funding: This research received no external financial funding.

Acknowledgments: The authors would like to thank Clare Chow and Angela Lau for their contribution in data collection.

Conflicts of Interest: The authors declare no conflict of interest.

References

1. Euromonitor International. Packaged Food in Australia. Available online: http://www.portal.euromonitor.com.ezproxy1.library.usyd.edu.au/portal/analysis/tab (accessed on 15 August 2019).
2. Watson, W.L.; Kury, A.; Wellard-Cole, L.; Hughes, C.; Dunford, E.K.; Chapman, K. Variations in serving sizes of Australian snack foods and confectionery. *Appetite* **2016**, *96*, 32–37. [CrossRef]
3. Poti, J.A.; Mendez, M.; Ng, S.W.; Popkin, B.M. Highly Processed and Ready-to-Eat Packaged Food and Beverage Purchases Differ by Race/Ethnicity among US Households. *J. Nutr.* **2016**, *146*, 1722–1730. [CrossRef] [PubMed]
4. Food Standards Australia New Zealand. *Safe Food Australia*; Food Standards Australia New Zealand: Canberra, Australia, 2001; p. 23.
5. Johnson, B.; Bell, L.K.; Zarnowiecki, D.; Rangan, A.; Golley, R.K. Contribution of Discretionary Foods and Drinks to Australian Children's Intake of Energy, Saturated Fat, Added Sugars and Salt. *Children* **2017**, *4*, 104. [CrossRef] [PubMed]
6. National Health and Medical Research Council. Australian Dietary Guidelines Summary. Available online: https://www.eatforhealth.gov.au/sites/default/files/content/The%20Guidelines/n55a_australian_dietary_guidelines_summary_131014_1.pdf (accessed on 15 August 2019).
7. Crino, M.; Sacks, G.; Dunford, E.K.; Trieu, K.; Webster, J.; Vandevijvere, S.; Swinburn, B.; Wu, J.H.Y.; Neal, B. Measuring the Healthiness of the Packaged Food Supply in Australia. *Nutrients* **2018**, *10*, 702. [CrossRef] [PubMed]
8. Bernstein, J.T.; Franco-Arellano, B.; Schermel, A.; Labonté, M.-E.; L'Abbé, M.R. Healthfulness and nutritional composition of Canadian prepackaged foods with and without sugar claims. *Appl. Physiol. Nutr. Metab.* **2017**, *42*, 1217–1224. [CrossRef] [PubMed]
9. World Health Organisation. *World Health Organization Global Action Plan for the Prevention and Control of Noncommunicable Diseases 2013–2020*; World Health Organisation: Geneva, Switzerland, 2013.
10. Vella, M.N.; Stratton, L.M.; Sheeshka, J.; Duncan, A.M. Functional food awareness and perceptions in relation to information sources in older adults. *Nutr. J.* **2014**, *13*, 44. [CrossRef] [PubMed]
11. Wu, J.H.Y.; Neal, B.; Trevena, H.; Crino, M.; Stuart-Smith, W.; Faulkner-Hogg, K.; Louie, J.C.Y.; Dunford, E. Are gluten-free foods healthier than non-gluten-free foods? An evaluation of supermarket products in Australia. *Br. J. Nutr.* **2015**, *114*, 448–454. [CrossRef] [PubMed]
12. Massey, M.; O'Cass, A.; Otahal, P. A meta-analytic study of the factors driving the purchase of organic food. *Appetite* **2018**, *125*, 418–427. [CrossRef]

13. Hoek, A.; Pearson, D.; James, S.; Lawrence, M.; Friel, S. Shrinking the food-print: A qualitative study into consumer perceptions, experiences and attitudes towards healthy and environmentally friendly food behaviours. *Appetite* **2017**, *108*, 117–131. [CrossRef]
14. Anastasiou, K.; Miller, M.D.; Dickinson, K. The relationship between food label use and dietary intake in adults: A systematic review. *Appetite* **2019**, *138*, 280–291. [CrossRef]
15. The Nielsen Company. *We Are What We Eat Healthy Eating Trends around the World*; The Nielsen Company: New York, NY, USA, 2015; pp. 3–26.
16. Definition of HEALTHY. Available online: https://www.merriam-webster.com/dictionary/healthy (accessed on 11 March 2019).
17. Lee, H.-J.; Yun, Z.-S. Consumers' perceptions of organic food attributes and cognitive and affective attitudes as determinants of their purchase intentions toward organic food. *Food Qual. Prefer.* **2015**, *39*, 259–267. [CrossRef]
18. Chapman, K.; Innes-Hughes, C.; Goldsbury, D.; Kelly, B.; Bauman, A.; Allman-Farinelli, M. A comparison of the cost of generic and branded food products in Australian supermarkets. *Public Health Nutr.* **2012**, *16*, 894–900. [CrossRef] [PubMed]
19. Chandon, P.; Wansink, B. The Biasing Health Halos of Fast-Food Restaurant Health Claims: Lower Calorie Estimates and Higher Side-Dish Consumption Intentions. *J. Consum. Res.* **2007**, *34*, 301–314. [CrossRef]
20. Bui, M.; Tangari, A.H.; Haws, K. Can health "halos" extend to food packaging? An investigation into food healthfulness perceptions and serving sizes on consumption decisions. *J. Bus. Res.* **2017**, *75*, 221–228. [CrossRef]
21. Talati, Z.; Norman, R.; Kelly, B.; Dixon, H.; Neal, B.; Miller, C.; Pettigrew, S. A randomized trial assessing the effects of health claims on choice of foods in the presence of front-of-pack labels. *Am. J. Clin. Nutr.* **2018**, *108*, 1275–1282. [CrossRef] [PubMed]
22. Fernan, C.; Schuldt, J.P.; Niederdeppe, J. Health Halo Effects from Product Titles and Nutrient Content Claims in the Context of "Protein" Bars. *Health Commun.* **2017**, *33*, 1425–1433. [CrossRef]
23. Iles, I.; Nan, X.; Verrill, L. Nutrient Content Claims: How They Impact Perceived Healthfulness of Fortified Snack Foods and the Moderating Effects of Nutrition Facts Labels. *Health Commun.* **2017**, *33*, 1308–1316. [CrossRef]
24. Machín, L.; Aschemann-Witzel, J.; Curutchet, M.R.; Giménez, A.; Ares, G. Traffic Light System Can Increase Healthfulness Perception: Implications for Policy Making. *J. Nutr. Educ. Behav.* **2018**, *50*, 668–674. [CrossRef]
25. Health Star Rating about Health Star Ratings. Available online: http://healthstarrating.gov.au/internet/healthstarrating/publishing.nsf/content/about-health-stars (accessed on 10 March 2019).
26. Huang, L.; Lu, J. The Impact of Package Color and the Nutrition Content Labels on the Perception of Food Healthiness and Purchase Intention. *J. Food Prod. Mark.* **2015**, *22*, 191–218. [CrossRef]
27. Kreuter, M.B.L.; Scharff, D.; Lukwago, S. Do Nutrition Label Readers Eat Healthier Diets? Behavioral Correlates of Adults' Use of Food Labels. *Am. J. Prev. Med.* **1997**, *13*, 277–283. [CrossRef]
28. Food Standards Australia New Zealand. Nutrition Content Claims and Health Claims. Available online: http://www.foodstandards.gov.au/consumer/labelling/nutrition/Pages/default.aspx (accessed on 18 August 2019).
29. Williams, S.L.; Mummery, K.W. Characteristics of consumers using 'better for you' front-of-pack food labelling schemes—An example from the Australian Heart Foundation Tick. *Public Health Nutr.* **2012**, *16*, 2265–2272. [CrossRef]
30. Schuldt, J.P. Does Green Mean Healthy? Nutrition Label Color Affects Perceptions of Healthfulness. *Health Commun.* **2013**, *28*, 814–821. [CrossRef]
31. Haws, K.; Reczek, R.W.; Sample, K.L. Healthy Diets Make Empty Wallets: The Healthy=Expensive Intuition. *J. Consum. Res.* **2017**, *43*, 992–1007. [CrossRef]
32. Sundar, A.; Kardes, F.R. The Role of Perceived Variability and the Health Halo Effect in Nutritional Inference and Consumption. *Psychol. Mark.* **2015**, *32*, 512–521. [CrossRef]
33. Hughes, C.; Wellard-Cole, L.; Lin, J.; Suen, K.L.; Chapman, K. Regulating health claims on food labels using nutrient profiling: What will the proposed standard mean in the Australian supermarket? *Public Health Nutr.* **2013**, *16*, 2154–2161. [CrossRef] [PubMed]
34. Dickie, S.; Woods, J.; Lawrence, M. Analysing the use of the Australian Health Star Rating system by level of food processing. *Int. J. Behav. Nutr. Phys. Act.* **2018**, *15*, 128. [CrossRef] [PubMed]
35. Lawrence, M.; Woods, J. Re: Jones et al., Nutrients 2018, 10, 501. *Nutrients* **2018**, *10*, 746. [CrossRef]

36. Lawrence, M.; Dickie, S.; Woods, J. Do Nutrient-Based Front-of-Pack Labelling Schemes Support or Undermine Food-Based Dietary Guideline Recommendations? Lessons from the Australian Health Star Rating System. *Nutrients* **2018**, *10*, 32. [CrossRef]
37. Jones, A.; Rädholm, K.; Neal, B. Defining 'Unhealthy': A Systematic Analysis of Alignment between the Australian Dietary Guidelines and the Health Star Rating System. *Nutrients* **2018**, *10*, 501. [CrossRef]
38. Nutrition and Health Claims. Available online: https://assets.publishing.service.gov.uk/government/uploads/system/uploads/attachment_data/file/204320/Nutrition_and_health_claims_guidance_November_2011.pdf (accessed on 11 March 2019).
39. Jones, G.; Richardson, M. An objective examination of consumer perception of nutrition information based on healthiness ratings and eye movements. *Public Health Nutr.* **2007**, *10*, 238–244. [CrossRef]
40. Gorton, D.; Ni Mhurchu, C.; Chen, M.-H.; Dixon, R. Nutrition labels: A survey of use, understanding and preferences among ethnically diverse shoppers in New Zealand. *Public Health Nutr.* **2009**, *12*, 1359–1365. [CrossRef] [PubMed]
41. Williams, P. Consumer Understanding and Use of Health Claims for Foods. *Nutr. Rev.* **2005**, *63*, 256–264. [CrossRef] [PubMed]
42. Ford, G.T.; Hastak, M.; Mitra, A.; Ringold, D.J. Can Consumers Interpret Nutrition Information in the Presence of a Health Claim? A Laboratory Investigation. *J. Public Policy Mark.* **1996**, *15*, 16–27. [CrossRef]
43. Rangan, A.; Tieleman, L.; Louie, J.C.Y.; Tang, L.M.; Hebden, L.; Roy, R.; Kay, J.; Allman-Farinelli, M. Electronic Dietary Intake Assessment (e-DIA): Relative validity of a mobile phone application to measure intake of food groups. *Br. J. Nutr.* **2016**, *115*, 2219–2226. [CrossRef] [PubMed]
44. Commonwealth of Australia. *Guide for Industry to the Health Star Rating Calculator (HSRC)*, 6th ed.; Commonwealth of Australia: Canberra, Australia. Available online: http://www.healthstarrating.gov.au/internet/healthstarrating/publishing.nsf/Content/guide-for-industry- (accessed on 18 August 2019).
45. Food Standards Australia New Zealand. *AUSNUT 2011–13 Food Nutrient Database*; Food Standards Australia New Zealand: Canberra, Australia, 2013.
46. Rodrigues, V.M.; Rayner, M.; Fernandes, A.C.; De Oliveira, R.C.; Proença, R.P.D.C.; Fiates, G.M. Comparison of the nutritional content of products, with and without nutrient claims, targeted at children in Brazil. *Br. J. Nutr.* **2016**, *115*, 2047–2056. [CrossRef] [PubMed]
47. Campos, S.; Doxey, J.; Hammond, D. Nutrition labels on pre-packaged foods: A systematic review. *Public Health Nutr.* **2011**, *14*, 1496–1506. [CrossRef]
48. Lambert, K.; Ficken, C. Cost and affordability of a nutritionally balanced gluten-free diet: Is following a gluten-free diet affordable? *Nutr. Diet.* **2015**, *73*, 36–42. [CrossRef]
49. Dunford, E.C.M.; Thomas, M.; Wu, J. *Technical Report: Alignment of NSW Health Food Provision Policy with the Health Star Ratings System*; NSW Ministry of Health: Sydney, Australia, 2015.
50. Dangour, A.D.; Lock, K.; Hayter, A.; Aikenhead, A.; Allen, E.; Uauy, R. Nutrition-related health effects of organic foods: A systematic review. *Am. J. Clin. Nutr.* **2010**, *92*, 203–210. [CrossRef]
51. Food Standards Australia New Zealand. *Australia New Zealand Food Standards Code—Standard 1.2.7—Nutrition, Health and Related Claims*; Food Standards Australia New Zealand: Canberra, Australia, 2018.
52. Ni Mhurchu, C.; Gorton, D. Nutrition labels and claims in New Zealand and Australia: A review of use and understanding. *Aust. N. Z. J. Public Health* **2007**, *31*, 105–112. [CrossRef]
53. Harris, J.L.; Thompson, J.M.; Schwartz, M.B.; Brownell, K.D. Nutrition-related claims on children's cereals: What do they mean to parents and do they influence willingness to buy? *Public Health Nutr.* **2011**, *14*, 2207–2212. [CrossRef]
54. Food Standards Australia New Zealand. *A Qualitative Consumer Study Related to Nutrition Content Claims on Food Labels*; Food Standards Australia New Zealand: Canberra, Australia, 2003.
55. Talati, Z.; Pettigrew, S.; Kelly, B.; Ball, K.; Dixon, H.; Shilton, T. Consumers' responses to front-of-pack labels that vary by interpretive content. *Appetite* **2016**, *101*, 205–213. [CrossRef] [PubMed]
56. Maubach, N.; Hoek, J.; Mather, D. Interpretive front-of-pack nutrition labels. Comparing competing recommendations. *Appetite* **2014**, *82*, 67–77. [CrossRef] [PubMed]
57. Hamlin, R.; McNeill, L.; Moore, V. The impact of front-of-pack nutrition labels on consumer product evaluation and choice: An experimental study. *Public Health Nutr.* **2014**, *18*, 2126–2134. [CrossRef] [PubMed]

58. Roberto, C.A.; Bragg, M.A.; Seamans, M.J.; Mechulan, R.L.; Novak, N.; Brownell, K.D. Evaluation of Consumer Understanding of Different Front-of-Package Nutrition Labels, 2010–2011. *Prev. Chronic Dis.* **2012**, *9*. [CrossRef] [PubMed]
59. Talati, Z.; Pettigrew, S.; Dixon, H.; Neal, B.; Ball, K.; Hughes, C. Do Health Claims and Front-of-Pack Labels Lead to a Positivity Bias in Unhealthy Foods? *Nutrients* **2016**, *8*, 787. [CrossRef]
60. Basha, M.B.; Mason, C.; Shamsudin, M.F.; Hussain, H.I.; Taheri, S. Consumers Attitude Towards Organic Food. *Procedia Econ. Financ.* **2015**, *31*, 444–452. [CrossRef]
61. Hamlin, R.; McNeill, L. Does the Australasian "Health Star Rating" Front of Pack Nutritional Label System Work? *Nutrients* **2016**, *8*, 327. [CrossRef]
62. Kim, D.H.; Liu, W.G.A.; Rangan, A.; Gemming, L. A comparison of the Health Star Rating and nutrient profiles of branded and generic food products in Sydney supermarkets, Australia. *Public Health Nutr.* **2019**, *22*, 2132–2139. [CrossRef]
63. Smith-Spangler, C.M.; Brandeau, M.L.; Hunter, G.E.; Bavinger, J.; Pearson, M.; Eschbach, P.J.; Sundaram, V.; Liu, H.; Schirmer, P.; Stave, C.; et al. Are Organic Foods Safer or Healthier Than Conventional Alternatives? *Ann Intern. Med.* **2012**, *157*, 348. [CrossRef]
64. Kriwy, P.; Mecking, R.-A. Health and environmental consciousness, costs of behaviour and the purchase of organic food. *Int. J. Consum. Stud.* **2011**, *36*, 30–37. [CrossRef]
65. Román, S.; Sanchez-Siles, L.M.; Siegrist, M. The importance of food naturalness for consumers: Results of a systematic review. *Trends Food Sci. Technol.* **2017**, *67*, 44–57. [CrossRef]

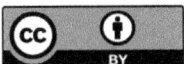 © 2020 by the authors. Licensee MDPI, Basel, Switzerland. This article is an open access article distributed under the terms and conditions of the Creative Commons Attribution (CC BY) license (http://creativecommons.org/licenses/by/4.0/).

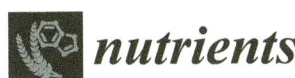

Article

The Nutritional Quality of Organic and Conventional Food Products Sold in Italy: Results from the Food Labelling of Italian Products (FLIP) Study

Margherita Dall'Asta [1,†], **Donato Angelino** [2,†], **Nicoletta Pellegrini** [3,*] and **Daniela Martini** [4,‡]

1. Department of Animal Science, Food and Nutrition, Università Cattolica del Sacro Cuore, 29122 Piacenza, Italy; margherita.dallasta@unicatt.it
2. Faculty of Bioscience and Technology for Food, Agriculture and Environment, University of Teramo, 64100 Teramo, Italy; dangelino@unite.it
3. Department of Agricultural, Food, Environmental and Animal Sciences, University of Udine, 33100 Udine, Italy
4. Department of Food, Environmental and Nutritional Sciences (DeFENS), Università degli Studi di Milano, 20133 Milan, Italy; daniela.martini@unimi.it
* Correspondence: nicoletta.pellegrini@uniud.it; Tel.: +39-0432-558183
† These authors contributed equally to this work.
‡ On behalf of the SINU Young Working Group are listed in Appendix A (Table A1).

Received: 18 March 2020; Accepted: 27 April 2020; Published: 30 April 2020

Abstract: The market for organic products is growing rapidly, probably attributable to the general customer perception that they are healthier foods, with a better nutritional profile than conventional ones. Despite this, the available studies show limited differences in the nutrient profile of organically and conventionally primary food products. Apart from this literature, no studies have focused on the nutrition profile of commercially prepacked foods. Thus, the aim of the present survey was to compare the nutritional quality intended as nutrition facts of organic and conventional prepacked foods sold in Italy. A total of 569 pairs of prepacked products (organic and their conventional counterparts) were selected from nine food categories sold by online retailers. By comparing organic and conventional products in the "pasta, rice and other cereals" category, the former were lower in energy, protein, and higher in saturates compared to the latter. Organic "jams, chocolate spreads and honey" products were lower in energy, carbohydrates, sugars and higher in protein than their regular counterparts. No differences were found for energy, macronutrients and salt for other categories. Therefore, based on the mandatory information printed on their packaging, prepacked organic products are not of a superior nutritional quality than conventional ones, with just a few exceptions. Consequently, the present study suggests that organic certification cannot be considered an indication of better overall nutritional quality. Further studies examining the nutritional quality of organic foods, taking into account the ingredients used, might better explain the results obtained.

Keywords: organic food; food labeling; nutrition facts; nutritional quality

1. Introduction

Organic production has become increasingly important worldwide, as a potential alternative to conventional intensive agriculture, due to great concerns about the environment, food safety, and human health [1–3]. In developed countries, demand for organic products is steadily rising and a relevant proportion of food consumed comes from organic sources [4]. Undoubtedly, the increase in production and consumption of organic foods is one of the major market trends of recent years [5].

Following the U.S., in 2017, the European organic food market was the second largest in the world in terms of sales with most of the organic food retailers mainly located in Germany, France and Italy [5]. In particular, a recent survey performed in Italy confirmed that the value of sales of the organic foods follows a positive trend [6].

As stated in Council Regulation (EC) No 834/2007 [7], organic products can be defined as food products deriving from "organic production", which means the use of the production method compliant with the rules established in the European Regulation, at all stages of production, preparation and distribution. Organic production must be based on the appropriate design and management of biological processes based on ecological systems using natural resources while restricting the use of external inputs [7].

Considering the definition and the principles of organic production, the consumption of organic foods may reduce exposure to nitrate and pesticide residues due to the strict limitation of the use of chemically synthesized inputs [3,8]. However, the significance of these differences is questionable, because actual levels of contamination in organic and conventional foods are generally well below acceptable limits [9] and in general the proximity to sources of contamination (e.g., traffic, chemical industries) seems to have a crucial role in the occurrence of environmental pollutants in foodstuffs [10]. This may partially explain why evidence on the association between the consumption of organic foods and the risk of developing chronic diseases is generally weak [11,12].

Conversely, the definition given by Council Regulation (EC) No 834/2007 [7] does not include any mention of possible differences in terms of the nutritional quality and healthiness of organic and conventional products. Despite this, evidence suggests that people tend to perceive organic foods as healthier than standard, non-organic foods [13–15], with healthiness primarily understood as nutritional value [16,17]. This is probably due to the so called "health halo effect", which induces the consumer to overestimate the healthfulness of a food with a specific attribute [18]. For instance, compared to conventional products, organic foods are perceived as of lower calorific value and more palatable to consumers who also generally show more intention to pay for organic products [13,15,19–21].

In this scenario, several studies have investigated the possible differences between several categories of organic and conventional foods [22,23], including fruit and vegetables [24,25], meat [26], milk [27] and dairy foods [28]. Only small differences in nutrient content between organic and conventional products have been evidenced, mostly related to differences in production methods [22]. For instance, different agricultural managements have been shown to play a role on the polyphenol content in vegetables, plausibly because a higher polyphenolic content is observed when less nitrogen fertilizer is added to the soil [29]. However, no conclusive data have clearly evidenced neither a higher nutritional quality of organic products when compared with the conventional alternatives [22,30], nor nutrition-related health effects for organic products [31]. However, most of the studies have been focused on the nutritional quality of primary products. Conversely, the possible differences between processed and prepacked organic and conventional products have been barely investigated.

Based on these premises, the aim of the present study was to investigate and compare the nutritional quality of pairs of organic and conventional prepacked foods currently sold in Italy with the same brand name, by collecting the nutritional data on their packaging. This study was performed as part of the Food Labelling of Italian Products (FLIP) Study that aims at systematically investigating the overall quality of prepacked foods sold on the Italian market.

2. Materials and Methods

2.1. Data Collection

The online search for information was conducted from January 2019 until July 2019 on the home-shopping website of the major retailers present on the Italian market (Auchan, Bennet, Carrefour, Conad, Coop Italia, Crai, Despar, Esselunga, Il Gigante, Iper, Pam Panorama, Selex, Sidis).

The systematic search was performed by specifically focusing on the selection of all potential pairs of products (organic and conventional) of the same brand considered if available in at least one online shop. We included all the prepacked foods (regardless of the level of processing) for which, as stated in the Council Regulation (EC) no. 1169/2011 [32], mandatory food information shall appear directly on the package or on a label attached thereto. Products were considered eligible as organic food if the Community logo referred to in Article 25(1) Regulation 834/2007 [7] as regards pre-packaged food was present on the packaging.

The exclusion criteria for product selection were: (i) not prepacked; (ii) organic foods with no conventional counterparts of the same brand; (iii) incomplete images of all the sides of the pack; (iv) unclear images of nutrition declaration or list of ingredients; (v) nine products that were marked as "product currently unavailable" in all the online stores which were selected throughout the data collection period.

2.2. Data Extraction

Data from the complete images of all the sides of the pack were collected for all the selected products. For each food item, as previously described [33], the quali-quantitative and specifically regulated (mandatory) information was documented: company name, brand name, descriptive name, energy (kcal/100 g or 100 mL), total fat (g/100 g or 100 mL), saturates (g/100 g or 100 mL), carbohydrate (g/100 g or 100 mL), sugars (g/100 g or 100 mL), protein (g/100 g or 100 mL), and salt (g/100 g or 100 mL). Moreover, the number of nutrition claims (NC) as listed in the Council Regulation (EC) No 1924/2006 [34] was collected.

Data were extracted once (by DM) but the accuracy of the extracted data was double-checked by two researchers (MDA, DA) and inaccuracies were resolved through secondary extractions made by a third researcher (DM).

A dataset was created with all the collected data and items were sub-grouped for specific comparisons by considering the descriptive name reported and the presence/absence of organic declaration. Based on the descriptive name, the food items were classified in the following categories: (i) sweet cereal-based foods; (ii) bread and substitutes; (iii) pasta, rice and other cereals; (iv) milk, dairy foods and plant based-drinks; (v) fruit juices, nectars and iced teas; (vi) jams, chocolate spreads and honey; (vii) fruit and vegetable-based foods; (viii) legumes; (ix) oils, fats and dressings.

2.3. Statistical Analysis

Statistical analysis was carried out using IBM SPSS Statistics® (Version 25.0, IBM corp., Chicago, IL, USA) and performed at $p < 0.05$ of significance level. The normality of data distribution was firstly verified through the Kolmogorov-Smirnov test and rejected. Therefore, variables were expressed as median (interquartile range). Data of energy and nutrient contents per 100 grams or 100 mL of products for each item were analyzed with the Mann-Whitney non-parametric test for two independent samples (for differences between organic and conventional products).

3. Results

3.1. Number and Categories of Products

A total of 569 pairs of products were selected through the online store search. The number and the type of pair items for each category is reported in Table 1. The largest category was "milk, dairy foods and plant based-drinks" ($n = 123$), of which 74% of the items were yogurts and cheese. The second largest category was "pasta, rice and other cereals" one ($n = 104$ pairs), while the smallest ones were "bread and substitutes" ($n = 42$) and "sweet cereal based-foods" ($n = 28$). The number of organic and conventional products with at least one NC was also analyzed. Overall, the number of items with an NC was relatively similar for all categories of organic and their conventional counterparts, except for "pasta, rice and other cereals", which had a greater number of products with claims for organic products ($n = 60$) than for non-organic ones ($n = 7$).

Table 1. Categories, total number of pairs, subcategories of products considered within each category and number of organic and conventional products with at least a Nutrition Claim (NC).

Category	Number of Pairs	Subcategories (Number of Pairs)	Number of Products with at Least a NC (Organic/Conventional)
Sweet cereal based-foods	28	Cookies (13), breakfast cereals (9), snacks (6)	8/13
Bread and substitutes	42	Wraps (11), crackers (10), breadsticks (9), bread (6), rusks (6)	12/10
Pasta, rice and other cereals	104	Pasta (77), rice and other cereals (12), wheat flour (12), gnocchi (3)	60/7
Milk, dairy foods and plant-based drinks	123	Yogurt (46), cheese (45), milk (27), plant-based drinks (5)	19/22
Fruit juices, nectars and iced teas	54	Fruit juices and nectars (52), iced teas (2)	7/12
Jams, chocolate spreads and honey	61	Jam and jelly (44), honey (14), chocolate spreads (3)	0/0
Fruit and vegetable-based foods	51	Tomato-based sauces (21), dried fruit (15), frozen vegetables (15)	6/2
Legumes	55	Dry legumes (21), canned and frozen legumes (34)	12/16
Oils, fats and dressings	51	Olive oil, other vegetable oils (32), animal fats and margarine (10), vinegar (9)	12/14

3.2. Nutritional Comparison Among Organic and Conventional Products

The mandatory nutrition information indicated by Council Regulation (EU) no. 1169/2011 [32], across the considered categories of products, is reported in Table 2. Overall, results showed that there are slight differences in terms of nutritional quality between the organic and their conventional counterparts, with only significant differences for two out of the nine food categories investigated. Concerning the "pasta, rice and other cereals" category, the data show a slightly, but significant, lower median of energy of organic products ($p < 0.001$) compared to the conventional ones. These results may be explained by the significantly higher median protein content in this conventional food category compared to the organic one. Conversely, in the organic "pasta, rice and other cereals" category, a significantly higher saturates median value was found compared to conventional products ($p = 0.007$). More appreciable differences were found for the category "jams, chocolate spreads and honey", where organic products, compared with their conventional counterparts, were characterized by a lower ($p < 0.001$) median of energy, total carbohydrates and sugars. On the contrary, in this category, a significantly higher median protein content was found in organic products compared conventional ones ($p = 0.002$). The statistical significant differences observed in the categories "pasta, rice and other cereals" and "jams, chocolate spreads and honey" may be attributable to significant differences in the subcategories "pasta" (Figure 1) and "jam and jelly" (Figure 2), respectively. No other differences were found for other categories, including "Sweet cereal based-foods", "Bread and substitutes", "Milk, dairy foods and plant-based drinks", "Fruit juices, nectars and iced teas", "Fruit and vegetable-based products, "Legumes", and "Oils, fats and dressings".

Table 2. Energy, macronutrients, and salt across the considered categories.

Category		Number of Items	Energy kcal/100 g or 100 mL	Total Fat g/100 g or 100 mL	Saturates g/100 g or 100 mL	Total Carbohydrates g/100 g or 100 mL	Sugars g/100 g or 100 mL	Protein g/100 g or 100 mL	Salt g/100 g or 100 mL
Sweet cereal based-foods	Total	56	419 (377–455)	14.0 (2.4–17.0)	2.3 (0.8–4.1)	65.5 (61.9–76.9)	21.3 (17.0–30.0)	7.8 (6.8–8.5)	0.6 (0.5–0.8)
	Conventional	28	419 (375–453)	14.0 (2.4–16.9)	2.2 (0.6–3.5)	67.4 (63.0–76.9)	23.0 (19.5–31.0)	7.3 (6.5–8.0)	0.6 (0.5–0.8)
	Organic	28	421 (380–455)	14.0 (2.4–17.0)	2.3 (1.1–5.1)	64.6 (60.5–78.3)	21.0 (16.5–27.4)	8.0 (7.2–8.8)	0.6 (0.3–0.9)
Bread and substitutes	Total	84	401 (305–427)	9.4 (6.2–12.0)	1.5 (0.8–2.0)	61.7 (47.1–68.0)	2.0 (1.6–3.5)	10.7 (8.2–12.3)	1.6 (1.3–1.9)
	Conventional	42	408 (303–429)	8.6 (6.5–11.5)	1.4 (1.0–2.4)	63.1 (47.1–69.9)	2.0 (1.5–4.0)	10.0 (8.1–12.0)	1.7 (1.3–1.8)
	Organic	42	395 (306–426)	9.6 (5.8–12.0)	1.7 (0.8–2.0)	59.5 (46.0–67.0)	2.0 (1.6–3.0)	11.4 (8.5–12.5)	1.5 (1.3–2.0)
Pasta, rice and other cereals	Total	208	351 (346–356)	1.5 (1.3–1.7)	0.3 (0.3–0.5)	71.0 (67.5–73.0)	2.9 (1.6–3.2)	12.0 (11.0–12.7)	0.0 (0.0–0.0)
	Conventional	104	354 (348–358)a	1.5 (1.3–1.5)	0.3 (0.3–0.4)b	71.5 (69.2–73.1)	2.9 (1.4–3.2)	12.5 (11.0–13.0)a	0.0 (0.0–0.0)
	Organic	104	350 (346–354)b	1.5 (1.2–1.9)	0.3 (0.3–0.5)a	71.0 (66.6–72.5)	2.9 (1.7–3.2)	11.0 (11.0–12.0)b	0.0 (0.0–0.0)
Milk, dairy foods and plant-based drinks	Total	246	100 (65–238)	3.7 (3.0–19.0)	2.6 (2.0–13.0)	4.8 (2.1–5.6)	4.6 (1.7–5.1)	3.7 (3.3–12.0)	0.1 (0.1–0.6)
	Conventional	123	100 (65–236)	3.6 (3.0–19.0)	2.6 (2.0–13.0)	4.9 (2.3–5.6)	4.8 (1.7–5.1)	3.7 (3.3–12.0)	0.1 (0.1–0.6)
	Organic	123	101 (64–240)	3.7 (2.3–19.0)	2.6 (1.2–13.0)	4.8 (2.1–5.6)	4.5 (1.7–5.1)	3.8 (3.2–13.0)	0.1 (0.1–0.6)
Fruit juices, nectars and iced teas	Total	108	57 (49–59)	0.0 (0.0–0.0)	0.0 (0.0–0.0)	13.3 (11.4–14.0)	13.0 (10.2–14.0)	0.2 (0.0–0.4)	0.1 (0.0–0.1)
	Conventional	54	57 (51–60)	0.0 (0.0–0.1)	0.0 (0.0–0.0)	13.7 (11.6–14.2)	13.2 (10.2–14.0)	0.2 (0.0–0.4)	0.0 (0.0–0.0)
	Organic	54	56 (47–59)	0.0 (0.0–0.0)	0.0 (0.0–0.0)	13.1 (11.2–14.0)	13.0 (11.2–13.7)	0.2 (0.1–0.4)	0.0 (0.0–0.0)
Jams, chocolate spreads and honey	Total	122	190 (168–320)	0.0 (0.0–0.2)	0.0 (0.0–0.0)	45.0 (40.0–60.0)	44.0 (37.0–59.0)	0.4 (0.0–0.6)	0.1 (0.0–0.1)
	Conventional	61	206 (187–320)a	0.0 (0.0–0.1)	0.0 (0.0–0.0)	50.0 (45.0–60.0)a	50.0 (43.0–59.0)a	0.4 (0.0–0.5)b	0.1 (0.0–0.1)
	Organic	61	168 (160–320)b	0.0 (0.0–0.3)	0.0 (0.0–0.0)	40.0 (38.0–59.0)b	37.0 (35.0–56.0)b	0.5 (0.3–0.6)a	0.1 (0.0–0.1)
Fruit and vegetable-based products	Total	102	54 (30–352)	0.5 (0.1–32)	0.1 (0.0–3.8)	6.0 (4.2–8.8)	3.8 (2.2–4.5)	2.5 (1.4–4.8)	0.1 (0.0–0.3)
	Conventional	51	53 (30–352)	0.5 (0.1–32.0)	0.1 (0.0–3.8)	6.0 (4.1–9.2)	3.9 (2.4–4.5)	2.7 (1.4–4.9)	0.1 (0.0–0.4)
	Organic	51	55 (30–429)	0.5 (0.1–41.0)	0.1 (0.0–4.6)	6.0 (4.2–8.7)	3.7 (1.6–4.5)	2.4 (1.3–4.7)	0.0 (0.0–0.3)
Legumes	Total	110	106 (87–310)	1.0 (0.5–1.9)	0.1 (0.1–0.3)	15.4 (12.2–44.0)	1.1 (0.6–2.6)	6.9 (5.5–20.1)	0.6 (0.0–0.8)
	Conventional	55	124 (89–323)	1.0 (0.5–1.9)	0.2 (0.1–0.3)	16.2 (13.2–44.8)	0.8 (0.6–2.6)	7.0 (5.6–20.9)	0.7 (0.0–1.0)
	Organic	55	97 (87–304)	0.9 (0.4–2.0)	0.1 (0.1–0.3)	14.2 (12.0–42.8)	1.2 (0.5–2.5)	6.9 (5.6–20.8)	0.6 (0.0–0.8)
Oils, fats and dressings	Total	102	822 (747–824)	91.5 (83.0–91.8)	13.7 (11.0–15.2)	0.0 (0.0–0.1)	0.0 (0.0–0.1)	0.0 (0.0–0.1)	0.0 (0.0–0.0)
	Conventional	51	822 (751–824)	91.3 (83.0–92.0)	13.5 (11.0–15.2)	0.0 (0.0–0.1)	0.0 (0.0–0.1)	0.0 (0.0–0.1)	0.0 (0.0–0.0)
	Organic	51	823 (739–824)	91.6 (82.0–91.8)	14.0 (11.0–15.2)	0.0 (0.0–0.1)	0.0 (0.0–0.1)	0.0 (0.0–0.1)	0.0 (0.0–0.0)

Values are expressed as median (25th–75th percentile). For each category, different letters in the same column indicate significant differences among conventional and organic products (Mann–Whitney non-parametric test for two independent samples). $p < 0.05$.

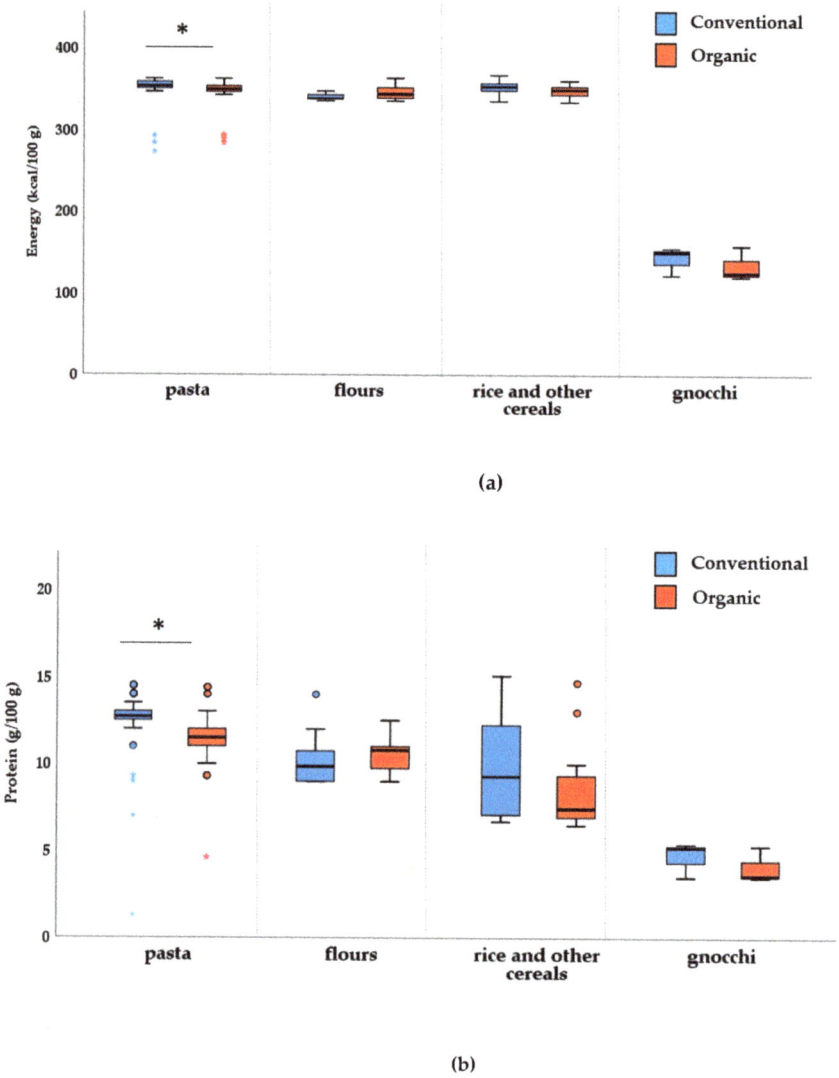

Figure 1. Box plot for energy (kcal/100 g) (**a**) and protein (g/100 g) (**b**) of "pasta, rice and other cereals" category. * $p < 0.05$, Mann–Whitney non-parametric test for two independent samples.

To better evaluate the nutritional quality of both organic and non-organic paired products within the different categories, data related to the single types belonging to the nine categories are reported in Supplementary Table S1. Organic pasta products presented significantly lower median energy ($p < 0.001$) and significantly lower amounts of carbohydrates ($p = 0.001$) than in conventional pasta. Moreover, saturates were present in significantly lower amounts in non-organic products than organic ones ($p = 0.003$). Protein displayed significantly higher in non-organic pasta than organic pasta products ($p < 0.001$); on the contrary, a lower median salt amount was found in organic pasta compared to non-organic ones ($p = 0.049$). By analyzing the type of nutrition claim for "pasta" subcategory, 53 organic items out of the 77 pairs of products presented the claim related to fiber content, while only two items were present in regular counterparts. Within the same category of products, organic flours differed from the regular ones only for the higher amount of sugar content ($p = 0.012$).

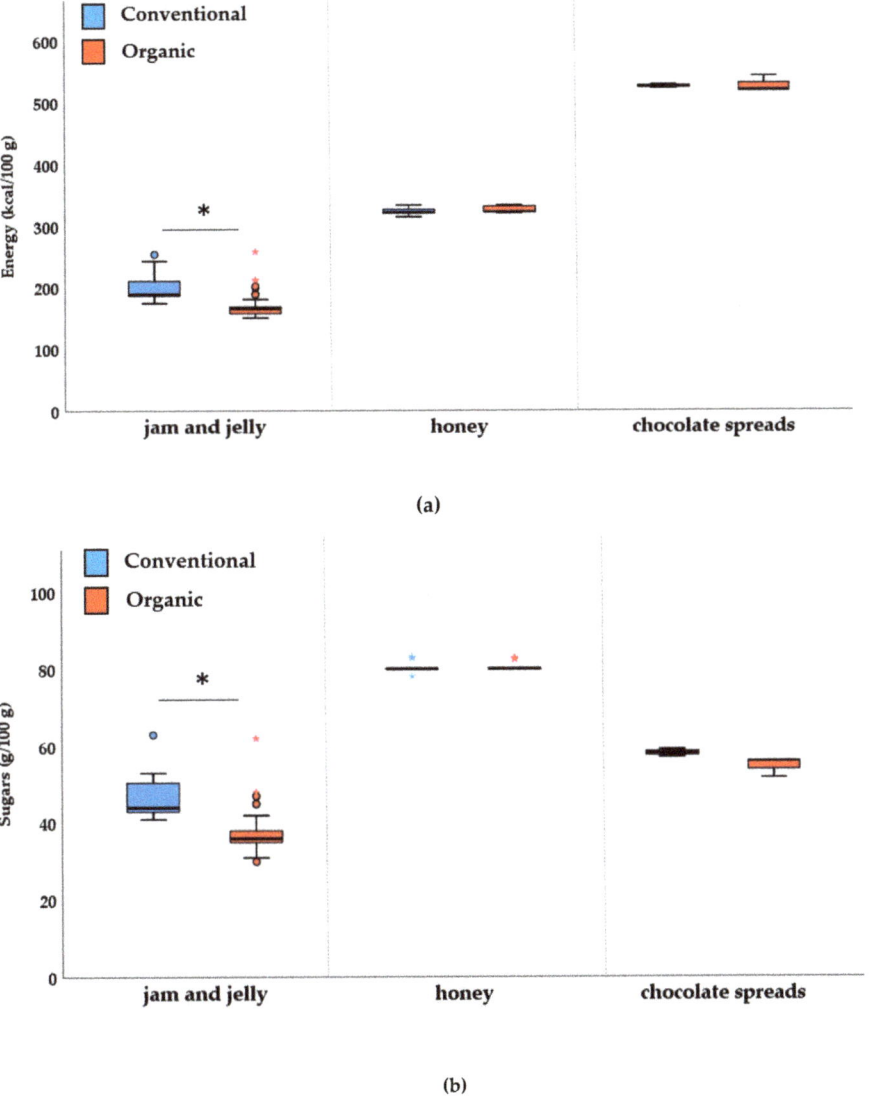

Figure 2. Box plot for energy (kcal/100 g) (**a**) and sugars (g/100 g) (**b**) of "jams, chocolate spreads and honey" category. * $p < 0.05$, Mann–Whitney non-parametric test for two independent samples.

Organic jam and jelly presented a significantly lower median value energy than conventional products ($p < 0.001$). Total carbohydrates, almost totally represented by sugars, were significantly higher in non-organic jam and jelly items compared to organic ones ($p < 0.001$ as for total carbohydrates and sugars). Finally, protein were lower in conventional products than in organic counterparts ($p = 0.011$).

Among bread and substitutes, organic wraps were higher in sugars ($p = 0.010$), but lower in salt ($p = 0.002$) than conventional ones. On the contrary, organic crackers were lower in sugars than non-organic ones ($p = 0.023$).

Organic yogurts were slightly higher in salt than conventional ones ($p < 0.001$). Interestingly, organic plant based-drinks had significantly lower median energy values than conventional ones ($p = 0.016$) mainly attributable to their significantly lower amount total carbohydrates ($p = 0.008$) and sugars ($p = 0.016$) than non-organic products.

4. Discussion

To our knowledge, this is the first study to provide a snapshot of the nutritional quality of organic prepacked products sold on the home-shopping website of the major retailers present on the Italian market, by selecting pairs of products (organic and conventional ones) of the same brand present in at least one shop and considering the legally required data regarding nutritional content, printed on the packaging. There are two main reasons why only organic products for which a non-organic counterpart is available from the same brand were chosen. Firstly, although this inclusion criterion might have lowered the number of products screened, it avoids the weakness of the statistical comparison of data from categories with substantial differences in terms of number of organic and non-organic items. Furthermore, this approach may allow us to take into account the relevant role of a brand in customers' intention-to-buy. In fact, it has been ascertained that consumers tend to perceive the brand as "a first sign of quality" and then to consider other evaluation criteria [35].

The results obtained from 569 pairs of items indicated an overall comparable nutritional profile of the two alternatives. Only two out of the nine analyzed categories presented statistically significant differences, based on both energy and nutritional content. Organic "pasta, rice and other cereals" had a lower energy density and protein content in 100 g of the product than the conventional alternatives. Moreover, a higher amount of saturates was evidenced for organic products than regular ones within such a category, even if this difference can be considered of marginal nutritional significance due to the generally low amount of saturates in these types of products. Within this category, the subcategory "pasta" had most likely contributed to these significant differences. This might be due to the fact that organic pasta had a higher number of products with a nutrition claim related to the fiber content compared to conventional ones and this may in turn influence the content of the other analyzed nutrients. Furthermore, the lower energy, carbohydrate and sugar contents observed in organic "jams, chocolate spreads and honey" may be attributed to significant nutrient changes observed in the subcategory "jam and jelly". In this case, differences cannot be explained by the presence of several nutrition claims, because no claims were found neither among organic nor among conventional items.

Although no significant differences were found for other food categories, further analysis of subcategories showed some interesting differences. The most remarkable difference was the higher sugar content in conventional plant-based drinks compared to organic alternatives. However, on the whole, organic foods do not seem to be of a higher nutritional quality than conventional foods from the same brand.

The focus of this research was to investigate the nutritional quality of products, which is not only the result of the organic production methods applied in the food chain, but depends also on the ingredients selected for the product formulation. For this reason, a comparison of the results obtained in the present survey with previous studies appears tricky, since the majority of the studies focused on components that were not considered in the present survey. Indeed, previous literature suggested that there were differences in the nutritional profile of organic products and non-organic ones, particularly for polyunsaturated fatty acids, vitamins, minerals, and bioactive compounds, such as polyphenols [23,27,36–39], although the information available is not exhaustive. Therefore, it is not to be excluded that the products considered in the present survey could present different amounts of some components, i.e., bioactive compounds or micronutrients, but this was out of the scope of this study, which only focused on the mandatory information to be included in the nutrition declaration compliant to Regulation (EC) 1169/2011 [32].

Only few studies reported the nutritional quality of organic prepacked foods compared to conventional counterparts. For instance, sugar content in German breakfast cereals, both generic and specific for children, was significantly lower in organic products than in the conventional ones [40]. In contrast, another study conducted in the U.S. investigating the nutritional quality of ready-to-eat breakfast cereals did not support the higher nutritional value of the organic products in comparison with conventional ones, when taking into account macronutrients and micronutrients and bioactive compounds [41]. Interestingly, in a study performed in the UK, organic yogurts were compared to all the other types of yogurts, and they showed to be higher in sugar content compared to the other types, except for desserts [42]. Finally, a study analyzing the front-of-pack declarations and the critical nutrients (free sugar, total fats, saturated fats, trans fat, and sodium) of a wide range of products sold in Brazil showed that products presenting claims related to environment, such as "organic", were more unlikely to present high content of such nutrients [43].

Therefore, the evidence to date cannot support the view that organic products have a higher nutritional quality than conventional ones, also because studies concerning the health effects of organic foods in humans are still scarce and sometimes inconclusive [2,11,44–46]. Apart from the direct effects attributed to organic products, it is noteworthy that other factors may play a role in defining the beneficial effect of consuming organic products. Interestingly, there is evidence that people who purchase organic foods generally have a healthier lifestyle, including a healthier diet, than those who don't buy them, thus potentially reducing the risk of several major diseases, independently of the potential additional health effects brought by organic foods [47–49]. Indeed, comparisons of diets containing organic and non-organic foods have been challenged because consumers of organic food most frequently maintain a healthy lifestyle [2]. For these reasons, there is still insufficient evidence to recommend organic over conventional products [25], at least from a nutritional point of view.

This study has some limitations worth highlighting. The first is in regards to the methodology of product selection, as it did not include other retail outlets, such as discount warehouses, which would be worthy of future investigation. Secondly, the present study focused on the evaluation of nutritional quality based only on mandatory information, which does not include other nutritional components, such as fiber, vitamins, minerals and bioactive compounds. Moreover, it is important to note that, considering the Regulation 1169/2011 [32], nutrition declaration can be formulated either from direct analysis of food or from data extrapolated from reference databases of food composition, which do not take into account potential differences between organic and non-organic ingredients. Another limitation is the low number of pairs for some sub-categories that may have limited the statistical significance of some results. Finally, some of the major brands of either organic or conventional products do not produce the counterparts and therefore have not been considered in the present survey. Thus, comparing the nutritional quality of all organic foods to all conventional foods would provide a valuable addition to the findings of the present study. However, it is worth remarking that the aim of the study was to compare items of the same brand, which can be considered a strength of the study. In this way, the brand name cannot act as a possible cause of bias in the results because it represents one of the most relevant factors driving the consumer's intention to buy at the time of purchase. Another strength of the present work belongs to the fact that the studies covered several categories and subcategories of products, leading to a high number of pairs selected for the study. Moreover, collecting information from online shops results the best way to ensure that the study covers the majority of products sold by the same brand, for which both the conventional and organic alternatives exist.

The present work was conceived in the frame of the Food Labelling of Italian Products (FLIP) project, which primarily focused on systematically evaluating the nutritional quality of commercial foods sold on the Italian market, and specifically took into account the different declarations present on the packaging. As for the other declarations present on the packaging (e.g., nutrition and health claims), the presence of organic certification on the food pack seems to not be indicative of the overall quality of the products.

5. Conclusions

Based on the mandatory information reported on the packaging, this original survey indicated that, with few exceptions, organic labelled prepacked products sold in Italy were not characterized by a better nutritional profile than conventional ones. Consequently, the "organic" claim should not be interpreted by consumers as proxy of "healthier" food than regular food. However, future studies are needed to broaden the analysis to other food groups not considered within the present survey. Certainly, there is the need to better investigate the nutritional quality of the single ingredients (i.e., types and amount) used for the formulation of organic products, which might sometimes be formulated taking into account the healthier perception of organic products by consumers. Moreover, further research could be aimed at analyzing data by considering the type of producers of organic/non-organic products (i.e., transnational food companies versus small companies).

Supplementary Materials: The following are available online at http://www.mdpi.com/2072-6643/12/5/1273/s1: Table S1: Energy, macronutrients, and salt for all the types of products analyzed.

Author Contributions: M.D., D.A. and D.M. were involved in the protocol design, data analyses, interpretation of results, and drafted the manuscript; N.P. participated in the protocol design and critically reviewed the manuscript; D.M. conceived the study, supervised the data collection, and had primary responsibility for the final content. Other members of the Italian Society of Human Nutrition (SINU) Young Working Group were involved in the data analysis. All authors have read and agreed to the published version of the manuscript.

Funding: This research received no external funding.

Acknowledgments: The authors wish to thank all students who participated to the development of the dataset.

Conflicts of Interest: The present publication has been conceived within the Italian Society of Human Nutrition (SINU) Young Group, and it has been made without any funding from food industries or other entities. The authors declare no conflict of interest.

Finally: In this context, there remains a strong need to define the real impact of organic production on the nutritional quality of ingredients with well-designed studies, taking also into account the potential impact of the formulation of processed foods on nutrient quality and quantity.

Appendix A

Table A1. SINU Young Working Group.

Name	Affiliation
Marika Dello Russo	Institute of Food Sciences, National Research Council, Avellino, Italy
Stefania Moccia	Institute of Food Sciences, National Research Council, Avellino, Italy
Daniele Nucci	Veneto Institute of Oncology IOV-IRCCS, Padova, Italy
Gaetana Paolella	Department of Chemistry and Biology A. Zambelli, University of Salerno, Fisciano, Italy
Veronica Pignone	Department of Epidemiology and Prevention, IRCCS Neuromed, Pozzilli, Italy
Alice Rosi	Department of Food and Drug, University of Parma, Parma, Italy
Emilia Ruggiero	Department of Epidemiology and Prevention, IRCCS Neuromed, Pozzilli, Italy
Carmela Spagnuolo	Institute of Food Sciences, National Research Council, Avellino, Italy
Giorgia Vici	University of Camerino, Camerino, Italy

References

1. Gomiero, T.; Pimentel, D.; Paoletti, M.G. Environmental impact of different agricultural management practices: Conventional vs. organic agriculture. *Crit. Rev. Plant Sci.* **2011**, *30*, 95–124. [CrossRef]
2. Brantsæter, A.L.; Ydersbond, T.A.; Hoppin, J.A.; Haugen, M.; Meltzer, H.M. Organic food in the diet: Exposure and health implications. *Annu. Rev. Public Health* **2017**, *38*, 295–313. [CrossRef] [PubMed]

3. Smith-Spangler, C.; Brandeau, M.L.; Hunter, G.E.; Bavinger, J.C.; Pearson, M.; Eschbach, P.J.; Sundaram, V.; Liu, H.; Schirmer, P.; Stave, C.; et al. Are organic foods safer or healthier than conventional alternatives? A systematic review. *Ann. Intern. Med.* **2012**, *157*, 348–366. [CrossRef] [PubMed]
4. Baudry, J.; Méjean, C.; Allès, B.; Péneau, S.; Touvier, M.; Hercberg, S.; Lairon, D.; Galan, P.; Kesse-Guyot, E. Contribution of organic food to the diet in a large sample of French adults (the Nutrinet-Santé cohort study). *Nutrients* **2015**, *7*, 8615–8632. [CrossRef] [PubMed]
5. IFOAM Research Institute of Organic Agriculture & Organics International. The World of Organic Agriculture. Statistic and Emerging Trends 2019. Available online: https://www.ifoam.bio/en/news/2019/02/13/world-organic-agriculture-2019 (accessed on 13 April 2020).
6. Nielsen. Osservatorio Immagino Nielsen GS1 Italy. Le Etichette dei Prodotti Raccontano i Consumi Degli. Italiani. 2019. Available online: https://osservatorioimmagino.it/ (accessed on 13 April 2020).
7. European Union. Council Regulation (EC) No 834/2007 on organic production and labelling of organic products with detailed rules on production, labelling and control. *Off. J. Eur. Union* **2007**, *L189*, 20–27.
8. Barański, M.; Srednicka-Tober, D.; Volakakis, N.; Seal, C.; Sanderson, R.; Stewart, G.B.; Benbrook, C.; Biavati, B.; Markellou, E.; Giotis, C.; et al. Higher antioxidant and lower cadmium concentrations and lower incidence of pesticide residues in organically grown crops: A systematic literature review and meta-analyses. *Br. J. Nutr.* **2014**, *112*, 794–811. [CrossRef]
9. Magkos, F.; Arvaniti, F.; Zampelas, A. Organic food: Buying more safety or just peace of mind? A critical review of the literature. *Crit. Rev. Food Sci. Nutr.* **2006**, *46*, 23–56. [CrossRef]
10. González, N.; Marquès, M.; Nadal, M.; Domingo, J.L. Occurrence of environmental pollutants in foodstuffs: A review of organic vs. conventional food. *Food Chem. Toxicol.* **2019**, *125*, 370–375. [CrossRef]
11. Bradbury, K.E.; Balkwill, A.; Spencer, E.A.; Roddam, A.W.; Reeves, G.K.; Green, J.; Key, T.J.; Beral, V.; Pirie, K.; Million Women Study, C. Organic food consumption and the incidence of cancer in a large prospective study of women in the United Kingdom. *Br. J. Cancer* **2014**, *110*, 2321–2326. [CrossRef]
12. Baudry, J.; Assmann, K.E.; Touvier, M.; Allès, B.; Seconda, L.; Latino-Martel, P.; Ezzedine, K.; Galan, P.; Hercberg, S.; Lairon, D. Association of frequency of organic food consumption with cancer risk: Findings from the NutriNet-Santé prospective cohort study. *JAMA Intern. Med.* **2018**, *178*, 1597–1606. [CrossRef]
13. Schouteten, J.J.; Gellynck, X.; Slabbinck, H. Influence of organic labels on consumer's flavor perception and emotional profiling: Comparison between a central location test and home-use-test. *Food. Res. Int.* **2019**, *116*, 1000–1009. [CrossRef] [PubMed]
14. Prada, M.; Garrido, M.V.; Rodrigues, D. Lost in processing? Perceived healthfulness, taste and caloric content of whole and processed organic food. *Appetite* **2017**, *114*, 175–186. [CrossRef] [PubMed]
15. Besson, T.; Lalot, F.; Bochard, N.; Flaudias, V.; Zerhouni, O. The calories underestimation of "organic" food: Exploring the impact of implicit evaluations. *Appetite* **2019**, *137*, 134–144. [CrossRef] [PubMed]
16. Ditlevsen, K.; Sandøe, P.; Lassen, J. Healthy food is nutritious, but organic food is healthy because it is pure: The negotiation of healthy food choices by Danish consumers of organic food. *Food Qual. Pref.* **2019**, *71*, 46–53. [CrossRef]
17. Lazaroiu, G.; Andronie, M.; Uță, C.; Hurloiu, I. Trust management in organic agriculture: Sustainable consumption behavior, environmentally conscious purchase intention, and healthy food choices. *Front. Public Health* **2019**, *7*, 340. [CrossRef]
18. Sundar, A.; Kardes, F.R. The role of perceived variability and the health halo effect in nutritional inference and consumption. *Psychol. Mark.* **2015**, *32*, 512–521. [CrossRef]
19. Sörqvist, P.; Hedblom, D.; Holmgren, M.; Haga, A.; Langeborg, L.; Nöstl, A.; Kågström, J. Who needs cream and sugar when there is eco-labeling? Taste and willingness to pay for "eco-friendly" coffee. *PLoS ONE* **2013**, *8*, e80719. [CrossRef]
20. Batte, M.T.; Hooker, N.H.; Haab, T.C.; Beaverson, J. Putting their money where their mouths are: Consumer willingness to pay for multi-ingredient, processed organic food products. *Food Policy* **2007**, *32*, 145–159. [CrossRef]
21. Schleenbecker, R.; Hamm, U. Consumers' perception of organic product characteristics. A review. *Appetite* **2013**, *71*, 420–429. [CrossRef]
22. Dangour, A.D.; Dodhia, S.K.; Hayter, A.; Allen, E.; Lock, K.; Uauy, R. Nutritional quality of organic foods: A systematic review. *Am. J. Clin. Nutr.* **2009**, *90*, 680–685. [CrossRef]

23. Bernacchia, R.; Preti, R.; Vinci, G. Organic and conventional foods: Differences in nutrients. *Ital. J. Food Sci.* **2016**, *28*, 565–578.
24. Worthington, V. Nutritional quality of organic versus conventional fruits, vegetables, and grains. *J. Altern. Complement. Med.* **2001**, *7*, 161–173. [CrossRef]
25. Hoefkens, C.; Sioen, I.; Baert, K.; De Meulenaer, B.; De Henauw, S.; Vandekinderen, I.; Devlieghere, F.; Opsomer, A.; Verbeke, W.; Van Camp, J. Consuming organic versus conventional vegetables: The effect on nutrient and contaminant intakes. *Food. Chem. Toxicol.* **2010**, *48*, 3058–3066. [CrossRef] [PubMed]
26. Średnicka-Tober, D.; Barański, M.; Seal, C.; Sanderson, R.; Benbrook, C.; Steinshamn, H.; Gromadzka-Ostrowska, J.; Rembiałkowska, E.; Skwarło-Sońta, K.; Eyre, M.; et al. Composition differences between organic and conventional meat: A systematic literature review and meta-analysis. *Brit. J. Nutr.* **2016**, *115*, 994–1011. [CrossRef] [PubMed]
27. Średnicka-Tober, D.; Barański, M.; Seal, C.J.; Sanderson, R.; Benbrook, C.; Steinshamn, H.; Gromadzka-Ostrowska, J.; Rembiałkowska, E.; Skwarło-Sońta, K.; Eyre, M.; et al. Higher PUFA and n-3 PUFA, conjugated linoleic acid, α-tocopherol and iron, but lower iodine and selenium concentrations in organic milk: A systematic literature review and meta- and redundancy analyses. *Br. J. Nutr.* **2016**, *115*, 1043–1060. [CrossRef]
28. Palupi, E.; Jayanegara, A.; Ploeger, A.; Kahl, J. Comparison of nutritional quality between conventional and organic dairy products: A meta-analysis. *J. Sci. Food Agric.* **2012**, *92*, 2774–2781. [CrossRef]
29. Heimler, D.; Romani, A.; Ieri, F. Plant polyphenol content, soil fertilization and agricultural management: A review. *Eur. Food Res. Technol.* **2017**, *243*, 1107–1115. [CrossRef]
30. Bourn, D.; Prescott, J. A comparison of the nutritional value, sensory qualities, and food safety of organically and conventionally produced foods. *Crit. Rev. Food Sci. Nutr.* **2002**, *42*, 1–34. [CrossRef]
31. Dangour, A.D.; Lock, K.; Hayter, A.; Aikenhead, A.; Allen, E.; Uauy, R. Nutrition-related health effects of organic foods: A systematic review. *Am. J. Clin. Nutr.* **2010**, *92*, 203–210. [CrossRef]
32. European Union. Council Regulation (EC) No. 1169/2011 on the provision of food information to consumers. *Off. J. Eur. Union* **2011**, *L304*, 18–63.
33. Angelino, D.; Rosi, A.; Dall'Asta, M.; Pellegrini, N.; Martini, D. Evaluation of the nutritional quality of breakfast cereals sold on the Italian market: The Food Labelling of Italian Products (FLIP) study. *Nutrients* **2019**, *11*, 2827. [CrossRef]
34. European Union. Council Regulation (EC) No 1924/2006 on nutrition and health claims made on foods. *Off. J. Eur. Union* **2006**, *L404*, 9–26.
35. Vranešević', T.; Stančec, R. The effect of the brand on perceived quality of food products. *Br. Food J.* **2003**, *105*, 811–825. [CrossRef]
36. Crinnion, W.J. Organic foods contain higher levels of certain nutrients, lower levels of pesticides, and may provide health benefits for the consumer. *Altern. Med. Rev.* **2010**, *15*, 4–12. [PubMed]
37. Hunter, D.; Foster, M.; McArthur, J.O.; Ojha, R.; Petocz, P.; Samman, S. Evaluation of the micronutrient composition of plant foods produced by organic and conventional agricultural methods. *Crit. Rev. Food Sci. Nutr.* **2011**, *51*, 571–582. [CrossRef] [PubMed]
38. Lairon, D. Nutritional quality and safety of organic food. A review. *Agron. Sustain. Dev.* **2010**, *30*, 33–41. [CrossRef]
39. Magkos, F.; Arvaniti, F.; Zampelas, A. Organic food: Nutritious food or food for thought? A review of the evidence. *Int. J. Food Sci. Nutr.* **2003**, *54*, 357–371. [CrossRef]
40. Germer, S.; Hilzendegen, C.; Ströbele-Benschop, N. Sugar content of German breakfast cereals for children—Recommendations and reality. *Ernahr. Umsch.* **2013**, *60*, 89–95.
41. Woodbury, N.J.; George, V.A. A comparison of the nutritional quality of organic and conventional ready-to-eat breakfast cereals based on NuVal scores. *Public Health Nutr.* **2014**, *17*, 1454–1458. [CrossRef]
42. Moore, J.B.; Horti, A.; Fielding, B.A. Evaluation of the nutrient content of yogurts: A comprehensive survey of yogurt products in the major UK supermarkets. *BMJ Open* **2018**, *8*, e021387. [CrossRef]
43. Duran, A.C.; Ricardo, C.Z.; Mais, L.A.; Martins, A.P.B.; Taillie, L.S. Conflicting Messages on Food and Beverage Packages: Front-of-Package Nutritional Labeling, Health and Nutrition Claims in Brazil. *Nutrients* **2019**, *11*, 2967. [CrossRef] [PubMed]
44. Sun, Y.; Liu, B.; Du, Y.; Snetselaar, L.G.; Sun, Q.; Hu, F.B.; Bao, W. Inverse association between organic food purchase and diabetes mellitus in US adults. *Nutrients* **2018**, *10*, 1877. [CrossRef] [PubMed]

45. Mie, A.; Andersen, H.R.; Gunnarsson, S.; Kahl, J.; Kesse-Guyot, E.; Rembiałkowska, E.; Quaglio, G.; Grandjean, P. Human health implications of organic food and organic agriculture: A comprehensive review. *Environ. Health* **2017**, *16*, 111. [CrossRef] [PubMed]
46. De Lorenzo, A.; Noce, A.; Bigioni, M.; Calabrese, V.; Della Rocca, D.G.; Di Daniele, N.; Tozzo, C.; Di Renzo, L. The effects of Italian Mediterranean organic diet (IMOD) on health status. *Curr. Pharm. Des.* **2010**, *16*, 814–824. [CrossRef]
47. Baudry, J.; Allès, B.; Péneau, S.; Touvier, M.; Méjean, C.; Hercberg, S.; Galan, P.; Lairon, D.; Kesse-Guyot, E. Dietary intakes and diet quality according to levels of organic food consumption by French adults: Cross-sectional findings from the Nutrinet-Santé cohort study. *Public Health Nutr.* **2017**, *20*, 638–648. [CrossRef]
48. Petersen, S.B.; Rasmussen, M.A.; Strøm, M.; Halldorsson, T.I.; Olsen, S.F. Sociodemographic characteristics and food habits of organic consumers-a study from the Danish national birth cohort. *Public Health Nutr.* **2013**, *16*, 1810–1819. [CrossRef]
49. Eisinger-Watzl, M.; Wittig, F.; Heuer, T.; Hoffmann, I. Customers purchasing organic food - do they live healthier? Results of the German national nutrition survey ii. *Eur. J. Nutr. Food Saf.* **2014**, *5*, 59–71. [CrossRef]

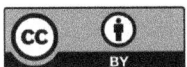

© 2020 by the authors. Licensee MDPI, Basel, Switzerland. This article is an open access article distributed under the terms and conditions of the Creative Commons Attribution (CC BY) license (http://creativecommons.org/licenses/by/4.0/).

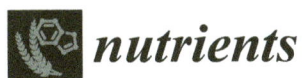

Article

Sugar Content in Processed Foods in Spain and a Comparison of Mandatory Nutrition Labelling and Laboratory Values

María José Yusta-Boyo [1,*], Laura M. Bermejo [2,3], Marta García-Solano [1], Ana M. López-Sobaler [2,3], Rosa M. Ortega [2,3], Marta García-Pérez [1], María Ángeles Dal-Re Saavedra [1] and on behalf of the SUCOPROFS Study Researchers [†]

1. Spanish Food Safety and Nutrition Agency, Alcala, 56., 28014 Madrid, Spain; mgarcias@mscbs.es (M.G.-S.); mgarciape@mscbs.es (M.G.-P.); mdalre@mscbs.es (M.Á.D.-R.S.)
2. Nutrition and Food Science Department, Faculty of Pharmacy, Complutense University of Madrid, 28040 Madrid, Spain; mlbermej@ucm.es (L.M.B.); asobaler@ucm.es (A.M.L.-S.); rortega@ucm.es (R.M.O.)
3. VALORNUT Research Group, Faculty of Pharmacy, Complutense University of Madrid, 28040 Madrid, Spain
* Correspondence: mjyusta@mscbs.es; Tel.: +34-913380062
† For more information see Acknowledgments Section.

Received: 21 February 2020; Accepted: 10 April 2020; Published: 13 April 2020

Abstract: To reduce the sugar content of processed foods through reformulation, the first step is to determine the content of the largest sources of sugars in each country's diet. The aim of this work was to describe the sugar content in the most commonly consumed processed foods in Spain and to compare that sugar's labelling and laboratory analysis values (LVs and AVs, respectively) to confirm its adequacy. A sample of the 1173 most commonly consumed processed foods in Spain (28 groups; 77 subcategories) was collected. For each product, the total sugar content was compared according to its AV and LV. The median (25th –75th percentiles, interquartile range) sugar content by group was calculated for the total sample, and the groups were classified as "high sugar content" when this value was above 22.5 g/100g of product. The adequacy of the LV, according to the European Union (EU) tolerance requirements, was then evaluated, and each subcategory median was compared with the AV to determine its appropriateness via a median test for independent samples ($p < 0.05$). In total, 10 out of 28 groups presented high sugar content. Moreover, 98.4% of the products met the EU tolerance ranges. Finally, only one subcategory ("cured ham") presented significant differences between the AV and LV median values (0.4 g vs. 0.1 g sugar/100g, $p < 0.05$). The groups of food products whose sugar content reduction could have the greatest impact on public health were identified. In addition, our study showed the high adequacy of LV with the EU labeling tolerance requirements, as well as the LV's appropriateness as a tool to implement actions aimed at reducing sugar consumption.

Keywords: nutrition labeling; food labeling; food processing; nutrition policy; Spain; food analysis; dietary sugars; reformulation

1. Introduction

The prevalence of overweight, obesity, and related non-communicable diseases (cardiovascular diseases, diabetes, and cancer) remains high in all European countries, including Spain [1].

The impact of dietary risk factors on the mortality and morbidity associated with non-communicable diseases highlights the importance of implementing measures to improve the quality of citizens' diets within national health policies [2].

Diets must meet energy needs and provide a variety of foods of a high nutritional quality that are safe to consume. Moreover, these diets should be sustainable, affordable, accessible, and culturally acceptable [3].

The European Union (EU) has long promoted initiatives to tackle obesity and to improve nutrition in European countries. One of the main initiatives of the European Commission was the adoption of the White Paper of 30 May 2007 entitled 'A Strategy for Europe on Nutrition, Overweight and Obesity related health issues' [4], focusing on actions that can be taken at the local, regional, national, and European levels. One of the initiatives included in this document is for the food industry (including retailers) to reformulate its products, particularly by reducing the content of salt, sugar, and fats.

In this regard, the High Level Group on Nutrition and Physical Activity (HLGNPA), composed of representatives of EU Member States and the European Commission, launched two EU Frameworks for the reformulation of food products: the EU Framework for National Initiatives on salt reductions [5] and the EU Framework for National Initiatives on Selected Nutrients [6] with two annexes: Annex I on saturated fats [7] and Annex II on added sugars [8]. These EU frameworks and annexes establish benchmarks and timelines for nutrient content reduction, focusing their action on certain food categories while taking into account the priorities, health needs, baseline nutrient contents, traditions, and pattern of consumption of each member state.

For more than a decade, the Ministry of Health in Spain, through the NAOS Strategy (Strategy for Nutrition, Physical Activity and the Prevention of Obesity) of the Spanish Agency for Food Safety and Nutrition (Spanish acronym AESAN, formerly Spanish Agency for Consumption, Food Safety and Nutrition, AECOSAN) has promoted reformulation initiatives for food and beverages, following the recommendations outlined in the HLGNPA Frameworks. To establish these initiatives, different studies have been carried out to determine the nutrient consumption and main food sources of the population and to ascertain the nutrient content (mainly fats and salt) of processed products [9–13]. The results of these studies have facilitated measures to reduce fats and salt in the main processed foods in Spain. Among these initiatives are the agreements between AESAN and food sector associations to achieve nutrient reduction targets, which were committed to all companies that belong to the sector association [14]. A successful example of public–private collaboration to achieve the reduction of salt content is the agreement (legal document) between AECOSAN, the Spanish Confederation of Bakers (CEOPAN by its Spanish acronym), and the Spanish Association of Manufacturers of Frozen Dough (ASEMAC by its Spanish acronym) signed in 2004, in which a salt reduction from 22 g NaCl/Kg in bread flour in 2004 to a maximum of 18 g NaCl/kg by 2008 was agreed upon. The average NaCl content measured in 2008 was 16.3 g of NaCl/Kg in bread-making flour [14]. In addition, a new study conducted in 2014 concluded that the salt content in bread in Spain has remained stable since 2008 [15].

However, no study has yet been conducted to ascertain the sugar content in processed products in Spain in order to establish reference values for addressing public health food policies, such as the reformulation or improvement of processed food and beverage composition.

For this reason, at the end of 2016, AESAN conducted the present study to describe the sugar content in the food groups included in the Annex II of added sugar [8] and in the most commonly consumed processed foods in Spain, especially by children and adolescents [16]. In addition, the other secondary objectives were to compare the label value (LV) with the laboratory analysis value (AV) in order to assess the adequacy of the LV based on the EU labelling requirements, and to study the appropriateness of using the label values as reference data to monitor the reformulation of sugar and other nutrients or for strategies such as front-of-pack labelling or marketing restrictions.

2. Materials and Methods

2.1. Sample Selection

We selected 28 food and beverage groups of processed foods to perform the present study (Table 1), starting with the 11 groups recommended in the Annex II (on added sugar) in the HLGNPA [8]. Some of these 11 groups were divided due to the diversity of products included in each of them. For example, "Sugary dairy products and other similar products" was divided into six groups: flavoured milk drinks, drinking yoghurt, yoghurt, dairy-based desserts, cheeses, and soy drinks. Moreover, according to the results observed in the ENALIA study (National Dietary Survey on the Child and Adolescent Population), the groups "milk", "juices", "nectars", and "meat products" were included because these groups represent an important source of energy for children and adolescents in Spain [16].

Table 1. Selected food and beverage groups for this study.

Food Groups to Focus Action on Added Sugar Reduction, According to Annex II of the High Level Group on Nutrition and Physical Activity (HLGNPA)	Selected Groups for this Study (HLGNPA Groups + other Highly Consumed Groups by Spanish Children)
Sugar sweetened Beverages	Sugar sweetened beverages
Sugar sweetened dairy and dairy imitates	Flavoured milk drinks
	Drinking yoghurt
	Yoghurt
	Dairy-based desserts
	Cheese
	Soy drinks
Breakfast cereals	Breakfast cereals and cereal bars
Bread and bread products	Special packaged bread
Bakery products (e.g., cakes and cookies)	Baking and pastries
	Biscuits
Confectionaries	Sweets
	Chocolates
	Other sweets (chewing gum, marshmallow, etc.)
Ready meals (including ready to prepare products like dry soups, dried mashed potatoes, rice mixture)	Ready meals
Savoury snacks	Savoury snacks
	Crisps
Sauces (including ketchup)	Sauces
Sugar sweetened desserts, ice cream and topping	Desserts
	Ice creams
	Jam
	Confitures
Canned fruits and vegetables	Canned pineapple
	Other Fruits in syrup
	Milk
	Fruit juices
	Nectars
	Meat products

The 28 processed food groups selected were classified into 77 subcategories according to their composition and legal denomination. For some analyses, classification by subcategory was used; this type of classification is considered more appropriate than classification by group due to the variability within a group. The number of products to be analyzed in each food subcategory was established by consensus among researchers. Food products were selected from among those with the greatest presence in the national market at that time (including both brand names and retailer brands), according to data published in the report on the Alimarket study in 2015 [17]. This report provided the most important economic and financial variables by sector in Spain, including information about 9286 companies in the food sector.

2.2. Data Collection

Once the groups and subcategories to be studied were selected, the total number of processed product samples was 1173. The study was awarded through public tender to "AENOR Laboratorio Alimentacion" (AENOR Food laboratory), which carried out the plans to purchase the products. All samples were acquired in October 2016 and transported under adequate storage conditions to "AENOR Laboratorio Alimentacion" to proceed with the storage and subsequent determination of the total sugar AV of each processed product. In addition, the total sugar LV declared in the mandatory nutrition labelling (MNL) was recorded.

The Luff–Schoorl method was used to measure the total sugar AV. This method is the official method to control sugars intended for human consumption in Spain [18] according to the European legislation First Commission Directive of 26 July 1979, which outlines the community methods for testing certain sugars intended for human consumption (79/786/EEC) [19]. This method involves the elimination of all reducing materials other than sugars present in the sample by drying; subsequently, the sugar content is assessed based on the reducing action in a cupro–alkaline solution.

In order to collect the total sugar LV, we considered the proposed methodology for the monitoring and food reformulation initiatives of the Joint Action on Nutrition and Physical Activity (JANPA) of the European Commission [20]. In this methodology, the MNL was accepted as the data source to collect nutritional information.

2.3. Statistical Analysis

The data collected were recorded in a database designed ad hoc (for this study). This procedure was carried out in other countries as a tool for the reformulation and monitoring of processed food and beverage composition (Oqali database) [21]. Statistical analyses were performed using the SPSS software (SPSS, version 25.0; SPSS, Chicago, IL, USA).

For a descriptive study of the total sugar AV and LV, the median (25th–75th percentiles, interquartile range) were calculated for each food group, in the total sample ($n = 1173$), and in the two subsamples, according to the presence of nutrition claims about sugar content (light, low sugar content, no added or zero sugar, etc.) on the label ($n = 64$) vs. the absence of a sugar-based nutritional claim ($n = 1109$). Moreover, an adequacy study of the LV based on the EU labelling requirements, using the tolerance of the values declared on the labelling [22], was conducted. The final sample used to study adequacy of the LV included 1074 products (excluding products with nutritional claims and without a LV). A product met the tolerance range ("Meets") when its LV < 10 g/100g of product and its deviation from the AV was ±2 g; when its LV was 10–40 g/100 g and its deviation from the AV was ±20%; or when its LV > 40 g/100 g and deviation from the AV was ±8 g. Any product outside of these tolerance ranges was classified as "Does not meet".

Finally, an appropriateness study of LV as reference data for reformulation, monitoring, and other strategies was conducted. For the sample consisting of 1074 products, the LV and AV medians of each product subcategory were compared using the SPSS Median Test for 2 Independent Medians ($p < 0.05$).

3. Results

A flowchart with the sample selection and the different analyses carried out in the present study is detailed in Figure 1.

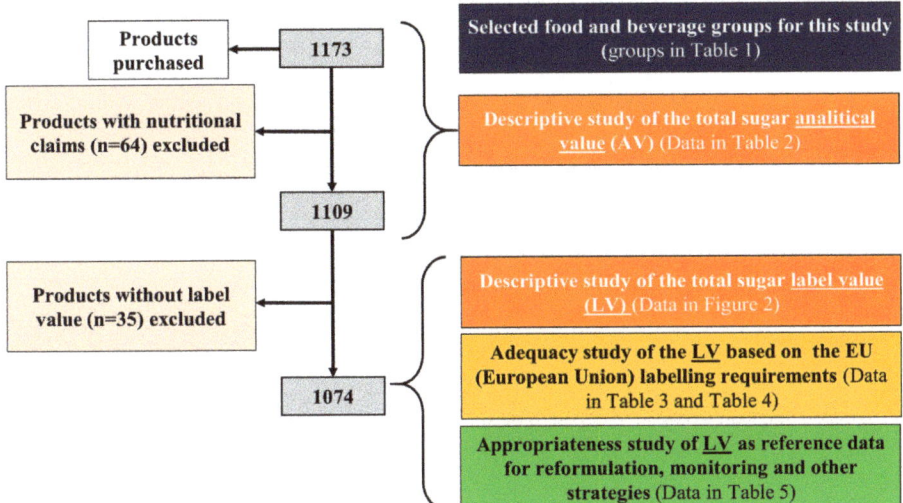

Figure 1. Flow diagram. Sample selection and the different analyses carried out.

3.1. Descriptive Study of the Total Sugar AV and LV

Table 2 provides the results of the AV statistical analysis median (25th–75th percentiles, interquartile range) of the total sample analyzed ($n = 1173$). In addition, the analysis of the subsamples according to the presence or absence of a nutrition claim about sugar content showed that the total sugar AV was higher in products without a nutritional claim ($n = 1109$) than in those with such a claim ($n = 64$).

Figure 2 presents the median content of the total sugar LV for each group of products studied in the total sample. The 25th-75th percentiles and interquartile ranges (IQRs) are also shown.

Table 2. Analytical value (AV) of the total sugar content (g/100g of product) in the different groups of products, in the total sample, and in the two subsamples according to the presence or absence of nutritional claims related to sugar content.

Groups	All Products (n = 1173)			Products with Nutritional Claims (n = 64)			Products without Nutritional Claims (n = 1109)		
	n	Median	(P25–P75) IQR	N	Median	(P25–P75) IQR [2]	n	Median	(P25–P75) IQR
Baking and pastries	61	27.3	(19.8–31.5) 11.7	1	–	4.6	60	27.4	(19.9–31.7) 11.9
Biscuits	45	24.9	(20.9–34.0) 13.1	2	–	(0.3, 0.6)	43	25.3	(21.0–34.1) 13.1
Breakfast cereals and cereal bars	107	25.8	(19.3–31.4) 12.1	1	–	0.1	106	25.9	(19.3–31.4) 12.1
Canned pineapple	10	11.7	(11.4–12.2) 0.8	–	–	–	10	11.7	(11.4–12.2) 0.8
Cheeses	30	4.4	(2.8–4.9) 2.1	–	–	–	30	4.4	(2.8–4.9) 2.1
Chocolate	92	52.0	(47.3–58.0) 10.7	2	–	(0.6, 13.5)	90	52.6	(47.8–58.0) 10.2
Confitures	30	42.5	(26.3–46.7) 20.4	11	5.5	(2.2–35.0) 32.8	19	46.5	(42.6–47.0) 4.4
Crisps	30	0.7	(0.4–0.8) 0.4	–	–	–	30	0.7	(0.4–0.8) 0.4
Dairy-based desserts	65	15.9	(14.1–19.3) 5.2	–	–	–	65	15.9	(14.1–19.3) 5.2
Desserts [1]	29	23.2	(12.7–33.8) 21.1	4	9.8	(6.7–23.1) 16.4	25	26.7	(15.6–39.1) 23.5
Drinking yoghurt	10	13.1	(11.6–13.2) 1.6	2	–	(4.0, 4.7)	8	13.2	(12.7–13.4) 0.7
Flavoured milk drinks	20	11.3	(10.4–12.0) 1.6	2	–	(4.6, 5.8)	18	11.6	(10.9–12.0) 1.1
Fruit juices	44	10.0	(9.0–11.0) 2.1	–	–	–	44	10.0	(9.0–11.0) 2.1
Ice creams	45	24.2	(21.0–27.1) 6.1	–	–	–	45	24.2	(21.0–27.1) 6.1
Jam	5	51.2	(43.2–58.8) 15.6	1	–	2.9	4	55.0	(47.2–59.5) 12.3
Meat products	90	0.7	(0.1–1.2) 1.1	–	–	–	90	0.7	(0.1–1.2) 1.1
Milk	51	4.7	(4.6–4.8) 0.2	–	–	–	51	4.7	(4.6–4.8) 0.2
Nectars	18	9.5	(4.3–10.7) 6.4	7	4.2	(4.1–6.0) 1.9	11	10.4	(9.6–11.1) 1.5
Other Fruits in syrup	20	14.3	(13.7–16.4) 2.7	3	5.3	(5.2–5.8) 0.6	17	15.6	(14.0–16.7) 2.7
Other sweets	27	49.4	(0.1–66.9) 66.8	10	0.1	(0.1–0.1) 0.0	17	61.6	(54.8–67.1) 12.3
Ready meals	55	2.1	(1.0–3.2) 2.2	–	–	–	55	2.1	(1.0–3.2) 2.2
Sauces	63	6.4	(2.4–17.0) 14.6	4	3.7	(2.5–7.6) 5.1	59	6.4	(2.4–18.9) 16.5

Table 2. Cont.

Groups	All Products (n = 1173)			Products with Nutritional Claims (n = 64)			Products without Nutritional Claims (n = 1109)		
	n	Median	(P25–P75) IQR	N	Median	(P25–P75) IQR [2]	n	Median	(P2–P75) IQR
Savoury snacks	45	1.2	(0.4–2.8) 2.4	–	–	–	45	1.2	(0.4–2.8) 2.4
Soy drinks	5	2.1	(1.0–2.7) 1.7	–	–	–	5	2.1	(1.0–2.7) 1.7
Special packaged bread	45	4.4	(3.9–5.1) 1.2	–	–	–	45	4.4	(3.9–5.1) 1.2
Sugar Sweetened Beverages	47	7.2	(4.7–10.1) 5.4	4	4.6	(4.0–5.8) 1.9	43	7.6	(6.0–10.2) 4.2
Sweets	34	70.2	(62.8–76.1) 13.3	5	0.1	(0.1–0.1) 0.0	29	71.4	(66.3–81.7) 15.4
Yoghurt	50	12.3	(5.8–13.5) 7.7	5	4.9	(4.9–5.2) 0.3	45	12.6	(10.5–13.6) 3.1
Total	1173	11.6	(3.7–26.9) 23.2	64	4.2	(0.2–5.8) 5.6	1109	12.2	(4.0–28.1) 24.1

Including non-dairy desserts (jello, "tocino de cielo" (pudding made with egg yolks and syrup), and chocolate cake) and powders for dessert preparation (flan powder, cake powder, and chocolate cake powder). [2] For groups with 1 or 2 items, the median was not calculated, and the data are presented in the IQR column separated by a comma; IQR = Interquartile range.

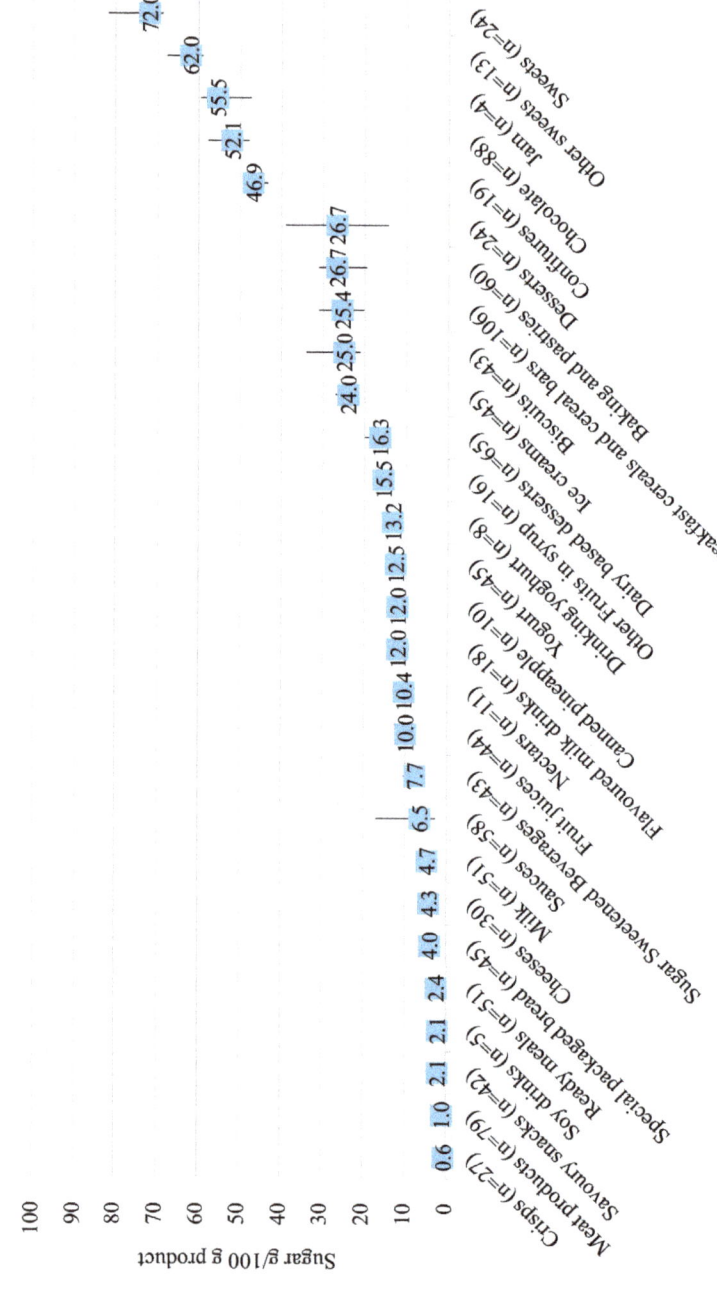

Figure 2. Median and 25th and 75th percentiles of label values (LV) for total sugar for the most consumed groups of products in Spain.

Moreover, according to data from the AV of products without nutritional claims ($n = 1109$), the food groups were classified as high total sugar content groups ($n = 10$) and no high total sugar content groups ($n = 18$), with the value 22.5 g/100 g as the cut-off point according to the criterion used for the front of the pack in the UK (25% of the recommended intake in Annex XIII of the EU regulation 1169/2011) [23] and in Chile's Law on Food Labelling and Advertising [24]. There were a total of 10 groups with high total sugar content (in descending order): sweets, other sweets, jam, chocolate, confitures, baking and pastries, desserts, breakfast cereals and cereal bars, biscuits, and ice creams. For the dispersion within each group, the estimated interquartile range was greater than 15 g/100 g in three groups (desserts, sauces, and sweets), between 15 and 10 g/100 g in six groups (biscuits, other sweets, jam, breakfast cereals and cereal bars, baking and pastries, and chocolate), and lower than 10 g/100g in 19 groups.

3.2. Adequacy Study of the LV Based on the EU Labelling Requirements for the Tolerance of the Values Declared on the Label

An adequacy study of the LV compared to the EU labelling requirements was conducted considering the tolerance for the values declared on the label [22]. Tolerance refers to the acceptable difference between the nutritional values declared on the label and those established over the course of official controls in relation to the "nutritional information" or "nutritional labeling" described in Regulation (EU) No. 1169/2011 on the provision of food information provided to consumers [25].

For this study, 64 products with nutritional claims related to sugar content were excluded (Table 2) since their sugar content was reduced to comply with the requirements of Regulation (EC) No. 1924/2006 on the nutritional and health claims made for foods [26], the tolerance requirements for these products are different and are beyond the scope of this study, which focuses instead on products that can be reformulated. In addition, 35 products without LV data (0.09% of the total samples analyzed) were also excluded (11 meat products, five sweets, four ready meals, four from other sweets, three crisps, three savoury snacks, two chocolates, one sauce, one dessert, and one fruit in syrup). Notably, the obligation to show the mandatory nutrition labelling (MNL) (according to Regulation (EU) No. 1169/2011 on the food information provided to the consumer) has been in force since 13 December 2016 [25], but the sampling for this study took place earlier (October 2016). Therefore, the final sample included 1074 products. Therefore, the final sample analyzed was 1074 products.

Of the aforementioned 1074 products, 1057 (98.4%) met the tolerance ranges, while 17 products did not, among which only five (0.45% of the total sample) declared a total sugar LV in the NML that was lower than an AV: one in the "baking and pastries" group ($n = 60$; 1.7% of the group's products), one in the "breakfast cereals and cereal bars" group (n = 106; 0.9%), one in the "special packaged bread" group ($n = 45$; 2.2%), one in the "desserts" group (n = 24; 4.2%), and one in the "dairy-based desserts" group ($n = 65$; 1.5%), while the remaining 12 (1.1% of the total sample) declared a value in their NML greater than the AV (Table 3).

Table 4 shows the 17 products that did not meet the tolerance ranges.

Table 3. Products that meet or do not meet the EU tolerance ranges.

		Meets n (%)	Does not Meet (n (%))	
	n		Label Value (LV) >Analytical Value (AV)	Label value (LV) <Analytical value (AV)
Baking and pastries	60	59 (98.3)	0 (0)	1 (1.7)
Biscuits	43	43 (100)	0 (0)	0 (0)
Breakfast cereals and cereal bars	106	102 (96.2)	3 (2.8)	1 (0.9)
Canned pineapple	10	10 (100)	0 (0)	0 (0)
Cheese	30	29 (96.7)	1 (3.3)	0 (0)
Chocolate	88	88 (100)	0 (0)	0 (0)
Confitures	19	19 (100)	0 (0)	0 (0)
Crisps	27	27 (100)	0 (0)	0 (0)
Dairy-based desserts	65	64 (98.5)	0 (0)	1 (1.5)
Desserts	24	23 (95.8)	0 (0)	1 (4.2)
Drinking yoghurt	8	8 (100)	0 (0)	0 (0)
Flavoured milk drinks	18	18 (100)	0 (0)	0 (0)
Fruit juices	44	44 (100)	0 (0)	0 (0)
Ice creams	45	45 (100)	0 (0)	0 (0)
Jam	4	4 (100)	0 (0)	0 (0)
Meat products	79	78 (98.7)	1 (1.3)	0 (0)
Milk	51	51 (100)	0 (0)	0 (0)
Nectars	11	10 (90.9)	1 (9.1)	0 (0)
Other fruits in syrup	16	16 (100)	0 (0)	0 (0)
Other sweets	13	13 (100)	0 (0)	0 (0)
Ready meals	51	51 (100)	0 (0)	0 (0)
Sauces	58	57 (98.3)	1 (1.7)	0 (0)
Savoury snacks	42	39 (92.9)	3 (7.1)	0 (0)
Soy drinks	5	5 (100)	0 (0)	0 (0)
Special packaged bread	45	44 (97.8)	0 (0)	1 (2.2)
Sugar Sweetened Beverages	43	41 (95.3)	2 (4.7)	0 (0)
Sweets	24	24 (100)	0 (0)	0 (0)
Yoghurt	45	45 (100)	0 (0)	0 (0)
Total	1074	1057 (98.4)	12 (1.1)	5 (0.5)

Table 4. Individual label values (LVs) and analytical values (AVs) of the products that did not meet EU tolerance ranges.

Groups	Product	LV (g/100g)	AV (g/100g)	LV-AV (g/100 g)
Baking and pastries	Children's industrial bakery	20	38.6	−18.6
Breakfast cereals and cereal bars	Breakfast cereals with honey	49	35	14
	Cereal bars	36	21	15
	Integral breakfast cereals with fruit	23	30.5	−7.5
	Muesli	20.2	12.9	7.3

Table 4. *Cont.*

Groups	Product	LV (g/100g)	AV (g/100g)	LV-AV (g/100 g)
Cheeses	Spread and melted cheeses	7	4.7	2.3
Dairy-based desserts	Custard	4.5	15.2	−10.7
Desserts	Chocolate cake	15.2	21.9	−6.7
Meat products	Chopped	3.5	0.8	2.7
Nectars	Nectar	14.4	10	4.4
Sauces	Mustard	5.9	3.5	2.4
Savoury snacks	Microwave popcorn 1	3.8	0.4	3.4
	Microwave popcorn 2	3.8	0.8	3
	Microwave popcorn 3	3.4	0.4	3
Special packaged bread	Integral tin loaf bread	3	6.2	−3.2
Sugar Sweetened Beverages	Sugar sweetened beverage 1	6.3	4.1	2.2
	Sugar sweetened beverage 2	5.2	3.1	2.1

3.3. Appropriateness Study of Using the LV as Reference Data for Reformulation, Monitoring, and other Strategies

Table 5 shows the medians and the 25th and 75th percentiles of the LV and AV data obtained for each group and subcategory of products. Of the 28 groups studied, only the "meat products" group presented significant differences between both medians, with the LV being greater than the AV (LV: 1.0 (0.0–5.0) g vs. AV: 0.7 (0.1–4.2) g, $p < 0.05$). In addition, in the study by subcategories, within the group of meat products, "cured ham" was the only subcategory that presented significant differences (LV: 0.4 g vs. AV: 0.1 g, $p < 0.05$).

Table 5. Comparison of the label value (LV) and analytical value (AV) medians of the total sugar for each group and subcategory of products (appropriateness study).

Groups	Subcategories	n	Label Value (LV) (g/100 g)	Analytical Value (AV) (g/100 g)
			Median (P25–P75)	Median (P25–P75)
Baking and pastries	Industrial croissants and similar	11	12.0 (12.0–13.0)	12.4 (12.1–13.0)
	Industrial pastries for children	21	32.0 (24.6–39.0)	32.0 (26.5–38.0)
	Muffins	15	29.0 (26.4–30.0)	29.1 (26.9–31.3)
	Other (donuts, etc.)	13	24.4 (19.0–30.0)	24.4 (19.8–29.9)
	Total	60	26.7 (19.5–31.0)	27.4 (19.9–31.7)
Biscuits	Filled biscuits	18	37.0 (32.0–41.0)	37.3 (33.1–40.7)
	Sweet biscuit	21	22.0 (21.0–24.0)	23.6 (20.9–24.6)
	Other unfilled biscuits (digestives, cookies, etc.)	4	18.0 (17.2–18.0)	18.0 (17.2–18.2)
	Total	43	25.0 (21.0–34.0)	25.3 (21.0–34.1)

Table 5. Cont.

Groups	Subcategories	n	Label Value (LV) (g/100 g) Median (P25–P75)	Analytical Value (AV) (g/100 g) Median (P25–P75)
Breakfast cereals and cereal bars	Breakfast Cereals with honey	16	30.5 (26.7–36.0)	31.0 (27.5–35.1)
	Cereal bars	16	30.7 (28.0–36.0)	30.4 (27.5–34.5)
	Chocolate filled Breakfast Cereals	6	33.3 (29.0–36.0)	34.3 (29.4–36.8)
	Chocolate flavoured Breakfast Cereals	14	28.9 (28.0–34.0)	29.7 (28.7–34.0)
	Cornflakes cereals	14	7.0 (5.0–8.0)	7.1 (4.9–8.0)
	Muesli	16	22.2 (20.2–25.7)	22.4 (18.9–24.3)
	Sugared breakfast cereals	12	25.0 (24.1–30.5)	24.4 (23.4–30.0)
	Other breakfast cereals	12	19.0 (2.8–23.5)	18.8 (2.8–23.5)
	Total	106	25.4 (20.2–31.0)	25.9 (19.3–31.4)
Canned pineapple	Canned pineapple Total	10	12.0 (11.6–12.0)	11.7 (11.4–12.2)
Cheeses	Spread and melted cheeses Total	30	4.3 (3.0–5.2)	4.4 (2.8–4.9)
Chocolates	Chocolate bars	15	49.5 (44.0–51.1)	48.9 (46.3–51.7)
	Chocolate eggs and similar	5	57.7 (57.6–58.0)	58.0 (56.9–58.2)
	Chocolate large bars (dark, with milk, white)	31	53.8 (46.0–55.9)	54.0 (46.3–56.1)
	Chocolate like bean (carob) and similar	5	53.8 (43.7–64.1)	53.5 (44.4–62.4)
	Chocolate spreads	5	58.0 (57.0–59.0)	58.0 (56.8–58.1)
	Chocolates	20	49.6 (47.1–51.9)	50.3 (46.7–51.8)
	Cocoa powder	7	70.0 (67.0–75.7)	69.9 (68.1–75.4)
	Total	88	52.1 (47.9–57.7)	52.0 (47.7–58.0)
Confitures	Confitures Total	19	46.9 (43.2–47.0)	46.5 (42.6–47.0)
Crisps	Crisps Total	27	0.6 (0.5–0.9)	0.7 (0.4–0.8)
Dairy-based desserts	Custard	15	16.0 (15.0–16.8)	15.9 (15.0–16.6)
	Flan	15	20.8 (16.0–24.3)	19.7 (15.9–23.3)
	Flavoured fromage frais	13	13.4 (13.0–14.0)	13.1 (12.3–13.8)
	Others (chocolate cups, mousse, etc.)	22	17.4 (16.0–20.0)	17.4 (15.0–19.9)
	Total	65	16.3 (14.9–20.0)	15.9 (14.1–19.3)
Desserts	Non-dairy desserts	16	19.6 (14.4–35.0)	21.0 (14.3–36.0)
	Powder for dessert preparation [1]	8	29.0 (13.3–70.4)	28.9 (13.6–69.9)
	Total	24	26.7 (14.4–39.0)	26.9 (14.3–39.6)

Table 5. Cont.

Groups	Subcategories	n	Label Value (LV) (g/100 g) Median (P25–P75)	Analytical Value (AV) (g/100 g) Median (P25–P75)
Drinking yoghurt	Drinking yoghurt Total	8	13.2 (12.7–13.8)	13.2 (12.7–13.4)
Flavoured milk drinks	Flavoured milk drinks Total	18	12.0 (11.0–12.0)	11.6 (10.9–12.0)
Fruit juices	Fruit juices Total	44	10.0 (9.2–11.0)	10.0 (9.0–11.0)
Ice creams	Ice cream to share (bars, frozen cakes, etc.)	25	24.0 (22.6–26.0)	23.8 (21.0–26.2)
	Individual ice cream	20	25.4 (21.5–29.0)	25.0 (21.1–28.4)
	Total	45	24.0 (22.0–27.0)	24.2 (21.0–27.1)
Jam	Jam Total	4	55.5 (47.4–59.5)	55.0 (47.2–59.5)
Meat products	Chopped	9	1.0 (0.5–2.5)	0.8 (0.1–0.9)
	Cooked ham	10	1.1 (1.0–1.3)	0.9 (0.7–1.4)
	Cured ham	15	0.4 (0.1–0.5)	0.1 (0.1–0.4)*
	Cured sausage (chorizo)	9	0.5 (0.3–1.0)	0.4 (0.1–1.0)
	Cured sausage (salchichon)	9	3.0 (1.6–3.5)	3.0 (1.7–3.8)
	Sausages	18	1.0 (0.5–1.0)	0.7 (0.4–1.2)
	Turkey	9	1.0 (0.4–2.0)	0.5 (0.1–1.5)
	Total	79	1.0 (0.5–1.6)	0.7 (0.1–1.3)*
Milk	Whole milk	15	4.6 (4.6–4.7)	4.7 (4.6–4.8)
	Semi-skimmed milk	15	4.7 (4.7–4.8)	4.7 (4.6–4.7)
	Skimmed milk	15	4.8 (4.7–4.8)	4.7 (4.7–4.8)
	Lactose free milk	6	4.8 (4.7–4.8)	4.7 (4.6–4.8)
	Total	51	4.7 (4.7–4.8)	4.7 (4.6–4.8)
Nectar	Nectar Total	11	10.4 (10.0–11.6)	10.4 (9.6–11.1)
Other fruits in syrup	Peach	8	16.2 (14.0–17.0)	15.9 (13.9–17.1)
	Pineapple	3	15.0 (14.0–16.4)	14.2 (14.1–16.7)
	Other fruits	5	14.0 (14.0–16.0)	14.3 (13.8–15.6)
	Total	16	15.5 (14.0–16.4)	15.0 (13.9–16.4)
Other sweets	Other sweets [2] Total	13	62.0 (59.0–67.8)	62.0 (59.3–67.5)
Ready meals	Lasagna /cannelloni	11	2.7 (1.2–3.4)	2.7 (1.0–3.4)
	Pizza	20	2.4 (1.7–3.5)	2.7 (1.7–3.4)
	Others	20	2.0 (1.0–3.0)	1.9 (0.8–2.8)
	Total	51	2.4 (1.2–3.1)	2.3 (1.3–3.3)

Table 5. Cont.

Groups	Subcategories	n	Label Value (LV) (g/100 g) Median (P25–P75)	Analytical Value (AV) (g/100 g) Median (P25–P75)
Sauces	Ketchup	14	21.4 (19.3–22.8)	20.8 (19.1–22.8)
	Mayonnaise	14	1.6 (1.4–3.0)	1.4 (1.0–1.9)
	Tomato sauce	13	7.4 (6.7–8.1)	7.2 (7.1–7.8)
	Other sauces	17	3.0 (2.6–5.9)	3.2 (2.6–4.9)
	Total	58	6.5 (2.6–17.0)	6.4 (2.4–17.0)
Savoury snacks	Corn snacks	15	2.2 (1.0–4.1)	2.1 (0.8–4.2)
	Microwave popcorn	8	1.1 (0.4–3.6)	0.4 (0.4–0.9)
	Other savoury snacks [3]	19	1.8 (0.7–5.1)	1.9 (0.1–4.9)
	Total	42	2.1 (0.8–3.8)	1.4 (0.4–3.7)
Soy drinks	Soy drinks Total	5	2.1 (0.7–2.8)	2.1 (1.0–2.7)
Special packaged bread	White tin loaf bread	14	3.2 (2.9–4.0)	4.0 (3.5–4.5)
	Integral tin loaf bread	16	3.0 (2.7–4.2)	4.2 (3.4–4.8)
	Toasted bread	15	5.1 (4.3–5.6)	5.5 (4.4–5.9)
	Total	45	4.0 (3.0–5.0)	4.4 (3.9–5.1)
Sugar sweetened beverages	Beverages with fruits	3	11.0 (4.6–11.9)	10.8 (4.6–11.9)
	Sugar Sweetened beverages	40	7.5 (6.3–10.2)	7.5 (6.1–10.1)
	Total	43	7.7 (6.3–10.5)	7.6 (6.0–10.2)
Sweets	Sweets Total	24	72.0 (68.8–81.8)	71.9 (67.2–81.9)
Yoghurt	Plain yoghurt	9	4.0 (4.0–4.3)	4.0 (3.9–4.8)
	Flavoured yoghurt	18	12.8 (11.0–14.0)	12.8 (11.4–13.5)
	Fruit Yoghurt	12	14.1 (12.8–15.0)	14.3 (12.8–15.1)
	Sugar sweetened yoghurt	6	12.5 (12.3–13.3)	12.4 (12.2–13.4)
	Total	45	12.5 (10.1–14.0)	12.6 (10.5–13.6)

* Significant differences between the labelling value (LV) and laboratory analysis value (AV) (median test for unpaired samples); [1] Powder for dessert preparation (flan powder, cake powder, chocolate cake powder, etc.); [2] Sweet gels, liquorice, marshmallow, chewing gum; [3] Wheat rinds, pork rinds, potato sticks, crackers.

4. Discussion

To study the content of total sugar, we presented the AVs of 28 groups of processed food products that are most frequently consumed by the Spanish population. The groups whose reformulation could have the greatest impact on public health were identified by their high sugar content and dispersion, which indicates that there is room for the reduction of their sugar content and that reformulation is, therefore, possible.

The most commonly consumed groups, especially by children and adolescents, should also be distinguished and prioritized (compared to those consumed more rarely) based on their energy contribution to the diet (cereals and meats and derivatives, among others), added sugar contribution to the diet (sugar sweetened beverages, chocolate, and nectars), or both (dairy products, baking and pastries, and breakfast cereals, among others) [16,27,28]. In Europe, high sugar consumption, especially in children and adolescents [29], has become a major public health concern, which is highlighted by scientific reports and studies associating high sugar consumption with an increased risk of dental caries [30], overweight [31], cardiometabolic risk factors [32], and adult cardiovascular mortality [33].

This study, promoted by the Observatory of Nutrition and Study of Obesity of AESAN in the framework of the NAOS Strategy, answers the call to action of the EU from the Council Conclusions of June 2016 for the improvement of food to develop a national reformulation initiative (the "Collaboration Plan for the improvement of the composition of food and beverages and other measures 2020" [34]), which is in line with the EU Plan of Action against Childhood Obesity 2014–2020 [35] and the WHO European Action Plan for Food and Nutrition 2015–2020 [36].

One of the limitations of this study is its small sample size, which was mainly due to our limited budget. For some subcategories, this reduced sample size was due to other specific reasons. For "pineapple in syrup", the market is dominated by a single brand, and for "beverages with fruits" (included in the group "sugar sweetened beverages"), we decided to create a new subcategory, resulting in only three products; sugar content in fruit is very different from that in the rest of the group, so the groups could not all be considered together. For this reason (sample size) and to prevent the influence of the most distal values, the median was used as a measure of the central tendency. Moreover, to produce a snapshot of sugar availability in our food environment and to estimate the potential impact of reformulation, market shares should have been considered. In our more feasible approach, the products in each subcategory were selected according to the results of a food market study that identified the most commonly consumed food products.

Our results provide novel information on the presence of total sugars in our food environment. This study quantifies the total sugar content in the main groups of processed products on the Spanish market, assesses the adequacy of label values based on the tolerance ranges for sugar according to EU labelling requirements, and assesses the appropriateness of using the LV as reference data. These are relevant aspects for designing and implementing actions aimed at reducing sugar consumption, which will help tackle obesity and its consequences for health.

Reformulation policies aimed at reducing the content of certain nutrients are some of the measures recommended by international institutions and organizations (European Union, WHO, OECD) to improve the quality of diets, reduce the consumption of foods high in salt, fats, and sugars, and prevent obesity and its related non-communicable diseases [37].

The Annex II on added sugars [8] proposes that the Member States should set a general benchmark for a minimum of 10% added sugar reduction in food products against their baseline levels or to move towards a 'best in class' level of sugar content.

In Spain, in order to establish the sugar reduction objectives of the "Collaboration plan for the improvement of the composition of food and beverages and other measures 2020" [34], AESAN opted in 2017 to deploy the first strategy mentioned in Annex II, which entails the reduction of a percentage of sugar from the basal median content, which was considered a viable and realistic method. Thus, all companies in the sector related to each food subcategory made a commitment to follow this plan. The evaluation of this plan, after its completion in 2020, will allow us to determine the degree of compliance with the objectives and to draw pertinent conclusions about the contribution of this initiative and its possible "drag effect" on other subsequent initiatives.

This work shows that most of the analyzed processed products (98.4%) meet the European Union tolerances for nutrient values declared on the labels. A very low percentage of products in our study did not meet the tolerance values because they had a lower LV than AV (0.45%). A study conducted with a sample of products that contribute the most to sodium intake in the United States [38] concluded that the majority of the labeling and analytical values agree with each other; thus, label under-declaration is limited. However, the authors observed that the differences in total sugars were greater and more systematic and that 19% products did not meet tolerance requirements because their labelled total sugars were lower than their analytical data. In our study, each of the five products that did not meet tolerance levels (due to a lower LV than AV) belonged to a different group (baking and pastries, breakfast cereals, special packaged bread, desserts, and dairy-based desserts), which also included a considerable number of other products that did meet the tolerance requirements.

To our best knowledge, this is the first time that the LVs and AVs of the studied processed products groups were compared in Spain, showing that the total sugar values are similar under both methods for most of the products and subcategories, according to the tolerance requirements for the nutritional information established by the European Union. Of the 28 food and beverage groups and the 77 subcategories analyzed, only the "meat products" group and, specifically, the "cured ham" subcategory, showed significant differences between their median AV and LV data. Taking into account the low sugar content of cured ham and the specific characteristics of its manufacturing and maturation process, such as the infiltration variability of additives depending on the part of the product (fat, bone, etc.), these differences are not considered relevant.

In light of these findings, we conclude first that a reduction in sugar content is feasible in a wide range of products. We recommend setting benchmarks at the subcategory level because this level includes similar products to which the same quality standards apply and allows one to compare the nutrient content of each product within a subcategory to its median, thus facilitating the identification of products with the greatest potential for reformulation.

Moreover, our results show a remarkably high compliance with the tolerance requirements and the appropriateness of the declared total sugar content in the MNL for most sold packaged processed products in Spain.

Thus, the MNL provides an accessible and efficient tool for various aims: to inform consumers truthfully, to conduct studies on the sugar content or other nutrients in labeled products, to establish and monitor reformulation initiatives, to implement front-of-pack initiatives, to apply nutritional profiles for different objectives, and for food advertising policies, among others. Regulation (EU) No. 1169/2011 [25] establishes (starting from 13 December 2016) the mandatory obligation to provide a nutritional declaration on the labels of most processed food products. This declaration must include the energy values and six nutrients, one of them being the sugar content.

Briefly, the groups identified to boost reformulation policies based on their sugar content, the differences in sugar content between similar products, and their contributions to energy, added sugars, or both to the diet are the following: sweets, other sweets, jam, chocolate, confitures, desserts, baking and pastries, breakfast cereals and cereals bars, biscuits, ice cream, sauces, meat products, sugar sweetened beverages, nectars, and dairy products [16,27,28].

The results obtained from this research may help make the nutritional composition of food products more visible, to better explore the feasibility of improving nutrition and evaluate related actions.

5. Conclusions

The results of the present study will help identify the groups of food products whose sugar content reduction could have the greatest impact on public health. In addition, we showed the adequacy of labelling values with the EU labelling tolerance requirements; labelling values are, therefore, an adequate tool to implement and evaluate actions aimed at reducing sugar consumption.

Author Contributions: Conceptualization and methodology, M.J.Y.-B., L.M.B., A.M.L.-S., R.M.O., M.Á.D.-R.S., and SUCOPROFS; formal analysis, M.J.Y.-B., L.M.B., M.G.-S., and A.M.L.-S.; original draft preparation, M.J.Y.-B., L.M.B., M.G.-S., and A.M.L.-S.; writing—review and editing, M.J.Y.-B., L.M.B., A.M.L.-S., M.G.-S., R.M.O., M.G.-P., M.Á.D.-R.S., and SUCOPROFS; funding acquisition and contract design, M.J.Y.-B., M.Á.D.-R.S., and SUCOPROFS. All authors have read and agreed to the published version of the manuscript.

Funding: This research received funding from the Spanish Food Safety and Nutrition Agency.

Acknowledgments: Technical support was provided by Estefania Labrado Mendo. Sample collection and analytics were done by the AENOR Laboratory. **SUCOPROFS (Sugar content in processed foods in Spain) Study researchers.** AGENCIA ESPAÑOLA DE SEGURIDAD ALIMENTARIA Y NUTRICIÓN. VOCALÍA ASESORA PARA LA ESTRATEGIA NAOS: Napoleón Pérez Farinós, Sara Santos Sanz, Carmen Villar Villalba, Mª Araceli García López, Teresa Robledo de Dios. UNIVERSIDAD COMPLUTENSE DE MADRID. FACULTAD DE

FARMACIA. DEPARTAMENTO DE NUTRICIÓN Y CIENCIA DE LOS ALIMENTOS: Esther Cuadrado Soto, Aránzazu Aparicio Vizuete.

Conflicts of Interest: The authors declare no conflict of interest.

References

1. Blundell, J.E.; Baker, J.L.; Boyland, E.; Blaak, E.; Charzewska, J.; de Henauw, S.; Frühbeck, G.; Gonzalez-Gross, M.; Hebebrand, J.; Holm, L.; et al. Variations in the prevalence of obesity among european countries, and a consideration of possible causes. *Obes. Facts* **2017**, *10*, 25–37. [CrossRef] [PubMed]
2. Health Effects of Dietary Risks in 195 Countries, 1990–2017: A Systematic Analysis for the Global Burden of Disease Study 2017—The Lancet. Available online: https://www.thelancet.com/article/S0140-6736(19)30041-8/fulltext (accessed on 21 January 2020).
3. High Level Panel of Experts (HLPE). *Nutrition and Food Systems. A Report by the High Level Panel of Experts on Food Security and Nutrition of the Committee on World Food Security*; Committee on World Food Security: Rome, Italy, 2017.
4. *White Paper on a Strategy for Europe on Nutrition, Overweight and Obesity Related to Health Issues*; COM(2007) 279 Final; Commission of the European Communities: Brussels, Belgium, 2007.
5. EU Framework for National Salt Initiatives. 2008. Available online: https://ec.europa.eu/health/ph_determinants/life_style/nutrition/documents/salt_initiative.pdf (accessed on 14 February 2020).
6. EU Framework for National Initiatives on Selected Nutrients. 2009. Available online: https://ec.europa.eu/health/sites/health/files/nutrition_physical_activity/docs/euframework_national_nutrients_en.pdf (accessed on 14 February 2020).
7. Annex I Saturated Fats. EU Framework for National Initiatives on Selected Nutrients. 2012. Available online: https://ec.europa.eu/health/sites/health/files/nutrition_physical_activity/docs/satured_fat_eufnisn_en.pdf (accessed on 14 February 2020).
8. Annex II Added Sugars. EU Framework for National Initiatives on Selected Nutrients. 2015. Available online: https://ec.europa.eu/health/sites/health/files/nutrition_physical_activity/docs/added_sugars_en.pdf (accessed on 14 February 2020).
9. Ortega, R.M.; López-Sobaler, A.M.; Ballesteros, J.M.; Pérez-Farinós, N.; Rodríguez-Rodríguez, E.; Aparicio, A.; Perea, J.M.; Andrés, P. Estimation of salt intake by 24 h urinary sodium excretion in a representative sample of Spanish adults. *Br. J. Nutr.* **2011**, *105*, 787–794. [CrossRef] [PubMed]
10. Pérez-Farinós, N.; Dal Re Saavedra, M.Á.; Villar Villalba, C.; Robledo de Dios, T. Trans-fatty acid content of food products in Spain in 2015. *Gac. Sanit.* **2016**, *30*, 379–382. [CrossRef] [PubMed]
11. Contenido de sal en los Alimentos en España. 2012. Agencia Española de Consumo, Seguridad Alimentaria y Nutrición; Ministerio de Sanidad, Servicios Sociales e Igualdad. Madrid; 2015. Available online: http://www.aecosan.msssi.gob.es/AECOSAN/docs/documentos/nutricion/estudio_contenido_sal_alimentos.pdf (accessed on 22 January 2020).
12. Trans Fatty Acid Content in Foods in Spain 2010. Spanish Agency for Consumer Affairs, Food Safety and Nutrition; Ministry of Health, Social Services and Equality. Madrid; 2014. Available online: http://www.aecosan.msssi.gob.es/AECOSAN/docs/documentos/nutricion/Informe_ingles_Contenido_AGT_alimentos_2010_ingles.pdf (accessed on 22 January 2020).

13. Trans Fatty Acid Content in Food in Spain 2015. Spanish Agency for Consumer Affairs, Food Safety and Nutrition; Ministry of Health, Social Services and Equality. Madrid; 2016. Available online: http://www.aecosan.msssi.gob.es/AECOSAN/docs/documentos/nutricion/Informe_AGT2015_Ingles.pdf (accessed on 22 January 2020).
14. Reformulacion de Alimentos. Convenios y Acuerdos; Aecosan—Agencia Española de Consumo, Seguridad Alimentaria y Nutrición. Available online: http://www.aecosan.msssi.gob.es/AECOSAN/web/nutricion/ampliacion/reformulacion_alimentos.htm (accessed on 22 January 2020).
15. Pérez Farinós, N.; Santos Sanz, S.; Dal Re, M.Á.; Yusta Boyo, J.; Robledo, T.; Castrodeza, J.J.; Campos Amado, J.; Villar, C. Salt content in bread in Spain, 2014. *Nutr. Hosp.* **2018**, *35*, 650–654. [CrossRef] [PubMed]
16. Estudio ENALIA 2012–2014: Encuesta Nacional de Consumo de Alimentos en Población Infantil y Adolescente. Agencia Española de Consumo, Seguridad Alimentaria y Nutrición; Ministerio de Sanidad, Servicios Sociales e Igualdad. Madrid; 2017. Available online: http://www.aecosan.msssi.gob.es/AECOSAN/docs/documentos/seguridad_alimentaria/gestion_riesgos/Informe_ENALIA2014_FINAL.pdf (accessed on 22 January 2020).
17. García, M. Informe 2015 del Mercado de Supermercados—Informes y Reportajes de Alimentación en Alimarket, Información Económica Sectorial. Available online: http://www.alimarket.es/alimentacion/informe/182798/informe-2015-del-mercado-de-supermercados (accessed on 22 January 2020).
18. Orden de 18 de Julio de 1989 por la que se Aprueban los Métodos Oficiales de Análisis para el Control de Determinados Azúcares Destinados al Consumo Humano. Available online: https://www.boe.es/buscar/doc.php?id=BOE-A-1989-17511 (accessed on 22 January 2020).
19. *Laying Down Community Methods of Analysis for Testing Certain Sugars Intended for Human Consumption*; The Commission of the European Communities: Brussels, Belgium, 1979; 79/78 6/EEC.
20. Joint Action on Nutrition and Physical Activity (JANPA). *Work Package 5 Nutritional Information Monitoring and Food Reformulation Prompting*; European Commission 3rd Health Programme (2014-2020): Brussels, Belgium, 2014.
21. Menard, C.; Dumas, C.; Goglia, R.; Spiteri, M.; Gillot, N.; Combris, P.; Ireland, J.; Soler, L.G.; Volatier, J.L. OQALI: A French database on processed foods. *J. Food Compos. Anal.* **2011**, *24*, 744–749. [CrossRef]
22. *Guidance Document for Competent Authorities for the Control of Compliance with EU Legislation with Regard to the Setting of Tolerances for Nutrients Values Decslred on a Label*; European Commission: Brussels, Belgium, 2012.
23. *Guide to Creating a Front of Pack (FoP) Nutrition Label for Pre-Packed Products Sold through Retail Outlets*; Department of Health and Food Standard Agency: London, UK, 2016.
24. Aprobación de Nueva ley de Alimentos en Chile: Resumen del Proceso. Organización de las Naciones Unidas para la Alimentación y la Agricultura Organización Panamericana de la Salud Santiago. 2017. Available online: http://www.dinta.cl/wp-content/uploads/2018/11/FAO-Ley-etiquetado-Chile-Resumen-2017.pdf (accessed on 22 January 2020).
25. EUR-Lex—32011R1169—EN—EUR-Lex. Available online: https://eur-lex.europa.eu/legal-content/EN/ALL/?uri=CELEX%3A32011R1169 (accessed on 22 January 2020).
26. EUR-Lex—32006R1924—EN—EUR-Lex. Available online: https://eur-lex.europa.eu/legal-content/en/ALL/?uri=CELEX%3A32006R1924 (accessed on 22 January 2020).
27. Ruiz, E.; Ávila, J.M.; Valero, T.; del Pozo, S.; Rodriguez, P.; Aranceta-Bartrina, J.; Gil, Á.; González-Gross, M.; Ortega, R.M.; Serra-Majem, L.; et al. Energy intake, profile, and dietary sources in the spanish population: Findings of the anibes study. *Nutrients* **2015**, *7*, 4739–4762. [CrossRef] [PubMed]
28. Ruiz, E.; Rodriguez, P.; Valero, T.; Ávila, J.M.; Aranceta-Bartrina, J.; Gil, Á.; González-Gross, M.; Ortega, R.M.; Serra-Majem, L.; Varela-Moreiras, G. Dietary intake of individual (free and intrinsic) sugars and food sources in the spanish population: Findings from the ANIBES study. *Nutrients* **2017**, *9*, 275. [CrossRef] [PubMed]
29. Azaïs-Braesco, V.; Sluik, D.; Maillot, M.; Kok, F.; Moreno, L.A. A review of total & added sugar intakes and dietary sources in Europe. *Nutr. J.* **2017**, *16*, 6. [PubMed]
30. Moynihan, P. Sugars and dental caries: evidence for setting a recommended threshold for intake. *Adv. Nutr.* **2016**, *7*, 149–156. [CrossRef] [PubMed]
31. Te Morenga, L.; Mallard, S.; Mann, J. Dietary sugars and body weight: Systematic review and meta-analyses of randomised controlled trials and cohort studies. *BMJ* **2012**, *346*, e7492. [CrossRef] [PubMed]

32. Te Morenga, L.A.; Howatson, A.J.; Jones, R.M.; Mann, J. Dietary sugars and cardiometabolic risk: Systematic review and meta-analyses of randomized controlled trials of the effects on blood pressure and lipids. *Am. J. Clin. Nutr.* **2014**, *100*, 65–79. [CrossRef] [PubMed]
33. Yang, Q.; Zhang, Z.; Gregg, E.W.; Flanders, W.D.; Merritt, R.; Hu, F.B. Added sugar intake and cardiovascular diseases mortality among US adults. *JAMA Intern. Med.* **2014**, *174*, 516–524. [CrossRef] [PubMed]
34. Collaboration PLAN for the Improvement of the Composition of Food and Beverages and Other Measures 2020. Spanish Agency for Consumer Affairs, Food Safety and Nutrition; Ministry of Health, Social Services and Equality. Madrid; 2018. Available online: http://www.aecosan.msssi.gob.es/AECOSAN/docs/documentos/nutricion/Plan_Colaboracion_INGLES.pdf (accessed on 22 January 2020).
35. EU Action Plan on Childhood Obesity 2014–2020. Available online: https://ec.europa.eu/health/sites/health/files/nutrition_physical_activity/docs/childhoodobesity_actionplan_2014_2020_en.pdf (accessed on 14 February 2020).
36. European Food and Nutrition Action Plan 2015–2020. World Health OrganizationRegional Office for Europe. Available online: http://www.euro.who.int/__data/assets/pdf_file/0003/294474/European-Food-Nutrition-Action-Plan-20152020-en.pdf?ua=1 (accessed on 22 January 2020).
37. Federici, C.; Detzel, P.; Petracca, F.; Dainelli, L.; Fattore, G. The impact of food reformulation on nutrient intakes and health, a systematic review of modelling studies. *BMC Nutr.* **2019**, *5*, 2. [CrossRef] [PubMed]
38. Ahuja, J.K.C.; Li, Y.; Nickle, M.S.; Haytowitz, D.B.; Roseland, J.; Nguyen, Q.; Khan, M.; Wu, X.; Somanchi, M.; Williams, J.; et al. Comparison of label and laboratory sodium values in popular sodium-contributing foods in the United States. *J. Acad. Nutr. Diet.* **2019**, *119*, 293–300. [CrossRef] [PubMed]

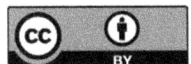

© 2020 by the authors. Licensee MDPI, Basel, Switzerland. This article is an open access article distributed under the terms and conditions of the Creative Commons Attribution (CC BY) license (http://creativecommons.org/licenses/by/4.0/).

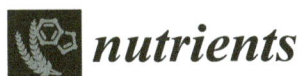

Article

Consumers' Perceptions of the Australian Health Star Rating Labelling Scheme

Fiona E. Pelly [1,*], Libby Swanepoel [1], Joseph Rinella [1] and Sheri Cooper [2]

[1] University of the Sunshine Coast, Sunshine Coast, QLD 4558, Australia; lswanepo@usc.edu.au (L.S.); joseph.rinella@gmail.com (J.R.)
[2] Southern Cross University, Gold Coast, QLD 4558, Australia; sheri.cooper@scu.edu.au
* Correspondence: fpelly@usc.edu.au

Received: 6 February 2020; Accepted: 4 March 2020; Published: 6 March 2020

Abstract: The objective of this study was to explore consumers' use and perception of the Australian Health Star Rating (HSR). A purposive sample of fifteen Australian grocery shoppers was recruited into four focus groups using a supermarket intercept strategy. Focus group discussions were recorded, transcribed and analysed using an iterative approach to thematic analysis. Three key themes emerged from analysis. The HSR was seen as simple, uncluttered, easy to understand and useful for quick comparison across products. The nutrition information was viewed positively; however, there was little confidence in the HSR due to a perceived lack of transparency in the criteria used to determine the number of stars. Highly processed foods were generally seen as having inflated ratings and participants expressed concern that this would increase consumption of these products. Finally, there was a belief that the HSR had a lack of negative imagery limiting the dissuasive impact on consumers when presented with low-rated foods. Consumers saw benefits in the HSR but were sceptical about how the ratings were derived. Transparency about the development and education on the application may assist with consumers' perception of the HSR.

Keywords: front-of-pack labelling; health star rating; nutrition labelling; consumer perception; qualitative research

1. Introduction

Nutrition labelling on food allows consumers to be informed about the nutritional composition of the products they are purchasing [1]. Nutrition labelling on packaging has been demonstrated to improve consumers' ability to assess product healthiness and encourage healthier food choices [2]. The display of nutrition information on packaged goods is mandatory in many countries [3] and typically comes in the form of a nutrition information panel (NIP) and ingredients list. The NIP displays numerical nutrition information on the side or back of a package, which is not always obvious to the consumer. In contrast, front-of-pack nutrition labels (FoPLs) are more likely to facilitate exposure to nutrition information as they are visible at the moment of choice [4].

FoPLs can be categorised according to factual information versus a continuum proposed by Kleef and Dagevos [5]. At one end of this continuum, the 'purely reductive' FoPL presents factual information condensed from the NIP and leaves the evaluation up to the consumer. The impact is therefore likely determined by the consumer's understanding of the facts provided. At the other end of the continuum are the 'purely evaluative' FoPLs that are binary in nature because they depict whether a product meets a particular nutrition standard through the presence or absence of the label, typically with a simple graphic such as a tick or stamp. The impact is reliant upon the consumer's awareness of the meaning of the graphic and the evaluation of the nutrition standard that is being met.

In the middle of the continuum are 'hybrid' FoPLs that present a combination of information from the NIP and an evaluation of that information. A preference for the appearance and use of hybrid compared to purely reductive FoPLs has been found in previous research [2,6,7]. It has been suggested that consumers are generally able to perform tasks related to identifying healthier food products when using a hybrid FoPL compared to a purely reductive version [8,9].

In 2014, the Health Star Rating (HSR) [10] was introduced for use on packaged foods in Australia. The hybrid scheme displays an evaluative component based on an algorithm-derived star rating from half a star (least healthy) to five stars (most healthy). Foods high in energy, saturated fat, sodium or total sugar are assigned lower star ratings than similar foods with fewer of these components. The star rating is increased based on the amount of fruits, nuts, vegetables, legumes, and in some cases protein and dietary fibre in the food. The HSR also presents a reductive component, that is, numeric nutrient information per 100 g or 100 mL for energy, sugar, saturated fat and sodium and one additional positive nutrient [10]. The HSR is a voluntary scheme that has recently undergone a formal review after a five-year implementation period. The recommendations from the report suggest some changes should be made to the appearance and calculation of the HSR, but with continued support of the system [11].

The aim of this study was to undertake an in-depth exploration of consumers' perceptions of the HSR considering the visual layout, nutrient information provided and application to a select number of food products. A secondary aim was to explore how consumers' use nutrition labelling to inform decisions around the healthiness of packaged food.

2. Materials and Methods

This study was underpinned by descriptive phenomenology given that the underlying aim was to explore and describe consumers' experiences of the HSR. A qualitative approach with focus group discussions was used to gain a rich understanding and comparison of consumers' perceptions of the HSR. Participants were recruited by the third author (male) using supermarket intercept convenience sampling from two major supermarket chains in regional locations in Queensland, Australia. Two additional participants were recruited through snowball sampling. Participants were considered eligible for the study if they were over 18 years and reported to do at least half of the shopping for themselves or their household. Those with nutrition education were excluded from the study. No prior relationship existed between the researchers and participants. All participants gave their informed consent prior to participation. This study was approved by the Human Research Ethics Committee of the University of the Sunshine Coast (S/14/709).

Four semi-structured focus group discussions involving 15 participants were conducted and moderated by the third author who was previously trained in focus group facilitation. Focus group discussions were guided by an interview protocol designed by the research team based on inquiry logic that was informed by the literature and the study aims (Table 1). A pilot focus group was conducted, feedback sought and the order and wording of some questions were modified accordingly. Participants were asked if they consider the healthiness of food when grocery shopping, and if so, how this is determined. All other questions were delivered following the presentation of props, beginning with four A4 pages (297 × 210 mm) showing different examples of the full HSR format which includes the HSR, and the energy and nutrient icons [12]. This approach invited participants' initial impression of the visual layout and the nutrient information provided by the HSR outside of the context of a food package. Five pairs of nutritionally equivalent packaged products (breakfast cereal, artificially sweetened carbonated beverage, cordial, crackers and sweet biscuits) that differed in their FoPL scheme were used as food props. First, products labelled with the Daily Intake Guide (%DI) were presented, and this was followed by those labelled with the HSR. The %DI is a reductive scheme that represents the energy or nutrient content per serve as a percentage of a standard reference value [13]. This allowed for comparisons between labelling formats and also facilitated discussion about perceptions of the HSR within the context of food products. The food props were purchased from a major supermarket in regional Australia and were selected based on availability of HSR-labelled products prior to commencement of the first focus group. Focus group discussions lasted between 35 and 65 min and were audio recorded and transcribed with permission from the participants.

Table 1. Questions from the focus group questionnaire on the Health Star Rating.

1. When you are purchasing food, do you consider the healthiness of the food product? If so, how do you work out if a food product is healthy? 2. [Show A4 printouts of the HSR] What are your first impressions of the HSR?
3. How do you feel about the look and design of the HSR?
(a) Which parts do you like and why? (b) Which parts don't you like and why?
4. How do you feel about the nutrition information presented on the HSR?
(a) What information is useful and why? (b) What information is not useful and why? (c) What information do you wish was on there and why?
5. [Shows food products with the %DI label] How do you perceive the healthiness of this product?
6. [Shows food products with the HSR label] How do you perceive the healthiness of these same food products now?
7. How could the HSR be improved? In what ways do you feel this would be an improvement?
8. Is there anything else that you'd like to discuss regarding the HSR?
9. Could you summarise your perceptions around the HSR?

Focus group transcripts were thematically analysed by two members of the research team (LS and JR) using an iterative approach as described by Srivastava and Hopwood [14]. Analysis followed the process described by Green et al. [15], where researchers initially immersed themselves in the data, then conceptualised the parts of the data that addressed the research questions into codes. Similar codes were then grouped into broader categories and connections between categories were examined. Categories that emerged were considered important based on length, depth of discussion, order of emergence as well as tendency to appear in more than one focus group. Explanations and interpretations of categories as themes were discussed and agreed upon by the research team in a process of peer debriefing [16] in order to increase the trustworthiness of findings. As all researchers had expertise in nutrition and health, bracketing was employed to further improve the trustworthiness of the data, whereby the researchers attempted to suspend their own perspectives and biases in order to focus on the participants' descriptions of their experience during the focus groups [17]. Focus group recruitment ceased when no new relevant information emerged.

3. Results

Three men and twelve women participated in the focus groups. Nine were over the age of 50, three were aged between 35 and 49 and three were aged between 25 and 34; four participants reported to be educated at a postgraduate level, four at a bachelor level and the remainder had high school, diploma or trade training. Participants' purchasing behaviours were influenced by various factors including individual health conditions, personal nutritional priorities, allergies, food safety, weight control, taste and price. The NIP was used by most participants to help determine the healthiness of a product, rather than use of any particular FoPL. Sugar, fat, saturated fat and food additives were the nutrients of most interest.

3.1. Themes

Three key themes relating to participants' perceptions of the HSR emerged in the focus group discussions: (1) Practicality of the HSR; (2) Lack of confidence in the HSR; and (3) Lack of dissuasive impact of the HSR, as described below.

3.1.1. Theme One: Practicality of the HSR

Participants' first impression of the HSR was that it appeared simple, uncluttered and easy to understand. The stars were a commonly recognized symbol that most participants understood to relate to the healthfulness of the product on a scale of half a star to five.

> "I think it's really straightforward, really obvious, really easy to get a quick glance at something of how many stars it is that's a really common visual reference for many people of one out of five stars or five out of five stars being good or bad so it's quite easy to read."
>
> (Participant 9)

In each of the four focus groups, participants related the HSR to the energy rating used on electrical appliances in Australia [18]. This familiarity made it easier to understand how to utilize the label without guidance.

> "I think the stars are good in that people are already familiar with appliances, so you don't have to fully educate them on what the concept is."
>
> (Participant 4)

The explanatory text was also pointed out as being a useful visual aid as it provided context to the numerical information on the HSR. Most participants believed that the HSR would facilitate comparisons between similar products at a glance. In this way, participants felt that the HSR would influence them to purchase higher-rated products.

> "Yeah if I went in and saw my regular chips that I was going to get and they were like 1 star and these ones were right next to them and they're 3 stars, yeah sure I'd try them."
>
> (Participant 10)

Most participants felt that higher-rated products still required supporting information and verification that was only available by checking the NIP and ingredients list. Most participants preferred the NIP and the ingredients when making purchasing decisions as they were viewed to be more transparent, thorough and credible sources of nutrition information.

> "I think I'd still look at the table on the back and then make my own assessment from that. There's no spin or there's no kind of magic numbers."
>
> (Participant 5)

The HSR was seen by most participants to be aimed towards people who were time poor.

> "A busy mum with three kids who's doing a weekly shop isn't necessarily going to have time to thoroughly read the label."
>
> (Participant 6)

3.1.2. Theme Two: Lack of Confidence in the HSR

There was a general lack of confidence in the HSR. Many participants viewed there to be a lack of transparency in the process used to determine the ratings. Participants felt there was an incongruence between their perceptions of the healthiness of a food product and the respective star rating. A number of participants were sceptical of the food industry, with concerns that food companies would change the nutritional makeup of their products to increase their HSR. These participants felt that rather than making the food products healthier, the reformulation would be superficial and exploitative.

> "...companies will just manipulate it. They will make subtle changes. Add things, take things out for their product to exploit the algorithm."
>
> (Participant 4)

Participants were interested in the governing body behind the HSR and the nutrition science used to develop the algorithm. Although most participants trusted the HSR governance, there was suspicion around the evidence base underpinning the algorithm, with some participants voicing concern around the food industries involvement in boosting ratings.

"The sceptic in me says that those scientists are lobbied by the food industry to present things that will be favourable towards agricultural, you know, whatever."

(Participant 2)

Other participants felt that consumers needed to be aware of how the algorithm works because an informed consumer is less able to be manipulated.

"I support any measure that helps people make more informed choices on the nutritional value of food absolutely, I just want to be able to trust that that is, that people understand what's behind, how these things are rated."

(Participant 5)

Participants voiced more concern around the ratings of foods towards the lower end of the scale. They felt that ratings seemed to be inflated for some foods they deemed to be 'junk foods' with little or no health value. These foods were products with ratings ranging from one and a half to two stars and included the cordial, sweet biscuits and the artificially sweetened carbonated beverages. It was generally the high proportions of sugar in the first two products and the additives in the third that led to dissonance with the ratings.

"I still think that that rating is very high with all that sugar in it. I've got a problem with how they've come up with this rating, this number."

(Participant 15)

Participants appeared to have more confidence in the HSR when rating foods at the higher end of the scale. This view is shown through the following quote relating to the five-star rating of a breakfast cereal.

"Well five stars is pretty unequivocal, it's pretty clear. You're not going to get away with claiming 5 stars unless you can back it up."

(Participant 4)

3.1.3. Theme Three: Lack of Dissuasive Impact of the HSR

Many participants expressed concerns that the HSR did not appropriately dissuade consumers from purchasing lower-rated products. This view is illustrated in the following quote relating to a product with a rating of two stars:

"Ok that's less than 50% so logic would tell you that it's not so healthy but even so, 2 is sounding reasonable."

(Participant 15)

It was suggested that low ratings could be accompanied by a symbol reinforcing the negative. Incorporating traffic light colouring into the HSR was also suggested in two of the four focus groups to address this perceived limitation.

"Even like a colour scheme wouldn't be a bad thing if that one over there had a green star and this one's got a red star you're like "Woah, that's bad.""

(Participant 10)

The framing of the label as a 'Health Star Rating' was also viewed as potentially confusing, as participants felt that this indicates that there is an absolute health value to any food with a rating.

4. Discussion

This study explored consumers' perceptions of the HSR. Three key themes emerged from the results, namely the practicality of the HSR, the lack of confidence in the HSR and the lack of dissuasive impact of the labelling scheme. The HSR was considered useful for quick comparisons across similar products at a glance due to its summary indicator, which was predicted to be particularly useful in the grocery shopping environment. The nutrient information provided on the HSR was considered to be important and useful to the participants in this study. Participants responded positively to the simplistic visual design of the HSR, contrary to a global study that found the HSR was perceived to have little visual appeal and 'not stand out' [19]. Elements that were identified as simple by the participants were as follows: (1) the explanatory text, (2) the uncluttered design, (3) the picture-based interpretation and (4) the familiarity of the stars. A study by Talati et al. [20] found similar results from focus group discussions, with the HSR being preferred over both the %DI and, to a lesser extent, the traffic light system due to the speed with which an evaluation could be made from the summary indicator saving time and effort while shopping. Similarly, simple FoPLs [21] or graphically representative FoPLs [22] have been shown to be liked by consumers and are considered easier to understand than labels with a lot of numbers and words. Many consumers evaluate as little information as possible to make their purchase decisions [23], and although nutrition content may be considered, it is often a lower priority when grocery shopping than factors such as price, taste and food safety [21,24].

Lack of confidence in the HSR was a key theme that emerged from this study. The provision of information on governance was considered essential to our participants. Transparency in the organisation behind the FoPL is known to increase credibility and trust [21], with well-known and trusted organisations being most credible for consumers [25]. The perception by some participants that labelling schemes are not backed by credible organisations may have influenced their confidence in the HSR by association. This finding suggests that consumers need to be educated about the governing body of the HSR as well as how its application onto products is regulated and monitored. The review of the HSR has suggested that there has been improved transparency in the information provided to consumers through the HSR system website, but greater confidence would be apparent if transferred to Food Standards Australia New Zealand [11].

Participants reacted differently to the idea that the implementation of the HSR may influence the food industry in reformulating their products. Some were concerned that reformulation efforts would be superficial and provide limited health benefits to consumers, whereas others felt that these changes would tangibly improve the nutritional profile of food products. Product reformulation of foods following the implementation of an FoPL has previously been successful [26,27]. The implementation of the HSR has the potential of encouraging food companies to reformulate their products by reducing levels of sugar, sodium and saturated fat, and also by increasing nutrients such as dietary fibre. This has been recently demonstrated in the reformulation of children's packaged foods [28].

Participants in this study also wanted to know how the star ratings were calculated before they could have confidence in the rating. Scepticism of the algorithm was highest when participants were presented with discretionary foods (artificially sweetened carbonated beverage, cordial and sweet biscuits), which they felt were rated too highly. Participants felt that, in these cases, the mechanics of the algorithm may be flawed, which is concurrent with previous studies indicating transparent labelling criteria to instil consumer trust [2,5,21]. This supports the recommendation to better align the HSR with the Australian Dietary Guidelines through changes to the calculator [11]. Consumers use food labels to make judgements about the food product as well as the food supply system behind the product [29]. Health and nutrition content claims on the front of the pack are often viewed by consumers as 'just an advertising tool' [30]. This was the case in our study, where participants felt distrust for the HSR, linking this to the food supply system by making judgements about the credibility of the food manufacturer. On the other hand, the NIP and ingredients list on the side or back of the pack (BoP) were viewed by our participants as highly trustworthy sources of information, which may reflect their confidence in how this BoP nutrient information is determined.

The participants in this study felt that the HSR had a limited ability to dissuade consumers to purchase lower-rated products due to its positively framed imagery. All foods eligible for the HSR scheme obtain, at worst, a half star rating, with the only negative communication being the optional explanatory text indicating a 'high' level of one of the key nutrients. It was suggested across several of our focus groups that incorporating some negative framing such as red colouring could help to address this. Similarly, traffic light colouring has been proposed to reduce the complexity of numerical information presented on the HSR [20], and interpretive aids such as colour are viewed favourably by consumers [19]. There is preliminary research to suggest that the inclusion of the traffic light colouring would be an effective way of modifying the HSR [31]. However, the recent review of the HSR did not support the use of the traffic light system [11].

While our recruitment strategy and methodology allowed for a rich understanding into consumers' perceptions of the HSR, it also led to some limitations in our findings. We conducted four focus groups at which point we reached data saturation, whereby no new themes emerged from the data, giving a high indication of the trustworthiness of our findings [32]. Data saturation is the optimal guide for sample size in qualitative research; however, it is known that a sample size of two or three focus groups will likely capture at least 80% of themes on a topic [33]. The qualitative exploratory nature of our study allowed participants to discuss issues around health, nutrition and labelling with high levels of passion, confidence and articulation, which suggests the findings from this study provide authentic insight into consumers' perception of the HSR, but they may not be generalisable to the wider Australian population. Our participant demographics also showed some variance when compared with the general grocery shopper population in Australia. Eight out of 15 (53%) participants had a bachelor or postgraduate education, compared to approximately 33% of Australian adults in the general population [34]. A further limitation of this study was the small range of HSR-labelled food products that were available for use as food props in the focus groups at the time of this study. An increasing number of products currently display the HSR, and it is recommended that future studies select foods that reflect the full range of products that consumers are exposed to in the supermarket environment.

This study provides an insight into consumers' perceptions of the HSR. The HSR was perceived as simple and easy to understand, and as being most useful when comparing across similar products at a glance. It was perceived as less useful for analysing single products in isolation and particularly for lower-rated products due to its positively framed communication design. While our results cannot be generalised to the wider Australian grocery shopper population, this sample of participants indicated that there was a lack of confidence in the HSR. This was due to a variety of reasons including a lack of familiarity, a lack of transparency on how the ratings are calculated and a disagreement with the product ratings.

5. Conclusions

There is a need to improve consumer confidence in the HSR to ensure accurate guidance when navigating the modern food environment. Campaigns to promote the use of the HSR should focus on improving consumer understanding and the evidence base underpinning the HSR.

Author Contributions: All authors were involved in the study design. Authors are listed in order of contribution. F.E.P. was the researcher leader on this study. J.R. transcribed the audio recordings following focus group training, and J.R. and L.S. conducted the thematic analysis. F.E.P., L.S., S.C., and J.R. contributed to the interpretation of the results and research write-up. The researcher held no assumptions and did not know the participants before the focus groups. All authors have read and agreed to the published version of the manuscript.

Funding: This research received no external funding

Conflicts of Interest: The authors declare no conflict of interest.

References

1. Campos, S.; Doxey, J.; Hammond, D. Nutrition labels on pre-packaged foods: a systematic review. *Public Health Nutr.* **2011**, *14*, 1496–1506. [CrossRef] [PubMed]
2. Dana, L.M.; Chapman, K.; Talati, Z.; Kelly, B.; Dixon, H.; Miller, C.; Pettigrew, S. Consumers' Views on the Importance of Specific Front-of-Pack Nutrition Information: A Latent Profile Analysis. *Nutrients* **2019**, *11*. [CrossRef] [PubMed]
3. Kanter, R.; Vanderlee, L.; Vandevijvere, S. Front-of-package nutrition labelling policy: global progress and future directions. *Public Health Nutr.* **2018**, *21*, 1399–1408. [CrossRef] [PubMed]
4. Egnell, M.; Talati, Z.; Hercberg, S.; Pettigrew, S.; Julia, C. Objective Understanding of Front-of-Package Nutrition Labels: An International Comparative Experimental Study across 12 Countries. *Nutrients* **2018**, *10*, 1542. [CrossRef]
5. Kleef, E.V.; Dagevos, H. The growing role of front-of-pack nutrition profile labeling: a consumer perspective on key issues and controversies. *Crit. Rev. Food Sci. Nutr.* **2015**, *55*, 291–303. [CrossRef]
6. Maubach, N.; Hoek, J. A qualitative study of New Zealand parents' views on front-of-pack nutrition labels. *Nutr. Diet.* **2010**, *67*, 90–96. [CrossRef]
7. Signal, L.; Lanumata, T.; Robinson, J.A.; Tavila, A.; Wilton, J.; Mhurchu, C.N. Perceptions of New Zealand nutrition labels by Maori, Pacific and low-income shoppers. *Public Health Nutr.* **2008**, *11*, 706–713. [CrossRef]
8. Hawley, K.L.; Roberto, C.A.; Bragg, M.A.; Liu, P.J.; Schwartz, M.B.; Brownell, K.D. The science on front-of-package food labels. *Public Health Nutr.* **2013**, *16*, 430–439. [CrossRef]
9. Newman, C.L.; Burton, S.; Andrews, J.C.; Netemeyer, R.G.; Kees, J. Marketers' use of alternative front-of-package nutrition symbols: An examination of effects on product evaluations. *J. Acad. Mark. Sci.* **2018**, *46*, 453–476. [CrossRef]
10. Australian Government. The Health Star Rating System. 2019. Available online: http://www.healthstarrating.gov.au/internet/healthstarrating/publishing.nsf/Content/Calculator (accessed on 6 February 2020).
11. The Australia and New Zealand Ministerial Forum on Food Regulation. *The Australia and New Zealand Ministerial Forum on Food Regulation response to the Health Star Rating System five year review December 2019*; Commonwealth of Australia: Canberra, Australia, 2019.
12. Australian Government. The Health Star Rating System. How to use Health Star Ratings. 2019. Available online: http://www.healthstarrating.gov.au/internet/healthstarrating/publishing.nsf/Content/How-to-use-health-stars (accessed on 6 February 2020).
13. The Australian Food and Grocery Council. Daily Intake Guide. 2011. Available online: http://www.mydailyintake.net/ (accessed on 6 February 2020).
14. Srivastava, P.; Hopwood, N. Reflection/Commentary on a Past Article: "A Practical Iterative Framework for Qualitative Data Analysis". *Int. J. Qual. Methods* **2018**, *17*. [CrossRef]
15. Green, J.; Willis, K.; Hughes, E.; Small, R.; Welch, N.; Gibbs, L.; Daly, J. Generating best evidence from qualitative research: the role of data analysis. *Aust. New Zealand J. Public Health* **2007**, *31*, 545–550. [CrossRef] [PubMed]
16. Lincoln, Y.S.; Guba, E.G. *Naturalistic Inquiry*; Sage Publications: Beverly Hills, CA, USA, 1985; p. 416.
17. Tufford, L.; Newman, P. Bracketing in Qualitative Research. *Qual. Social Work* **2012**, *11*, 80–96. [CrossRef]
18. Australian Government Department of Industry, Energy and Resources. *The E3 Program*; 2020. Available online: https://www.energyrating.gov.au/about-e3-program#toc1 (accessed on 6 February 2020).
19. Talati, Z.; Egnell, M.; Hercberg, S.; Julia, C.; Pettigrew, S. Consumers' Perceptions of Five Front-of-Package Nutrition Labels: An Experimental Study Across 12 Countries. *Nutrients* **2019**, *11*, 1934. [CrossRef] [PubMed]
20. Talati, Z.; Pettigrew, S.; Kelly, B.; Ball, K.; Dixon, H.; Shilton, T. Consumers' responses to front-of-pack labels that vary by interpretive content. *Appetite* **2016**, *101*, 205–213. [CrossRef]
21. Grunert, K.G.; Wills, J.M. A review of European research on consumer response to nutrition information on food labels. *J. Public Health Heidelb.* **2007**, *15*, 385–399. [CrossRef]
22. Viswanathan, M.; Hastak, M.; Gau, R. Understanding and Facilitating the Usage of Nutritional Labels by Low-Literate Consumers. *J. Public Policy Mark.* **2009**, *28*, 135–145. [CrossRef]
23. Wood, W. Attitude change: Persuasion and social influence. *Annu. Rev. Psychol.* **2000**, *51*, 539–570. [CrossRef]
24. Pettigrew, S.; Pescud, M. The Salience of Food Labeling Among Low-income Families With Overweight Children. *J. Nutr. Educ. Behav.* **2013**, *45*, 332–339. [CrossRef]

25. Feunekes, G.I.; Gortemaker, I.A.; Willems, A.A.; Lion, R.; Van Den Kommer, M. Front-of-pack nutrition labelling: testing effectiveness of different nutrition labelling formats front-of-pack in four European countries. *Appetite* **2008**, *50*, 57–70. [CrossRef]
26. Young, L.; Swinburn, B. Impact of the Pick the Tick food information programme on the salt content of food in New Zealand. *Health Promot Int.* **2002**, *17*, 13–19. [CrossRef]
27. Vyth, E.L.; Steenhuis, I.H.; Roodenburg, A.J.; Brug, J.; Seidell, J.C. Front-of-pack nutrition label stimulates healthier product development: a quantitative analysis. *Int. J. Behav. Nutr. Phys. Act.* **2010**, *7*, 65. [CrossRef] [PubMed]
28. Morrison, H.; Meloncelli, N.; Pelly, F.E. Nutritional quality and reformulation of a selection of children's packaged foods available in Australian supermarkets: Has the Health Star Rating had an impact? *Nutr. Diet* **2019**, *76*, 296–304. [CrossRef] [PubMed]
29. Tonkin, E.; Wilson, A.M.; Coveney, J.; Webb, T.; Meyer, S.B. Trust in and through labelling—A systematic review and critique. *Br. Food J.* **2015**, *117*, 318–338. [CrossRef]
30. Singer, L.; Williams, P.G.; Ridges, L.; Murray, S.; McMahon, A. Consumer reactions to different health claim formats on food labels. *Food Aust.* **2006**, *58*, 92–97.
31. Pettigrew, S.; Dana, L.; Talati, Z. Enhancing the effectiveness of the Health Star Rating via presentation modifications. *Aust. N. Z. J. Public Health* **2019**, *44*, 20–21. [CrossRef]
32. Hennink, M.M.; Kaiser, B.N.; Weber, M.B. What Influences Saturation? Estimating Sample Sizes in Focus Group Research. *Qual. Health Res.* **2019**, *29*, 1483–1496. [CrossRef]
33. Guest, G.; Namey, E.; McKenna, K. How Many Focus Groups Are Enough? Building an Evidence Base for Nonprobability Sample Sizes. *Field Methods* **2017**, *29*, 3–22. [CrossRef]
34. Australian Bureau of Statistics. Education and Work, Australia. 2019. Available online: http://www.abs.gov.au/ausstats/abs@.nsf/mf/6227.0 (accessed on 6 February 2020).

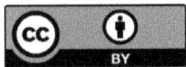

© 2020 by the authors. Licensee MDPI, Basel, Switzerland. This article is an open access article distributed under the terms and conditions of the Creative Commons Attribution (CC BY) license (http://creativecommons.org/licenses/by/4.0/).

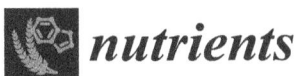

Article

How Much Sugar is in My Drink? The Power of Visual Cues

Bethany D. Merillat * and Claudia González-Vallejo

Ohio University, Athens, OH 45701, USA; gonzalez@ohio.edu
* Correspondence: bl872911@ohio.edu; Tel.: (440) 829-7634

Received: 29 December 2019; Accepted: 30 January 2020; Published: 2 February 2020

Abstract: Despite widespread attempts to educate consumers about the dangers of sugar, as well as the advent of nutritional labeling, individuals still struggle to make educated decisions about the foods they eat, and/or to use the Nutrition Facts Panel. This study examined the effect of visual aids on judgments of sugar quantity in popular drinks, and choices. 261 volunteers at four different locations evaluated 11 common beverages. Key measures were estimates of sugar in the drinks, nutrition knowledge, and desire to consume them. In the experimental condition, participants viewed beverages along with test tubes filled with the total amount of sugar in each drink; the control condition had no sugar display. Both groups were encouraged to examine the Nutrition Facts Panel when making their evaluations. Correlational analyses revealed that consumers exposed to the visual aid overestimated sugar content and the length of time needed to exercise to burn off the calories; they also had lower intentions to consume any of the beverages. Individuals asserting to use the Nutrition Facts Panel (NFP) in general were also less likely to admit using it in this particular study ($r = -2, p = 0.001$). This study suggests that a simple visual aid intervention affected judgments and choices towards curtailing sugar intake. This has implications for labeling format implementation.

Keywords: nutrition facts panel; food label; consumer behavior; food decision making; food packaging; food choice; nutrition and health claims; food label; sugar; nutrition

1. Introduction

" ... sugar is cheap, sugar tastes good and sugar sells, so companies have little incentive to change [1] (p.29)."

A U.S. citizen consumes an average of 216 L of soda per year, of which 58% contains sugar [1]. The obesity problem in the U.S. is well documented, with obesity rates as high as 25% in 41 states, and above 20% in every state [2]. Importantly, child obesity has increased in the 1999–2016 period as a recent report shows [3]. Researchers have attributed the obesity problem, in part, to consumption of nutrient poor processed foods, containing high amounts of sugar, sodium, and saturated fats [4,5].

Added sugars alone are linked to a wide range of non-communicable diseases, including tooth decay, gout, heart disease, diabetes, obesity, and metabolic syndrome which is characterized by higher blood pressure, blood sugar, and triglycerides, and lower "good" cholesterol [6]. The health care costs associated with metabolic syndrome is estimated to be $150 billion annually [1]. Furthermore, the United Nations World Health Organization places non-communicable diseases as the leading cause of deaths globally, responsible for about 68% of deaths worldwide in 2012 [7]. Given the relationship between added sugar consumption and metabolic syndrome, researchers have gone as far as to call sugar a toxin, and have proposed stricter regulations for added sugars similar to those controlling alcohol [1].

While the American Heart Association recommends that the population limit added sugar to six teaspoons a day for women and nine for men [6,7], the average sugar consumption in the form of fructose is at an all-time high with current estimates at around 57.7g/day (or approximately 14.42 teaspoons-4g per teaspoon) accounting for 10.2% of total caloric intake. A study also placed sugar-sweetened beverages as the most important contributor of fructose intake (30.1%) [8].

1.1. Strategies to Promote Healthier Eating

Increasing the availability of healthy foods, and/or restricting specific types of foods, such as soft drinks in school settings, have proven effective methods to curtail poor nutritional consumption by both the Food and Agricultural Organization of the United Nations (FAO) [9,10] and the Centers for Disease control [11] (see also [12–14]. Curbing choices via pricing has also proven effective [15] (see the Chilean experience in Jacobs [16]). The FAO further notes that education-only interventions appeared less successful than those including environmental changes [10]. This poses a challenge for promoting better food choices outside school settings because price adjusting and/or limiting the supply of certain foods is more difficult to implement [16].

In a positive light, a number of prominent health campaigns are targeting the consumption of sugary drinks in many states (e.g., California's Kick the Can campaign; the Kansas' Just Add Water! public health intervention). However, a report from the Food and Agriculture Organization of the United Nations [10] concludes that public awareness campaigns, which take many different forms all over the world, have received mixed support regarding their effectiveness.

Another strategy to encourage healthy eating is by means of nutrition labelling. To address the issue of unhealthy eating, the US Nutritional Labeling and Education Act of 1990 [17] mandated the use of a standardized nutrition label (the Nutrition Facts Panel, NFP). The aim of the law was to provide consumers with nutritional information that was accurate and easy to read and encourage healthier food choices [18]. Studies by the US Agriculture Department found that the percentage of adults who reported using the NFP 'always or most of the time' went from 34% in 2007–08 to 42% in 2009–10 [19] and 77% in 2014 [20].

However, the assumption that the NFP indeed helps consumers to judge the nutritional quality of the foods and to make better decisions is debatable. In the 2014 survey, half of those who reported rarely or never using the NFP said they did not feel they needed to use the label [20], and several studies indicate that there has been no aggregate improvement of American nutrient consumption since the implementation of the NFP [21,22]. People may think that they do not need to use the label, but their health may be suffering because with the myriad of products in the market today, understanding of, and the ability to use the NFP can make a significant difference in one's ability to judge the healthfulness of food and drink options.

Current studies find positive and significant correlation between judgments of nutrition quality of foods based on the NFP, and a nutrition quality expert standard, but the levels of agreement are low [23,24]. More broadly, these studies and others investigating a host of other ecological factors, including those related to dietary choices, necessitate viewing the role of the NFP through the context of a multi-factored public health issue.

The FAO's 2013 report reveals a greater understanding of nutritional information form label usage, but not necessarily improvements in consumption [10]. Additionally, nutrient lists, which is the format used by the U.S. Nutrition Facts Panel (NFP), are often found to be confusing, and may disproportionally affect individuals having lower knowledge about nutrition and health. Why? While a number of factors certainly contribute to the problem, research has found that both those of lower socio-economic status and individuals with lower knowledge concerning nutrition and health are less likely to use such labels [25]. While more generally, research shows that the process by which food marketing affects food decisions is not well understood [26], and although a number of suggestions on how to improve consumer choice have been proposed, few are supported with empirical research [27]. Further investigation of packaged label use is still needed to determine whether they have a positive effect on nutritional understanding and decision making [28].

However, there are a number of other interventions which have both real-world applicability and have been proven to improve consumer choices. For example, research by Donnelly et al. found that evocative, graphic warning labels, as compared to text warning labels (calorie labels and no labels) significantly reduced the share of sugary drinks purchased in a cafeteria [29]. These graphic labels also served to heighten negative affect (toward unhealthy options) while promoting deeper thought concerning the health consequences of consuming sugary options [29]. We point this out to highlight that for an intervention to have success in changing consumer behavior, it must be both effective in research studies, and have the capability of being implemented and accepted in the broader consumer market (including both consumers and retailers).

While these studies have certainly played an important role in our understanding of the power of visual aids, it is important to consider that they may have limited real-world applicability because of the difficulty of adopting them in the market, and making them visible/available to consumers on a wide-scale.

1.2. The Present Study

The central and negative role of sugar in human health has been identified in numerous sources (e.g., Williams and Nestle [30]) and in conjunction with the current debates on designing successful interventions via NFP changes [31], a direct examination of judgments of nutrients from label information is in demand. In particular, the current study contrasts perceptions of sugar content in beverages when consumers use the current NFP vs. using the NFP with the addition of a simple visual aid.

A study by Viskaal-van Dongen, de Graaf, Siebelink, and Kok [32] exemplified the importance of visualizing nutrition content in order to properly judge it. In that study, participants consumed either a meal with visibly fatty food, (e.g., bread with butter on top), or invisible fat (e.g., bread baked with extra oil). Unbeknownst to the participants, both meals contained the exact same amount of energy, fat, carbohydrates and proteins, but participants ate 9% more calories when the fat was hidden than when it was visible. Hence, judging the hidden nutritional make up of food is not simple and can lead to overconsumption. More generally, psychological research has shown that judgments are fallible in many domains [33,34].

Following the work of Viskaal-van et al. [32] we coin the term the hidden sugar hypothesis to propose that individuals are not able to make accurate judgments of sugar content in beverages because the solid sugar, like many other nutrients, is invisible or abstract, even when numerical information is available via the NFP, without any visible cues. We hypothesize that participants underestimate the amount of sugar and the number of calories in a drink when the sugar is hidden. In contrast, we expect different and more accurate perceptions when the amount of sugar is explicitly present. Better perceptions of amount would also lead to better judgments of other related variables, such as the amount of time needed to walk to burn off the calories in the drink. We also assumed that variability in judgments would relate to consumption intentions.

One aspect pertaining to the effectiveness of interventions on food consumption is nutrition knowledge. Studies have shown that greater nutrition knowledge is associated with increased intake of fruits and vegetables and greater adherence to recommendations on fat intake [35]. These researchers developed the Nutrition Knowledge Questionnaire (NKQ) and found that a lack of nutritional knowledge impacted the relationship between diet and disease (e.g., between high fat and salt intake and cardiovascular disease) [35]. Similarly, individuals high in motivation and obesity knowledge, termed the 'nutrition elite' were found to have appropriate evaluations of nutrient claims that impacted consumption intentions [36].

We thus measured participants on several individual-level measures including the participant's health, nutrition knowledge, education, and other demographic information that could impact their judgments and choices. We predicted that higher scores on the NKQ, indicating greater nutrition knowledge, would be associated with more accurate ratings of the healthfulness of beverages, and more accurate estimates of the amount of sugar contained in the drinks and walking estimates. Additionally, we predicted that for individuals with diabetes, accuracy of evaluations would be greatest irrespective of the display manipulation. Following past research as reviewed above, we also expected relations of self-report of NFP usage with variables such as nutrition knowledge, education, and income.

2. Materials and Methods

2.1. Participants

Participants ($n = 261$) were volunteers who came to shop at four different locales in Ohio. They were predominantly female (54.8%), and not currently dieting (75.1%), with 43.7% reporting that they were employed, and 6.9% were on disability. While the sample was largely Caucasian (87.70%), it also included African Americans (3.80%), Hispanics (1.10%), and Asians (2.70%). The mean age was 45.80 (SD = 17.02), and the average BMI for this group was 28.41 (SD = 6.89), which is considered overweight (BMIs 25–29.9) by the U.S. Department of Agriculture and U.S. Department of Health and Human Services Report (2010). Seventy percent of the sample reported an annual income of less than $49,000 per year. With relation to health, 37.5 % reported having health issues or other dietary restrictions that influenced their food choices. 52% reported eating out at least once a week or more, and over half the sample (58.5%) said they used the NFP 70% of the time.

Of the participants, 146 completed the survey in the sugar/tube and NPF condition (referred to as the Sugar group in what follows); these participants saw test tubes filled with the exact amount of sugar in each drink attached to each of the beverages, with the NFP visible as well. 115 participants completed the survey in the NFP alone condition (referred to as the No-Sugar group or control group). Participants in the No-Sugar condition only saw the beverage—no test tubes were attached but the NFP was visible. There were no significant differences between the two conditions for gender, dieting, employment, race, age, BMI, income, health issues, eating out or use of the NFP.

2.2. Procedure

For the study, the researchers set up a small folding station at five different locations in Ohio: Lottridge Ridge Food Pantry, Save-A-Lot, the Athens Farmers Market, and the Solon Community Center (Table 1). Participants were randomly assigned to the control (No-Sugar) and experimental (Sugar) groups. The stand was set on different days with randomized days to conditions so as to obtain approximately equal number of participants from each location in each experimental condition.

Table 1. Sample Size in Different Locations by Experimental Condition.

Location	Sugar	No-sugar	Total
Lottridge Ridge Food Center	25	23	48
Save-A-Lot	38	41	79
Athens Farmers Market	42	21	63
Solon Community Center	41	30	71
Total	146	115	261

On the table, there were 11 popular beverages (see Table 2). In the No-Sugar condition, the beverages were presented alone; in the experimental Sugar condition, sugar bottles (test tubes) filled with the exact grams of sugar contained in the entire beverage were attached to the drink with rubber bands. Figure 1 shows one such display.

Table 2. Study Drinks with Key Information.

Drink Name	NuVal Score	Serving Size (Ounces)	Serving Per Container	Calories Per Serving	Total Calories Per Bottle	Total Sugar (Grams) Per Bottle	Number of Teaspoons Sugar (1 tsp = 4 g)	Number of Sugar Bottles	Minutes to Burn Calories
Organic Horizon Low-Fat Chocolate Milk	32	8	1	150	150	22	5.5	1.375	30
Pepsi	1	12	1	150	150	41	10.25	2.5625	30
Monster Energy Drink	3	8	2	110	220	54	13.5	3.375	44
Starbucks Frappuccino Mocha (Low-Fat)	23	9.5	1	180	180	31	7.75	2	36
Diet Snapple Lemonade Iced Tea Half n' Half	40	16	1	10	10	0	0	0	2
Coca Cola	1	12	1	140	140	39	9.75	2.5	28
Odwalla Mango Tango Fruit Smoothie Blend	31	12	1	220	220	44	11	2.75	44
Sprite Lemon Lime Soda	1	12	1	140	140	38	9.5	2.375	28
Simply Orange (Florida's Natural 100% Orange Juice)	30	13.5	1	190	190	41	10.25	2.5625	38
Red Bull Cola	1	8.4	1	110	110	27	6.75	1.6875	22
Gatorade Lemon-Lime G2 Thirst Quencher	1	12	2.5	30	75	17.5	4.375	1.09375	15

tsp = teaspoons.

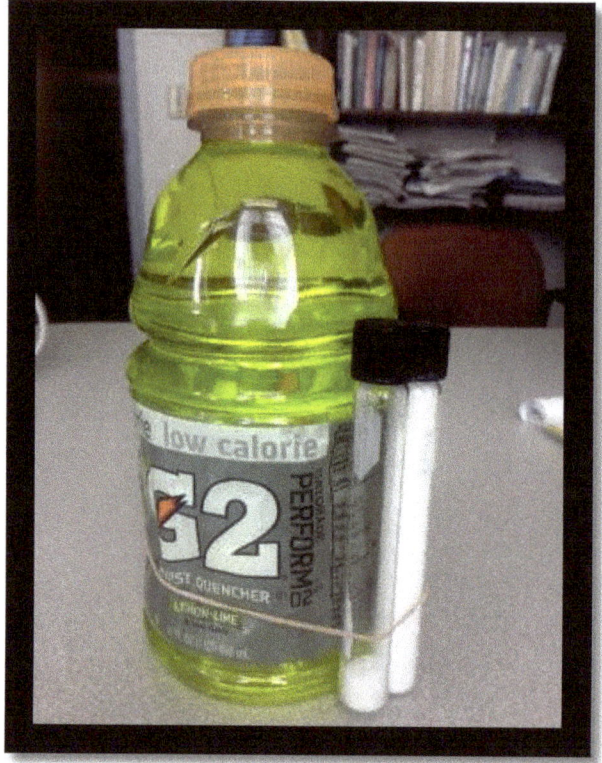

Figure 1. A drink with its sugar content displayed.

Participants were solicited for the study as they walked by the booth. They were asked if they would be willing to complete a short survey in exchange for the chance to win a $50 Visa gift card. If they agreed, they were read the informed consent statement and signed that they understood and were willing to participate. Participants were given a survey packet and writing utensil and completed the survey as they stood by the table which contained unopened bottles of all 11 drinks. They were told that they should answer the questions to the best of their knowledge, and were encouraged to use the NFP and all other information about the drinks to help answer the questions.

Participants, after answering a series of questions for each drink, completed a demographic questionnaire, a nutrition quiz, and follow-up questions concerning their affective state and experience participating in the study. All measures are found in Supplementary Materials Figures S1–S4. After completing the survey, they were thanked for their time and debriefed.

2.3. Measures

Expert Nutrition Quality Scores: NuVal® is a Nutrition Scoring System developed by medical and nutritional experts which summarizes the overall nutrition of a food on a scale from 1 to 100 (with higher scores indicating more nutritious food) [37]. It utilizes an Overall Nutritional Quality Index (ONQI) algorithm to convert the complex nutritional information from the Nutrition Facts Panel into a single score. For this study, NuVal scores were used as the "gold standard" with which to determine how accurately participants could judge the healthfulness of a food. NuVal ratings for the beverages used in this study can be found in Table 2.

Beverage Questions: For each of the 11 beverages in the study, participants were asked to, "Please answer the following questions based on what you observed today at the nutrition and sugar display." On each page of the packet, a picture of the beverage from the display was shown, along with the drink's name, and the participant was asked to answer seven questions concerning the drink: "If you consume (drink name) how many times a week do you drink it (put 0 if you never consume it or don't like it)?"; "What proportion of this beverage is sugar (e.g., if a drink contains 1/2 a cup of sugar, and 1/2 cup of milk, the beverage would be 1/2 or 50% sugar)?"; "How HEALTHY is this beverage?" (on a scale from 0 to 100, with 100 being the healthiest); "How well does the beverage meet nutritional requirements/how NUTRITIOUS is the drink?" (on a scale from 0 to 100, with 100 "meets them extremely well"); "How many teaspoons of sugar are in this drink?"; "How many minutes of brisk walking (3.5 mph) would it take to burn off the calories from consuming this drink (assume you are drinking the ENTIRE bottle, which may contain more than one serving size)?", and "How confident are you in your answer?" (for the walking estimate). They completed all of these questions for each of the 11 drinks found in Table 2.

Demographic Questions: Participants answered a comprehensive set of questions concerning their height, weight, age, gender highest level of education and employment. Information was also gathered concerning their eating habits, medical history, and use of packaging/NFP when making purchases. Participants also rated the importance of the various nutrients in the NFP in general, and in relation to their use in this study. Finally, they were asked qualitative questions concerning their participation in the study, and factors they believed would influence their choice of healthy vs. unhealthy foods, as well as their knowledge of health guidelines.

Nutrition Knowledge Questionnaire (NKQ): The NKQ [38] was designed to provide a comprehensive measure of nutritional knowledge in adult populations. The scale consists of items concerning dietary advice, dieting and disease in five main areas: understanding of health terminology (e.g., fiber and cholesterol); awareness of dietary recommendations; knowledge of food sources related to the recommendations (e.g., which foods contain which nutrients); using dietary information to make dietary choices, and awareness of the association between diet and disease. For the present study, a modified 12-item survey was created using items from the original scale. Participants were asked to decide whether or not they believed a health statement was true or false (e.g., "Butter is higher in calories than regular margarine"). Higher scores or more correct answers reflect better nutrition knowledge.

Choices. Participants were asked which beverages they would consume right now, given the choice, and how thirsty they were at the present time.

2.4. Analyses

Data was analyzed using SPSS. A Chi-squared test, correlational statistics, and a MANOVA were run.

3. Results

3.1. NFP Usage

Self-report of NFP usage was assessed in three different questions. Individuals could check yes or no to viewing the NFP in food packages in general, when they shop for food. Results showed that 61.1% (n = 159 of 260 participants who provided answers) affirmed using the NFP. In contrast, participants were less likely to report using the NFP in the current study (n = 100 of 258, 38.76%) (It is important to note that there are slight discrepancies in the total respondents for several questions, as not all participants answered all of the questions. Therefore the n value will vary slightly). This relatively low rate of NFP usage in the present study is surprising given that participants were encouraged to do so. Nevertheless, individuals in the No-Sugar condition reported using the NFP to evaluate the drinks at a higher rate (49.12%, n = 56 out of 114 individuals with no missing values) than those in the Sugar condition (30.5%, n = 44 of 144 individuals) (X^2 (1) = 9.24, p = 0.002). This is expected because the only way to judge content accurately would be from the label, but again we note the rates are not high. This result contrasts to no significance difference in reporting general NFP usage between the two groups (X^2 (1) = 0.184, p = 0.668).

The third assessment of NFP usage pertained to self-report frequency, or how often the participant states using the NFP when considering to purchase or consume a food item. A total of 151 participants (58.52%, n = 258), across both experimental conditions reported using the NFP 70% of the time or more. There were no differences in the pattern of responses to this question between the Sugar and No-Sugar individuals (X^2 (13) = 16, p = 0.249).

In terms of predicted relations of self-report of NFP usage with demographics, we found positive and significant correlations (all ps < 0.0001) with: nutrition knowledge (r = 0.325), education (r = 0.361), self-report of being healthy (r = 0.22), income (r = 0.25), self-report of eating healthy (r =0.5), eating regular meals (r = 0.46), being concerned with healthy eating (r = 0.56). Surprisingly, individuals asserting to use the NFP in general were less likely to admit using it in this particular study (r = −2, p = 0.001).

3.2. Accuracy of Sugar Estimates

The relationship (correlation) between the subjective and the objective amount of sugar in the beverages was examined in order to assess the degree to which individuals discriminated high versus low sugary drinks. This achievement measure derives from judgment analysis [39], a theory and methodology based on Brunswik's lens model [40]. Using the number of teaspoons of sugar as the unit, Pearson's correlation coefficient was computed for the judged and actual number of teaspoons of sugar across the 11 drinks for each person who had judged at least six drinks. As expected the judgment achievement of the Sugar group was higher (a median correlation equal to 0.6, which is strong and positive) than that of the No-sugar group with a median equal to 0.44. In other words, one half of the participants in the Sugar group had correlation equal to 0.6 or higher. Contrasting the mean correlation of the groups (mean r = 0.55 for the Sugar group, and mean r = 0.42 for the No-Sugar group), they are significantly different (using Fisher z transformation and unequal variance correction, t (244.36) = 3.48, p < 0.01). Thus, a simple display that makes the hidden sugar explicit allowed consumers to give estimates that more closely related to the actual amounts of sugar across the drinks.

In terms of raw estimates of the number of sugar teaspoons, the proportion of sugar in each drink, and the amount of walking needed to burn the calories in the drink, the Sugar group tended to produce greater overestimation (greater error) in all cases. A MANOVA using the mean absolute error, computed as a difference between subjective and objective quantities (computed for each person) revealed a main effect of condition (F (3,251) = 2.72, Wilks' Lambda = 0.97, p = 0.045) with larger means for the Sugar group with means equal to: 9.95 (SE = 1.89) for the teaspoon judgment; 40.04 min (SE = 3.47) for the walking judgment, and 28.58% for the proportion of sugar in the drink judgment (SE = 1.1). The corresponding means for the No-Sugar group were: 9.50 (SE = 2.15) for the teaspoon sugar judgment; 25.62 min for the walking estimate (SE = 3.95), and 26.68% for the proportion (SE = 1.26).

We note that the differences were first computed; the sign of the average differences were positive for both groups but greater for the Sugar group (raw mean differences equal to 4.3 for the Sugar group and 2.06 for the No-sugar participants; the mean of the Sugar group is significantly larger (t (252) = 1.86, p = 0.03) (three outliers with means 2 standard deviations above the mean were removed for this test). The proportion of participants with positive means (displaying overestimation) was greater in the Sugar than the No-Sugar group (81 of 144, 56.25%, participants in the Sugar condition; 48 of 113, 42.47%, in the No-sugar condition), X^2 (1) = 4.8, p = 0.028. In combination, using either the absolute or the raw differences, results point to greater overestimation by the Sugar than the No-Sugar group.

Comparing the judgments of healthiness of the beverages with the beverages' NuVal showed similarity of the two groups. The median correlation for the Sugar group was 0.63 and that of the No-sugar group was equal to 0.61. Comparing the mean correlations resulted in no significant mean difference (mean correlations equal to 0.58 and 0.55, for the Sugar and No-sugar groups, respectively; $p = 0.34$). Thus, the sugar visualization did not affect judgments of nutrition quality of the drinks. Focusing on judgments errors with regards to judging healthiness, the groups did not differ either. However, absolute judgment errors in this variable tended to be smaller for individuals with higher nutrition knowledge ($r = -124, p = 0.023$) and education ($r = -27, p = 0.00$). Furthermore, individuals reporting higher nutrition knowledge also reported having better health ($r = 0.134, p = 0.015$) (all ps one-tail tests).

3.3. Participants with Diabetes

Focusing on participants who reported having diabetes ($n = 43, 16.4\%$), this group had higher BMI (28.71) and lower income (median \$20k and below annually) when compared to the rest of the participants (BMI = 26.24, median income \$20–\$29k annually). They were also older (median age 54; median age 46 for others). Results showed greater overestimation of sugar content by these individuals. The mean absolute error overestimating teaspoons of sugar was equal to 15.42 (with raw mean difference equal to 11.01). Without including the three outliers (one who was in the diabetics group), the mean of the absolute error describing overestimation for the diabetic group (mean = 9.9) is significantly larger than that of the rest of the participants (mean = 6.7), $t(74.37) = 1.68, p = 0.049$.

3.4. Person Level Factors that Relate to Judgment Accuracy

Regression analysis was employed to predict the accuracy measures from person-level characteristics. In particular, we hypothesized that nutrition knowledge and concern for healthy eating would result in greater accuracy. Because of the special health concern of diabetics, we also expected greater accuracy for this sub-group.

With regards to the correlation between the judged vs. objective total number of teaspoons in the drinks results showed that indeed the availability of sugar affected discrimination accuracy in the expected direction ($\beta = 0.203, p < 0.01$), but additionally individuals with higher levels of education and higher BMI had greater accuracy ($\beta = 0.28, p < 0.01$, for Education; $\beta = 0.16, p < 0.01$, for BMI; $F(3, 242) = 12.62, p < 0.0001$, adj $R^2 = 0.12$). Surprisingly, higher nutrition knowledge, or higher concern for healthy eating did not predict this accuracy criterion. Of great interest is that individuals reporting having diabetes had no greater accuracy in judging relative sugar content than did individuals not having such a health issue. No other individual level variables were significant predictors of the relationship between subjective and objective amounts of sugar.

In terms of the average difference between judged and objective amounts of sugar (both in terms of proportion and of number of teaspoons), we found that nutrition knowledge was not predictive of these variables. In terms of the accuracy of judging amount of walking to be done to burn the calories, a model with condition, nutrition knowledge, diabetes and income as predictors resulted in, $F(4, 240) = 2.72, p = 0.03$, adj $R^2 = 0.027$, but with significant beta weights for only the condition experimental manipulation ($\beta = 0.17$) with greater overestimation for those viewing the sugar display (i.e., the Sugar group).

Individuals with diabetes had greater overestimation of the amount of sugar present in the drinks as earlier stated. Additionally, the group of diabetics gave greater importance to sugar when judging the overall nutrition of foods (means = 51.63 and 42.83 for diabetics and controls, respectively). A MANOVA with both measures as dependent variables and group (diabetes vs. control) as independent variable revealed a significant group effect ($F(2, 237) = 3.77, p = 0.024$, Wilks' Lambda = 0.97) (this analysis does not include the three outliers who produced very large estimates; results do not change when included).

3.5. Choice of Drink as a Function of the Visual Aid

The great majority of participants stated not wanting to consume any of the sugary drinks being judged at the moment (88.4% response rate towards not wanting to consume across participants and across the 10 drinks containing sugar). The condition manipulation, nevertheless, lowered the intentions of consuming any of the drinks; the mean number of drinks individuals felt like consuming was equal to 1.165 drinks for the No-Sugar group and equal to 0.89 for the Sugar group and this difference was statistically significant, t (255) = 2.077, $p = 0.02$ (one-tail). Another way to look at this is that in the No-Sugar group, across all participants and drinks, the average selection of sugary drinks was 14.9%, and this proportion was equal to only 8.8% in the Sugar group—a 40.93% decrease. These proportions are significantly different by z-test ($z = 4.8$, $p < 0.0001$).

We must note that on average people stated not being very thirsty with means equal to 39.33 and 36.89 for the Sugar and No-sugar groups, respectively, using the 0–100 scale with 100 denoting maximum thirst (these means are not statistically significantly different). Additionally, the open-ended question about drinks showed that the choices available in the study were not common drink options for participants. Orange juice was the most selected drink and this was stated by only 22 participants in the entire sample (8.4%). The next most popular drink was coke, but with only 5 selections. Besides these, water, coffee, and milk were more commonly listed as beverages consumers drink. Thus, the effect of the manipulation is likely to be stronger than observed if the individuals were thirstier and the sugary drinks were their habitual choices.

The results of this study also suggested that self-report of NFP usage both in general and for this study, as well as knowledge of nutrition and concern for healthy eating, did not play a significant role in predicting the total number of sugary drinks that participants reported they would hypothetically consume. However, it is important to note that these factors could be linked to habitual choices which would remain regardless of the intervention, and may be difficult to change. Other variables predictive of the choices, once the effect of the experimental manipulation was accounted for, were degree to which the person eats healthy ($\beta = -18$, $p = 0.009$), and education ($\beta = -18$, $p = 0.006$), F (5, 247) = 4.33, $p < 0.0001$, adj. $R^2 = 0.138$.

Finally, we also found that in terms of estimating sugar in drinks, individuals were generally off, overestimating sugar by three spoons or more. This was true even for individuals with higher levels of education, nutrition knowledge, and concern for healthy eating. The simplest explanation is that, in general, people have no concept of the correlation between grams (the measure on the NFP) and teaspoons. Grams, for US participants, is also a more abstract concept. This would suggest that the NFP is of little benefit whether or not it is used, in helping to determine overall quantities of sugar. Strong positive correlations among self-report of NFP usage in daily life with concerns for eating healthy, education, income, nutrition knowledge suggests a "wealthier get wealthier" scenario, in that those who are aware of the value of, and are concerned with, health knowledge, are better prepared to make nutritional judgments than those who are not. This will be further elaborated on in the discussion.

4. Discussion

The evidence from medical and health care research is mounting to support the link between sugar consumption and cardiovascular disease and mortality [41]. The politics behind the high availability of sugary drinks and food products containing added sugars is complex [42]. In the center of these realities lies the psychological machinery that reacts positively to sugar and does not perceive the world in a purely objective way. It is the judgment and decision-making processes that ultimately determine the degree to which consumers are able to judge information effectively and use it to make smart food selections.

Our work focuses on understanding the psychological judgment processes with the hope that interventions, other than those based on pricing and/or availability of products, can be developed to support effective decision making. How well can individuals judge how much of a nutrient is present in a food product? What factors contribute to accurate perceptions and cognitions? Answers to these questions, we believe, are essential in determining support systems that result in calibrated perceptions and more optimal food choices.

The study was conducted mostly in rural Appalachia, but it also had individuals from a community center in Cleveland which allows our results to generalize to a range of income and education. We tested a simple intervention designed to make sugar explicit when considering amounts of sugar in a set of popular drinks. Two important findings from this study are: 1) estimation of nutrient content was difficult even when sugar amounts were made obvious via the test-tube sugar displays for each drink, and 2) both judgments and choices were influenced by the intervention. With a few exceptions, other person level characteristics, such as nutrition knowledge and concern for healthy eating, did not influence judgment accuracy.

In terms of estimating sugar content, such as number of teaspoons of sugar, individuals were better able to discriminate among drinks when sugar was made explicit. Additionally, higher levels of education and higher BMI related to higher accuracy, but contrary to our expectation, no relationship was found with nutrition knowledge and concern for healthy eating. Exact estimates, on the other hand, were no more accurate, but tended to move in the direction of overestimation. The overestimation also occurred with regards to amount of time walking needed to burn the calories.

From the perspective of the helpfulness of the NFP information we note that sugar amounts, as described in the label, did not translate into common units such as teaspoons, and individuals were generally off, overestimating sugar by three spoons or more. This was true even for individuals with higher levels of education, nutrition knowledge, and concern for healthy eating. Of great consequence is the fact that we found strong positive correlations among self-report of NFP usage in daily life with concerns for eating healthy, education, income, nutrition knowledge. However, NFP frequency related negatively to using the NFP in the current study and it did not predict judgment accuracy of any type, nor did it predict choice. Thus, our results cast doubts on the meaning and validity of high levels of NFP usage derived from self-report.

On the positive side, whatever information was used from the label, or from past experience, the judgments about the overall nutritional quality of the drinks produced relatively high discriminations as measured by the correlation between NuVal (the objective nutrition scores) and the subjective impressions. Accuracy with respect to NuVal also depended on nutrition knowledge and education.

In terms of drink selection, we found a low rate of preference for the options the study provided, yet the visual aid manipulation influenced choice. Using the total number of sugary-drinks a participant may drink as a measure of consumption intention, we found that the visual displayed produced lower rates of consumption. Beyond this manipulation effect, self-report of eating healthy and education were the only other predictors of choices. Interestingly, the status of being diabetic, having concern for healthy eating, or identifying sugar as an important nutrient did not predict choice.

Focusing on the group of 43 diabetics across locations, we noted that they reported giving great importance to sugar when judging nutrition as would be expected. In addition, their estimates of sugar content were greater than the rest of the participants by an average of approximately three teaspoons. But the group did not differ in terms of drink selections, as previously mentioned, which highlights the possible disconnect between beliefs and actions.

Finally, another interesting finding was that individuals who reported that they regularly used the NFP were less likely to admit to using it in the present study. As this did not vary as a function of condition (e.g., they were not more or less likely to use the NFP if the sugar tubes were present), other factors could be at work. More research is needed to determine if this was simply a function of being part of a research study, or their normal habitual behavior.

It is also possible that these individuals in general tended to adhere to the social desirability bias, and thus wanted to report that using the NFP was a regular habit, as it was the center of the study and known to be beneficial. They may also want to use it, but in general tend to forget, or get distracted when they do.

5. Conclusions

In the sugar debate, the psychology of sugar needs greater attention with emphasis on the perceptual and cognitive processes that determine judgments and choices. The human perception system is not a purely bottom up information processor reflecting objective quantities, and judgments are influenced as much from expectations and suggestions as they are from the sensory processes from which those judgments come from [43]. Greater attention to these psychological underpinnings is in demand in order to progress towards creating environments that support effective choices. Such environments may need to go beyond placing limits on food availability via pricing, or the lowering of supply, which present implementation challenges. Our findings demonstrate that nutrient visualization can support judgments and decisions and thus may be a viable tool for curtailing consumption of undesirable nutrients. Perhaps, labels that more obviously convey information, such as providing the exact number of teaspoons of sugar in the product, are in demand.

Supplementary Materials: The following are available online at http://www.mdpi.com/2072-6643/12/2/394/s1, Figure S1: Questions About Drinks; Figure S2: demographic questionnaire; Figure S3: Nutrition Questions; Figure S4: Overall Questions

Author Contributions: Conceptualization, B.D.M. and C.G.-V.; methodology, B.D.M. and C.G.-V.; validation, B.D.M. and C.G.-V.; formal analysis, B.D.M. and C.G.-V.; investigation, B.D.M. and C.G.-V.; resources, B.D.M. and C.G.-V.; data curation, B.D.M. and C.G.-V.; writing—original draft preparation, B.D.M. and C.G.-V.; writing—review and editing, B.D.M. and C.G.-V.; visualization, B.D.M. and C.G.-V.; supervision, C.G.-V.; project administration, B.D.M. and C.G.-V.; funding acquisition, B.D.M. and C.G.-V. All authors have read and agreed to the published version of the manuscript.

Funding: This research was funded by the Diabetes Institute at Ohio University via the Student Research Award.

Acknowledgments: The authors would like to thank the Diabetes Institute at Ohio University for support to this research via The Student Research Award, and NuVal® for providing the nutritional ratings for the food items used in this study.

Conflicts of Interest: The authors declare no conflict of interest.

References

1. Lustig, R.H.; Schmidt, L.A.; Brindis, C.D. The Toxic Truth about Sugar. *Nature* **2012**, *482*, 27–29. [CrossRef] [PubMed]
2. F As in Fat: How Obesity Threatens America's Future. Available online: https://www.rwjf.org/en/library/research/2012/09/f-as-in-fat--how-obesity-threatens-america-s-future-2012.html (accessed on 15 December 2019).
3. Skinner, A.C.; Ravanbakht, S.N.; Skelton, J.A.; Perrin, E.M.; Armstrong, S.C. Prevalence of obesity and severe obesity in US children, 1999–2016. *Pediatrics* **2018**, *141*, e20173459. [CrossRef] [PubMed]
4. Koplan, J.P.; Liverman, C.T.; Kraak, V.I. *Preventing Childhood Obesity: Health in the Balance*; National Academies Press: Washington, DC, USA, 2005.
5. McGinnis, J.M.; Gootman, J.A.; Kraak, V.I. *Food Marketing to Children and Youth: Threat or Opportunity*; National Academies Press: Washington, DC, USA, 2006.
6. Johnson, R.K.; Appel, L.J.; Brands, M.; Howard, B.V.; Lefevre, M.; Lustig, R.H.; Sacks, F.; Steffen, L.M.; Wylie-Rosett, J. Dietary sugar intake and cardiovascular health. A scientific statement from the American heart association. *Circulation* **2009**, *120*, 1011–1020. [CrossRef] [PubMed]
7. The American Heart Association. Sugar 101. Available online: http://www.heart.org/HEARTORG/GettingHealthy/NutritionCenter/HealthyEating/Sugar-101_UCM_306024_Article.jsp#.VjkMySs4v4A (accessed on 20 October 2019).
8. Vos, M.B.; Kimmons, J.E.; Gillespie, C.; Welsh, J.; Blanck, H.M. Dietary fructose consumption among US children and adults: The Third National Health and Nutrition Examination Survey. *Medscape J. Med.* **2008**, *10*, 160. [PubMed]
9. World Health Organization. *Global Status Report on Alcohol and Health: 2014*; World Health Organization: Geneva, Switzerland, 2014.
10. Food and Agriculture Organization (FAO). *State of Food and Agriculture 2013: Food Systems for Better Nutrition*; ESA/FAO: Rome, Italy, 2014.

11. Moran, A.; Krepp, E.M.; Johnson Curtis, C.; Lederer, A. An intervention to increase availability of healthy foods and beverages in new york city hospitals: The healthy hospital food initiative, 2010–2014. *Prev. Chronic Dis.* **2016**, *13*. [CrossRef]
12. Influence of Competitive Food and Beverage Policies on Children's Diets and Childhood Obesity. Available online: https://healthyeatingresearch.org/wp-content/uploads/2013/12/Competitive_Foods_Research_Review_HER_BTG_7-2012.pdf (accessed on 15 December 2019).
13. Hawkes, C. The worldwide battle against soft drinks in schools. *Am. J. Prev. Med.* **2010**, *38*, 457–461. [CrossRef]
14. Snelling, A.M.; Yezek, J. The effect of nutrient-based standards on competitive foods in 3 schools: Potential savings in kilocalories and grams of fat. *J School Health* **2012**, *82*, 91–96. [CrossRef]
15. French, S.A. Pricing effects on food choices. *J. Nutr.* **2003**, *133*, 841S–843S. [CrossRef]
16. Jacobs, A. Is Sweeping War on Obesity, Chile Slays Tony the Tiger. 2018. Available online: https://www.nytimes.com/2018/02/07/health/obesity-chile-sugar-regulations.html (accessed on 13 March 2016).
17. Greenberg, E.F. The Changing Food Label: The Nutrition Labeling and Education Act of 1990. *Loy. Consumer L. Rep.* **1990**, *3*, 10.
18. Kessler, D.A.; Mande, J.R.; Scarbrough, F.E.; Schapiro, R.; Feiden, K. Developing the "nutrition facts" food label. *Harvard Health Policy Rev.* **2003**, *4*, 13–24.
19. Changes in Eating Patterns and Diet Quality Among Working-Age Adults, 2005–2010. Available online: https://ageconsearch.umn.edu/record/262214/ (accessed on 15 December 2019).
20. Lin, C.J.; Zhang, Y.; Carlton, E.D.; Lo, S.C. *2014 FDA Health and Diet Survey*; Center for Food Safety and Applied Nutrition, United States Food and Drug Administration: Silver Spring, MA, USA, 2016.
21. Burton, S.; Garretson, J.A.; Velliquette, A.M. Implications of accurate usage of nutrition facts panel information for food product evaluations and purchase intentions. *J. Acad. Market Sci.* **1999**, *27*, 470–480. [CrossRef]
22. International Food Information Council Foundation. 2010 Food and Health Survey: Consumer Attitudes towards Food Safety, Nutrition, & Health. 2010. Available online: http://www.foodinsight.org/Content/3651/2010FinalFullReport.pdf (accessed on 17 October 2019).
23. Gonzalez-Vallejo, C.; Lavins, B.D. Evaluation of Breakfast Cereals with the current NFP and FDA NFP Proposal. *Public Health Nutr.* **2016**, *19*, 1047–1058. [CrossRef] [PubMed]
24. Gonzalez-Vallejo, C.; Lavins, B.D.; Carter, K.A. Analysis of Nutrition Judgments Using the Nutrition Facts Panel. *Appetite* **2016**, 105. [CrossRef]
25. Cowburn, G.; Stockley, L. Consumer Understanding and Use of Nutrition Labelling: A Systematic Review. *Public Health Nutr.* **2005**, *8*, 21–28. [CrossRef] [PubMed]
26. Harris, J.L.; Pomeranz, J.L.; Lobstein, T.; Brownell, K.D. A crisis in the marketplace: How food marketing contributes to childhood obesity and what can be done. *Annu. Rev. Public Health* **2009**, *30*, 211–225. [CrossRef] [PubMed]
27. Harris, J.L.; Bargh, J.A.; Brownell, K.D. Priming effects of television food advertising on eating behavior. *Health Psychol.* **2009**, *28*, 404–413. [CrossRef] [PubMed]
28. Andrews, J.C.; Lin, C.T.J.; Levy, A.S.; Lo, S. Consumer research needs from the food and drug administration on front-of-package nutritional labeling. *J. Public Policy Mark.* **2014**, *33*, 10–16. [CrossRef]
29. Donnelly, G.E.; Zatz, L.Y.; Svirsky, D.; John, L.K. The effect of graphic warnings on sugary-drink purchasing. *Psychol. Sci.* **2018**, *29*, 1321–1333. [CrossRef]
30. Williams, N.S.; Nestle, M. Editorial: 'Big Food': Taking a critical perspective on a global public health problem. *Crit. Public Health* **2015**, *25*, 245–247. [CrossRef]
31. US Food and Drug Administration. Nutrition Facts Label: Proposed Changes Aim to Better Inform Food Choices. FDA Consum Health Info 2014. Available online: http://www.fda.gov/downloads/ForConsumers/ConsumerUpdates/UCM387431.pdf (accessed on 15 December 2019).
32. Viskall-Van Dongen, M.; de Graff, C.; Siebelink, E.; Kok, F.J. Hidden fat facilitates passive overconsumption. *J. Nutr.* **2009**, *139*, 394–399. [CrossRef]
33. Thaler, R.H.; Sunstein, C.R. *Nudge: Improving Decisions about Health, Wealth, and Happiness*; Penguin Books: New York, NY, USA, 2008.
34. Kahneman, D.; Tversky, A. *A Judgment of Representativeness. The Concept of Probability in Psychological Experiments*; D. Reidel Publishing Company: Boston, MA, USA, 2012.

35. Parmenter, K.; Waller, J.; Wardle, J. Demographic variation in nutrition knowledge in england. *Health Educ. Res.* **2000**, *15*, 163–174. [CrossRef] [PubMed]
36. Andrews, J.C.; Netemeyer, R.G.; Burton, S. The nutrition elite: Do only the highest levels of caloric knowledge, obesity knowledge, and motivation matter in processing nutrition ad claims and disclosures? *JOF Public Policy Mark* **2009**, *28*, 41–55. [CrossRef]
37. NuVal ®LLC. The NuVal System: FAQ. Available online: http://www.nuval.com/How (accessed on 12 July 2013).
38. Parmenter, K.; Wardle, J. Development of a general nutrition knowledge questionnaire for adults. *Eur. J. Clin. Nutr.* **1999**, *53*, 298–308. [CrossRef] [PubMed]
39. Stewart, T.R. Judgment analysis: Procedures. In *Advances in Psychology, 54. Human Judgment: The SJT View*; Brehmer, B., Joyce, C.R.B., Eds.; North-Holland: Oxford, UK, 1988; pp. 41–74.
40. Hammond, K.R. Probabilistic functioning and the clinical method. *Psychol. Rev.* **1955**, *62*, 255–262. [CrossRef]
41. Yang, Q.; Zhang, Z.; Gregg, E.; Flanders, W.D.; Merritt, R.; Hu, F. Added sugar intake and cardiovascular diseases mortality among US adults. *JAMA Intern. Med.* **2014**, *174*, 516–524. [CrossRef]
42. Nestle, M. *Food Politics: How the Food Industry Influences Nutrition and Health*; University of California Press: Berkeley, CA, USA, 2013; Volume 3.
43. Wansink, B. *Mindless Eating—Why We Eat More Than We Think*; Bantam-Dell: New York, NY, USA, 2006.

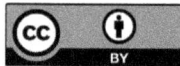

© 2020 by the authors. Licensee MDPI, Basel, Switzerland. This article is an open access article distributed under the terms and conditions of the Creative Commons Attribution (CC BY) license (http://creativecommons.org/licenses/by/4.0/).

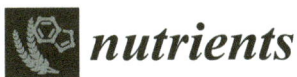 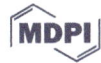

Article

The Color Nutrition Information Paradox: Effects of Suggested Sugar Content on Food Cue Reactivity in Healthy Young Women

Jonas Potthoff *, Annalisa La Face and Anne Schienle

Institute of Psychology, University of Graz, Universitaetsplatz 2, 8010 Graz, Austria;
annalisa.la-face@uni-graz.at (A.L.F.); anne.schienle@uni-graz.at (A.S.)
* Correspondence: jonas.potthoff@uni-graz.at; Tel.: +43-316-380-3883

Received: 12 December 2019; Accepted: 21 January 2020; Published: 24 January 2020

Abstract: Color nutrition information (CNI) based on a traffic light system conveys information about food quality with a glance. The color red typically indicates detrimental food characteristics (e.g., very high sugar content) and aims at inhibiting food shopping and consumption. Red may, however, also elicit cross-modal associations with sweet taste, which is a preferable food characteristic. We conducted two experiments. An eye-tracking study investigated whether CNI has an effect on cue reactivity (dwell time, saccadic latency, wanting/liking) for sweet foods. The participants were presented with images depicting sweets (e.g., cake). Each image was preceded by a colored circle that informed about the sugar content of the food (red = high, green = low, gray = unknown). It was tested whether the red circle would help the participants to direct their gaze away from the 'high sugar' item. A second experiment investigated whether colored prime circles (red, green, gray) without nutrition information would influence the assumed sweetness of a food. In Experiment 1, CNI had the opposite of the intended effect. Dwell time and saccadic latency were higher for food items preceded by a red compared to a green circle. This unintended response was positively associated with participants' liking of sweet foods. CNI did not change the wanting/liking of the displayed foods. In Experiment 2, we found no evidence for color priming on the assumed sweetness of food. Our results question whether CNI is helpful to influence initial cue reactivity toward sweet foods.

Keywords: nutrition facts; food cue reactivity; sugar; eye tracking; priming; color

1. Introduction

Food is a primary reinforcer that automatically captures visual attention. This evolutionary-based mechanism assists with the localization of food sources within the environment and, in turn, enables sufficient caloric uptake by the individual [1]. Studies utilizing neurophysiological measures and eye-tracking have shown that the human attention system very quickly identifies visual food cues and differentiates them from non-food objects [2–4]. Additionally, high-calorie food captures more attention than low-calorie food [5,6].

The increased attention to cues of high-calorie food has become problematic in Western countries because the exposure to such stimuli triggers the urge to eat [7]. Food cues and (high-calorie) foods are almost omnipresent in our everyday lives. Therefore, a link between individual food cue reactivity (FCR), overeating, and weight gain is not surprising [7].

In order to reduce the shopping and consumption of high-calorie food, effective interventions that are able to reduce FCR are urgently needed. It has already been demonstrated that nutritional knowledge is able to influence FCR [8]. A number of studies has found a positive correlation between nutritional knowledge and healthy dietary habits [9–14]. The knowledge transfer about the sugar content of food seems to be a promising starting point for such interventions because large proportions of calories are consumed in the form of sugar [15]. Moreover, the excessive consumption of sugary food is associated with an increased risk of cardiovascular disease, cancer, and diabetes [16]. However, findings regarding the relationship between individual knowledge about the sugar content of specific foods and actual consumption are heterogeneous [17–19]. Therefore, it seems likely that knowledge about the sugar content of food cannot always be accessed easily and quickly enough [20–23].

Therefore, color nutrition information (CNI) based on a traffic light system seems to be an efficient method to convey information about food quality. This system is already used in front of pack food labels [24]. The color red (as a stop signal) typically indicates detrimental food characteristics (e.g., very high sugar content), whereas green signals positive features [25–28].

However, even though the traffic light system is widely used, little is known about how CNI influences initial food cue reactivity. Furthermore, little is known about possible unintended effects of the commonly used colors (red, green). The color red may elicit cross-modal associations with sweet taste, which is a preferable food characteristic [29,30]. For example, cider was perceived as sweeter when served in a bottle with a red label compared to a green label [31]. The red-sweetness association seems to be stronger for drinks compared to solid foods. Lemos et al. [32] presented colored prime stimuli (red, green, amber cycles) that were followed by an image of a salty or sweet food item. The seven sweet food items used in this experiment were, on average, rated as more positive (hedonic valence) after the presentation of a red cycle compared to a green cycle. This effect was most pronounced for the only liquid (a carbonated soft drink) used as stimulus material. However, for half of the solid sweet foods, the hedonic valence was actually lower after the presentation of a red cycle compared to a green one. Based on this previous research, it remains unclear whether red color used in food labels as 'warning signals' implicitly primes sweet taste associations.

The aim of the present investigation was twofold. We investigated effects of colored nutrition information (traffic light symbols indicating the sugar content) on initial food cue reactivity (Experiment 1). In a second experiment, we investigated priming effects of the colors red and green on assumed sugar content/sweet taste (Experiment 2).

2. Materials and Methods

2.1. Sample

Experiments 1 and 2 were conducted following the rules of the Declaration of Helsinki of 1975, revised in 2013. The experiments were approved by the ethics committee of the University of Graz (ethical approval code: 39/31/63 ex 2018/19).

2.1.1. Sample Experiment 1

Fifty-one women (mean age: 22.0 years, SD = 2.99; range 18–33) with a body mass index (BMI) of $M = 22.5$ (SD = 3.85) took part in this study. We selected women because previous research has suggested that the use and understanding of nutrition information is related to demographic characteristics, notably social grade, age, and gender [33]. Participants had normal or corrected-to-normal vision and did not report any current medication or mental disorder. Forty-nine participants were university students, and the other were white-collar workers. Participants were recruited via email lists and postings at the university campus as well as dormitories. Psychology students ($N = 32$) received course credits for their participation. Sample characteristics are displayed in Table 1.

Table 1. Sample characteristics and rating data.

Measure	Mean (SD)
Age (years)	22.04 (2.99)
BMI	22.47 (3.85)
Hunger level (0–6)	1.47 (1.52)
General appetite (0–6)	1.86 (1.55)
Sweet food preference (1–4)	2.86 (1.02)
Specific appetite (0–6)	
low sugar	2.06 (1.34)
high sugar	2.11 (1.26)
unknown sugar	2.22 (1.38)
General liking (0–6)	
low sugar	3.51 (1.48)
high sugar	3.64 (1.29)
unknown sugar	3.77 (1.27)

2.1.2. Sample Experiment 2

A total of 99 participants (age: $M = 25.03$ years, $SD = 6.17$ years; BMI: $M = 22.61$ kg/m^2, $SD = 2.81$ kg/m^2) completed an online experiment. Of the participants, 55 had a high school diploma, 44 participants graduated from college. The majority of participants was female (female: $N = 74$, male: $N = 25$).

2.2. Stimuli and Design Experiment 1

We presented color nutrition information (CNI) that reflected the sugar content of a specific food item (green: Low sugar content, red: High sugar content, gray: Unknown sugar content; diameter: 354 pixels) and 48 pictures of sweet foods (e.g., cakes, ice cream, candies from the FoodPics database [34]). Each picture had a size of 600 × 450 pixels. Food images and CNI were presented on a white background on an LCD screen. We selected food products of which low sugar versions are commonly available on the market. We assigned 16 images to each category (low/high/unknown sugar content) and created three parallel versions of the experiment. Due to the parallel versions, each image was suggested to have a low, high, or unknown sugar-content for one-third of the participants. Participants were randomly assigned to one of the three parallel versions.

At the beginning of each trial, a circle was presented on either the center of the left or the right half of the screen. As soon as participants were gazing at it steadily for 1000 ms, the CNI disappeared and the allocated food image was presented for 1500 ms. Each pair of CNI and food image was shown in two trials: Once the food image appeared in the same location as the CNI (current gaze location: Figure 1), the other time the food image was presented on the opposite side of the screen (peripheral location), resulting in 96 trials (16 per suggested sugar content: Low, high, unknown; and position: Current gaze location, peripheral). Trials were followed by an intertrial interval of 200 ms. The trial order was randomized.

The participants were instructed to inspect the circles. Throughout the paradigm, two food items of each category were presented in the center of the screen. Participants were asked to rate these food items regarding their specific appetite ("How much would you like to taste this food right now?" 0: "Not at all", 6: "Very much") and general liking ("How much do you like this food in general?" 0: "Not at all", 6: "Very much").

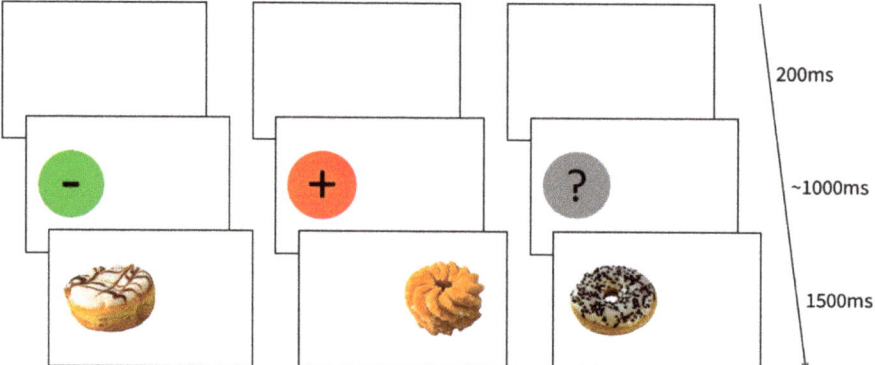

Figure 1. Example trials for (from left to right) low sugar label, high sugar label, and unknown sugar label. Each food image was presented twice: Once in the same location as the label (example: low sugar & unknown sugar) and once in the peripheral location (example: high sugar label). In 50% of trials, the label was presented on the left side of the screen. In the other 50%, the label was presented on the right side of the screen (not displayed here).

2.3. Procedure Experiment 1

After providing written informed consent, participants read a short info sheet about color-coded nutrition facts (high sugar/red symbol: Above 12.5 g sugar per 100 g food, low sugar/green symbol: Below 5 g sugar per 100 g food). Subsequently, participants rated their general appetite and hunger on a seven-point scale (appetite: 0: "I have no appetite at all.", 6: "I have an extreme urge to eat something right now."; hunger: 0: "I have no hunger at all.", 6: "I am extremely hungry."). Furthermore, participants rated their preference for sweet food ("How much do you like sweet food in general?", 0: "Not at all.", 4: "Very much."). Subsequently, the eye-tracking paradigm described above was conducted.

Following the eye-tracking paradigm, participants conducted a survey about their demographics and the following questionnaires.

2.4. Questionnaires Experiment 1

The participants completed the Eating Disorder Examination-Questionnaire (EDE-Q; [35]) and the Impulsivity Short Scale (I-8; [36]). The EDE-Q consists of 41 items (e.g., "Were you afraid to lose control over your eating?") that are answered on seven-point scales (0: "Not at all", 6: "Very much") and are concerned with the previous four weeks. Furthermore, the EDE-Q inquires weight and size (i.e., BMI). In the present sample, Cronbach's alpha for the EDE-Q was $\alpha = 92$. The I-8 consists of eight items (e.g., "I usually think carefully before I act."), which are answered on five-point scales (1: "Doesn't apply at all", 5: "Applies completely"; Cronbach's $\alpha = 75$ for the I-8).

The questionnaires were selected because disordered eating and impulsivity have been associated with elevated food cue reactivity in previous research [37].

2.5. Eye Movement Recording and Analysis Experiment 1

Two-dimensional eye movements were recorded using an SMI RED250mobile eye-tracker with a sampling rate of 250 Hz. Head movements were minimized by a chin rest. We calibrated both eyes and analyzed data from the eye that produced the better spatial resolution (typically more accurate than a 0.35° visual angle). Stimuli were presented on a white background on a 24-inch screen with a resolution of 1920 × 1080 pixels. The viewing distance was 60 cm, resulting in a size of 15.6° × 11.7° viewing angle for food images and a diameter of 9.2° viewing angle for CNIs. The experiment was controlled using the SMI Experiment Center (Version 3.6.53, SensoMotoric Instruments, Teltow,

Germany). For event detection, standard thresholds of the SMI BeGaze Software (Version 3.6.52, SensoMotoric Instruments, Teltow, Germany) for high speed eye-tracking data (recommended for sampling rate > 200 Hz) were used to detect saccades (velocity threshold: 40°/s). Data were exported using SMI BeGaze and customized Python scripts. Within BeGaze, we defined the food images as areas of interest (AOI). We conducted gaze data analysis exclusively for the food AOI of each trial. We defined the dependent variable, 'saccadic latency', as the time from stimulus onset to the start of the first saccade that ended outside of the food AOI. Saccadic latency was calculated only for trials with the participants' gaze position within the AOI at stimulus onset (CNI was presented in the same position as the subsequently presented food). Saccadic latency therefore measured how long it took participants to actively relocate their gaze away from a food item.

The second dependent variable, 'dwell time', was defined as the sum of fixation durations within the AOI. Other than saccadic latency, we computed dwell time for all trials (trials in which the food appeared at gaze location, as well as trials in which food appeared in the peripheral location).

2.6. Stimuli and Design Experiment 2

Thirty pictures of sweet food from Experiment 1 (size: 600 × 450 pixels) were presented in the center of the computer screen for 1500 ms each. Prior to the picture presentation, one of three colored circles (red, green, gray) was shown. The circles (diameter: 354 pixels) were displayed centrally on a white background for 1000 ms. The circles did not contain any text and were presented without any further instructions. We created three subsets of prime-stimulus combinations to ensure that each picture was preceded by a red, green, or gray circle. The participants were randomly assigned to one of the three color-food combinations (combination 1: $N = 28$, combination 2: $N = 38$, combination 3: $N = 33$). There was no significant difference between groups in mean age ($F(2,96) = 0.17$, $p = 0.84$, $\eta 2p = 0.004$), BMI ($F(2,67) = 1.64$, $p = 0.20$, $\eta 2p = 0.047$), hunger level ($F(2,96) = 0.83$, $p = 0.44$, $\eta 2p = 0.02$), or gender distribution (Chi^2 (2, $N = 99$) = 1.52, $p = 0.47$).

After the presentation of each food image, the participants rated the assumed sweetness of the food on a scale from 0% ("not sweet at all") to 100% ("extremely sweet"). Additionally, the valence of two food images per color was rated (0%: "Extremely unpleasant", 100%: "Extremely pleasant"). The trials were presented in random order.

2.7. Procedure Experiment 2

Participants were asked to conduct the experiment at home without distraction on a computer with a (hardware) keyboard and mouse. After giving informed consent, participants provided demographic data (age, education, gender). They reported their current hunger level ("How hungry are you right now?" 0: "Not hungry at all", 6: "Extremely hungry"), weight, and height. Subsequently, the participants were presented with 30 images of sweet food in randomized order. The experiment was conducted using Pavlovia and was programmed in Python using PsychoPy 3.2.2 [38].

2.8. Statistical Analysis

Repeated measures analyses of variance (ANOVAs) were computed to test the effect of CNI (low, high, unknown sugar content) on specific appetite, general liking of the displayed food items, and dwell time spent on food images, as well as saccadic latency away from food. For trials in which the food image was presented in the periphery of the current gaze, the repeated measures ANOVA was conducted only for dwell time (Experiment 1). In Experiment 2, ANOVAs were conducted to test the effect of color. If sphericity was violated (Mauchly's Test of Sphericity), Greenhouse–Geisser correction was applied. We reported the effect size as $\eta 2p$ (partial eta squared) and Holm adjusted p-values. The p-values smaller than 0.05 were considered statistically significant. Data are available online at OSF (OSF Project DOI: 10.17605/OSF.IO/FJ3UZ, Center for Open Science, Charlottesville, VA): www.osf.io/g4d7s/

3. Results

3.1. Results Experiment 1

3.1.1. Questionnaire Data

Participants obtained an average EDE-Q score of $M = 1.33$ (SD = 0.96), which did not differ significantly from the mean ($M = 1.44$) of the healthy norm sample (individuals without any current diagnosis of an eating disorder, $N = 409$, [35]), $t(50) = 0.80$, $p = 0.43$, $d = 0.11$. The mean I-8 score of the present sample of $M = 2.63$ (SD = 0.62) did not differ significantly from the average impulsivity of the female norm sample aged between 18 and 35 years ($M = 2.62$), $t(50) = 0.09$, $p = 0.93$, $d = 0.01$.

3.1.2. Appetite and General Liking of Presented Food Images

CNI had no statistically significant effect on reported appetite ($F(2,100) = 0.38$, $p = 0.68$, $\eta2p = 0.008$) and general liking of the depicted food items ($F(2,100) = 0.58$, $p = 0.56$, $\eta2p = 0.01$; see Table 1).

3.1.3. Eye Movements

Saccadic Latency: For gaze relocation (same position), the repeated measures ANOVA revealed a significant main effect of CNI on saccadic latency ($F(1.71,85.55) = 4.98$, $p = 0.012$, $\eta2p = 0.091$). The saccadic latency was significantly lower for food with a low sugar content compared to food with a high sugar content ($t(50) = 2.35$, $p = 0.045$, $d = 0.33$) and unknown sugar content ($t(50) = 2.63$, $p = 0.034$, $d = 0.37$). The saccadic latency did not differ between unknown and high sugar content ($t(50) = 0.24$, $p = 0.82$, $d = 0.03$; see Figure 2).

Dwell Time: The ANOVA revealed a significant main effect of CNI on the dwell time spent on the food images ($F(1.61,80.48) = 5.61$, $p = 0.009$, $\eta2p = 0.10$). The dwell time was shorter for food with a low sugar content compared to food with a high sugar content ($t(50) = 2.37$, $p = 0.043$, $d = 0.33$) and unknown sugar content ($t(50) = 2.83$, $p = 0.020$, $d = 0.40$). Dwell time did not differ between unknown and high sugar content ($t(50) = 0.44$, $p = 0.66$, $d = 0.06$; see Figure 2 and Table 2).

Table 2. Summary results of Experiments 1 and 2.

Measure	ANOVA	Green (SD)	Red (SD)	Gray (SD)
Experiment 1:				
Saccadic latency	$F(1.71,85.55) = 4.98$, $p = 0.012$, $\eta2p = 0.091$	276.3 ms (77.4 ms)	297.4 ms (58.6 ms)	398.8 ms (64.4 ms)
Dwell time current *	$F(1.61,80.48) = 5.61$, $p = 0.009$, $\eta2p = 0.10$	255.6 ms (67.3 ms)	272.5 ms (58.8 ms)	274.5 ms (52.9 ms)
Dwell time peripheral *	$F(2,100) = 1.70$, $p = 0.19$, $\eta2p = 0.03$	71.5 ms (61.1 ms)	58.4 ms (52.1 ms)	65.0 ms (49.1 ms)
Experiment 2:				
Sweetness	$F(2,196) = 0.22$, $p = 81$, $\eta2p = 0.002$	74.4% (10.9%)	74.0% (11.1%)	74.0% (10.8%)
Valence *	$F(2,196) = 3.16$, $p = 045$, $\eta2p = 0.031$	44.7% (21.1%)	43.1% (19.7%)	49.6% (22.2%)

In Experiment 1, green indicated low sugar, red indicated high sugar, and gray indicated no specific sugar content. For gaze data (Experiment 1), mean durations in milliseconds are given. Sweetness and valence were rated from 0% to 100%. Asterisks indicate significant main effects.

For gaze avoidance (peripheral position), there was no significant effect of CNI on dwell time ($F(2,100) = 1.70$, $p = 0.19$, $\eta2p = 0.03$). The dwell time did not differ significantly between low sugar content ($M = 71.5$, SD = 61.1), high sugar content ($M = 58.4$, SD = 52.1), and unknown sugar content ($M = 65.0$, SD = 49.1).

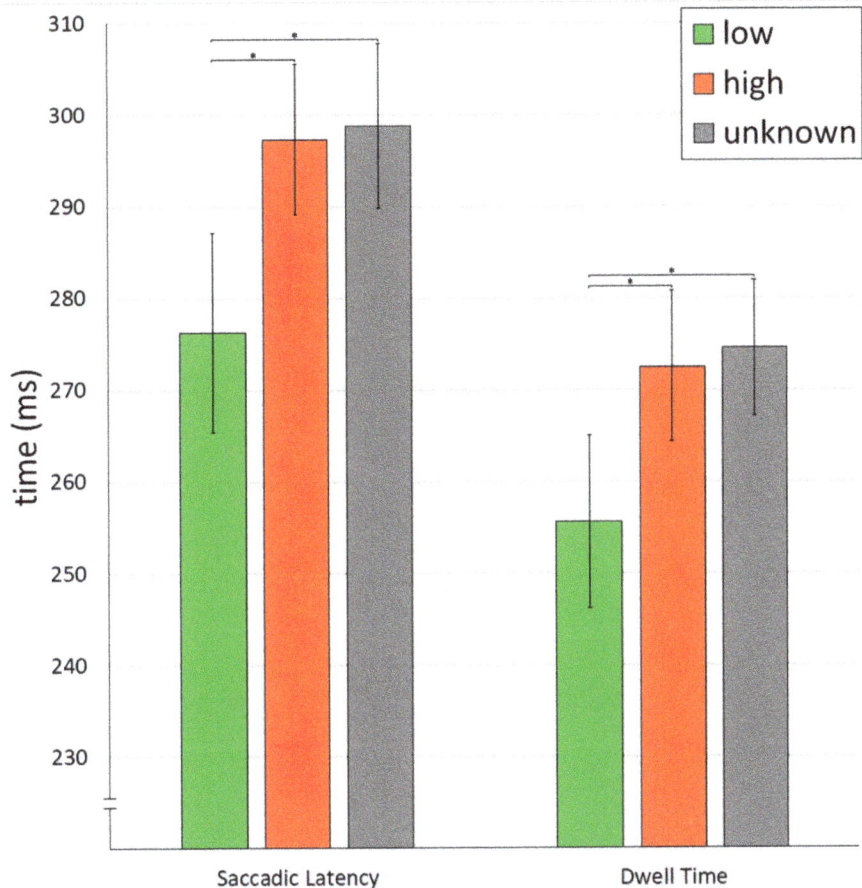

Figure 2. Mean saccadic latency and dwell time for trials in which food appeared in the current gaze location for three CNI conditions: Low (green CNI/low sugar), high (red CNI/high sugar), and unknown (gray CNI/unknown sugar). Whiskers indicate standard errors. Asterisks indicate Holm-adjusted $p < 0.05$.

3.1.4. Exploratory Analysis

To analyze if the general preference for sweet foods was correlated with CNI, we calculated Pearson correlations between liking of sweet foods and (1) the difference in saccadic latency between high and low sugar content (high sugar saccadic latency minus low sugar saccadic latency) and with (2) the difference in dwell time (high sugar dwell time minus low sugar dwell time). On average, the reported liking was $M = 2.86$ (SD = 1.02). We found positive correlations between liking and difference in saccadic latency ($r = 0.298$, $p = 0.034$) and dwell time ($r = 0.369$, $p = 0.008$).

The difference in saccadic latency was not correlated with the I-8 score ($r = 0.022$, $p = 0.879$), the EDE-Q score ($r = 0.217$, $p = 0.126$), the BMI ($r = 0.01$, $p = 0.95$), hunger ($r = 0.169$, $p = 0.236$), or appetite ($r = 0.055$, $p = 0.700$). Also, the difference in dwell time was not correlated with the I-8 score ($r = -0.081$, $p = 0.570$), the EDE-Q ($r = 0.247$, $p = 0.081$), the BMI ($r = 0.08$, $p = 0.58$), hunger ($r = 0.103$, $p = 0.474$), or appetite ($r = -0.003$, $p = 0.982$).

3.2. Results Experiment 2

We calculated two ANOVAs to test the effects of color (red, green, gray circles) on estimated sweetness and valence of the food stimuli. We found no significant color effect for sweetness $F(2,196) = 0.22$, $p = 0.81$, $\eta 2p = 0.002$ (Table 2). The effect for valence was significant, $F(2,196) = 3.16$, $p = 0.045$, $\eta 2p = 0.031$ (Table 2). The post-hoc pairwise comparisons were not significant (all $p > 0.08$). Food items preceded by a gray circle received marginally higher valence ratings compared to red circles.

4. Discussion

The shopping of food, including high-calorie sweet snack foods, is often impulsive. In order to influence this spontaneous shopping behavior, simple interventions are needed that are able to interrupt this process. The current eye-tracking study investigated the influence of provided information about a product's sugar content on visual food cue reactivity. It was tested whether a red circle that indicated a high sugar content of a product would be able to help the participants to direct their gaze away from the displayed food item. The results showed that the intervention had the opposite of the intended effect. The dwell time and the saccadic latency were lower for food items preceded by a green circle compared to a red and gray circle. Obviously, it was easier for the participants to ignore food cues if low sugar content was assumed relative to high or unknown sugar content. Thus, the participants showed a paradox reaction.

Similar paradox effects have been reported in studies that attempted to influence knowledge and beliefs about food [39,40]. A study by Berry et al. [39] examined how calorie information on menus in chain restaurants affected the food choice. The results indicated that calorie labeling even increased the calories ordered if the consumers were taste-oriented rather than health-oriented. Similarly, Provencher et al. [40] found that participants ate 30% more of the same cookies when labeled as healthy.

Whereas the current study contributes to the existing evidence that nutrition facts may be ineffective [39–42], other findings have indicated that nutrition fact information provided via food labels is a useful tool to target food cue reactivity and food choices [28,43,44]. Further research is needed to evaluate in which cases unintended effects of CNI on food cue reactivity might occur. Our exploratory analysis indicated that it was more difficult for participants with a high compared to a low preference for sweet foods to avoid 'high sugar' foods. Thus, individual preferences might overrule CNI [41].

Additionally, previous research has indicated that the color-coding itself may elicit unintended effects on FCR. Cross-modal associations between the color red and sweet taste have been reported in many studies. Cross-modal associations were observed primarily for fluids [30] and not for solid foods [45]. The present study (with exclusively solid foods) found no evidence for priming effects of red on estimated sweetness and pleasantness of the depicted food products. The food items even received marginally higher valence ratings after the presentation of a gray circle compared to a red circle. Thus, it is unlikely that the results of Experiment 1 were caused by cross-modal associations between priming color and visual food perception.

We need to mention the following limitations of the present study. In Experiment 1, we only studied female participants. The majority of the women were university students. Therefore, our findings cannot be generalized to other samples. However, it is important to note that we used an innovative gaze performance task to evaluate visual food cue reactivity without the possible effects of self-monitored gaze direction or social desirability (as opposed to free exploration paradigms and self-reports). The task was very easy and therefore should have been accomplished by this group of highly educated women. Nevertheless, to determine if the basic findings of the present study can be applied to other participants and circumstances (e.g., male and/or less-educated participants), a replication study is highly recommended. Experiment 2 was not conducted in the lab, but at home. Thus, we were not able to control unintended distractions during participation.

Author Contributions: Conceptualization, J.P., A.L.F. and A.S.; methodology, J.P., A.L.F. and A.S..; software, J.P.; validation, J.P. and A.S.; formal analysis, J.P. and A.S.; investigation, A.L.F. and J.P.; writing—original draft preparation, J.P., A.L.F. and A.S.; writing—review and editing, J.P. and A.S.; visualization, J.P.; supervision, A.S.; project administration, A.S. All authors have read and agreed to the published version of the manuscript.

Funding: This research received no external funding.

Acknowledgments: Open Access Funding by the University of Graz. The authors acknowledge the financial support by the University of Graz.

Conflicts of Interest: The authors declare no conflict of interest.

References

1. Nummenmaa, L.; Hietanen, J.K.; Calvo, M.G.; Hyönä, J. Food catches the eye but not for everyone: A BMI-contingent attentional bias in rapid detection of nutriments. *PLoS ONE* **2011**, *6*, e19215. [CrossRef] [PubMed]
2. Castellanos, E.H.; Charboneau, E.; Dietrich, M.S.; Park, S.; Bradley, B.P.; Mogg, K.; Cowan, R.L. Obese adults have visual attention bias for food cue images: Evidence for altered reward system function. *Int. J. Obes.* **2009**, *33*, 1063–1073. [CrossRef] [PubMed]
3. Sarlo, M.; Übel, S.; Leutgeb, V.; Schienle, A. Cognitive reappraisal fails when attempting to reduce the appetitive value of food: An ERP study. *Biol. Psychol.* **2013**, *94*, 507–512. [CrossRef] [PubMed]
4. Van der Laan, L.N.; De Ridder, D.T.D.; Viergever, M.A.; Smeets, P.A.M. The first taste is always with the eyes: A meta-analysis on the neural correlates of processing visual food cues. *Neuroimage* **2011**, *55*, 296–303. [CrossRef]
5. Doolan, K.J.; Breslin, G.; Hanna, D.; Murphy, K.; Gallagher, A.M. Visual attention to food cues in obesity: An eye-tracking study. *Obesity (Silver Spring)* **2014**, *22*, 2501–2507. [CrossRef]
6. Toepel, U.; Knebel, J.-F.; Hudry, J.; Le Coutre, J.; Murray, M.M. The brain tracks the energetic value in food images. *Neuroimage* **2009**, *44*, 967–974. [CrossRef]
7. Boswell, R.G.; Kober, H. Food cue reactivity and craving predict eating and weight gain: A meta-analytic review. *Obes. Rev.* **2016**, *17*, 159–177. [CrossRef]
8. Yegiyan, N.S.; Bailey, R.L. Food as risk: How eating habits and food knowledge affect reactivity to pictures of junk and healthy foods. *Health Commun.* **2016**, *31*, 635–642. [CrossRef]
9. Dallongeville, J.; Marécaux, N.; Cottel, D.; Bingham, A.; Amouyel, P. Association between nutrition knowledge and nutritional intake in middle-aged men from Northern France. *Public Health Nutr.* **2001**, *4*, 27–33. [CrossRef]
10. Fonseca, L.G.; Bertolin, M.N.T.; Gubert, M.B.; da Silva, E.F. Effects of a nutritional intervention using pictorial representations for promoting knowledge and practices of healthy eating among Brazilian adolescents. *PLoS ONE* **2019**, *14*, e0213277. [CrossRef]
11. Handu, D.J.; Monty, C.E.; Chmel, L.M. Nutrition education improved nutrition knowledge, behavior, and intention among youth in Chicago public schools. *J. Am. Diet. Assoc.* **2008**, *108*, A91. [CrossRef]
12. Klohe-Lehman, D.M.; Freeland-Graves, J.; Anderson, E.R.; McDowell, T.; Clarke, K.K.; Hanss-Nuss, H.; Cai, G.; Puri, D.; Milani, T.J. Nutrition knowledge is associated with greater weight loss in obese and overweight low-income mothers. *J. Am. Diet. Assoc.* **2006**, *106*, 65–75. [CrossRef] [PubMed]
13. Lee, J.W.; Lee, H.S.; Chang, N.; Kim, J.-M. The relationship between nutrition knowledge scores and dietary behavior, dietary intakes and anthropometric parameters among primary school children participating in a nutrition education program. *Korean J. Nutr.* **2009**, *42*, 338–349. [CrossRef]
14. Wardle, J.; Parmenter, K.; Waller, J. Nutrition knowledge and food intake. *Appetite* **2000**, *34*, 269–275. [CrossRef]
15. Langlois, K.; Garriguet, D. Sugar consumption among Canadians of all ages. *Health Rep.* **2011**, *22*, 23–27.
16. Lustig, R.H.; Schmidt, L.A.; Brindis, C.D. The toxic truth about sugar. *Nature* **2012**, *482*, 27–29. [CrossRef]
17. Nelson, M.C.; Lytle, L.A.; Pasch, K.E. Improving literacy about energy-related issues: The need for a better understanding of the concepts behind energy intake and expenditure among adolescents and their parents. *J. Am. Diet. Assoc.* **2009**, *109*, 281–287. [CrossRef]
18. Park, S.; Onufrak, S.; Sherry, B.; Blanck, H.M. Health-related knowledge and attitudes are associated with sugars-sweetened beverages intake among U.S. adults. *FASEB J.* **2013**, *27*, 622–624. [CrossRef]

19. Zoellner, J.; You, W.; Connell, C.; Smith-Ray, R.L.; Allen, K.; Tucker, K.L.; Davy, B.M.; Estabrooks, P. Health literacy is associated with healthy eating index scores and sugar-sweetened beverage intake: Findings from the rural Lower Mississippi Delta. *J. Am. Diet. Assoc.* **2011**, *111*, 1012–1020. [CrossRef]
20. Ni Mhurchu, C.; Eyles, H.; Jiang, Y.; Blakely, T. Do nutrition labels influence healthier food choices? Analysis of label viewing behaviour and subsequent food purchases in a labelling intervention trial. *Appetite* **2018**, *121*, 360–365. [CrossRef]
21. Graham, D.J.; Heidrick, C.; Hodgin, K. Nutrition label viewing during a food-selection task: Front-of-package labels vs nutrition facts labels. *J. Acad. Nutr. Diet.* **2015**, *115*, 1636–1646. [CrossRef] [PubMed]
22. Graham, D.J.; Jeffery, R.W. Location, location, location: Eye-tracking evidence that consumers preferentially view prominently positioned nutrition information. *J. Am. Diet. Assoc.* **2011**, *111*, 1704–1711. [CrossRef] [PubMed]
23. Ollberding, N.J.; Wolf, R.L.; Contento, I. Food label use and its relation to dietary intake among US adults. *J. Am. Diet. Assoc.* **2011**, *111*, S47–S51. [CrossRef] [PubMed]
24. Kanter, R.; Vanderlee, L.; Vandevijvere, S. Front-of-package nutrition labelling policy: Global progress and future directions. *Public Health Nutr.* **2018**, *21*, 1399–1408. [CrossRef]
25. Campos, S.; Doxey, J.; Hammond, D. Nutrition labels on pre-packaged foods: A systematic review. *Public Health Nutr.* **2011**, *14*, 1496–1506. [CrossRef]
26. Hawley, K.L.; Roberto, C.A.; Bragg, M.A.; Liu, P.J.; Schwartz, M.B.; Brownell, K.D. The science on front-of-package food labels. *Public Health Nutr.* **2013**, *16*, 430–439. [CrossRef]
27. Sinclair, S.E.; Cooper, M.; Mansfield, E.D. The influence of menu labeling on calories selected or consumed: A systematic review and meta-analysis. *J. Acad. Nutr. Diet.* **2014**, *114*, 1375–1388. [CrossRef]
28. Sonnenberg, L.; Gelsomin, E.; Levy, D.E.; Riis, J.; Barraclough, S.; Thorndike, A.N. A traffic light food labeling intervention increases consumer awareness of health and healthy choices at the point-of-purchase. *Prev. Med.* **2013**, *57*, 253–257. [CrossRef]
29. Spence, C. Multisensory flavor perception. In *Multisensory Perception: From Laboratory to Clinic*; Elsevier Academic Press: Cambridge, MA, USA, 2019; pp. 221–237. ISBN 9780128124925.
30. Spence, C. On the psychological impact of food colour. *Flavour* **2015**, *4*, 21. [CrossRef]
31. Sugrue, M.; Dando, R. Cross-modal influence of colour from product and packaging alters perceived flavour of cider. *J. Inst. Brew.* **2018**, *124*, 254–260. [CrossRef]
32. Lemos, T.C.; Almo, A.; Campagnoli, R.R.; Pereira, M.G.; Oliveira, L.; Volchan, E.; Krutman, L.; Delgado, R.; Fernández-Santaella, M.C.; Khandpur, N.; et al. A red code triggers an unintended approach motivation toward sweet ultra-processed foods: Possible implications for front-of-pack labels. *Food Qual. Prefer.* **2020**, *79*, 103784. [CrossRef]
33. Grunert, K.G.; Wills, J.M. A review of European research on consumer response to nutrition information on food labels. *J. Public Health* **2007**, *15*, 385–399. [CrossRef]
34. Blechert, J.; Meule, A.; Busch, N.A.; Ohla, K. Food-pics: An image database for experimental research on eating and appetite. *Front. Psychol.* **2014**, *5*, 617. [CrossRef] [PubMed]
35. Hilbert, A.; Tuschen-Caffier, B.; Karwautz, A.; Niederhofer, H.; Munsch, S. Eating disorder examination-questionnaire. *Diagnostica* **2007**, *53*, 144–154. [CrossRef]
36. Kovaleva, A.; Beierlein, C.; Kemper, C.; Rammstedt, B. Eine kurzskala zur messung von impulsivität nach dem UPPS-ansatz: Die skala impulsives-verhalten-8 (I-8). *Gesis Working Papers* **2012**, *20*, 1–31.
37. Schag, K.; Schönleber, J.; Teufel, M.; Zipfel, S.; Giel, K.E. Food-related impulsivity in obesity and binge eating disorder—A systematic review. *Obes. Rev.* **2013**, *14*, 477–495. [CrossRef]
38. Peirce, J.; Gray, J.R.; Simpson, S.; MacAskill, M.; Höchenberger, R.; Sogo, H.; Kastman, E.; Lindeløv, J.K. PsychoPy2: Experiments in behavior made easy. *Behav. Res. Methods* **2019**, *51*, 195–203. [CrossRef]
39. Berry, C.; Burton, S.; Howlett, E.; Newman, C.L. Understanding the calorie labeling paradox in chain restaurants: Why menu calorie labeling alone may not affect average calories ordered. *J. Public Policy Mark.* **2019**, *38*, 192–213. [CrossRef]
40. Provencher, V.; Polivy, J.; Herman, C.P. Perceived healthiness of food. If it's healthy, you can eat more! *Appetite* **2009**, *52*, 340–344. [CrossRef]
41. Hamlin, R.; McNeill, L. Does the Australasian "Health Star Rating" front of pack nutritional label system work? *Nutrients* **2016**, *8*, 327. [CrossRef]

42. Graham, D.J.; Lucas-Thompson, R.G.; Mueller, M.P.; Jaeb, M.; Harnack, L. Impact of explained v. unexplained front-of-package nutrition labels on parent and child food choices: A randomized trial. *Public Health Nutr.* **2017**, *20*, 774–785. [CrossRef] [PubMed]
43. Watson, W.L.; Kelly, B.; Hector, D.; Hughes, C.; King, L.; Crawford, J.; Sergeant, J.; Chapman, K. Can front-of-pack labelling schemes guide healthier food choices? Australian shoppers' responses to seven labelling formats. *Appetite* **2014**, *72*, 90–97. [CrossRef] [PubMed]
44. Thorndike, A.N.; Riis, J.; Sonnenberg, L.M.; Levy, D.E. Traffic-light labels and choice architecture: Promoting healthy food choices. *Am. J. Prev. Med.* **2014**, *46*, 143–149. [CrossRef] [PubMed]
45. Alley, R.L.; Alley, T.R. The influence of physical state and color on perceived sweetness. *J. Psychol.* **1998**, *132*, 561–568. [CrossRef] [PubMed]

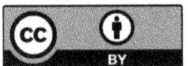

© 2020 by the authors. Licensee MDPI, Basel, Switzerland. This article is an open access article distributed under the terms and conditions of the Creative Commons Attribution (CC BY) license (http://creativecommons.org/licenses/by/4.0/).

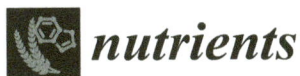 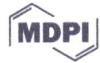

Article

Selected Predictors of the Importance Attached to Salt Content Information on the Food Packaging (a Study among Polish Consumers)

Paweł Bryła

Department of International Marketing and Retailing, Faculty of International and Political Studies, University of Lodz, Narutowicza 59a, 90-131 Lodz, Poland; pawel.bryla@uni.lodz.pl; Tel.: +48-4266-55830

Received: 20 December 2019; Accepted: 19 January 2020; Published: 22 January 2020

Abstract: This paper aims to identify selected antecedents of the importance attached to salt content information (ISCI) placed on food labels, on the basis of a representative survey of 1051 Polish consumers. The study was conducted with the use of the CAWI (Computer Assisted Web Interviews) method in 2018. Quota sampling was applied with reference to the following five criteria: sex, age, education, place of living (urban and rural areas), and region. In a multiple regression model, ISCI depends on the respondent's: sex, age, evaluation of the quantity of nutrition claims, importance attached to nutrition claims, willingness to pay a price premium for products with nutrition claims, attention paid to health and nutrition claims, agreeing with the opinion that unreliable nutrition claims are a serious problem, evaluation of healthiness of one's diet, self-rated knowledge about healthy nutrition, buying organic food, and reading front-of-package (FOP) labels during and after the purchase. The strongest effects on the importance attached to salt content information on the food packaging were displayed by the importance of nutrition claims, attention paid to nutrition and health claims, respondent's age, FOP label reading at home, and agreeing that the use of unreliable nutrition claims is a serious problem.

Keywords: salt information; salt content; salt label; sodium label; sodium information; nutritional information; nutritional labeling; salt information use; nutrition knowledge

1. Introduction

Consumer preferences for information vary widely and an optimal policy should provide different labels for different market segments. Increasing the amount of information may reduce its effectiveness among the low-income consumers it is intended to help [1]. Food consumers understand and value easily recognizable logos more than the information found on nutritional composition labels [2]. Front-of-package labels that include content descriptors are more effective in helping consumers to select lower-sodium products, and traffic light labels, which incorporate content descriptors and color coding, turned out most effective at helping participants select low-sodium products [3]. In a restaurant setting, traffic light and red stop sign warning labels significantly reduced sodium ordered compared with a control. Warning labels also increased knowledge about high sodium content [4]. More accurate use of the nutrition facts panel moderates the effect of product nutrition value on consumer evaluations [5]. Nutrition knowledge has a strong effect on general label use, degree of use, and on use of nutrient content [6]. A literature review demonstrated no consensus on the effect of age, income, or working status on nutritional label use. However, education and gender were found to positively affect label use. It also appears that consumers who are more concerned about nutrition and health are more likely to use nutritional labels. Consequently, consumers on a special diet, organic buyers, and those aware of the diet-disease relation are more likely to search for on-pack nutrition information than others [7]. Although consumers evaluate the nutrition table most positively, it receives little attention and does not stimulate healthy choices. Health goals of consumers increase attention to and use of nutrition labels, especially when these health goals concern specific nutrients [8]. In another study, age, education, income, household size, and nutrition knowledge had an impact on nutritional label use [9].

Excess sodium intake has an important, if not predominant, role in the pathogenesis of elevated blood pressure, one of the most important modifiable determinants of cardiovascular diseases. The strategies to reduce sodium intake include: (1) public education, (2) individual dietary counseling, (3) food labeling, (4) coordinated and voluntary industry sodium reduction, (5) government and private sector food procurement policies, and (6) regulations to modify sodium's generally regarded as safe (GRAS) status [10]. Globally, the average daily dietary salt intake is more than double the recommended level. Key sources of salt in the diet include commercially prepared or manufactured food products and discretionary salt added by consumers during cooking and consumption. Therefore, a significant lowering in the current salt intake requires a shift in both commercial foods and consumer behavior [11]. Regan et al. [12] called for a multi-actor approach that utilizes co-designed, participatory tools to facilitate the involvement of all stakeholders, especially consumers, in making decisions around how best to achieve population-level salt reduction. In 2011, 10 countries had front-of-pack salt labelling schemes [13]. However, emphasizing salt reduction by means of a front-of-pack label can have a negative effect on taste perception and salt use [14]. It is worth noting salt labeling rules differ across countries, e.g., in Malaysia, only 62% of instant noodles displayed the salt content on their food label [15]. In my opinion, it may be advisable to consider some basic standards of salt labeling at the global level. Providing information about the salt content is necessary to encourage a healthy choice, but the claims placed on the packaging seem to be insufficient, as they contribute to the avoidance of the product. Increasing consumer awareness of nutrition claims of foods is required [16]. Consumers' knowledge about their health is a precondition for changing related behavior, which entails objective knowledge about salt intake, sources of salt, and ultimately the salt information on food labels [17]. It is necessary to identify strategies to improve individuals' health and nutrition literacy, to develop strategies that help consumers comprehend and apply Nutrition Facts Label information, and to assess the impact of label usage on dietary behaviors [18]. Smartphone apps may be effective in supporting people, especially with cardiovascular diseases, to make lower salt food purchases [19]. Culture-specific awareness campaigns on salt intake and its association with health are needed [20].

There is a large variation of salt content information use across countries and over time as well as according to certain socio-demographic criteria. In the UK, in 2005, 38% of respondents looked at labelling to find out salt content, and 33% said that salt content would always affect their decision to buy a product [21]. In New Zealand, most participants did not know how to interpret the nutritional information, and many underestimated the salt content of the product by confusing it with sodium content [22]. Similarly, in Japan, few people could convert sodium content to salt, which suggested difficulty in using food labels to control their salt intake [23]. In Melbourne, 69% of respondents reported reading the salt content of food products when shopping. Salt label usage was significantly related to shoppers concern about the amount of salt in their diet and the belief that their health could improve by lowering salt intake. Approximately half of the sample was unable to accurately use labelled sodium information to pick low salt options [24]. In 2007, 70% of Australian consumers correctly identified that most dietary salt comes from processed foods but only a quarter regularly checked food labels for salt content. Even fewer reported that their food purchases were influenced by the salt level indicated (21%) [25]. In a more recent study, conducted in 2015, 89% of Australians were aware of the health risks associated with a high salt intake, 75% correctly identified salt from processed foods as being the main source of salt in the diet, but only 28% could correctly identify the maximum recommended daily intake for salt [26]. Brazilian consumers were concerned about the amount of salt (sodium chloride) in the products they consumed, regardless of educational levels, income, age, lifestyles, or health conditions. The majority of respondents rarely read the sodium content on food labels; however, men and older individuals were more likely to read label information on sodium content [27]. In China, only 5% of respondents understood the meaning of NRV% (Percentage of Nutrient Reference Values), 48% did not know the relationship between sodium and salt, and 13% reported they frequently read the label when shopping. Factors for why people were more likely to choose a product because of its low level of salt shown on the label included income level and their level of awareness of the link between salt and diet [28]. In Korea, the proportion of female college students who read the nutrition information reached 62% but it was only 32% for the sodium information. Their intention to buy low sodium foods increased up to 40% if sodium information was provided on the food label [29]. In Lebanon, only 38% of respondents checked for salt label content, 44% reported that their food purchases were influenced by salt content, and 39% tried to buy low-salt foods [30]. Among Pakistani women, a relationship was found between knowledge about low-salt foods and using low-salt labels [31]. In Pakistan, people of upper castes, people in large families, respondents who were advised to lower salt intake, and who checked salt/sodium labels were less likely to consume higher amounts of salt [32]. In the United States, 19% of respondents agreed they were confused about how to figure out how much sodium is in the foods they eat, and 47% reported they check nutrition labels for sodium content as a tactic to limit salt. Consumers with a high school education or less were more likely than college graduates to report they were confused about sodium content on labels and less likely to check labels for sodium as a tactic to limit salt intake [33]. In Denmark, most consumers are willing to purchase salt-reduced food products, even without having a salt reduction goal. Personal and social norms reveal the strongest influences on intention to change dietary habits, whereas personal norms, knowledge, and awareness of health consequences exert the strongest influences on willingness to purchase salt-reduced food products [34]. In Poland, even commodity science students could not correctly interpret information provided by the Guideline Daily Amount (GDA) system, despite their declarations of full or partial understanding of nutritional labeling [35]. According to Polish food processors and distributors, the information on the content of salt was the third most important type of nutritional information on the food packaging, following content of sugar and of fat [36], whereas among Polish consumers, the information on the salt content ranked fourth after the content of sugar, vitamins, and fats [37]. However, the fact that information about salt content information is missing in some product categories (e.g., cereal products) makes consumer choice more difficult [38]. In a large-scale international survey in Germany, Austria, USA, Hungary, India, China, South Africa, and Brazil, it was found that while salt reduction was seen to be healthy and important, over one third of participants were not interested in salt reduction and the majority were unaware of recommendations [39]. A recent review of 24 studies across 12 countries showed that while consumers were aware of the health implications of a high salt intake, fundamental knowledge regarding recommended dietary intake, primary food sources, and the relationship between salt and sodium was lacking. Moreover, many participants were confused by nutrition information panels, but food purchasing behaviors were positively influenced by front of package labelling [40].

This paper aims to identify selected antecedents of the importance attached to salt content information (ISCI) placed on food labels, on the basis of a large-scale, representative survey of Polish consumers. To the best of my knowledge, this is the first study to investigate the ISCI in a representative, nation-wide sample of Polish consumers. As the literature review showed large differences across nations, it is necessary to examine this issue in the biggest Central European country. The age-standardized estimated sodium intake for persons aged 20 and over was at the level of 3.84 g/day in Poland in 2010, which was similar to the global average of 3.95 g/day [41]. However, within the European Union, Central European countries, including Poland, rank at the top of the table of estimated salt intakes. Poland ranked fifth in the EU with the average salt intake of as much as 11.5 g/day, and five out of the six countries with the highest consumption of salt per capita in the European Union were from the Central European region (Czech Republic, Slovenia, Hungary, Poland, and Romania), with the exception of Portugal taking the fourth place [42]. A wide range of potential predictors were analyzed to see if they differentiated the ISCI in a statistically significant way.

Next, a multiple regression model was constructed to examine the simultaneous impact of various independent variables. Finally, a simplified model with only significant predictors was arrived at. The main contribution of this paper lies not only in studying the phenomenon in a new geographic context, but also identifying new predictors of the importance attached to salt content information, in particular concerning various aspects of the attitude to nutrition claims and the context of reading labels (at home rather than in the shop).

2. Materials and Methods

The study was conducted with the use of the CAWI (Computer Assisted Web Interviews) method in 2018. The online survey was administered by a specialized research agency commissioned by the University of Lodz. The author of this manuscript designed the questionnaire and set sampling criteria. The respondents were informed that the results would be used only for scientific purposes with the respect of the principle of anonymity. The sample size amounted to 1051 persons. Quota sampling was applied with reference to the following five criteria: sex (males and females), age (the following age intervals: 15–24, 25–34, 35–44, 45–54, 55–64 and 65 and more), education (primary, secondary, tertiary), place of living (urban and rural areas) and voivodeship (all 16 Polish regions). Thanks to this approach, the structure of the sample was similar to the general population of Polish consumers according to the aforementioned criteria.

The sample comprised of 560 women (53.3%) and 491 men (46.7%). Regarding the age structure, the sample was composed in the following way: 15–24 years—15.0%, 25–34—17.3%, 35–44—17.9%, 45–54—13.9%, 55–64—15.7%, 65 and more—20.2%. The mean age amounted to 45.0. As far as the household size is concerned, the structure was as follows: 1 person—9.5%, 2—31.7%, 3—24.6%, 4—19.1%, 5—7.7%, 6 and more—7.3%. Regarding the number of children in the household, the sample was structured in the following way: 0 children—52.4%, 1—25.1%, 2—16.9%, 3—3.8%, 4—1.2%, 5 and more—0.5%. The sample resembled the general population in terms of the education level, with 47.7% of respondents having primary and vocational education, 31.6%—secondary, and 20.7%—tertiary. Regarding professional activity, the sample had the following characteristics: white-collar workers—13.3%, blue-collar workers—28.0%, unemployed—4.7%, students—10.5%, not working and caring for the family—9.5%, old age pensioners and disability pensioners—29.7%. As far as the family monthly net income is concerned, the structure was as follows: under 2000 PLN—15.0%, 2001–3000—23.8%, 3001–4000—21.9%, 4001–5000—18.2%, 5001–6000—10.5%, over 6000—10.7%. 61.7% of the respondents lived in the urban areas, while 38.3% were rural inhabitants. Regarding the size of city, the structure was as follows: rural areas—38.3%, town up to 50,000 inhabitants—18.4%, city of 50,000–500,000—18.6%, city having more than 500,000 inhabitants—14.7%. All 16 Polish regions were represented in the sample, with the highest shares from the most populated regions—Mazowieckie (with the national capital Warsaw)—13.5% and Śląskie (Silesia)—11.4%.

The operationalization of the key variables used in this study is provided in Table 1.

In order to analyze the collected empirical material, t-tests, analyses of variance (ANOVAs), Pearson correlation coefficients, and multiple regression models were applied. The analyses were conducted in Statistica 12.0 (TIBCO Software Inc., Palo Alto, CA, USA).

Table 1. Operationalization of variables included in the regression models.

Variable	Operationalization
ISCI	Importance attached to salt content information (ISCI) on food packaging: very high—5, rather high—4, average—3, rather small—2, none—1
Sex	Woman—1, man—0
Age	In years
BMI	Body Mass Index—the body mass divided by the square of the body height
Special diet	Being on a special diet for health reasons: yes—1, no—0
Self-rated health	How do you evaluate your health status? Very good—5, rather good—4, average—3, rather poor—2, very poor—1
Education	Primary—0, vocational—1, secondary—2, tertiary—3
White-collar worker	Yes—1, no—0
Pensioner	Old age or disability pensioner: yes—1, no—0
Children	The number of children in the respondent's household
Quantity of nutrition claims	Evaluation of the quantity of nutrition claims on the packaging of food products: excessive—1, appropriate—2, insufficient—3
Understandability of nutrition claims	Very understandable—5, rather understandable—4, average—3, rather not understandable—2, completely not understandable—1
Importance of nutrition claims	Very big—5, rather big—4, average—3, rather small—2, none—1
Credibility of nutrition claims	Very credible—5, rather credible 4, average—3, rather not credible—2, definitely not credible—1
Nutrition information at first purchase	Indicating nutrition information as the most important type of information on the label (with the exception of price) when the respondent buys a food product for the first time (1 or 0)
Willingness to pay for nutrition claims	Willingness to pay a higher price for a product with nutrition claims compared to a similar product without such claims: definitely yes—5, rather yes—4, I don't know—3, rather not—2, definitely not—1
Attention to health and nutrition claims	Do you pay attention to health and nutrition claims? Definitely yes—5, rather yes—4, hard to say—3, rather not—2, definitely not—1
Unreliable nutrition claims	Agreement with the opinion that the use of unreliable nutrition claims is a serious problem in Poland: definitely yes—5, rather yes—4, hard to say—3, rather not—2, definitely not—1
Diet healthiness evaluation	How do you evaluate your diet? Very healthy—5, rather healthy—4, average—3, rather unhealthy—2, very unhealthy—1
Knowledge about healthy nutrition	How do you evaluate your knowledge about healthy nutrition? Very big—5, rather big—4, average—3, rather small—2, very small—1
Dietary supplements	Buying dietary supplements: yes—1, no and don't know—0
Organic food	Buying organic food: yes—1, no and don't know—0
Functional food	Buying functional food: yes—1, no and don't know—0
Fair trade products	Buying fair trade products: yes—1, no and don't know—0
FOP label reading in the shop	The share of food products during the purchase of which the respondent reads the Front-of-Package (FOP) label (%)
BOP label reading in the shop	The share of food products during the purchase of which the respondent reads the Back-of-Package (BOP) label (%)
FOP label reading at home	The share of food products after the purchase of which the respondent reads the Front-of-Package (FOP) label (%)
BOP label reading at home	The share of food products after the purchase of which the respondent reads the Back-of-Package (BOP) label (%)

3. Results

My dependent variable was the importance attached to salt content information on food packaging (ISCI). It was measured with the use of the following question: 'How important is the following information on the packaging of food products?—Salt content' with five answer options: very big, rather big, average, rather small, none, which were subsequently coded in the scale 5-1.

Sex differentiated the level of ISCI. Women attached higher importance to salt content information on food packaging than men (Mean: 3.896 versus 3.635, $t = 4.134$, $p < 0.001$).

Age correlated positively with the ISCI ($r = 0.137$, $p < 0.001$), meaning that older respondents declared a higher importance of this type of information.

The importance attached to salt content information on food packaging was analyzed with the use of ANOVAs based on selected characteristics of respondents: place of living (size of the city), household size, number of children in the household, respondent's education level, occupational status, household income, evaluation of the quantity of nutrition claims, and the most important information during the first purchase of a food product (Table 2).

The place of living, understood as the size of the respondent's city, did not affect in a significant way the importance attached to salt content information. The household size did not affect in a significant way the importance attached to salt content information.

The number of children in the respondent's household marginally affected the importance attached to salt content information. Respondents from families with no children and 1 child attached higher importance to this kind of information compared to those with 2 or more children.

The importance attached to salt content information depends on the level of education. The higher the education, the more importance is attached to this kind of information.

Occupational status influenced the level of importance attached to salt content information. The highest importance was declared by pensioners (including old age pensioners and disability pensioners) and white-collar workers, whereas the lowest was displayed by students, which is at least partly related to the age structure of these groups.

Income marginally affected the importance attached to salt content information on food packaging. The highest importance was observed in the group of respondents with middle income—3001–4000 PLN (approximately 700–900 EUR) of total monthly disposable income of their household. The lowest importance of this kind of information was indicated by respondents with extremely low and high income.

The evaluation of the quantity of nutrition claims on food packaging affected the importance attached to salt content information significantly. Respondents feeling that there were too many nutrition claims attributed less importance to salt content information than those who believed that this quantity was appropriate or insufficient.

The ISCI depended on which information was the most important for respondents when they bought a food product for the first time. Price was deliberately excluded from the catalogue of answers, and the respondents were asked to consider only non-price attributes. It turned out that the highest ISCI characterized those who indicated nutrition information as the most important type of information during the first purchase.

Being on a special diet for health reasons significantly increased the declared importance of salt content information (4.006 versus 3.728, $t = 3.271$, $p = 0.001$).

Body Mass Index (BMI) correlated positively with the level of importance attached to salt content information ($r = 0.378$, $p < 0.001$), meaning that people with higher BMI paid more attention to the salt content information.

Self-rated health correlated strongly with the ISCI ($r = 0.917$, $p < 0.001$). Respondents evaluating their health more favorably attributed more importance to the salt content information.

Table 2. The importance attached to salt content information on food packaging by selected characteristics of respondents (analyses of variance—ANOVAs).

Independent Variables	Groups	ISCI	ANOVAs
Place of living	Rural areas	3.799	$F = 0.555, p = 0.645$
	Town up to 50 thousand	3.731	
	City of 50–500 thousand	3.807	
	City of over 500 thousand	3.701	
Household size (1)	1	3.790	$F = 0.664, p = 0.651$
	2	3.826	
	3	3.795	
	4	3.697	
	5	3.779	
	6	3.612	
Number of children (2)	0	3.815	$F = 2.278, p = 0.059$
	1	3.833	
	2	3.624	
	3	3.625	
	4	3.308	
Level of education	Primary	3.605	$\mathbf{F = 4.619, p = 0.003}$
	Vocational	3.691	
	Secondary	3.804	
	Tertiary	3.968	
Occupational status	White-collar worker	3.950	$\mathbf{F = 5.350, p < 0.001}$
	Blue-collar worker	3.660	
	Unemployed	3.633	
	Student	3.555	
	Housekeeper	3.630	
	Pensioner	3.962	
Income (3)	Below 2000 PLN	3.690	$F = 1.985, p = 0.078$
	2001–3000 PLN	3.736	
	3001–4000 PLN	3.943	
	4001–5000 PLN	3.723	
	5001–6000 PLN	3.836	
	Over 6000 PLN	3.661	
Nutrition claims (4)	Excessive	3.305	$\mathbf{F = 17.550, p < 0.001}$
	Appropriate	3.729	
	Insufficient	4.014	
Type of information (5)	Country of origin	3.808	$\mathbf{F = 4.763, p < 0.001}$
	Nutrition information	3.984	
	Health information	3.864	
	List of ingredients	3.881	
	Expiry date	3.612	

Notes: (1) Households with over 6 members were not included in the ANOVA. They were represented by 2.7% of the respondents. (2) Households with over 4 children were not included in the ANOVA. They were represented by 0.5% of the respondents. (3) Average monthly disposable income of the respondent's household. (4) Evaluation of the quantity of nutrition claims on food packaging. (5) The most important information on the label (excluding price) during the first purchase of a food product. Respondents indicating 'other' and 'don't know' were excluded from the ANOVA. They accounted for 0.6% and 2.1% of the sample, respectively. Significant results indicated in bold.

The ISCI correlated strongly with understandability of nutrition claims ($r = 0.913$, $p < 0.001$), showing that understanding nutrition claims better increased the importance attached to salt content information.

There was a strong correlation of ISCI with the perceived credibility of nutrition claims ($r = 0.928$, $p < 0.001$), underlining the link between the importance attached to such information and trust in its accuracy.

The ISCI was strongly associated with the importance attached to nutrition claims on food packaging (r = 0.945, $p < 0.001$) as well as with the importance of other types of information placed on the packaging, such as: health claims (r = 0.944, $p < 0.001$), list of ingredients (r = 0.943, $p < 0.001$), expiry date (r = 0.932, $p < 0.001$), country of origin (r = 0.926, $p < 0.001$), culinary recipes (r = 0.914, $p < 0.001$), brand (r = 0.922, $p < 0.001$), organic label (r = 0.936, $p < 0.001$), quality signs (r = 0.938, $p < 0.001$), recommendations of scientific institutes (r = 0.930, $p < 0.001$), and price (r = 0.917, $p < 0.001$). As the importance of these types of information was highly correlated (correlation coefficients exceeding 0.9), I selected the importance attached to nutrition claims only for further analyses.

The ISCI was also strongly correlated with the importance ascribed to other types of nutrition information, such as: energy value (r = 0.954, $p < 0.001$), fat content (r = 0.968, $p < 0.001$), sugar content (r = 0.967, $p < 0.001$), protein content (r = 0.959, $p < 0.001$), vitamin content (r = 0.960, $p < 0.001$), roughage content (r = 0.961, $p < 0.001$), and Omega-3 fatty acids content (r = 0.961, $p < 0.001$). These results indicate that those attaching high importance to one type of nutrition information tend to appreciate highly also other types of such information. There are very strong correlations between these measures (correlation coefficients exceeding 0.95). Therefore, I excluded the importance attached to particular types of nutrition information from further analyses with the exception of the ISCI.

I also found strong correlations of the ISCI with the importance of all analyzed health claims, concerning the impact of the product on: lowering the cholesterol level (r = 0.942, $p < 0.001$), lowering the risk of heart diseases (r = 0.946, $p < 0.001$), strengthening bones (r = 0.947, $p < 0.001$), the digestive system (r = 0.948, $p < 0.001$), reducing tiredness and fatigue (r = 0.939, $p < 0.001$), maintaining proper vision (r = 0.943, $p < 0.001$), proper development of children (r = 0.929, $p < 0.001$), and proper functioning of the heart (r = 0.944, $p < 0.001$). Due to the very strong correlations among these variables (correlation coefficients above 0.9), they were not included in further analyses.

The ISCI was associated with the willingness to pay (WTP) a higher price for products with nutrition claims compared to similar products without such claims. The WTP was operationalized in two ways in my research. First, it was an answer to the question: 'Are you willing to pay more for products with nutrition claims (compared to similar products without such claims)?' The following answer options were proposed: definitely yes, rather yes, I don't know, rather not, and definitely not, and subsequently coded in the scale 5-1. The second operationalization of the WTP was numerical. Those respondents who answered 'definitely yes' or 'rather yes' to the above question were asked to estimate how much higher a price (on average) they would be willing to pay for products with nutrition claims (compared to similar products without such claims), expressed in percentage. It turned out that the ISCI correlated significantly with both types of WTP. For the former, the correlation coefficient amounted to 0.925 ($p < 0.001$), whereas for the latter it was 0.152 ($p = 0.001$). The former measure of the WTP was selected for further analyses.

Unsurprisingly, the ISCI was strongly correlated to paying attention to health and nutrition claims (r = 0.945, $p < 0.001$).

More surprising was a very strong correlation between the ISCI and the opinion that the use of unreliable nutrition claims is a serious problem in Poland (r = 0.928, $p < 0.001$). Paradoxically, respondents who confirmed the existence of this problem attached a higher importance to salt content information. They might have a better knowledge of this negative phenomenon, which did not prevent them from paying attention to nutrition claims.

Consumers evaluating their diet as more healthy indicated a higher importance of salt content information on the packaging (r = 0.944, $p < 0.001$).

The ISCI was also related to the self-evaluated knowledge on a healthy diet (r = 0.941, $p < 0.001$).

Consumers purchasing certain types of products were characterized by significantly higher importance attached to salt content information (Table 3). It applied to: dietary supplements, organic food, functional food, and fair trade products.

Table 3. The importance attached to salt content information on food packaging by purchasing certain products (*t* tests).

Purchasing	Yes	No	t	p
Dietary supplements	3.855	3.699	2.451	0.014
Organic food	4.023	3.482	8.790	<0.001
Functional food	3.987	3.658	5.013	<0.001
Fair trade products	3.906	3.725	2.557	0.011

Note: the category 'No' includes those who answered 'No' and 'Don't know'.

The ISCI was significantly related to reading food labels, both during the purchase in the point of sale, and at home after the purchase (Table 4). It was correlated with front-of-package and back-of-package labels in both contexts. Please not that this variable was operationalized as the percentage share of products during and after the purchase of which the respondent reads information placed on the packaging. This measurement approach reduces potential bias between heavy buyers and those who do not engage in food shopping frequently, as I focus on the relative, not absolute frequency of reading labels.

Table 4. Correlation coefficients between the importance attached to salt content information on food packaging and reading labels (the share of food products for which the respondent reads FOP or BOP labels in the shop or at home).

Reading Labels		r	p
Shop	FOP	0.071	0.022
	BOP	0.118	<0.001
Home	FOP	0.104	0.001
	BOP	0.116	<0.001

Note: FOP—front-of-package labels, BOP—back-of-package labels.

Variables which significantly affected the importance attached to salt content information in the *t* tests, correlation coefficients, and ANOVAs (with the exception of those that were highly correlated with similar independent variables) were included in a multiple regression model in order to test their simultaneous impact on the dependent variable (ISCI) (Table 5). The initial regression model included 27 independent variables, 11 out of which turned out to be statistically significant predictors of the ISCI at the level of $p < 0.05$. The whole model was highly significant ($p < 0.001$) and explained 32.8% of the variance of the dependent variable.

In order to arrive at a more parsimonious model, I gradually eliminated from the full model those predictors that failed to reach statistical significance ($p < 0.05$), starting with those that had the highest statistical significance in the initial model. The implementation of this procedure led to the emergence of the final multiple regression model (Table 6). It explains almost the same amount of the variance of the dependent variable ($R^2 = 0.320$, $p < 0.001$), with a considerably smaller set of predictors (12 variables). It is worth noting that all independent variables which were significant in the initial model remain significant in this modified model, and one variable which failed to reach statistical significance previously has now become significant (sex).

Table 5. Selected predictors of the importance attached to salt content information on food packaging (the initial multiple regression model).

Predictors	β	SE	t	p
Intercept	x	x	0.421	0.674
Sex	0.052	0.028	1.872	0.062
Age	0.139	0.041	3.419	**0.001**
BMI	−0.027	0.030	−0.889	0.374
Special diet	0.007	0.028	0.248	0.804
Self-rated health	−0.034	0.031	−1.078	0.281
Education	0.014	0.031	0.464	0.643
White-collar worker	0.018	0.030	0.606	0.544
Pensioner	0.011	0.039	0.281	0.779
Children	−0.026	0.028	−0.940	0.347
Quantity of nutrition claims	0.075	0.027	2.727	**0.006**
Understandability of nutrition claims	−0.020	0.030	−0.662	0.508
Importance of nutrition claims	0.225	0.031	7.284	**<0.001**
Credibility of nutrition claims	0.048	0.031	1.554	0.121
Nutrition information at first purchase	0.025	0.026	0.952	0.341
Willingness to pay for nutrition claims	0.069	0.031	2.204	**0.028**
Attention to health and nutrition claims	0.144	0.035	4.111	**<0.001**
Unreliable nutrition claims	0.106	0.027	3.920	**<0.001**
Diet healthiness evaluation	0.074	0.034	2.206	**0.028**
Knowledge about healthy nutrition	0.066	0.033	2.011	**0.045**
Dietary supplements	−0.020	0.026	−0.769	0.442
Organic food	0.062	0.029	2.109	**0.035**
Functional food	0.001	0.028	0.033	0.973
Fair trade products	−0.023	0.028	−0.796	0.426
FOP label reading in the shop	−0.098	0.034	−2.892	**0.004**
BOP label reading in the shop	0.033	0.035	0.949	0.343
FOP label reading at home	0.095	0.036	2.657	**0.008**
BOP label reading at home	0.038	0.037	1.026	0.305

Note: the operationalization of the variables is included in Table 1; SE—standard error. Significant values are shown in bold.

Table 6. Selected predictors of the importance attached to salt content information on food packaging (the final multiple regression model).

Predictors	β	SE	t	p
Intercept	x	x	−0.570	0.569
Sex	0.059	0.027	2.174	**0.030**
Age	0.156	0.027	5.857	**<0.001**
Quantity of nutrition claims	0.074	0.026	2.819	**0.005**
Importance of nutrition claims	0.237	0.030	8.026	**<0.001**
Willingness to pay for nutrition claims	0.070	0.030	2.313	**0.021**
Attention to health and nutrition claims	0.161	0.034	4.755	**<0.001**
Unreliable nutrition claims	0.105	0.026	3.972	**<0.001**
Diet healthiness evaluation	0.080	0.032	2.500	**0.013**
Knowledge about healthy nutrition	0.066	0.032	2.076	**0.038**
Organic food	0.057	0.029	1.988	**0.047**
FOP label reading in the shop	−0.086	0.032	−2.638	**0.008**
FOP label reading at home	0.111	0.033	3.400	**0.001**

Note: the operationalization of the variables is included in Table 1; SE—standard error. Significant values are shown in bold.

The importance attached to salt content information on food packaging depends on the respondent's: sex, age, evaluation of the quantity of nutrition claims, importance attached to nutrition claims, willingness to pay a price premium for products with nutrition claims, attention paid to health and nutrition claims, agreeing with the opinion that unreliable nutrition claims are a serious problem, evaluation of healthiness of one's diet, self-rated knowledge about healthy nutrition, buying organic food, and reading front-of-package labels during and after the purchase. Being a woman increases the ISCI. Older consumers attach more importance to salt content information. Evaluating the quantity of nutrition claims as appropriate and insufficient reinforces the ISCI. Higher importance attached to nutrition claims in general translates into a higher ISCI. Being more willing to pay a higher price for products with nutrition claims increases the ISCI. Paying more attention to health and nutrition claims increases the ISCI. Agreeing with the opinion that the use of unreliable nutrition claims constitutes an important problem boosts the ISCI. Evaluating one's diet as healthy contributes to a higher ISCI. Displaying better (self-rated) knowledge about healthy nutrition also improves the ISCI. Buying organic food is positively related to the ISCI. A bit surprisingly, reading front-of-package information in the shop actually reduces the ISCI, whereas reading the same kind of information on the label after the purchase at home increases it.

The multivariate model can be used for profiling consumer characteristics more prone to value ISCI. I estimated the predicted ISCI for a sensitive set of combination of covariates in the regression model (Table 7). The predictions for different levels of a given independent variable were made on the assumption that the remaining covariates were at their mean level observed in the sample.

On the basis of these calculations, we can notice, for instance, that the difference in the predicted ISCI between men and women is $3.831 - 3.710 = 0.121$. In relative terms, it is $0.121/3.710 = 0.0326$, i.e., 3.26%. The ISCI values for men and women actually observed in the sample were 3.635 and 3.896 respectively, which means a difference between sexes of 0.261 or 7.18%. Does it mean that the above predictions are inaccurate? Not necessarily, because we should bear in mind that the multiple regression takes into account the simultaneous impact of all predictors included in the model. For example, if women in the sample tend to be younger than men and age is positively correlated with ISCI, the impact of age is not reflected in the ISCI ANOVA for sex, but it is taken into account in the multiple regression with ISCI as the dependent variable and both sex and age included as predictors. Ceteris paribus, being older by 10 years leads to a higher predicted ISCI by 0.091. Ceteris paribus, those who consider the quantity of nutrition claims on the food packaging as insufficient have a higher predicted ISCI than those who think there are too many nutrition claims by 0.272. Ceteris paribus, those who attach very high importance to nutrition claims have a predicted ISCI higher than those who consider their importance as none by as much as 1.092. Ceteris paribus, those who declare they are definitely willing to pay more for products with nutrition claims than for analogous products without such claims have their predicted ISCI higher by 0.279 than those who definitely would not pay more. Ceteris paribus, those who definitively pay attention to health and nutrition claims have their predicted ISCI higher than those who definitively do not by 0.725. Ceteris paribus, those who definitively agree with the statement that the use of unreliable nutrition claims is a serious problem have their predicted ISCI higher by 0.497 than those who definitively do not agree with this opinion. Ceteris paribus, those who consider their diet as very healthy have their predicted ISCI higher than those who consider it very unhealthy by 0.484. Ceteris paribus, those who evaluate their knowledge about healthy nutrition as very big have their predicted ISCI higher than those who think it is very small by 0.383. Ceteris paribus, buying organic food leads to an increase in the predicted ISCI by 0.117. Ceteris paribus, those who declare they read FOP labels for 90% of food products in the shop have their predicted ISCI lower by 0.255 than those who declare reading such labels for 10% of food products in the point of purchase. Ceteris paribus, those who declare reading 90% of FOP labels at home have their predicted ISCI higher by 0.298 than those who read only 10% of such labels after shopping.

Table 7. ISCI predicted for different levels of independent variables in the final multiple regression model.

Predictors	Predictor Levels	ISCI Estimate	95% CI
Sex	Men	3.710	3.633–3.788
	Women	3.831	3.758–3.903
Age	20 years old	3.546	3.454–3.638
	30 years old	3.637	3.568–3.706
	40 years old	3.729	3.675–3.782
	50 years old	3.820	3.766–3.874
	60 years old	3.911	3.842–3.980
Quantity of nutrition claims	Excessive	3.612	3.487–3.736
	Appropriate	3.748	3.693–3.803
	Insufficient	3.884	3.792–3.976
Importance of nutrition claims	None	3.064	2.883–3.245
	Rather small	3.337	3.218–3.456
	Average	3.610	3.545–3.676
	Rather big	3.883	3.825–3.942
	Very big	4.156	4.050–4.263
Willingness to pay for nutrition claims	Definitely not	3.612	3.464–3.759
	Rather not	3.682	3.587–3.776
	Hard to say	3.751	3.696–3.807
	Rather yes	3.821	3.756–3.886
	Definitively yes	3.891	3.779–4.002
Attention to health and nutrition claims	Definitely not	3.327	3.134–3.518
	Rather not	3.508	3.386–3.629
	Hard to say	3.689	3.627–3.752
	Rather yes	3.871	3.806–3.936
	Definitively yes	4.052	3.927–4.178
Unreliable nutrition claims	Definitely not	3.415	3.229–3.600
	Rather not	3.539	3.412–3.666
	Hard to say	3.664	3.588–3.739
	Rather yes	3.788	3.736–3.840
	Definitively yes	3.912	3.827–3.998
Diet healthiness evaluation	Very unhealthy	3.491	3.263–3.720
	Rather unhealthy	3.612	3.475–3.750
	Average	3.733	3.673–3.794
	Rather healthy	3.854	3.773–3.936
	Very healthy	3.975	3.809–4.141
Knowledge about healthy nutrition	Very small	3.549	3.329–3.768
	Rather small	3.645	3.511–3.778
	Average	3.741	3.680–3.801
	Rather big	3.836	3.758–3.915
	Very big	3.932	3.774–4.090
Organic food	Purchasing	3.828	3.754–3.903
	Not purchasing	3.711	3.630–3.792
FOP label reading in the shop	10% of food products	3.919	3.800–4.038
	50% of food products	3.792	3.738–3.845
	90% of food products	3.664	3.567–3.761
FOP label reading at home	10% of food products	3.629	3.530–3.727
	50% of food products	3.778	3.726–3.830
	90% of food products	3.927	3.825–4.030

Notes: the operationalization of the variables is included in Table 1; CI—confidence interval.

4. Discussion

Only two out of the 12 statistically significant predictors of the importance attached to salt content information were demographic (sex and age), while the remaining 10 were behavioral and psychographic. The strongest effects on the importance attached to salt content information on the food packaging ($|\beta| > 0.1$) were displayed by the importance of nutrition claims, attention paid to nutrition and health claims, respondent's age, FOP label reading at home, and agreeing that the use of unreliable nutrition claims is a serious problem. Therefore, front-of-package labeling plays a key role in salt content communication, which is congruent with references [2–4,39]. Second, this study confirmed the impact of gender, age, buying organic food [7], and consumer knowledge [6,34] on the nutritional label use. Contrary to some previous studies [9,33], education, income, and household size did not affect the importance attached to salt content information in the multiple regression model. Contrary to a study conducted in Brazil [27], not men, but women attached more importance to the salt information.

The contribution of the current study is related to the fact that it enabled to focus on the importance attached to salt content information (regardless of its form on the label), rather than nutritional information in general on the one hand, and specific nutrition claims on the other hand. Furthermore, my findings indicate the importance of several new predictors of the ISCI, including various aspects of the attitude to nutrition claims and the context of reading FOP labels (at home rather than in the shop). Third, it is the first attempt to study this phenomenon in a representative sample of the inhabitants of Poland, the largest country in the Central European region, which is characterized by very unfavorable salt intake statistics within the European Union.

There are a few implications of my findings. First of all, there is a need to increase the importance attached to salt content information in certain segments of the population, especially among men and younger consumers. Second, it is advisable to conduct education campaigns stressing the importance of nutrition claims placed on food products, explaining the meaning of nutrition information presented on the labels, and increasing consumer knowledge about healthy nutrition. Third, it is recommended to augment consumers' attention to health and nutrition claims, e.g., by allocating a more prominent place on the packaging to this type of information, using bigger fonts of the typeface, using graphical symbols alongside textual information, and emphasizing them in other forms of marketing communications, in particular advertising. Fourth, it is recommended to run social marketing campaigns in favor of more healthy diets. Fifth, it is recommended to stimulate the development of the organic food market. Sixth, it may be beneficial to encourage consumers to read food labels after the purchase at home, e.g., by running loyalty programs requiring consumers to use promotion codes placed on the packaging. Seventh, the use of nutrition claims and other similar types of information on the food labels should be controlled by independent public authorities so as to minimize the concern about unreliable claims. Eighth, it may be advisable to consider the expansion of the obligation of salt content labeling to other food product categories.

It is worth noting that all measures used in this study were self-reported, rather than observed, which may be considered a limitation. Second, due to the intention-behavior gap, it is hard to translate the declarations of importance of particular information types into actual purchasing behaviors. However, our variable of interest was importance attached to salt content rather than just reading salt labels, which may be considered more accurate in predicting consumer behavior in my opinion.

Future research may focus on the perception of various types of salt content information by different segments of consumers. Second, structural equation modeling may be used to examine various paths of causal relationships, mediators, and moderators. Third, long-term purchasing data in consumer panels may be used to investigate the impact of socio-demographic variables on the preferences for low sodium products and the relationship between reading salt information, attaching importance to it, and implementing healthy diet practices.

Funding: This research was funded by the National Science Centre, Opus grant number 2015/17/B/HS4/00253. The APC was funded by the National Science Centre, Opus grant number 2015/17/B/HS4/00253.

Conflicts of Interest: The author declares no conflict of interest. The funder had no role in the design of the study; in the collection, analyses, or interpretation of data; in the writing of the manuscript, or in the decision to publish the results.

References

1. McCullough, J.; Best, R. Consumer preferences for food label information: A basis for segmentation. *J. Consum. Aff.* **1980**, *14*, 180–192. [CrossRef]
2. Sanz-Valero, J.; Sebastián-Ponce, M.I.; Wanden-Berghe, C. Interventions to reduce salt consumption through labeling. *Rev. Panam. Salud Publ.* **2012**, *31*, 332–337. [CrossRef] [PubMed]
3. Goodman, S.; Hammond, D.; Hanning, R.; Sheeshka, J. The impact of adding front-of-package sodium content labels to grocery products: An experimental study. *Public Health Nutr.* **2013**, *16*, 383–391. [CrossRef] [PubMed]
4. Musicus, A.A.; Moran, A.J.; Lawman, H.G.; Roberto, C.A. Online randomized controlled trials of restaurant sodium warning labels. *Am. J. Prev. Med.* **2019**, *57*, e181–e193. [CrossRef] [PubMed]
5. Burton, S.; Garretson, J.A.; Velliquette, A.M. Implications of accurate usage of nutrition facts panel information for food product evaluations and purchase intentions. *J. Acad. Mark. Sci.* **1999**, *27*, 470–480. [CrossRef]
6. Drichoutis, A.C.; Lazaridis, P.; Nayga, R.M. Nutrition knowledge and consumer use of nutritional food labels. *Eur. Rev. Agric. Econ.* **2005**, *32*, 93–118. [CrossRef]
7. Drichoutis, A.C.; Lazaridis, P.; Nayga, R.M. Consumers' use of nutritional labels: A review of research studies and issues. *Acad. Mark. Sci. Rev.* **2006**, *2006*, 1–25. Available online: http://www.amsreview.org/articles/drichoutis09-2006.pdf (accessed on 15 December 2019).
8. Van Herpen, E.; van Trijp, H.C.M. Front-of-pack nutrition labels. Their effect on attention and choices when consumers have varying goals and time constraints. *Appetite* **2011**, *57*, 148–160. [CrossRef]
9. Cannoosamy, K.; Pugo-Gunsam, P.; Jeewon, R. Consumer knowledge and attitudes toward nutritional labels. *J. Nutr. Educ. Behav.* **2014**, *46*, 334–340. [CrossRef]
10. Cobb, L.K.; Appel, L.J.; Anderson, C.A.M. Strategies to reduce dietary sodium intake. *Curr. Treat. Opt. Cardiovasc. Med.* **2012**, *14*, 425–434. [CrossRef]
11. Zandstra, E.H.; Lion, R.; Newson, R. Salt reduction: Moving from consumer awareness to action. *Food Qual. Prefer.* **2016**, *48*, 376–381. [CrossRef]
12. Regan, Á.; Kent, M.P.; Raats, M.M.; McConnon, Á.; Wall, P.; Dubois, L. Applying a consumer behavior lens to salt reduction initiatives. *Nutrients* **2017**, *9*, 901. [CrossRef] [PubMed]
13. Webster, J.L.; Dunfords, E.K.; Hawkes, C.; Neal, B.C. Salt reduction initiatives around the world. *J. Hypertens.* **2011**, *29*, 1043–1050. [CrossRef] [PubMed]
14. Liem, D.G.; Miremadi, F.; Zandstra, E.H.; Keast, R.S.J. Health labelling can influence taste perception and use of table salt for reduced-sodium products. *Public Health Nutr.* **2012**, *15*, 2340–2347. [CrossRef] [PubMed]
15. Tan, C.H.; Chow, Z.Y.; Ching, S.M.; Devaraj, N.K.; He, F.J.; Mac Gregor, G.A.; Chia, Y.C. Salt content of instant noodles in Malaysia: A cross-sectional study. *BMJ Open* **2019**, *9*, e024702. [CrossRef]
16. Gębski, J.; Jeżewska-Zychowicz, M.; Szlachciuk, J.; Kosicka-Gębska, M. Impact of nutritional claims on consumer preferences for bread with varied fiber and salt content. *Food Qual. Prefer.* **2019**, *76*, 91–99. [CrossRef]
17. Van Staden, J. Consumers' Attitudes Regarding the Use of the Salt Information on Food Labels. Master's Thesis, North-West University, van der Bair Park, South Africa, May 2018.
18. Davy, B.M.; Halliday, T.M.; Davy, K.P. Sodium intake and blood pressure: New controversies, new labels . . . new guidelines? *Nutr. Diabetes* **2015**, *115*, 200–204. [CrossRef]
19. Eyles, H.; McLean, R.; Neal, B.; Jiang, Y.; Doughty, R.N.; McLean, R.; Ni Mhurchu, C. A salt-reduction smartphone app supports lower-salt food purchases for people with cardiovascular disease: Findings from the SaltSwitch randomized controlled trial. *Eur. J. Prev. Cardiol.* **2017**, *24*, 1435–1444. [CrossRef]
20. Ismail, L.C.; Hashim, M.; Jarrar, A.H.; Mohamad, M.; Saley, S.T.; Jawish, N.; Bekdache, M.; Albaghli, H.; Kdsi, D.; Aldarweesh, D.; et al. Knowledge, attitude, and practice on salt and assessment of dietary salt and fat intake among University of Sharjah students. *Nutrients* **2019**, *11*, 941. [CrossRef]

21. Bussell, G.; Hunt, M. Improving the labelling of the salt content of foods. In *Reducing Salt in Food. Practical Strategies*; Kilcast, D., Angus, F., Eds.; Woodhead Publishing Limited: Cambridge, UK, 2007; pp. 134–154.
22. Gilbey, A.; Fifield, S. Nutritional information about sodium: Is it worth its salt? *N. Zeal. Med. J.* **2006**, *119*, U1934.
23. Okuda, N.; Nishi, N.; Ishokawa-Takata, K.; Yoshimura, E.; Horie, S.; Nakanishi, T.; Sato, Y.; Takimoto, H. Understanding of sodium content labeled on food packages by Japanese people. *Hypertens. Res.* **2014**, *37*, 467–471. [CrossRef] [PubMed]
24. Grimes, C.A.; Riddell, L.J.; Nowson, C.A. Consumer knowledge and attitudes to salt intake and labelled salt information. *Appetite* **2009**, *53*, 189–194. [CrossRef] [PubMed]
25. Webster, J.; Li, N.; Dunford, E.K.; Nowson, C.A.; Neal, B. Consumer awareness and self-reported behaviours related to salt consumption in Australia. *Asia Pac. J. Clin. Nutr.* **2010**, *19*, 550–554. [PubMed]
26. Grimes, C.A.; Kelley, S.-J.; Stanley, S.; Bolam, B.; Webster, J.; Khokhar, D.; Nowson, C.A. Knowledge, attitudes and behaviours related to dietary salt among adults in the state of Victoria, Australia 2015. *BMC Public Health* **2017**, *17*, 532. [CrossRef]
27. Rodrigues, J.F.; Pereira, R.C.; Silva, A.A.; Mendes, A.O.; Carneiro, J.S. Sodium content in foods: Brazilian consumers' opinions, subjective knowledge and purchase intent. *Int. J. Consum. Stud.* **2017**, *41*, 735–744. [CrossRef]
28. He, Y.; Huang, L.; Yan, S.; Li, Y.; Lu, L.; Wang, H.; Niu, W.; Zhang, P. Awareness, understanding and use of sodium information labelled on pre-packaged food in Beijing: A cross-sectional study. *BMC Public Health* **2018**, *18*, 509. [CrossRef]
29. Chang, S.-O. The amount of sodium in the processed foods, the use of sodium information on the nutrition label and the acceptance of sodium reduced ramen in the female college students. *J. Nutr. Health* **2006**, *39*, 585–591.
30. Nasreddine, L.; Akl, C.; Al-Shaar, L.; Almedawar, M.M.; Isma'eel, H. Consumer knowledge, attitudes and salt-related behavior in the Middle-East: The case of Lebanon. *Nutrients* **2014**, *6*, 5079–5102. [CrossRef]
31. Ahmadi, A.; Torkamani, P.; Sohrabi, Z.; Ghahremani, F. Nutrition knowledge: Application and perception of food labels among women. *Pak. J. Biol. Sci.* **2013**, *16*, 2026–2030. [CrossRef]
32. Ghimire, K.; Adhikari, T.B.; Rijal, A.; Kallestrup, P.; Henry, M.E.; Neupane, D. Knowledge, attitudes, and practices related to salt consumption in Nepal: Findings from the community-based management of non-communicable diseases project in Nepal (COBIN). *J. Clin. Hypertens.* **2019**, *21*, 739–748. [CrossRef]
33. Levings, J.L.; Maalouf, J.; Tong, X.; Cogswell, M.E. Reported use and perceived understanding of sodium information on US nutrition labels. *Prev. Chronic Dis.* **2015**, *12*, E48. [CrossRef] [PubMed]
34. Mørk, T.; Lähteenmäki, L.; Grunert, K.G. Determinants of intention to reduce salt intake and willingness to purchase salt-reduced food products: Evidence from a web survey. *Appetite* **2019**, *139*, 110–118. [CrossRef] [PubMed]
35. Halagarda, M.; Cichoń, Z. Znakowanie produktów spożywczych informacją o wartości odżywczej. *Zesz. Nauk. Uniw. Ekon. W Krakowie* **2011**, *874*, 19–36.
36. Bryła, P. Selected antecedents of the importance of nutrition claims for food processors and distributors. *J. Agribus. Rural. Dev.* **2019**, *2*, 103–110. [CrossRef]
37. Bryła, P. *Oświadczenia Zdrowotne I Żywieniowe na Rynku Produktów Żywnościowych*; Lodz University Press: Lodz, Poland, 2020; in press.
38. Winiarska-Mieczan, A.; Kwiatkowska, K.; Kwiecień, M.; Baranowska-Wójcik, E.; Wójcik, G.; Krusiński, R. Analysis of the intake of sodium with cereal products by the population of Poland. *Food Addit. Contam. Part. A* **2019**, *36*, 884–892. [CrossRef] [PubMed]
39. Newson, R.S.; Elmadfa, I.; Biro, G.; Cheng, Y.; Prakash, V.; Rust, P.; Barna, M.; Lion, R.; Meijer, G.W.; Neufingerl, N.; et al. Barriers for progress in salt reduction in the general population. An international study. *Appetite* **2013**, *71*, 22–31. [CrossRef]
40. Bhana, N.; Utter, J.; Eyles, H. Knowledge, attitudes and behaviours related to dietary salt intake in high-income countries: A systematic review. *Curr. Nutr. Rep.* **2018**, *7*, 183–197. [CrossRef]

41. Powles, J.; Fahimi, S.; Micha, R.; Khatibzadeh, S.; Shi, P.; Ezzati, M.; Engell, R.; Lim, S.; Danaei, G.; Mozaffarian, D. Global, regional and national sodium intakes in 1990 and 2020: A systematic analysis of 24 h urinary sodium excretion and dietary surveys worldwide. *BMJ Open* **2013**, *3*, e003733. [CrossRef]
42. Kloss, L.; Dawn Meyer, J.; Graeve, L.; Vetter, W. Sodium intake and its reduction by food reformulation in the European Union—A review. *NFS J.* **2015**, *1*, 9–19. [CrossRef]

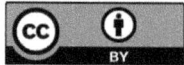

© 2020 by the author. Licensee MDPI, Basel, Switzerland. This article is an open access article distributed under the terms and conditions of the Creative Commons Attribution (CC BY) license (http://creativecommons.org/licenses/by/4.0/).

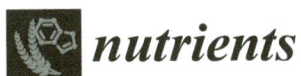 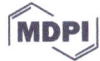

Article

Evaluation of the Nutritional Quality of Breakfast Cereals Sold on the Italian Market: The Food Labelling of Italian Products (FLIP) Study

Donato Angelino [1], Alice Rosi [2], Margherita Dall'Asta [2], Nicoletta Pellegrini [2,*] and Daniela Martini [1] on behalf of the Italian Society of Human Nutrition (SINU) Young Working Group

1. Human Nutrition Unit, Department of Veterinary Science, University of Parma, 43125 Parma, Italy
2. Human Nutrition Unit, Department of Food and Drug, University of Parma, 43125 Parma, Italy
* Correspondence: nicoletta.pellegrini@unipr.it; Tel.: +39-0521-903907

Received: 26 September 2019; Accepted: 14 November 2019; Published: 19 November 2019

Abstract: Breakfast cereals are present on the market as different types and, in general, are one of the food categories in which voluntary information, such as nutrition or health claims (NHC) or gluten free (GF) declarations, have the largest distribution. The aims of the present study were to compare (i) the nutritional declaration among different types of breakfast cereals, as well as among products with and without NHC or GF declarations; and (ii) the salt and sugar contents with the "Italian shared objectives for the improvement of the nutritional characteristics of food". To this aim, the nutrition declarations of 371 different breakfast cereal items, available in 13 retailers present on the Italian market, were analysed. Data showed an elevated inter-product variability, with cereal bars and muesli having the highest energy, total fat, and saturate contents per 100 g. Limited differences were found comparing products with and without NHC, as well as those with GF declaration. Most of the breakfast cereals were compliant to the shared objectives, although some items with NHC or GF declaration still have sugar or salt contents higher than these objectives. In conclusion, these data suggest that the different characteristics and the regulated information reported on the food label should not be considered as a marker of the overall nutritional quality. Thus, this study supports the importance of reading and understanding the information made on food label.

Keywords: breakfast cereals; food labelling; nutrition declaration; nutritional quality; gluten free; nutrition and health claims

1. Introduction

Breakfast is one of the most important meals of the day, as it comes after several hours of night fasting, and it literally "breaks the fast". Several epidemiological and intervention studies evidenced a pivotal role of breakfast consumption in the maintenance of cardiovascular health [1,2], improvement of cognitive functions [3], and positive influence on satiety-related hormones [4]. Despite this important role, there is no agreement in the scientific community on its definition because there is no standard breakfast meal due to different cultures, food choices, and behaviours [5]. However, several studies agree that certain criteria should be followed in order to have an appropriate breakfast [5]. For the Italian population, it has been proposed that a balanced breakfast should provide 15% to 25% of daily energy for adults [2]. At least three food groups should be considered: milk and milk-derived products (low-fat), fruit (fresh fruit or 100% fruit juices), and cereals (preferably whole-grain, unrefined) [2,6]. Cereals have been endorsed as the principal source of breakfast's carbohydrates [2] and allow the consumers to vary their breakfast meal with several different cereal-based products. Among these, breakfast cereals are nowadays available in numerous formulations and have been associated with the reduction of the risk of several chronic diseases in both adults and adolescents [7]. However, in Italy, breakfast cereals are still scarcely consumed—the total population has a median estimated intake close to 2 g/day, whereas adult habitual consumers (around 10% of the total population) have a median estimated intake of 15 g/day [8]. By comparing the intakes found in the European Prospective Investigation Cohort, the Italian intake is similar to those of other Mediterranean countries, such as Spain and Greece, and at least 20-fold lower compared to Scandinavian countries [9]. Other than a good source of available carbohydrates, breakfast cereals can be an important source of micronutrients (e.g., vitamins and minerals) and fibre, such as β-glucans, which play a key role in the prevention of cardiovascular risk, but also in the improvement in appetite control and increase of satiety [10,11]. However, breakfast cereals can also contain high amounts of added sugar and salt [12,13], ascertained risk factors of many chronic diseases when excessively ingested. For these reasons, there is a growing interest in the reformulation of breakfast cereal products. In Italy, as shown by the "Shared objectives for the improvement of the nutritional characteristics of food products" drafted by the Ministry of Health in collaboration with certain sectors of the food industry, the main reformulations for breakfast cereals were aimed to reduce sugar and salt up to mean contents of 30 g and 1 g per 100 g, respectively, by 2017 [14].

The first tool for the delivering of nutrition and health information to consumers is the food label. In Europe, mandatory and voluntary information made on food is regulated by specific laws including (i) the European Regulation (EU) no. 1169/2011, which regulates the mandatory information on foods, such as the list of ingredients and the nutritional declaration [15]; (ii) the European Regulation (CE) no. 1924/2006, concerning the voluntary Nutrition and Health Claims (NHC) [16]; and (iii) the European Implementing Regulation (EU) no. 828/2014, which regulates the information given to consumers on the absence or reduced presence of gluten in food [17]. Due to their nutritional composition, breakfast cereal is one of the food categories in which voluntary information, such as NHC, have the largest penetration [18,19]. However, on the basis of the so-called "health halo effect", consumers might be biased and lead to generalizing the healthiness of these foods simply from some information present on the labels, such as NHC, regardless of the whole nutritional quality of the product [20,21]. Thus, there is a great interest in understanding if this information made on food can be considered as a marker of the overall quality of breakfast cereals.

With these presumptions, the aims of the present work were (i) to investigate the nutritional quality of breakfast cereals by collecting their nutritional values as declared on the food labels; (ii) to compare the energy and nutrient content of the products, classified for different characteristics (type of product, presence/absence of nutrition or health claims, gluten free (GF) declaration); and (iii) to compare the salt and sugar contents of all the products with the mean contents expected in breakfast cereals in the "Shared objectives for the improvement of the nutritional characteristics of food products" (30 g/100 g and 1 g/100 g for sugar and salt, respectively) [14].

2. Materials and Methods

2.1. Food Product Selection on Online Stores

Breakfast cereal-based products considered for the present work were selected from the major retailers present on the Italian market that have a home-shopping website (Auchan, Bennet, Carrefour, Conad, Coop Italia, Crai, Despar, Esselunga, Il Gigante, Iper, Pam Panorama, Selex, Sidis).

The online search for the information was conducted from July 2018 until December 2018. The selection of products was performed by considering the eligibility of the extraction of all the breakfast cereal items that were present in each online shop.

The exclusion criteria for product selection were (i) non-prepacked foods, (ii) incomplete images of all the sides of the pack, (iii) unclear images of nutrition declaration or list of ingredients, (iv) products that were marked as 'product currently unavailable' on all the online stores selected during the whole data collection period.

2.2. Data Extraction

Data from the complete images of all the sides of the pack were collected for all included products. For each food item, the quali-quantitative and specifically regulated (mandatory) information was retrieved: company name, brand name, descriptive name, energy (kcal/100 g), total fat (g/100 g), saturates (g/100 g), carbohydrate (g/100 g), sugars (g/100 g), protein (g/100 g), and salt (g/100 g). Furthermore, other information, such as presence of NHC (presence or absence of at least one nutrition claim and presence or absence of at least one health claim) or GF declaration (presence or absence of gluten) was collected.

The precision of the extracted data was double-checked by two researchers and inaccuracies were solved through secondary extractions with the help of a third researcher.

A dataset was created with all the collected data and items were sub-grouped for specific comparisons by considering (i) descriptive name reported, (ii) presence/absence of GF declaration, and i(ii) presence/absence of NHC declaration. On the basis of the descriptive name, breakfast cereals were classified into six types: cereal bars, muesli, flakes, bran cereals, puffed cereals, and others (e.g., cereals with honey, cream-filled cereals). Definitions and examples of types and categories are provided in Table S1.

2.3. Data Analysis

The statistical analysis was carried out using the Statistical Package for Social Sciences software (IBM SPSS Statistics, Version 25.0, IBM corp., Chicago, IL, USA) and performed at a significance level of $p < 0.05$. The normality of data distribution was rejected through the Kolmogorov–Smirnov test and variables were expressed as median (interquartile range). Data of energy and nutrient contents per 100 grams of products were analysed using the Kruskal–Wallis non-parametric one-way ANOVA for independent samples with multiple pairwise comparisons (for differences among types) and using the Mann–Whitney non-parametric test for two independent samples (for differences between GF declaration categories, nutrition claim categories, and health claim categories). In addition, a principal component analysis (PCA) with varimax rotation was performed for all items, considering energy and nutrient contents per 100 g of products to better describe the inter-product nutritional variability.

Moreover, the sugar and salt content of the considered breakfast cereal products was compared with the mean amounts expected for 2017, as described in the "Shared objectives for the improvement of the nutritional characteristics of food products": 30 g of sugar per 100 g and 1 g of salt per 100 g [14].

3. Results

3.1. Nutritional Composition of Breakfast Cereals

A total of 415 breakfast cereals were identified during the research conducted in the online stores. After removing the products on the basis of the exclusion criteria, a total of 371 different items were retrieved (Table 1). Thus, almost ~90% of the products sold in the considered retailers were retrieved. The inter-rater agreement in excluding of products was 98% and the remaining 2% of disagreements were successfully resolved by the third researcher.

Table 1. Energy, macronutrients, and salt across breakfast cereal categories.

		Number of Items	Energy kcal/100 g	Total Fat g/100 g	Saturates g/100 g	Total Carbohydrates g/100 g	Sugars g/100 g	Protein g/100 g	Salt g/100 g
Category	Breakfast cereals	371	385 (372–417)	5.5 (2.5–13.5)	1.5 (0.5–3.8)	69.0 (61.0–79.0)	20.0 (8.6–27.0)	8.3 (7.0–10.8)	0.5 (0.2–0.8)
	Cereal bars	78	400 (383–448) [a]	11.4 (7.9–20.0) [a]	4.2 (2.5–5.9) [a]	64.2 (49.0–69.7) [b]	27.0 (21.6–31.1) [a]	7.8 (6.1–11.5) [b]	0.5 (0.3–0.7) [b,c]
	Muesli	54	443 (381–463) [a]	15.8 (7.9–18.0) [a]	4.5 (1.7–6.0) [a]	62.0 (60.0–65.0) [b,c]	21.0 (18.0–25.0) [b,c]	8.9 (8.0–9.5) [b]	0.3 (0.1–0.6) [c]
Type	Flakes	129	377 (371–385) [c]	2.0 (1.2–5.6) [c]	0.5 (0.3–1.3) [c]	78.0 (67.0–81.0) [a]	10.8 (6.0–17.7) [d]	8.4 (7.4–11.0) [b]	0.8 (0.3–1.1) [a]
	Bran cereals	14	318 (301–344) [d]	4.3 (3.9–7.3) [b,c]	0.9 (0.7–1.2) [b,c]	40.2 (34.0–48.0) [c]	3.4 (1.3–17.0) [d]	14.9 (13.0–16.0) [a]	0.2 (0.0–1.2) [a,b]
	Puffed cereals	29	381 (368–397) [b,c]	2.9 (1.9–4.0) [c]	0.6 (0.5–1.0) [c]	79.0 (75.9–84.0) [a]	15.0 (0.9–27.0) [c,d]	7.0 (6.9–9.9) [b]	0.0 (0.0–0.7) [c]
	Others	67	392 (382–437) [a,b]	4.4 (2.9–14.0) [b]	1.6 (1.0–3.1) [b]	73.0 (68.0–79.0) [a]	25.0 (20.0–29.7) [a,b]	8.0 (6.9–9.0) [b]	0.6 (0.3–0.8) [a,b]
Gluten free	No	338	385 (372–416)	5.5 (2.5–12.2)	1.4 (0.5–3.8)	69.0 (62.0–79.0)	20.0 (9.0–26.5)	8.4 (7.0–10.0)	0.5 (0.2–0.8)
	Yes	33	390 (375–448)	5.9 (2.5–17.0)	1.9 (0.6–3.8)	71.0 (51.0–81.0)	21.0 (7.7–30.0)	8.0 (7.1–11.0)	0.5 (0.1–0.8)
Nutrition claim	No	112	393 (378–449) [a]	5.3 (2.6–16.0)	1.8 (0.6–4.3)	72.0 (62.0–80.4)	22.0 (8.2–30.0) [a]	8.0 (7.0–10.0)	0.5 (0.1–1.0)
	Yes	259	382 (371–407) [b]	5.9 (2.5–11.2)	1.3 (0.5–3.5)	68.0 (60.3–78.7)	19.0 (9.0–25.0) [b]	8.4 (7.1–11.0)	0.5 (0.2–0.8)
Health claim	No	306	385 (372–422)	5.3 (2.3–14.0)	1.4 (0.5–3.8)	70.0 (62.0–79.5) [a]	20.0 (7.9–27.0)	8.1 (7.0–10.0) [b]	0.5 (0.2–0.8)
	Yes	65	383 (373–410)	6.9 (2.6–10.3)	1.6 (0.7–3.4)	65.0 (56.0–74.8) [b]	20.0 (14.0–27.0)	9.0 (7.4–12.5) [a]	0.7 (0.3–0.8)

Values are expressed as median (25th–75th percentile). For each category, different lowercase letters in the same column indicate significant differences among type (Kruskal–Wallis non-parametric one-way ANOVA for independent samples with multiple pairwise comparisons) or between groups (gluten free, nutrition claim, health claim; Mann–Whitney non-parametric test for two independent samples), $p < 0.05$.

Among these 371 items, products were mostly flakes (n = 129), followed by cereal bars (n = 78), muesli (n = 54), puffed cereals (n = 29), and lastly bran cereals (n = 14), whereas the remaining 67 items were classified as "others", being very heterogeneous. Overall, the median energy content of breakfast cereals was 385 (372–417) kcal/100 g, but widely differed among types ($p < 0.001$). Indeed, energy content ranged from a median of 318 (301–344) kcal/100 g for bran cereals to 443 (381–463) kcal/100 g for muesli. Considering macronutrients, contents of total fat and saturates differed among the types ($p < 0.001$ for both), with the highest contents in muesli (15.8 (7.9–18.0) and 4.5 (1.7–6.0) g/100 g for total fat and saturates, respectively) and cereal bars (11.4 (7.9–20.0) and 4.2 (2.5–5.9) g/100 g for total fat and saturates, respectively). Total carbohydrate content differed among the types ($p < 0.001$), with the highest values for flakes (78.0 (67.0–81.0) g/100 g), puffed cereals (79.0 (75.9–84.0) g/100 g), and other breakfast cereals 73.0 (68.0–79.0) g/100 g). When sugars were taken into account, differences among the types were found ($p < 0.001$), with cereal bars and other breakfast cereals reporting the highest sugar contents: 27.0 (21.6–31.1) and 25.0 (20.0–29.7) g/100 g, respectively. Differences in protein content were observed among the cereal types ($p < 0.001$), with the bran cereals showing the highest content (14.9 (13.0–16.0) g/100 g) compared with the others. Salt content varied among the types ($p < 0.001$), with the flakes group having the highest content (0.8 (0.3–1.1) g/100 g), and muesli (0.3 (0.1–0.6) g/100 g) and puffed cereals (0.0 (0.0–0.7) g/100 g) the lowest content.

No differences were identified when GF products were compared to the gluten counterparts.

Finally, breakfast cereals with at least nutritional claim resulted lower in total energy ($p < 0.001$) and sugars ($p = 0.005$) than their counterparts. Products carrying a health claim overall resulted as being lower in total carbohydrates ($p = 0.005$) and higher in protein content ($p = 0.017$) than the products without this declaration.

3.2. Inter-Product Variability of the Nutritional Composition of the Breakfast Cereals

Differences in the nutritional profile of the breakfast cereal types were explained by two Principal Components (PCs), which described 69% of the total variability (Figure 1). Energy, total fat, saturates, and sugars were the nutritional variables with the highest contribution to PC1, which explained 40% of the total variability. PC2 described 30% of the inter-product variability, being loaded positively by protein and negatively by salt and carbohydrates (Figure 1A). A high inter-product variability was observed for all breakfast cereal types (Figure 1B), in particular for cereal bars, muesli, and puffed cereals. Products belonging to the bran cereal type were the ones that grouped better (negative scores for PC1 and positive ones for PC2), and they were characterized by a high amount of protein and low quantities of energy and other nutrients. Even if flake products were heterogeneous, the majority of them were described by a high content of carbohydrates and salt (negative scores for both PCs).

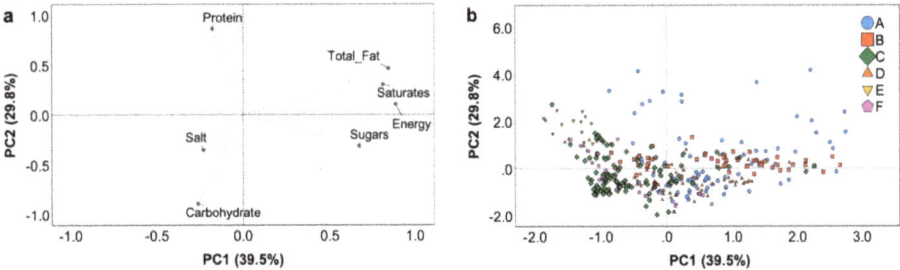

Figure 1. Principal component analysis (PCA) describing the inter-product variability based on the nutritional composition of products analysed (energy (kcal/100 g), total fat (g/100 g), saturates (g/100 g), carbohydrate (g/100 g), sugars (g/100 g), protein (g/100 g), and salt (g/100 g)). Loading plots of Principal Component (PC) 1 versus PC2 (**a**); score plots of the nutrition composition for each breakfast cereal product analysed from PC1 and PC2 (**b**). Legend: A, cereal bars; B, muesli; C, flakes; D, bran cereals; E, puffed cereals; F, others.

3.3. Comparison of the Sugar and Salt Contents of the Breakfast Cereals with the Italian Shared Objectives

In this survey, it emerged that most of the products matched the shared objectives for the improvement of the nutritional characteristics of products for both sugar (Figure 2a) and salt contents (Figure 2b) [14]. However, the percentage of products having a sugar content lower than 30 g/100 g ranged from 65% of the cereal bars to 98% of flakes and 100% of bran cereals. Although the number of GF and gluten-containing breakfast cereals was different (33 vs. 338, respectively), 72% and 88% of the products, respectively, had sugars lower than 30 g/100 g. Considering products with >30 g sugar/100 g, all GF products were cereal bars, whereas, among non GF products, ~50% were cereal bars and ~17% were puffed cereals (data not shown).

Similarly, products carrying or not carrying NHC had more than 75% of the products matching the objective of <30 g sugars/100 g, reaching 91% for products carrying at least a nutrition claim. Once again, most of the products with >30 g sugar/100 g were cereals bars (e.g., 16 out of 23 items with nutrition claims and 5 out of 7 items with health claims, data not shown).

Similarly to sugars, for all the breakfast cereal types, most of the products have a salt content lower than the objective of 1 g/100 g, ranging from 68% of the flakes to 100% of muesli products (Figure 2b). Both GF and gluten-containing breakfast cereals included more than 80% of the products below the objective of 1 g salt/100 g. It is worth noting that 4 out of 5 GF items and 33 out of 48 non-GF items with salt >1 g/100 g were flakes (data not shown).

Finally, 88% of products carrying nutrition claims, 79% of products without them, and 86% of products both with and without health claims were below the objective value for salt. Again, products above the threshold for salt were mostly flakes (e.g., 19/30 and 4/9 among items with nutrition and health claims, respectively) (data not shown).

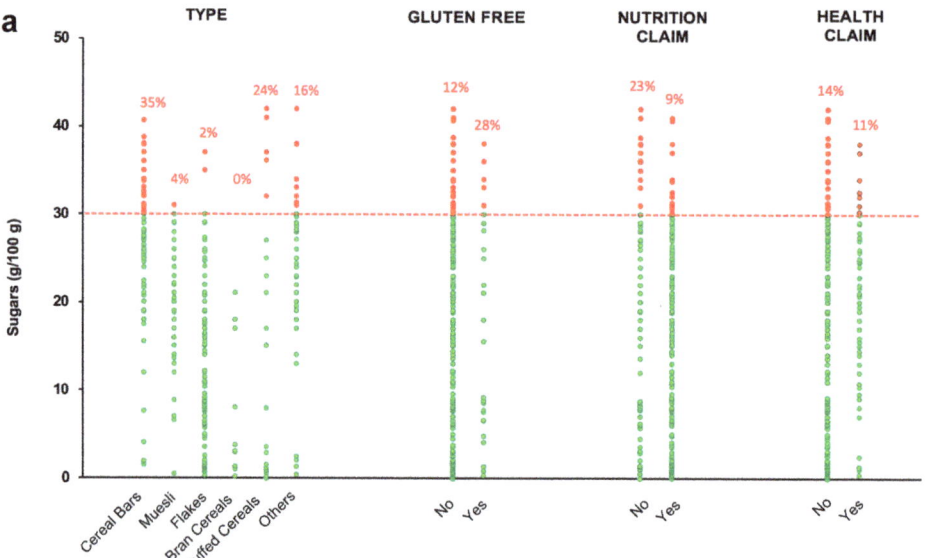

Figure 2. *Cont.*

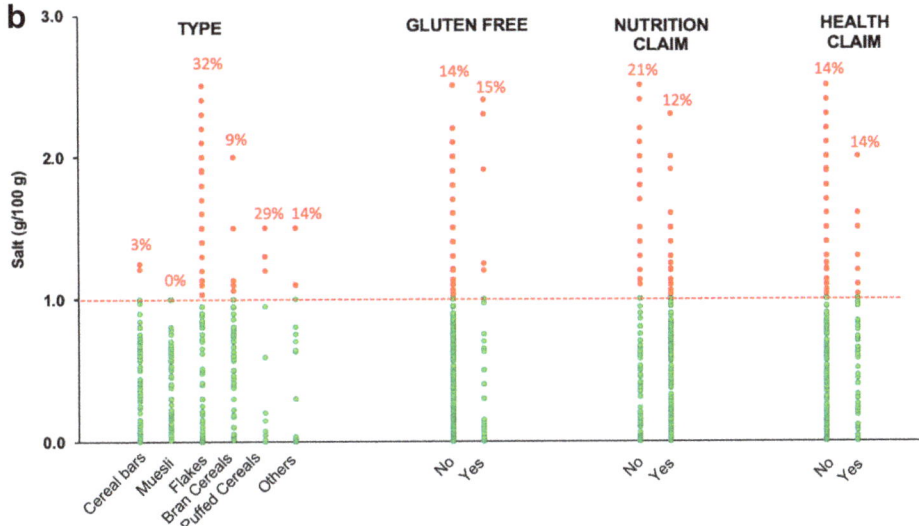

Figure 2. Sugar (**a**) and salt (**b**) content of the considered breakfast cereal products, classified per type, containing or not containing gluten, and carrying or not carrying nutrition and a health claim. Red dashed lines refer to the shared objectives for sugars (30 g/100 g, (**a**)) and salt (1 g/100 g, (**b**)) set by the Italian Ministry of Health [14]. Green and red dots represent the referring values of the product lower and higher, respectively, than the mean contents expected in the Italian Ministry of Health shared objectives. Percentage values on the top of each bar indicate the percentage number of the products with an amount of sugar (**a**) or salt (**b**) higher than the shared objectives.

4. Discussion

The inclusion in the breakfast of cereal-based products has been demonstrated to be a valid choice for increasing the nutritional quality of one's diet [22,23]. Despite their health effects, breakfast cereals are a heterogeneous category of food products and different international surveys report a great variability in their nutritional composition, mostly for sugar and salt content [12,24]. The present survey was aimed at giving an overview of the nutritional quality of the breakfast cereals sold on the Italian market, with particular focus on the differences among types, as well as among products with or without NHC and gluten declarations. Results evidenced a great variability of the nutritional values among the different types of products. Muesli products have shown the highest median energy as well as the highest total fat and saturate median contents. These values are in line with the ones of the items sold in French [25,26] and New Zealand [13] markets, as well as with the data shown in a comparative survey among muesli sold in Austria, France, and Romania [27]. Conversely, bran cereals sold in Italy have the highest content of protein but the lowest amount of energy and sugars compared to the other five Italian breakfast types. These median data of energy are slightly lower than those previously reported for the bran products, where total energy content of brans was on average around 348 kcal/100 g [13]. Intriguingly, the mean sugar content for these products sold in the New Zealand market was notably higher than the one found in the Italian products (22.5 g/100 g vs. 3.4 g/100 g), but it is worth noting that we found a greater inter-product variability, with a maximum value of 21 g/100 g. Similar results in terms of variability of sugar and total fat contents have been found for flakes, which are characterized by a high carbohydrate and salt content. These findings are in line with the ones found in a recent comparative survey among three European countries for oat flakes [27].

Taking into account the great difference in terms of numbers of items sold on the Italian market, there are no significant differences among the energy, macronutrient, and salt contents of breakfast cereals containing or not containing gluten. Previous surveys investigating the nutritional profiles of breakfast cereals with or without gluten often found opposite results. For instance, our data are partially contrasting with the ones of a U.K. survey that found lower sugar and salt contents in GF breakfast cereals compared to their gluten counterpart [28]. A lower salt content in GF cereal bars compared to the regular ones was also found in an Australian survey, whereas energy and sugars were lower in the products containing gluten [29]. Again, it is worth underlining that the present data are not sufficient for a thorough evaluation of the nutritional quality of GF breakfast cereals, as some other aspects such as the ingredient list and micronutrient contents should be considered [30].

Regarding the presence of NHC, a strict regulation on front/back-of-pack label information could be useful to deliver the correct nutritional and health information, as also suggested by García et al. in 2019 [31]. This is particularly important considering that NHC may play a role on the customer's intention to buy [32]. The EU Project "Food Labelling to Advance Better Education for Life" concluded that, even before the release of the European Regulation (EU) no. 1169/2011 concerning the mandatory information on foods [15], that breakfast cereals were the products with the highest penetration of nutrition information within the 27 EU countries [19]. In fact, by considering 6275 breakfast cereal products, nutritional information (i.e., NHC, labelling schemes such as traffic lights, guideline daily amounts other than nutrition declaration) were present on the back-of-pack of 94% of the items and on the front-of-pack of 70% of the items [19]. In this scenario, a recent Canadian study showed that, despite breakfast cereals being marked as "healthy food choices" and often boasting NHC on the front-of-pack, customers mainly find unhealthy products promoted in Canadian supermarkets [33]. Our findings concerning products depicting NHC confirm that there are no deep differences in terms of nutritional profile compared to breakfast cereals with no NHC. Breakfast cereals carrying nutrition claims showed only a 3% lower median energy content compared to the products not claiming nutrition, mainly due to a lower sugar content. Items boasting health claims were slightly, but significantly, lower in total carbohydrates and higher in protein contents than those not presenting a claim. However, it is worth noting that the number of items carrying a health claim was five-fold lower compared to the number of items without, which represents one of the main limitations of this study. These findings support the evidence of several surveys in the United Kingdom, USA, and New Zealand, which concretely demonstrated that products, in particular breakfast cereals, boasting nutrition and/or health claims do not necessarily have an overall better nutritional profile [31,34–36]. The absence of clear and marked differences among products with and without NHC may be because food items with NHC do not have to comply with any nutrient profile. In this scenario, it is worth noting that the Article 4 of the EU Regulation 1924/2006 stated that the European Commission should have established by 19 January 2009 specific nutrient profiles that foods or certain groups of foods should have respected in order to bear nutrition and health claims [16]. However, in 2016, the European parliament voted to scrap nutrient profile. As a consequence, manufacturers currently do not have to follow specific nutrient profile regulations to formulate products bearing NHC.

Despite this, food companies should formulate food products with the highest nutritional quality possible. The World Cancer Research Fund International considered that the nutritional reformulation of products is one of the main tools necessary to drastically reduce obesity and non-communicable diseases [37]. As already mentioned, the Italian Ministry of Health, in collaboration with food companies, initiated a process for the improvement of the nutritional characteristics of food products [14]. It is worth underlying that the shared objectives with manufacturers are just a first and not resolutive step for the production of nutritionally balanced breakfast cereal products. For example, by considering an expected mean content of 30 g sugars/100 g of breakfast cereals [14] and a reference serving size of 30 g, one portion of breakfast cereals provides on average ~9 g sugars. Considering that no more than 15% of the daily energy intake should come from sugars [38], ~9 g sugars from breakfast cereals corresponds to 12% of the daily amounts of sugar for a 2000 kcal-diet.

Similarly, 1 g salt per 100 g product means ~300 mg salt in a 30 g cereal serving, which is roughly 6% of the daily salt intake, considering 5 g per day as the suggested dietary target [39]. Again, these values suggest that further steps are needed in order to reach lower values for sugar and salt contents in breakfast cereal products.

In the present survey, it has been found that, despite the high variability in terms of the nutritional profile of the six breakfast cereal types, and regardless of whether they contained gluten or carried an NHC, most of the products were below the suggested targets for sugars and salt. However, at least 25% and 13% of the 371 considered products have a salt and sugar content higher than the objectives, respectively. This information supports that further reformulation is desirable for offering the consumers products with an improved nutrient profile.

5. Conclusions

The present work clearly highlighted the high variability in the nutritional profile among different types of breakfast cereals sold on the Italian market. On the whole, results showed that the boasting of NHC or declarations on gluten on the labels did not necessarily indicate a better nutritional quality of the product. Most importantly, these results support the need of an informative labelling on food products to help consumers to make informed food choices. Moreover, the results support the importance of a nutritional education towards a better understanding of food labels as a key point to help the consumer in making healthy food choices. In addition, one of the aspects of the present work was the evaluation of the nutritional profile of the products, mainly focusing on sugars and salt. In Italy, an initial step for the reformulation of different product categories—among which are breakfast cereals—has been jointly enacted by the Italian Ministry of Health and manufacturers. However, for a complete, accurate, and science-based reformulation process, it would be worthy to set-up a durable working group involving all the stakeholders, that is, industries, institutions, and scientific societies.

However, because this study considered only breakfast cereals, future surveys focused on other food groups are needed to draw a more accurate nutritional profile of food products currently on the Italian market. Moreover, in the present study, other retail channels, such as discounts, were not considered and would be worthy of future investigation. This would further increase the number of items in the study to better understand the potential role of food declarations as markers of the overall quality of food products. Lastly, it is advisable to replicate this research study on a regular basis in order to investigate the impact of reformulation on the nutritional quality of breakfast cereals.

Supplementary Materials: The following are available online at http://www.mdpi.com/2072-6643/11/11/2827/s1: Table S1: Definitions and examples of the categorization of the breakfast cereals.

Author Contributions: D.A. was involved in the protocol design, data analyses, in the interpretation of results, and drafted the manuscript; M.D.A. and A.R. performed data analyses, were involved in the protocol design and in the interpretation of the results, and contributed to the drafting of the manuscript; N.P. participated in the protocol design and critically reviewed the manuscript; D.M. conceived and designed the protocol of the study, was involved in the interpretation of the results, critically reviewed the manuscript, and had primary responsibility for the final content. Other members of the Italian Society of Human Nutrition (SINU) Young Working Group were involved in the protocol design and critically reviewed the final manuscript. All authors read and approved the final manuscript.

Funding: This research received no external funding.

Acknowledgments: The authors wish to thank all students who participated to the development of the dataset.

Conflicts of Interest: The present publication has been conceived within the Italian Society of Human Nutrition (SINU) Young Group, and it has been made without any funding from food industries or other entities. The authors declare no conflict of interest.

SINU Young Working Group

Marika Dello Russo	Institute of Food Sciences, National Research Council, Avellino, Italy
Stefania Moccia	Institute of Food Sciences, National Research Council, Avellino, Italy
Daniele Nucci	Veneto Institute of Oncology IOV-IRCCS, Padova, Italy
Gaetana Paolella	Department of Chemistry and Biology A. Zambelli, University of Salerno, Fisciano, Italy
Veronica Pignone	Department of Epidemiology and Prevention, IRCCS Neuromed, Pozzilli, Italy
Emilia Ruggiero	Department of Epidemiology and Prevention, IRCCS Neuromed, Pozzilli, Italy
Carmela Spagnuolo	Institute of Food Sciences, National Research Council, Avellino, Italy

References

1. Deedwania, P.; Acharya, T. Hearty breakfast for healthier arteries. *J. Am. Coll. Cardiol.* **2017**, *70*, 1843–1845. [CrossRef] [PubMed]
2. Marangoni, F.; Poli, A.; Agostoni, C.; Di Pietro, P.; Cricelli, C.; Brignoli, O.; Fatati, G.; Giovannini, M.; Riva, E.; Marelli, G.; et al. A consensus document on the role of breakfast in the attainment and maintenance of health and wellness. *Acta Biomed.* **2009**, *80*, 166–171. [PubMed]
3. Galioto, R.; Spitznagel, M.B. The effects of breakfast and breakfast composition on cognition in adults. *Adv. Nutr.* **2016**, *7*, 576S–589S. [CrossRef] [PubMed]
4. Clayton, D.J.; James, L.J. The effect of breakfast on appetite regulation, energy balance and exercise performance. *Proc. Nutr. Soc.* **2016**, *75*, 319–327. [CrossRef]
5. O'Neil, C.E.; Byrd-Bredbenner, C.; Hayes, D.; Jana, L.; Klinger, S.E.; Stephenson-Martin, S. The role of breakfast in health: Definition and criteria for a quality breakfast. *J. Acad. Nutr. Diet.* **2014**, *114*, S8–S26. [CrossRef]
6. Giovannini, M.; Verduci, E.; Scaglioni, S.; Salvatici, E.; Bonza, M.; Riva, E.; Agostoni, C. Breakfast: A good habit, not a repetitive custom. *J. Int. Med. Res.* **2008**, *36*, 613–624. [CrossRef]
7. Williams, P.G. The benefits of breakfast cereal consumption: A systematic review of the evidence base. *Adv. Nutr.* **2014**, *5*, 636S–673S. [CrossRef]
8. Leclercq, C.; Arcella, D.; Piccinelli, R.; Sette, S.; Le Donne, C. The Italian National Food Consumption Survey INRAN-SCAI 2005–06: Main results in terms of food consumption. *Public Health Nutr.* **2009**, *12*, 2504–2532. [CrossRef]
9. Wirfält, E.; McTaggart, A.; Pala, V.; Gullberg, B.; Frasca, G.; Panico, S.; Bueno-de-Mesquita, H.; Peeters, P.; Engeset, D.; Skeie, G.; et al. Food sources of carbohydrates in a European cohort of adults. *Public Health Nutr.* **2002**, *5*, 1197–1215. [CrossRef]
10. Rebello, C.J.; O'Neil, C.E.; Greenway, F.L. Dietary fiber and satiety: The effects of oats on satiety. *Nutr. Rev.* **2016**, *74*, 131–147. [CrossRef]
11. Geliebter, A.; Grillot, C.L.; Aviram-Friedman, R.; Haq, S.; Yahav, E.; Hashim, S.A. Effects of oatmeal and corn flakes cereal breakfasts on satiety, gastric emptying, glucose, and appetite-related hormones. *Ann. Nutr. Metab.* **2015**, *66*, 93–103. [CrossRef] [PubMed]
12. Pombo-Rodrigues, S.; Hashem, K.M.; He, F.J.; MacGregor, G.A. Salt and sugars content of breakfast cereals in the UK from 1992 to 2015. *Public Health Nutr.* **2017**, *20*, 1500–1512. [CrossRef] [PubMed]
13. Chepulis, L.; Hill, S.; Mearns, G. The nutritional quality of New Zealand breakfast cereals: An update. *Public Health Nutr.* **2017**, *20*, 3234–3237. [CrossRef] [PubMed]
14. Italian Ministry of Health. Shared Objectives for Improving the Nutritional Characteristics of Food Products, with a Particular Focus on Children (3–12 Years). Available online: http://www.salute.gov.it/imgs/C_17_pubblicazioni_2426_ulteriorialleggati_ulterioreallegato_0_alleg.pdf (accessed on 25 July 2019).
15. European Union. Regulation No. 1169/2011 on the provision of food information to consumers. *Off. J. Eur. Union* **2011**, *L304*, 18–63.
16. European Union. Regulation No. 1924/2006 on nutrition and health claims made on foods. *Off. J. Eur. Union* **2006**, *L404*, 9–25.
17. European Union. Regulation No. 828/2014 on the requirements for the provision of information to consumers on the absence or reduced presence of gluten in food. *Off. J. Eur. Union* **2014**, *L228*, 5–8.

18. Maschkowski, G.; Hartmann, M.; Hoffmann, J. Health-related on-pack communication and nutritional value of ready-to-eat breakfast cereals evaluated against five nutrient profiling schemes. *BMC Public Health* **2014**, *14*, 1178. [CrossRef]
19. Storcksdieck genannt Bonsmann, S.; Celemín, L.F.; Larrañaga, A.; Egger, S.; Wills, J.M.; Hodgkins, C.; Raats, M.M. Penetration of nutrition information on food labels across the EU-27 plus Turkey. *Eur. J. Clin. Nutr.* **2010**, *64*, 1379–1385. [CrossRef]
20. Roth, Y. Do brands serve as reliable signals of nutritional quality? The case of breakfast cereals. *J. Food Prod. Mark.* **2017**, *23*, 1–23. [CrossRef]
21. Dean, M.; Lampila, P.; Shepherd, R.; Arvola, A.; Saba, A.; Vassallo, M.; Claupein, E.; Winkelmann, M.; Lähteenmäki, L. Perceived relevance and foods with health-related claims. *Food Qual. Prefer.* **2012**, *24*, 129–135. [CrossRef]
22. McKevith, B.; Jarzebowska, A. The role of breakfast cereals in the UK diet: Headline results from the National Diet and Nutrition Survey (NDNS) year. *Nutr. Bull.* **2010**, *35*, 314–319. [CrossRef]
23. Drewnowski, A.; Rehm, C.; Vieux, F.; Drewnowski, A.; Rehm, C.D.; Vieux, F. Breakfast in the United States: Food and nutrient intakes in relation to diet quality in National Health and Examination Survey 2011–A Study from the International Breakfast Research Initiative. *Nutrients* **2018**, *10*, 1200. [CrossRef]
24. Nieto, C.; Rincon-Gallardo Patiño, S.; Tolentino-Mayo, L.; Carriedo, A.; Barquera, S. Characterization of breakfast cereals available in the Mexican market: Sodium and sugar content. *Nutrients* **2017**, *9*, 884. [CrossRef]
25. Goglia, R.; Spiteri, M.; Ménard, C.; Dumas, C.; Combris, P.; Labarbe, B.; Soler, L.G.; Volatier, J.L. Nutritional quality and labelling of ready-to-eat breakfast cereals: The contribution of the French observatory of food quality. *Eur. J. Clin. Nutr.* **2010**, *64*, S20–S25. [CrossRef]
26. Julia, C.; Kesse-Guyot, E.; Ducrot, P.; Péneau, S.; Touvier, M.; Méjean, C.; Hercberg, S. Performance of a five category front-of-pack labelling system–the 5-colour nutrition label–to differentiate nutritional quality of breakfast cereals in France. *BMC Public Health* **2015**, *15*, 179. [CrossRef]
27. Vin, K.; Beziat, J.; Seper, K.; Wolf, A.; Sidor, A.; Chereches, R.; Luc Volatier, J.; Ménard, C. Nutritional composition of the food supply: A comparison of soft drinks and breakfast cereals between three European countries based on labels. *Eur. J. Clin. Nutr.* **2019**. [CrossRef]
28. Fry, L.; Madden, A.M.; Fallaize, R. An investigation into the nutritional composition and cost of gluten-free versus regular food products in the UK. *J. Hum. Nutr. Diet.* **2018**, *31*, 108–120. [CrossRef]
29. Wu, J.H.Y.Y.; Neal, B.; Trevena, H.; Crino, M.; Stuart-Smith, W.; Faulkner-Hogg, K.; Yu Louie, J.C.; Dunford, E. Are gluten-free foods healthier than non-gluten-free foods? An evaluation of supermarket products in Australia. *Br. J. Nutr.* **2015**, *114*, 448–454. [CrossRef]
30. Morreale, F.; Angelino, D.; Pellegrini, N. Designing a Score-Based Method for the Evaluation of the nutritional quality of the gluten-free bakery products and their gluten-containing counterparts. *Plant Foods Hum. Nutr.* **2018**, *73*, 154–159. [CrossRef]
31. García, A.L.; Morillo-Santander, G.; Parrett, A.; Mutoro, A.N. Confused health and nutrition claims in food marketing to children could adversely affect food choice and increase risk of obesity. *Arch. Dis. Child.* **2019**, *104*, 541–546. [CrossRef]
32. Hamlin, R.P.; McNeill, L.S.; Moore, V. The impact of front-of-pack nutrition labels on consumer product evaluation and choice: An experimental study. *Public Health Nutr.* **2015**, *18*, 2126–2134. [CrossRef]
33. Potvin Kent, M.; Rudnicki, E.; Usher, C. Less healthy breakfast cereals are promoted more frequently in large supermarket chains in Canada. *BMC Public Health* **2017**, *17*, 877. [CrossRef]
34. Schwartz, M.B.; Vartanian, L.R.; Wharton, C.M.; Brownell, K.D. Examining the nutritional quality of breakfast cereals marketed to children. *J. Am. Diet. Assoc.* **2008**, *108*, 702–705. [CrossRef]
35. Devi, A.; Eyles, H.; Rayner, M.; Ni Mhurchu, C.; Swinburn, B.; Lonsdale-Cooper, E.; Vandevijvere, S. Nutritional quality, labelling and promotion of breakfast cereals on the New Zealand market. *Appetite* **2014**, *81*, 253–260. [CrossRef]
36. Schaefer, D.; Hooker, N.H.; Stanton, J.L. Are front of pack claims indicators of nutrition quality? Evidence from 2 product categories. *J. Food Sci.* **2016**, *81*, H223–H234. [CrossRef]
37. World Cancer Research Fund International. Diet, Nutrition, Physical Activity and Cancer: A Global Perspective - The Third Expert Report. Available online: https://www.wcrf.org/dietandcancer (accessed on 25 July 2019).

38. Italian Society of Human Nutrition (SINU). *Livelli Di Assunzione Di Riferimento Di Nutrienti Ed Energia Per La Popolazione Italiana, IV Revisione*; SICS: Milan, Italy, 2014; pp. 1–655.
39. World Health Organization (WHO). *Prevention of Cardiovascular Disease: Guidelines for Assessment and Management of Cardiovascular Risk*; World Health Organization: Geneva, Switzerland, 2007; pp. 1–92.

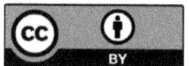

© 2019 by the authors. Licensee MDPI, Basel, Switzerland. This article is an open access article distributed under the terms and conditions of the Creative Commons Attribution (CC BY) license (http://creativecommons.org/licenses/by/4.0/).

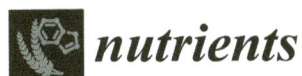

Review

Consumer Understanding, Perception and Interpretation of Serving Size Information on Food Labels: A Scoping Review

Klazine Van der Horst [1,2], Tamara Bucher [3,4], Kerith Duncanson [3,4], Beatrice Murawski [4,5] and David Labbe [2,*]

1. Department of Health Professions, Bern University of Applied Sciences, 3005 Bern, Switzerland; klazine.vanderhorst@bfh.ch
2. Société des Produits Nestlé S.A., Nestlé Research, Institute of Material Science, 1000 Lausanne, Switzerland
3. School of Health Sciences, Faculty of Health and Medicine, The University of Newcastle, Callaghan, NSW 2308, Australia; tamara.bucher@newcastle.edu.au (T.B.); kerith.duncanson@newcastle.edu.au (K.D.)
4. Priority Research Centre for Physical Activity and Nutrition, The University of Newcastle, Callaghan, NSW 2308, Australia; beatrice.murawski@newcastle.edu.au
5. School of Medicine and Public Health, Faculty of Health and Medicine, The University of Newcastle, Callaghan, NSW 2308, Australia
* Correspondence: david.labbe@rdls.nestle.com

Received: 18 July 2019; Accepted: 5 September 2019; Published: 11 September 2019

Abstract: The increase in packaged food and beverage portion sizes has been identified as a potential factor implicated in the rise of the prevalence of obesity. In this context, the objective of this systematic scoping review was to investigate how healthy adults perceive and interpret serving size information on food packages and how this influences product perception and consumption. Such knowledge is needed to improve food labelling understanding and guide consumers toward healthier portion size choices. A search of seven databases (2010 to April 2019) provided the records for title and abstract screening, with relevant articles assessed for eligibility in the full-text. Fourteen articles met the inclusion criteria, with relevant data extracted by one reviewer and checked for consistency by a second reviewer. Twelve studies were conducted in North America, where the government regulates serving size information. Several studies reported a poor understanding of serving size labelling. Indeed, consumers interpreted the labelled serving size as a recommended serving for dietary guidelines for healthy eating rather than a typical consumption unit, which is set by the manufacturer or regulated in some countries such as in the U.S. and Canada. Not all studies assessed consumption; however, larger labelled serving sizes resulted in larger self-selected portion sizes in three studies. However, another study performed on confectionary reported the opposite effect, with larger labelled serving sizes leading to reduced consumption. The limited number of included studies showed that labelled serving size affects portion size selection and consumption, and that any labelled serving size format changes may result in increased portion size selection, energy intake and thus contribute to the rise of the prevalence of overweight and obesity. Research to test cross-continentally labelled serving size format changes within experimental and natural settings (e.g., at home) are needed. In addition, tailored, comprehensive and serving-size-specific food literacy initiatives need to be evaluated to provide recommendations for effective serving size labelling. This is required to ensure the correct understanding of nutritional content, as well as informing food choices and consumption, for both core foods and discretionary foods.

Keywords: serving size; portion size; food labeling; nutrition facts label; back of pack; front of pack; health framing

1. Introduction

The food environment in which people select, prepare and consume food has changed considerably in recent years. Improvements to agricultural practices, food transportation, food processing, and food storage have contributed to an increase in food availability and variety [1]. A decrease in home-prepared foods and increased purchasing and consumption of packaged foods has led to increased reliance on food package labels including information about the composition of foods purchased and consumed [2–4]. In parallel, an increase in portion size for packaged food and beverages has been identified as a potential factor contributing to the rise of the prevalence of obesity between 1977 and 2006 in the United States of America (USA) [5]. The influence of the changing food environment on weight status resulted in increased investigation of this association in the literature [6]. The factors that influence food choice as a behavior in this abundant food environment are likely to be mediated by attitudes and beliefs at an individual level, as described by Ajzen's Theory of Planned Behavior [7,8].

In this context, the importance of nutritional information labelling including serving sizes is paramount for consumer awareness and understanding of their food purchasing and in guiding them toward informed food choices and portion size selection.

The term "serving size" pertains to the labelled serving size found on a food label [9], unlike "portion size", which describes the actual amount of food that has been consumed [10]. However, the terms "serving size" and "portion size" are often used interchangeably, which may lead consumers to believe they mean the same thing, despite this distinct difference. This misconception has led to confusion related to serving sizes on labels, which was originally intended to guide food selection and portion sizes [11–13].

In 35 countries (including European countries, USA, China, Brazil, Japan, Australia), a nutritional information panel on food packages is mandatory, and legislation requires or recommends the listing of nutritional information on a serving size basis [14]. Serving size information, which should represent the amount customarily consumed, is either regulated (e.g., USA, Canada) [15] or determined by the food manufacturers (e.g., in Australia and in European countries) [14]. Thus, serving sizes can vary between products in the same food category and with the same volume [16,17]. At a conceptual level, the "per serving" information is useful for consumers to estimate how much of a nutrient they are consuming. For example, if an individual with cardiovascular disease is monitoring fat consumption, they may use the "per serving" amount to help calculate their daily total fat intake from packaged foods [18].

In May 2016, the U.S. Food and Drug Administration (FDA) announced a new nutrition facts label for packaged foods to reflect new scientific information, including the link between diet and chronic diseases such as obesity and heart disease [15]. This new regulation included updates on serving sizes and labelling requirements for certain package sizes. As the portion sizes consumed have increased within the last decade [19], these regulations were updated. For packaged foods that contain up to 200% of the reference amount customarily consumed (RACC), such as a 20 ounce (600 mL) soda or a 15 ounce (425 g) can of soup, calories and other nutrients will now be required to be labelled as one serving, because a person typically consumes this amount in one sitting. These specified serving sizes tend to be similar to serving sizes in the national level food guidance systems, but are not exactly identical, which adds another layer of complexity and confusion for consumers. The confusion regarding the current standards for serving sizes used on packages as well as the advice provided to guide portion sizes (i.e., how much should be consumed) among consumers is partially due to the heterogeneity in rules and regulations surrounding serving sizes as well as inconsistencies in the terminology used.

The literature provides mixed information on consumer understanding and use of food labels. Several reviews are available that explore the consumer understanding of labelling. These reviews report that most consumers looked at nutrition labels "often" or "sometimes", with some participants indicating that labels influence their food purchases [20]; that consumers lack understanding with regard to some nutrition label terms [20–22]; or that there is a potential positive effect of front-of-pack labeling in guiding consumers' choices towards healthier products [23,24]. Low health literacy is associated with less food label use and poorer diet quality [25], as well as less accurate estimates of serving sizes [26]. The heterogeneity in presenting serving sizes, and hence nutritional information for similar foods, compromises its efficiency in guiding consumers toward informed food choices [14,16]. Additionally, a tendency has been identified whereby foods with a higher calorie density are displayed using smaller serving sizes. This further increases the complexity and limits the usefulness of nutritional information from a consumer perspective [17], while consumers also feel conflicted with inconsistent messages about what and how much they should eat [27]. The evidence shows that consumers obtain information regarding portion sizes from a number of sources including dietitians and food packages, much of which can be contradictory or inconsistent [27]. Consumers describing the burden of deciphering food labels and how this causes misinterpretations of portion size guidance also tend to perceive the serving sizes provided (e.g., cereal) as too small and not relatable to the amounts consumed [27]. One suggestion of how healthy portion size choices and consumption could be promoted concerns the manipulation of labelled serving sizes [28]. This type of manipulation is called "health framing" and capitalizes on consumers' perceptions of serving sizes. For example, food items with smaller serving sizes and nutritional information listed consequently might be considered healthier than a larger serving size of a similar food item [29]. The influence of labelled serving size information on attitudes, beliefs and resulting food choice behaviors in the current food environment has not been described within the current, abundant food environment.

The aim of this review is to provide an overview of the recent field of investigation related to consumers' interpretation of labelled serving size information and how this influences product perception and consumption. With complex food environments and consumer confusion surrounding serving size labels [27], this knowledge is needed to inform changes to simplify food labelling and assist consumers in choosing healthy portion sizes (e.g., through improved understanding of product nutritional information).

2. Material and Method

The current scoping review followed a five-stage framework [30]. These stages were used to structure and guide the processes of (1) identifying a research question; (2) identifying relevant studies; (3) selecting studies; (4) charting the data; and (5) collating, summarizing and reporting the results. With the aim of addressing the research questions of how consumers interpret the labelled serving size information and how this influences product perception and consumption, the following objectives were defined.

2.1. Search Strategy

Seven electronic databases were used to search for relevant papers published in English: MEDLINE, The Cochrane Library, EMBASE (Excerpta Medica Database), CINAHL (Cumulative Index to Nursing and Allied Health), Scopus, PsycInfo and Business Source Ultimate. The search comprised truncated key words used individually and in combination, including "point of sale", "point of purchase", "nutrition/food/health/front of pack (FOP)/back of pack (BOP)" and "label/rating/symbol/information or logo", "menu/food" and "label", "nutrition and guideline/panel/table/profile/summary or score", or "nutrition fact label", "portion size", "serve", "serving" or "serves" (see Supplementary Materials for the full search strategy). Publications were limited to human subjects only and, where possible, a number of terms describing various diseases were excluded. Record retrieval was limited to studies published between 2010 and April 2019. These publication dates were selected to ensure currency in relation to the food environment and to calibrate somewhat in relation to serving size labelling. For example, mandatory labelling was introduced in Australia in 2002 [31] and in Europe by 2011 [32].

2.2. Record Screening

Results of the search were exported to EndNote X8 (Clarivate Analytics, Philadelphia, PA, US), where duplicates were removed using the inbuilt function in Endnote, which enables the automatic identification of duplicates. In addition, the identified duplicates were checked manually prior to removal. The remaining titles and abstracts were uploaded to Covidence (Veritas Health Innovation, Melbourne, Australia; available at www.covidence.org), where members of the research team were able to undertake all screening processes. The screening of titles and abstracts was shared between three reviewers, with any studies categorized as "retrieve" or "unclear" included for full-text screening. Full-text screening was conducted by two reviewers, with a third reviewer independently assessing any conflicts.

2.3. Selection Criteria

To guide publication selection, a set of eligibility criteria were established that aligned with the research question defined in Stage 1 (research question identification). A publication was eligible if it provided information on how consumers perceive, understand or interpret labelled serving sizes (e.g., recommended vs. usual portion), if it provided information on how the labelled serving size on food labels influences product perception, choice or consumption, or if it provided information on whether consumers differentiate between the FOP-labelled serving size and portion guidance (which is sometimes found on BOP labels) and relate to dietary recommendations such as serve sizes.

Publications were excluded if they reported information on calorie labelling on menus or the general impact of FOP labelling on consumers (i.e., not focused on serving size). Publications were also excluded if this information was not provided in the form of an on-pack label format (e.g., printed or displayed elsewhere) or did not make reference to this, or if serving size per se was not addressed on the label. Any reports on the association between physical activities and portion size on calorie-related outcomes were beyond the scope of this review, as were publications focused on any forms of portion size education other than what was provided on the label (unless strictly relating to education on serving size labelling). Publications were excluded if there was no parameter relating to consumer behavior (i.e., perception, interpretation, food choice, intake), or if the publication was merely descriptive in nature (e.g., an overview of different types of labels on the market). Publications examining packaging waste were also deemed irrelevant for this review.

2.4. Data Extraction

Relevant data, including the study design (e.g., study type, sample size and setting), sample characteristics (e.g., age, gender and weight), description of labels, study outcomes (including perception, interpretation and behavior) and conclusions were extracted by one reviewer into an Excel spreadsheet. A second reviewer checked the data extracted from each publication for consistency. Conflicts on study inclusion and exclusion were discussed and resolved between all authors. Extracted data were further grouped into the following sub-sections, each of which were summarized in table format:

Publication selection: authors (year); country; study type and design; sample size; description of study arms/conditions; study setting; participant age; gender ratio; and weight status.

Description of included publications: authors (year); food type; food label type; main findings relating to perception and interpretation; main findings relating to behavior; and implications.

3. Results

3.1. Publication Selection

A total of 3738 publications were identified as part of the electronic database searches (MEDLINE ($k = 644$), The Cochrane Library ($k = 36$), EMBASE ($k = 720$), CINAHL ($k = 169$), Scopus ($k = 859$), PsycINFO ($k = 222$), Business Source Ultimate ($k = 191$)). Duplicates were removed (1363), which left 2375 titles and abstracts to be screened, and among them, 1793 publications were deemed irrelevant based on title and abstract screening, with disagreement resolved by a third reviewer. The remaining 72 full-text reports were assessed for inclusion by two reviewers, with conflicts resolved by discussion and consensus. Fourteen publications were included for the final synthesis (Figure 1).

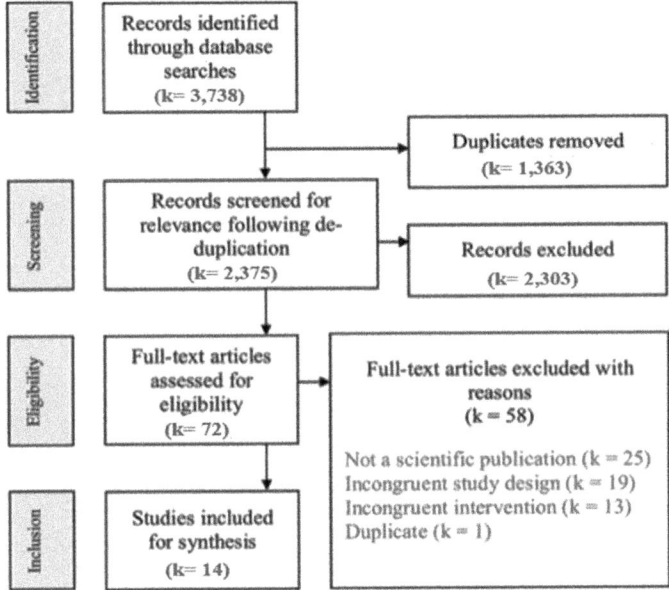

Figure 1. Flow diagram of study selection.

The 14 papers reporting findings from 29 studies (nested experiments) were published between 2012 and 2019. Studies took place in four different countries, including ten from the USA [33–41], two from Canada [42,43], one from Australia [44], and one from the United Kingdom [45]. Sample sizes across these studies ranged from $n = 51$ [39] to $n = 16,048$ [40], including nine studies with less than 1000 participants and four studies reporting results from 1000+ participants. Observations were either made in the form of online surveys ($m = 8$), in university settings ($m = 5$), at laboratories ($m = 8$), or held in local community settings such as at college basketball game ($m = 4$) or completed at home via postal survey ($m = 3$). Table 1 provides a summary of descriptive data for each of the included studies.

Table 1. Food label serving size information scoping review: summary of included studies.

Publication	Study Design & Sample	Study/Expt.	Setting	Study Conditions/Objective	Age (Years) M	Age (Years) SD	Gender (% m/f) a	BMI (kg/ht²) M	BMI (kg/ht²) SD
Baxter et al. (2018) [43]	Three-arm experimental design with random allocation (60 Canadian University students)	1	Laboratory (n = 20)	Consumer interpretation of nutrition facts table using single serving (i.e., smaller) pack size containing multi serving (SSMS)	20	3.0	55/45	24.7	3.9
		2	Laboratory (n = 20)	Consumer interpretation of nutrition facts table using single serving (i.e., smaller) pack size containing one serving (SSSS)	20	2.0	41/60	24.9	4.9
		3	Laboratory (n = 20)	Consumer interpretation of nutrition facts table using multi serving (i.e., larger) pack size containing multi serving (MSMS)	19	6.0	53.8/45.2	23.6	3.5
Dallas et al. (2015) [33]	Nested experimental design (273 U.S. adults)	1	Online (n = 101)	Consumer interpretation of the meaning of SS information	32.5	10.8	55.3/44.7	26.2	5.78
		2	College Basketball game (n = 51)	Influence of exposure to current vs. proposed SS on food portions participants serve themselves	34.0	11.3	58.8/41.2	25.4	4.74
		3	University marketing course (n = 60)	Influence of exposure to current SS labelling on food portions, served and purchased for others	20.0	1.4	53.3/46.7	21.7	3.45
		4	University marketing course (n = 61)	Influence of exposure to proposed SS labelling on food portions, served and purchased for others	19.7	1.5	51.8/48.2	22.0	3.39
Elshiewy et al. (2016) [45]	Cross-sectional analysis using purchase transaction data (n = 20 million transactions)		N/A	N/A	N/A		N/A	N/A	
Hydock et al. (2016) [35]	Nested experimental design (753 U.S. University students)	1	Laboratory (n = 208)	Current vs. proposed (double) SS on five different food packages in relation to perceived healthfulness and accuracy of SS depicted	32	12	54/46	N/A	
		2	Laboratory (n = 347)	Virtual portioning (for self) of six foods vs. label viewing to estimate own consumption, perceived healthfulness, calorie content and consumption guilt	31	10	54/46	N/A	
		3	Laboratory (n = 198)	Nutrition label showing current or larger SS vs. confectionery portion to assess the impact on consumption	20	1	53/47	N/A	
Jones et al. (2015) [42]	Nested experimental design with random group allocation (2011 Canadian adults)	1	Online	Beverage energy content estimation vs. per serving/per container/dual-column to test if participants correctly identify energy content	Range 16-24		50/50	22% were overweight or obese	
		2	Online	Cracker energy content vs. single serving small font/single serving large font/number of servings per bag to test if participants correctly identify energy content	Range 16-24		50/50	22% were overweight or obese	

Table 1. Cont.

Publication	Study Design & Sample	Study/Expt.	Setting	Study Conditions/Objective	Age (Years) M/SD	Gender (% m/f) a	BMI (kg/ht²) M/SD
Lando et al. (2012) [36]	Ten-arm experimental design with random group allocation (9493 U.S. Adults)		Online	Serving format: Two servings per container as single column vs. two servings per container as dual column vs. one serving per container as single-column Label format: Current Nutrition Facts label (control) vs. current label, without "calories from fat" vs. current label, without "calories from fat" and larger font vs. changed wording to emphasize there were two servings per container and "removed calories from fat" vs. dual listing for calories, with calories per serving and per container given, but remaining nutrients given only per serving and "calories from fat" removed Label content: Provision of all nutritional information per serving and per container in separate columns vs. same dual column, without "calories from fat" vs. dual column with only the calories and % DVs per serving and per container in separate columns (without "calories from fat"). Further, there were two label formats in the one serving, single-column grouping, both using a single, large serving either like the control label, but without "calories from fat" vs. one like the control label, but without "calories from fat" and larger font	46 / 15.5	51/49	28.5 / 7.1
Lewis et al., 2018 [46]	Two-arm experimental design with random group allocation (1221 US adults)	1	Public area (n = 80)	Impact of portion size information (1 serving vs. 11 pieces) on tortilla chips consumption intention	20.54/5.10	50/50	N/A
		2a	Public area (n = 79)	Impact of portion size information (1 serving vs. 15 pieces) on gummies consumption intention and consumption	21.37/5.21	46.8/33.2	N/A
		2b	Public area (n = 79)	Impact of portion size information (1 serving vs. 9 pieces) on mini rice cakes consumption intention and consumption	21.27/3.34	50.6/49.4	N/A
		3	Online (n = 200)	Impact of portion size information (1 serving vs. 16 pieces) on gummies consumption intention and perceived food size	32.4/9.03	52.5/47.5	NR
		4	Online (n = 160)	Impact of portion size information (1 serving vs. 16 pieces) on gummies and baby carrots consumption intention and self-regulation (with dieters)	32.23/10.84	52/48	NR
		5	Online (n = 300)	Impact of portion size information (1 serving vs. 16 pieces) on self-regulation facilitation (with dieters) with a measure of regulatory struggle	34.13/11.66	54.7/55.3	NR
		6	Laboratory (n = 323)	Impact of portion size information (1 serving vs. x pieces) on consumption intention, perceived food size and actual intake of carrots, gummies, potato chips, plain M&Ms, roasted and salted almonds, and seedless green grapes	34.62/16.66	31.3/68.7	N/A

Table 1. *Cont.*

Publication	Study Design & Sample	Study/Expt.	Setting	Study Conditions/Objective	Age (Years) M	Age (Years) SD	Gender (% m/f) [a]	BMI (kg/ht^2) M	BMI (kg/ht^2) SD
Miller et al. (2017) [37]	Pre-post experimental design (358 U.S. Community members)		Postal survey	Product pair comparison (8 items) for healthfulness, with pairs differing in SS vs. product pairs with consistent serving size to test the accuracy of serving size estimations in the context of product healthfulness	Range 20–78		40/60	N/A	
Mohr et al. (2012) [38]	Experimental between-subjects design with random allocation (151 U.S. Adults)	3b	Online	Comparison of provision of health frame (smaller SS) vs. no frame (larger SS) to examine product choice Comparison of discretionary weight (low/high) vs. product category (pizza vs. soup) with measured moderator (dietary concern, guilt) to examine product choice	46	N/A	N/A	N/A	
Persoskie et al. (2017) [34]	Repeat cross-sectional design (3165 US adults)		Postal survey	Consumer understanding of nutritional information labelling for ice-cream	N/A	N/A	48.3/51.7	N/A	N/A
Roberto et al. (2012) [41]	Three-arm RCT (216 U.S. University students)		University classroom	Original smart choices label (servings per package) vs. modified label (incl. SS) vs. no calorie label	26	10	37/63	23.2	4.5
Spanos et al. (2015) [44]	Four-arm pilot RCT (100 Australian University students)		Laboratory-based	Portion size: 200 g Pizza in 12 pieces or 400 g Pizza in 24 pieces (equal grams) Label formats: 3 × 200 g pizza (either stating "Contains 2 servings" or "Contains 4 servings" or no serving size given) and 1x 400 g pizza (no serving size given)	21	2.3	0/100	21.5	2.95
Tal et al. (2017) [39]	Observational study (51 U.S. University students)	1	University course	Comparison of FOP image with actual reported SS of 158 common cereals	N/A		N/A	N/A	
	Experimental study (51 U.S. University students)	2	University course	Comparison of varied SS (exaggerated, multiple SS vs. recommended single-SS) for two cereals in relation to pouring cereal.	22.3	N/A	31/69	N/A	
Zhang et al. (2014) [40]	Repeat cross-sectional design (16,048 U.S. adults)		Community-based surveys	Consumer understanding and use of SS information on nutrition facts in three large national surveys.	N/A		N/A	N/A	

Note. M = Mass; SD = Standard deviation; BMI = Body mass index (kilograms/height in metres^2); BOP = Back of pack; FOP = Front of pack; NR = Not reported; RCT = Randomized controlled trial; SS = Serving size; SSMS = Single serving pack size containing multi serving; SSSS = Single serving pack size containing one serving; MSMS = Multi serving pack size containing multi serving; a: % ratio of males/females; b: Studies 1 and 2 of this publication were deemed irrelevant for synthesis.

3.2. Description of Included Studies

Participants: Studies recruited adult volunteers either from the general public ($k = 8$) or university students ($k = 5$), and one study used purchase transaction data from a food retailer ($k = 1$). All but one sample [44] were mixed gender. One study [40] did not report a gender ratio but examined gender as a moderator. The average participant age per sample ranged from 18.0 years [34,44,46] to 75.0 years [34]. Measures of body mass index (BMI) or weight status were provided for six of the samples, which ranged from 21.5 to 28.5 [33,36,41–44]. For the remaining eight samples, no weight status was reported. None of the studies excluded individuals from participating based on this criterion.

Study designs: Various study designs were employed to answer respective research questions, with experimental studies involving between two and 10 comparator conditions. A non-randomized experimental design was used in three studies, none of which had a control group [33,35,37]. An experimental survey design (random allocation, no control group) was used in four studies [36,38,42,46]. A randomized controlled trial (RCT) design was chosen for three studies, either using three study arms [41,43] or four study arms [44]. A cross-sectional design was used in four studies [34,39,40,45].

Test conditions, comparator conditions and measurement of consumer perception, interpretation and behaviors: All of the included studies involved consumers reporting on serving size information on food packaging via a paper-based [34,37,43] or online survey [33,36,38,42,46] with the use of food models described in five of the papers [33–35,39,46]. Eight experiments/surveys specifically provided BOP nutrition facts and serving size labelling [33,34,36,37,40,42–44], and three provided both FOP and BOP nutrition facts and serving size labelling [35,38,39]. Seven papers reported having selected discretionary foods to be studied [34–37,41,42,44], five used both discretionary and core foods [33,38,39,45,46], and two studies involved the use of generic food labels [40,43].

Consumer perception and interpretation (including understanding, beliefs and concerns) about nutrition facts and serving sizes on existing labels were investigated in three studies [34,36,38] with a focus on the influence of health framing on consumer perception; i.e., how serving size affects nutritional information and related anticipated guilt after eating the product [38]. Seven studies investigated consumer understanding of proposed or modified nutrition facts labelling and serving size information in comparison to existing ones [33,35,37,39–42]. How consumers interpreted nutrition facts according to the number of servings per pack and the size of the pack was considered in one study [43].

Five articles investigated consumer behaviors in relation to proposed or modified nutrition facts labelling and serving sizes [33,35,39,41,44]. The influence of health framing on purchasing intention was also investigated [38], as were purchasing behaviors before and after the introduction of recommended serving sizes on nutrition labels [45], and the impact of varying granularity (i.e., fine-grained vs. gross-grained labels) of serving size information on intended and actual consumption and portion size perception [46].

3.3. Description of Study Findings

The 14 publications selected for inclusion in this scoping review related to a range of research questions and hypotheses. However, the studies were sufficiently consistent in design and measures to be consolidated into a set of study findings, as they were concerned with either the perception and interpretation, or behaviors (purchase, consumption) in relation to the labelled serving size. Table 2 summarizes the findings by study.

Table 2. Food label serving size information scoping review: summary of findings and implications.

Publication	Study/Expt.	Food Types	Label Types	Perception and Interpretation	Behaviour	Implications
Baxter et al. (2018) [43]		N/A	Nutrition facts table, incl. SS	Understanding nutrition facts per serving was improved for one serving per pack that appeared as a single serving (SSSS) or for a multiple serve in a multiple serve pack (MSMS) compared to a counter-intuitive small pack with multiple servings (SSMS).	N/A	"Multi serving packs lead to mathematical challenges to determine nutritional information if it seems to be a single serve". "Small package size of multiple serve packs led participants to interpret these products as single servings, underestimating nutrient and caloric content"
	1	Chicken vegetable Soup	BOP nutrition facts, incl. SS	78% believed SS related to how much food can or should be consumed in one sitting as part of a healthy diet, but the proportion of participants identifying correct meaning of serving size, incorrect meaning and "other" did not differ by condition	N/A	"Increased serving sizes may lead people who use this information as a reference to serve more food to themselves and others."
Dallas et al. (2015) [33]	2	Chocolate chip cookies	BOP nutrition facts, incl. SS	N/A	Modified (larger amount) label vs. current led consumers to serve themselves 41% more cookies	N/A
	3	Crackers	BOP nutrition facts, incl. SS	N/A	Modified (larger amount) label (vs. current) led consumers to serve 27% more cheese crackers to another person	N/A
	4	Lasagne	BOP nutrition facts, incl. SS	N/A	Modified (larger amount) label (vs. current) led consumers to buy 43% more lasagne for others and divide a lasagne into 22% larger slices	N/A
Elshiewy et al. (2016) [45]		Yoghurt (healthful) and cookies (unhealthful)	Guideline Daily Amount (FOP), incl. SS	N/A	Reduced SS specification increases sales volumes after label introduction in healthier category (yoghurt), but not in the unhealthy category (cookies). For example, a reduction in SS by 50% will increase sales volume by an average of 4% (yoghurt only)	"Consumers may overlook and misinterpret nutrition label information, which can result in increased consumption (health halo). Therefore, the use of FOP labels fails to promote healthy purchase behaviour."

Table 2. Cont.

Publication	Study/Expt.	Food Types	Label Types	Perception and Interpretation	Behaviour	Implications
Hydock et al. (2016) [35]	1	Pizza; pasta; fruit loops; sliced cheese; ham	FOP and BOP nutrition facts, incl. SS	Larger SS rated lower for health perceptions *, but more representative of serving size depicted *	N/A	"Providing consumers with easier to comprehend and more accurate information on all foods served in all contexts could reduce overeating. Decreasing caloric intake, through changing perceptions of health or increasing guilt, could improve public health. Updating serving sizes on nutrition labels could help promote better dietary choices and help curb the obesity epidemic in the United States."
	2	Macaroni cheese; chili; lasagne; rice snacks; soup; frozen fish		Larger serving sizes led consumers to perceive foods as less healthy * and estimate that their portion contained 18% more calories * and anticipate more guilt *	N/A	
	3	Confectionery		N/A	Consumers who viewed larger SS (proposed) ate less confectionery than those presented with the current SS *	
Jones et al. (2015) [42]	1	Chocolate milk	BOP nutrition facts, incl. SS	Nutrition label with per container or dual column is better for correctly identifying energy content than per serving **	N/A	"Per container and dual column increased understanding of energy content compared to per serving. This may help decrease individual consumption of DF by influencing perceptions of food health. Font size and display order of same information did not influence correct energy estimation."
	2	Crackers	N/A	No association between SS display format and correct energy estimation. 62% preferred SS size format including servings per package	N/A	
Lando et al. (2012) [36]		Frozen meal; crisps	BOP nutrition facts, incl. SS	Single-serving per contained and dual-column formats performed better and scored higher on most outcome measures	N/A	"For products that contain 2 servings, but are usually consumed in single eating occasion, a single-serving or dual-column labelling approach is recommended."
Lewis et al., (2018) [46]	1	Tortilla chips	1 serving vs. 11 pieces	Fine-grained label (11 pieces) decreased consumption intention vs. gross-grained labels (1 serving)		"Fine-grained label leads participants to decrease their consumption intentions and actual intake because portions are perceived to be bigger than portions described as with the gross-grained label." "Finally, granularity facilitates self-regulation of consumption," "Highlighting for consumers the concrete number they should consume could decrease consumption of those unhealthy foods. On the other hand, it may be fruitful to do the opposite for healthy foods that people struggle to begin eating."
	2 part a	Gummies	1 serving vs. 15 pieces	Fine-grained label decreased consumption intention vs. gross-grained labels	Fine-grained label decreased food consumption vs. gross-grained labels	
	2 part b	Mini rice cakes	1 serving vs. 9 pieces	Fine-grained label decreased consumption intention vs. gross-grained labels	Fine-grained label decreased food consumption vs. gross-grained labels	
	3	Gummies	1 serving vs. 16 pieces	Fine-grained label decreased consumption intention and increased perceived food size vs. gross-grained labels	N/A	

Table 2. Cont.

Publication	Study/Expt.	Food Types	Label Types	Perception and Interpretation	Behaviour	Implications
	4	Gummies and baby carrots	1 serving vs. 16 pieces	Fine-grained label reduced consumption intention vs. gross-grained labels for both foods Self-regulation is facilitated by fine-grained label vs. gross-grained label for gummies (unhealthy) whereas for baby carrots (healthy), label did not impact self-regulation	N/A	
	5	Candies	1 serving vs. 16 pieces	Fine-grained label reduced consumption intention vs. gross-grained labels Level of difficulty in dieting influenced consumption intention in the gross-grained condition only whereas the reducing impact of fine-grained on consumption intention was present at all levels of difficulty in dieting.		
	6	Carrots, gummies, potato chips, plain M&Ms, roasted and salted almonds, and seedless green grapes	1 serving vs. x pieces (number of pieces differed between foods)	Fine-grained label vs. gross-grained labels reduced consumption intention and perceived food size for all foods	Fine-grained label vs. gross-grained labels reduced intake for all foods	
Miller et al. (2017) [37]		Frozen pizza; snacks	BOP nutrition facts, incl. SS	Overall accuracy (i.e., ability to identify the healthiest product) was low (50–55%) across all age groups Numeracy, nutrition knowledge and self-reported food label use supported accuracy, but did not influence age differences in accuracy. Detailed instructions improve accuracy, even for difficult comparisons in which per serving and per package information is inconsistent Accuracy is compromised by poorer numeracy (all ages) and poor attention skills and with less instructions (older adults)	N/A	"Accuracy limited by lack of consideration for multiple servings rather than too many columns to evaluate or numeracy skills."
Mohr et al. (2012) [38]		Frozen pizza; vegetable soup	FOP and BOP nutrition facts, incl. SS	Health framing manipulation reduced guilt about consumption * for consumers who were more concerned about their diet People with high dietary concern are influenced more by health framing	Health frame dietary concern affects purchase intention * and guilt mediated the influence of health framing on purchase intention for participants with high concern *	"Prevention-focused health communication influenced participants towards selection of health-framed product whereas prompting to consider calories consumed influenced choice specifically towards listed calorie count. Health communication that encouraged participants to be diligent about their diet, but wary of health framing resulted in adjustment for serving sizes and selection of product with lowest negative nutrients."

Table 2. Cont.

Publication	Study/Expt.	Food Types	Label Types	Perception and Interpretation	Behaviour	Implications
Persoskie et al. (2017) [34]		Bulk ice-cream in container	Nutrition Facts Panel for one serving	Understanding nutrition fact information was poor, i.e., deriving calorie content in one serving for the entire container. Participants with healthier dietary habits performed better.		"To help consumers better understand serving size, dual column labels (nutritional information per serving and for the entire pack) can help". "Schools also have a role to play in teaching students the skills they need to understand the labels and make informed dietary decisions."
Roberto et al. (2012) [41]		Rainbow treasures cereal	FOP Smart Choices label, incl. SS	N/A	There were no significant differences between label conditions on the total amount of cereal and milk consumed	N/A
Spanos et al. (2015) [44]		Cheese pizza	BOP, incl. SS	N/A	Labelling pizza with a higher number of servings decreased food intake relative to labelling the pizza with a lower number of servings *	"Providing SS labelling on a food product can reduce the portion-size effect on consumer food intake."
Tal et al. (2017) [39]	1	Breakfast cereals	FOP food image (photo) and BOP nutrition facts, incl. SS	Portion size depictions on front of cereal boxes 64.7% larger than recommended portions on NFL.	N/A	"Biases in SS depicted on cereal packaging are prevalent and may lead to over-serving, which may consequently lead to overeating."
	2	Breakfast cereals	FOP food image (photo) and BOP nutrition facts, incl. SS	N/A	Boxes that depicted exaggerated SS resulted in 17.8% more cereal portioned compared to boxes that depicted a single-size portion of cereal matching suggested SS and 42% more than suggested SS	
Zhang et al. (2014) [40]		Generic	BOP, incl. SS	Majority of respondents misinterpreted the meaning of SS (Surveys 2 and 3). Women and obese individuals more likely to misinterpret SS meaning. A small subsample of participants expressed distrust of SS information	Use of SS information (often or sometimes) increased from 54% to 64% from 1994 to 2008 (Survey 1). Women and obese individuals more likely to use SS often or sometimes	"The increasing use, widespread misunderstanding and distrust of SS indicates need for change to both NFL education and information."

Note. Expt. = Experiment; BOP = Back of pack; FGS = Food guidance system; FOP = Front of pack; NFL = Nutrition facts label; OR = Odds ratio; SS = Serving size; SSMS = single serving pack size containing multi serving; SSSS = single serving pack size containing one serving; MSMS = multi serving pack size containing multi serving; N/A = Not applicable or data not available; * Mean values differed significantly from those of the comparator/control condition ($p < 0.05$); ** $p < 0.01$.

Consumer health perception of labelled serving size: Consumer health perceptions towards serving size labelling were measured in different ways in the studies that reported on this influence. In one study, serving size decreased product-related health perception ($p < 0.001$) and increased guilt associated with consumption ($p < 0.05$) but was perceived as more representative of portions typically consumed ($p < 0.05$ all foods) [35].

Two studies reported a negative impact in relation to consumer perception of serving size labelling. In a study specifically related to the health framing of labelling, the manipulation of serving size (and nutritional) information through health framing (i.e., reducing serving size) reduced consumption guilt ($p < 0.05$) for consumers who were more concerned about their diet [38]. These findings were consistent with the study that used a real-world setting in which a reduction of the labelled recommended serving size by 50% increased sales volume by an average of 4% in the yogurt category, with an even more pronounced effect when the serving-size specification was particularly small [45]. In the open response section of a large national cross-sectional survey reported, a small subsample of participants expressed distrust of serving size information [40].

Consumer understanding and interpretation of labelled serving size: Improved accuracy in serving size estimations is associated with higher numeracy, nutrition knowledge, and self-reported food label use and is enhanced by the provision of detailed instructions, even for difficult comparisons in which per serving and per package information was inconsistent [37]. Conversely, serving size estimation in this study was compromised by poorer numeracy (all ages), poor attention skills, and fewer instructions (older adults only).

Three studies investigated consumer interpretation of labelled serving size and identified that consumers interpret serving size as a recommended serving rather than as a typical serving [33,37,40]. A discrepancy between the understanding of serving size and portion size was reported, with 78% of participants believing that serving size related to how much food can or should be consumed in one sitting as part of a healthy diet [33]. In a cross-sectional study ($n = 16,280$) the majority of respondents misinterpreted the meaning of serving size, particularly women and obese individuals [40]. Indeed, about half the respondents reported that serving size is "the amount of this food that people should eat" rather than an amount that "people usually eat" or "that makes it easier to compare foods." In a recent experimental study, it was shown that reported accuracy in serving size interpretation was also low (50–55%) across all age groups [37].

In two studies that compared existing to modified versions of serving size labelling, accuracy in calorie estimation was improved with a nutrition label that contained both serving size per serving and per-container (dual column information) [42]. Dual column information has also been shown to improve accuracy for complex calorie estimation tasks [36]. Participants of another study had difficulties in estimating total nutrients and calorie content present in a four-serve ice-cream container based on nutrition facts provided for one serving. The authors recommended dual column nutritional information to improve understanding of nutritional information [34]. In the same study, participants with higher scores on nutritional information understanding consumed less soda. While there was no association between different serving size display formats (e.g., font size or order) and correct energy estimation, the majority (62%) of participants preferred a serving size format that included servings per package [42]. In a study that investigated food image depiction on the front of packages, the authors identified that portion size depictions (i.e., the image of the cereal bowl on cereal boxes) were 64.7% larger than the portions recommended on the nutrition facts label [39].

When a product was presented as a single serving pack, but actually contained multiple servings, participants made significantly more serving size assumption errors compared to when a pack was not misleading (i.e., a single pack containing a single serving and a multi serving pack containing multiple servings [43]).

Consumer behavior in relation to labelled serving size: The behaviors specific to labelled serving sizes exhibited by participants in the included studies were influenced by a range of factors, including understanding of food labelling, health framing, and intentional modification to labelling. Three articles reported increased portion sizes as a result of using larger serving sizes [33,39,44]. Modified (larger amount) serving sizes on labels relative to existing serving sizes led consumers to serve themselves 41% more cookies, serve 27% more cheese crackers to another person, buy 43% more lasagne for others and divide a lasagne into 22% larger slices [33]. Similarly, cereal boxes that depicted exaggerated serving sizes (i.e., a cereal bowl with a large portion on the package illustration) resulted in 17.8% more cereal being portioned compared to boxes that depicted a single-size portion and 42% more than the suggested serving size [39]. Labelling pizza with a higher number of servings decreased food intake relative to labelling the pizza with a lower number of servings ($p < 0.05$) [44]. In contrast, consumers who viewed larger serving sizes ate less confectionery than those presented with the current serving sizes ($p < 0.05$), and larger serving sizes led to an overestimation of calories and greater anticipated guilt ($p < 0.05$) [35].

Health framing influenced behaviors as well as perception and serving size interpretation [38]. Health framing seemed to reduce the anticipated guilt associated with consuming calories, enabling consumers who were concerned about their diet to form stronger purchase intentions ($p < 0.05$). FOP labels assisted consumers to better estimate calories per serving, but this improved knowledge did not influence perceptions of healthfulness, taste, purchase intent, or the amount of cereal poured or consumed [41]. A notable finding was a trend towards a significant positive effect of unhealthier purchases in terms of calories per 100 g after label introduction, indicating that consumers react differently to the health framing of nutritional information depending on the "healthiness" of products [45].

High granularity (e.g., 15 pieces of chips) in describing serving sizes relative to low granularity (e.g., one serving of chips) decreased both the intended and the actual intake of the labelled food [46]. High granularity serving size description increased the perceived food size (i.e., people considered the food as larger, weighing more, costing more, and containing more calories), which reduced intake. Low granularity serving size description showed the reverse.

Definitions of serving size: Different interpretations of serving and portion sizes were used across the studies. For example, Dallas, Liu and Ubel [33] reported that "the correct definition of serving size is the amount that people typically consume in one sitting" and an "incorrect definition of serving size is the amount of the product that can or should be consumed in one sitting as part of a healthy diet" [33]. This study was included as it was apparent that the influence of the labelled serving size was examined, although the working definition used in this study was unfitting. A further example of differing terminology was evident in a study demonstrating that "portion size depictions on FOP of breakfast cereal boxes are 64.7% larger than recommended portions on the nutrition facts label" [39]. The terminology used in two studies [33,39] differed from each other and from all other included studies, in that serving size referred to the manufacturer-set amount listed in conjunction with nutrition facts on labels, and portion size was the commonly consumed amount. It should also be noted that the study on breakfast cereal [39] referred to portion size images in terms of photographs of a cereal bowl, which is part of packaging design rather than a FOP label.

4. Discussion

This scoping review was undertaken to identify how consumers interpret labelled serving size information and how this influences product perception and consumption. The study aim was to provide recommendations for effective serving size display to ensure the correct understanding of product nutrition information and inform product choices, leading to a healthier diet.

The results of this scoping review highlight some key points for consideration in relation to the serving size labelling of food products and their relationship to usual consumption (portion size). Consumers tended to interpret the labelled serving size as a recommended serving size rather than a typical portion size [33,37,40] and to inaccurately estimate nutritional content per serving [34,36,42]. The incorrect or inaccurate interpretation of serving size was exacerbated by demographic characteristics (age, sex, education level) and weight status [37,40]. Findings showed that serving size estimation accuracy was enhanced by the provision of detailed instructions, even for difficult and inconsistent servings and per package information. This provides an indication that improvements to consumer food label literacy are an important focus for serving size labelling [37]. Overall, consumers interpreted recommended serving size information as indicative of nutrient consumption without following recommendations to inform portion size [41]. The theoretical interpretation of the findings of this review are highly consistent with Ajzen's Theory of Planned Behavior [7]. It is evident that the beliefs of the individual regarding recommended serving size information influenced their behavior, resulting in a larger portion being served. Labelling a product with both serving size and dual column information (per serving and for the whole pack) was preferred by consumers [42] and avoided confusion to extrapolate nutrition facts for one serving to the entire content of a multi serve pack product [34]. A dual column format is commonly used and widely accepted in food labelling [47] and has previously been reported to improve understanding by providing a contextual cue [48]. For this combination of labelling to be relevant and useful to consumers, appropriate serving size information against which to benchmark nutrient levels is necessary.

In general, the perceptions of consumers could be influenced by the manipulation or framing of serving size information, with evidence of demographic influences on susceptibility to misleading serving size information. Larger serving sizes were generally perceived as more realistic portions than smaller serving sizes, as these were perceived as unrealistic. This finding provides support for the changes to legislation such as those that have been implemented in North America [15] from the perspective of consumer approval and support. However, this may encourage consumers to eat more if serving size is understood as the recommended portion.

The impact of serving size information on consumer portion size varied between studies and between study foods and whether these were considered discretionary or core foods. These findings suggest that different reference information or conditions may need to be applied to core and discretionary foods. Further investigation is also needed to explore the influence of the health framing that results from the application of serving size information to other parts of BOP and FOP labelling; of particular importance is improving the understanding of the impact of health framing on "healthier" compared to "unhealthier" foods, especially in relation to food purchasing behaviors [45]. Moreover, alternative portion guidance labels could have a potential health framing and consumption effect, as was found in the five-a-day portion guidance label for fruit and vegetables. A study revealed significantly lower subsequent fruit and vegetables consumption using smoothies displaying the "3 of your 5-a-day" label compared to the "1 of your 5-a-day" label. This highlights the importance of examining actual product consumption and also indicates that the daily intake of certain food groups might be influenced by labelling [49]. From a theoretical perspective, the influence of health framing on perceptions about the healthfulness of foods aligns with the attitudes component of the Theory of Planned Behavior. Food choice behavior is mediated by the attitude of the consumer, which has been influenced by how the product has been framed [8].

While FOP labelling was considered helpful to consumers, it performed better for tasks that related to product choice based on perceived healthfulness rather than serving size estimation [37]. FOP serving size labelling could therefore be considered to be relevant for product selection; for instance, using a pictorial serving size recommendation instead of an amount in grams to more efficiently inform consumers with poor numerical literacy [50]. Providing more granularity in serving size information on FOP labels for unhealthy and countable food items could also have a positive influence on consumption, whereas less granularity in serving size information could promote the consumption of healthier foods [46]. BOP serving size information can subsequently be used to inform customers about how much to purchase and consume based on dual column information.

Further research in ecological environments (e.g., at point of sale, in the home) is required to provide recommendations for effective serving size labelling to ensure the correct understanding of nutritional content and informed food choice and consumption. It is important for future research to investigate the impact of the labelled serving size on consumption of specific core foods and on discretionary foods. There is a need to determine whether improved consumer serving size literacy can help overcome health framing effects for discretionary foods (e.g., a smaller serving size can increase perceived healthfulness and lead to increased intake, due to a lower calorie content per serving displayed on the pack) or if other measures are required to offset the influence of health framing, particularly for susceptible consumer groups. Promising strategies to increase serving size literacy reported in the scoping review include comparative information on nutrition facts labels, realistic serving sizes and a comparison to standard reference amounts; for example, from national food guidance systems or the use of international food volume units [51].

5. Limitations

The results of this scoping review need to be evaluated while taking into account several limitations. As 12 out of the 14 papers were conducted in North America, the results need to be contextualized to consider the change in serving size labelling legislation [15] in North America in May 2016, as most studies were conducted in the preceding four years or immediately after this time-point. These changes were intended to ensure that consumers were aware of the nutritional composition of foods they were consuming, using a more standardized and realistic food amount than previously indicated on serving size labels. Therefore, cross-cultural research is required including countries where serving size labelling is not regulated.

The majority of included studies for which weight status was measured predominantly involved participants with a healthy weight status. This is important as overweight and obesity have the potential to influence serving size perception, interpretation and behaviors, and thus, the weight status of study populations needs to be accounted for [52]. Studies were mainly conducted in lab environments, and it would be useful for future research on influences of serving size labelling on food choice and consumption to be conducted in more ecologically valid settings such as at the point of sale or in the home. This is increasingly feasible in the current research environment with the increasing availability of technologies such as wearable cameras that can monitor behaviors [53]. Therefore, the results of the scoping review are synthesized in light of the rapidly changing food labelling landscape, different serving size legislation between countries, changes to labelling legislation in some countries during the selected search period (2010–2019), and the possible implications of increasing or standardizing serving sizes and the environments in which studies were conducted.

The terms "serving size" and "portion size" appear to be used inconsistently in the scientific literature. The present review may have excluded a number of findings from research that used the term "portion size" but in fact examined how different "serving sizes" influence consumer perception or behaviors. However, it was not possible to identify such reports with sufficient consistency.

Supplementary Materials: The following are available online at http://www.mdpi.com/2072-6643/11/9/2189/s1: detailed overview of search strings per database.

Author Contributions: K.V.d.H. and D.L. initiated the project, with all authors contributing to define the database search criteria. T.B., B.M., and K.D. performed the article search. All authors contributed to article screening, data analyses, and the writing of the manuscript. All authors approved the final manuscript.

Funding: This research was funded by Société des Produits Nestlé grant number (G1701336) And The APC was funded by Société des Produits Nestlé.

Acknowledgments: We thank D.B. for her help with the database searches and X.Y.K. for assistance with screening papers and abstracts. T.B. was supported by the School of Health Sciences and the Faculty of Medicine of the University of Newcastle, Australia.

Conflicts of Interest: The authors declare no conflict of interest.

References

1. Southgate, D.D.; Graham, D.H.; Tweeten, L.G. *The World Food Economy*, 2nd ed.; John Wiley & Sons: Chichester, UK, 2010.
2. Diabetes Prevention Working Party for the National Public Health Partnership. *Prevention of Type 2 Diabetes: A Background Paper*; Diabetes Prevention Working Party for the National Public Health Partnership: Auckland, New Zealand, 2005.
3. National Heart Foundation of Australia. National Heart Foundation of Australia Position statement on dietary fat and overweight/obesity. *Nutr. Diet.* **2003**, *60*, 174–176.
4. World Cancer Research Fund. *Summary: Food, Nutrition, Physical Activity and the Prevention of Cancer: A Global Perspective*; American Institute of Cancer Research: Washington, DC, USA, 2008.
5. Duffey, K.J.; Popkin, B.M. Energy density, portion size, and eating occasions: Contributions to increased energy intake in the United States, 1977–2006. *PLoS Med.* **2011**, *8*, e1001050. [CrossRef] [PubMed]
6. Holsten, J.E. Obesity and the community food environment: A systematic review. *Public Health Nutr.* **2009**, *12*, 397–405. [CrossRef] [PubMed]
7. Ajzen, I. From intentions to actions: A theory of planned behavior. In *Action Control*; Springer: Berlin/Heidelberg, Germany, 1985; pp. 11–39.
8. Shepherd, R. Social determinants of food choice. *Proc. Nutr. Soc.* **1999**, *58*, 807–812. [CrossRef] [PubMed]
9. Taylor, C.L.; Wilkening, V.L. How the Nutrition Food Label Was Developed, Part 1: The Nutrition Facts Panel. *J. Am. Diet. Assoc.* **2008**, *108*, 437–442. [CrossRef] [PubMed]
10. Hackett, R. The IGD Industry Nutrition Strategy Group report–portion size: A review of existing approaches. *Nutr. Bull.* **2009**, *34*, 210–213. [CrossRef]
11. Bucher, T.; Rollo, M.E.; Smith, S.P.; Dean, M.; Brown, H.; Sun, M.; Collins, C. Position paper on the need for portion-size education and a standardised unit of measurement. *Health Promot. J. Aust. Off. J. Aust. Assoc. Health Promot. Prof.* **2017**, *28*, 260–263. [CrossRef] [PubMed]
12. Hogbin, M.B.; Hess, M.A. Public confusion over food portions and servings. *J. Acad. Nutr. Diet.* **1999**, *99*, 1209. [CrossRef]
13. Faulkner, G.P.; Livingstone, M.B.E.; Pourshahidi, L.K.; Spence, M.; Dean, M.; O'Brien, S.; Gibney, E.R.; Wallace, J.M.; McCaffrey, T.A.; Kerr, M.A. An evaluation of portion size estimation aids: Precision, ease of use and likelihood of future use. *Public Health Nutr.* **2016**, *19*, 2377–2387. [CrossRef]
14. Kliemann, N.; Kraemer, M.V.S.; Scapin, T.; Rodrigues, V.M.; Fernandes, A.C.; Bernardo, G.L.; Uggioni, P.L.; Proença, R.P.C. Serving Size and Nutrition Labelling: Implications for Nutrition Information and Nutrition Claims on Packaged Foods. *Nutrients* **2018**, *10*, 891. [CrossRef]
15. U.S. Food and Drug Administration. Changes to the Nutrition Facts Label. Available online: http://www.webcitation.org/6uMtBmqez (accessed on 21 October 2017).
16. Yang, S.; Gemming, L.; Rangan, A. Large Variations in Declared Serving Sizes of Packaged Foods in Australia: A Need for Serving Size Standardisation? *Nutrients* **2018**, *10*, 139. [CrossRef]
17. Chan, J.Y.M.; Scourboutakos, M.J.; L'Abbé, M.R. Unregulated serving sizes on the Canadian nutrition facts table–an invitation for manufacturer manipulations. *BMC Public Health* **2017**, *17*, 418. [CrossRef] [PubMed]
18. Food Standards Australia New Zealand. Nutrition Information Panels. Available online: http://www.webcitation.org/6uNPHpfV6 (accessed on 21 October 2017).
19. Hollands, G.J.; Shemilt, I.; Marteau, T.M.; Jebb, S.A.; Lewis, H.B.; Wei, Y.; Higgins, J.P.; Ogilvie, D. Portion, package or tableware size for changing selection and consumption of food, alcohol and tobacco. *Cochrane Database Syst. Rev.* **2015**. [CrossRef] [PubMed]
20. Cowburn, G.; Stockley, L. Consumer understanding and use of nutrition labelling: A systematic review. *Public Health Nutr.* **2005**, *8*, 21–28. [CrossRef] [PubMed]
21. Feunekes, G.I.J.; Gortemaker, I.A.; Willems, A.A.; Lion, R.; van den Kommer, M. Front-of-pack nutrition labelling: Testing effectiveness of different nutrition labelling formats front-of-pack in four European countries. *Appetite* **2008**, *50*, 57–70. [CrossRef] [PubMed]
22. Campos, S.; Doxey, J.; Hammond, D. Nutrition labels on pre-packaged foods: A systematic review. *Public Health Nutr.* **2011**, *14*, 1496–1506. [CrossRef]
23. Cecchini, M.; Warin, L. Impact of food labelling systems on food choices and eating behaviours: A systematic review and meta-analysis of randomized studies. *Obes. Rev.* **2016**, *17*, 201–210. [CrossRef] [PubMed]

24. Egnell, M.; Kesse-Guyot, E.; Galan, P.; Touvier, M.; Rayner, M.; Jewell, J.; Breda, J.; Hercberg, S.; Julia, C. Impact of front-of-pack nutrition labels on portion size selection: An experimental study in a French cohort. *Nutrients* **2018**, *10*, 1268. [CrossRef] [PubMed]
25. Cha, E.; Kim, K.H.; Lerner, H.M.; Dawkins, C.R.; Bello, M.K.; Umpierrez, G.; Dunbar, S.B. Health literacy, self-efficacy, food label use, and diet in young adults. *Am. J. Health Behav.* **2014**, *38*, 331–339. [CrossRef]
26. Huizinga, M.M.; Carlisle, A.J.; Cavanaugh, K.L.; Davis, D.L.; Gregory, R.P.; Schlundt, D.G.; Rothman, R.L. Literacy, numeracy, and portion-size estimation skills. *Am. J. Prev. Med.* **2009**, *36*, 324–328. [CrossRef]
27. Spence, M.; Livingstone, M.B.; Hollywood, L.E.; Gibney, E.R.; O'Brien, S.A.; Pourshahidi, L.K.; Dean, M. A qualitative study of psychological, social and behavioral barriers to appropriate food portion size control. *Int. J. Behav. Nutr. Phys. Act.* **2013**, *10*, 92. [CrossRef] [PubMed]
28. Van Assema, P.; Martens, M.; Ruiter, R.A.; Brug, J. Framing of nutrition education messages in persuading consumers of the advantages of a healthy diet. *J. Hum. Nutr. Diet. Off. J. Br. Diet. Assoc.* **2001**, *14*, 435–442. [CrossRef]
29. Bryant, A.; Hill, R.P. A Whole or Two Halves: Serving Size Framing Effects and Consumer Healthfulness Perceptions. *J. Consum. Aff.* **2018**, *52*, 452–465. [CrossRef]
30. Arksey, H.; O'Malley, L. Scoping studies: Towards a methodological framework. *Int. J. Soc. Res. Methodol.* **2005**, *8*, 19–32. [CrossRef]
31. Curran, M.A. Nutrition labelling: Perspectives of a bi-national agency for Australia and New Zealand. *Asia Pac. J. Clin. Nutr.* **2002**, *11*, S72–S76. [CrossRef] [PubMed]
32. Commission, E. Regulation (EU) No 1169/2011 of the European Parliament and of the Council of 25 October 2011 on the provision of food information to consumers, amending Regulations (EC) No 1924/2006 and (EC) No 1925/2006 of the European Parliament and of the Council, and repealing Commission Directive 87/250/EEC, Council Directive 90/496/EEC, Commission Directive 1999/10/EC, Directive 2000/13/EC of the European Parliament and of the Council, Commission Directives 2002/67/EC and 2008/5/EC and Commission Regulation (EC) No 608/2004. *Off. J. Eur. Union* **2011**, *54*, 18–61.
33. Dallas, S.K.; Liu, P.J.; Ubel, P.A. Potential problems with increasing serving sizes on the Nutrition Facts label. *Appetite* **2015**, *95*, 577–584. [CrossRef]
34. Persoskie, A.; Hennessy, E.; Nelson, W.L. US Consumers' Understanding of Nutrition Labels in 2013: The Importance of Health Literacy. *Prev. Chronic Dis.* **2017**, *14*, e86. [CrossRef]
35. Hydock, C.; Wilson, A.; Easwar, K. The effects of increased serving sizes on consumption. *Appetite* **2016**, *101*, 71–79. [CrossRef]
36. Lando, A.M.; Lo, S.C. Single-Larger-Portion-Size and Dual-Column Nutrition Labeling May Help Consumers Make More Healthful Food Choices. *J. Acad. Nutr. Diet.* **2013**, *113*, 241–250. [CrossRef]
37. Miller, L.M.; Applegate, E.; Beckett, L.A.; Wilson, M.D.; Gibson, T.N. Age differences in the use of serving size information on food labels: Numeracy or attention? *Public Health Nutr.* **2017**, *20*, 786–796. [CrossRef] [PubMed]
38. Mohr, G.S.; Lichtenstein, D.R.; Janiszewski, C. The Effect of Marketer-Suggested Serving Size on Consumer Responses: The Unintended Consequences of Consumer Attention to Calorie Information. *J. Mark.* **2012**, *76*, 59–75. [CrossRef]
39. Tal, A.; Niemann, S.; Wansink, B. Depicted serving size: Cereal packaging pictures exaggerate serving sizes and promote overserving. *BMC Public Health* **2017**, *17*, 169.
40. Zhang, Y.; Kantor, M.A.; Juan, W. Usage and Understanding of Serving Size Information on Food Labels in the United States. *Am. J. Health Promot.* **2016**, *30*, 181–187. [CrossRef] [PubMed]
41. Roberto, C.A.; Shivaram, M.; Martinez, O.; Boles, C.; Harris, J.L.; Brownell, K.D. The smart choices front-of-package nutrition label. Influence on perceptions and intake of cereal. *Appetite* **2012**, *58*, 651–657. [CrossRef] [PubMed]
42. Jones, A.C.; Vanderlee, L.; White, C.M.; Hobin, E.P.; Bordes, I.; Hammond, D. 'How many calories did I just eat?' An experimental study examining the effect of changes to serving size information on nutrition labels. *Public Health Nutr.* **2016**, *19*, 2959–2964. [CrossRef]
43. Baxter, V.M.; Andrushko, J.W.; Teucher, U. Size Matters: Package Size Influences Recognition of Serving Size Information. *Can. J. Diet. Pract. Res.* **2018**, *79*, 200–202. [CrossRef]
44. Spanos, S.; Kenda, A.S.; Vartanian, L.R. Can serving-size labels reduce the portion-size effect? A pilot study. *Eat. Behav.* **2015**, *16*, 40–42. [CrossRef]

45. Elshiewy, O.; Jahn, S.; Boztug, Y. Seduced by the Label: How the Recommended Serving Size on Nutrition Labels Affects Food Sales. *J. Consumer Res.* **2016**, *1*, 104–114. [CrossRef]
46. Lewis, J.N.A.; Earl, A. Seeing More and Eating Less: Effects of Portion Size Granularity on the Perception and Regulation of Food Consumption. *J. Personal. Soc. Psychol.* **2018**, *114*, 786–803. [CrossRef]
47. Food Standards Australia New Zealand. *Nutrition Information User Guide to Standard 1.2.8—Nutrition Information Requirements*; Food Standards Australia New Zealand: Canberra, Australia, 2013.
48. Antonuk, B.; Block, L.G. The effect of single serving versus entire package nutritional information on consumption norms and actual consumption of a snack food. *J. Nutr. Educ. Behav.* **2006**, *38*, 365–370. [CrossRef]
49. Appleton, K.; Pidgeon, H. 5-a-day fruit and vegetable food product labels: Reduced fruit and vegetable consumption following an exaggerated compared to a modest label. *BMC Public Health* **2018**, *18*, 624. [CrossRef] [PubMed]
50. Versluis, I.; Papies, E.K.; Marchiori, D. Preventing the pack size effect: Exploring the effectiveness of pictorial and non-pictorial serving size recommendations. *Appetite* **2015**, *87*, 116–126. [CrossRef] [PubMed]
51. Bucher, T.; Weltert, M.; Rollo, M.E.; Smith, S.P.; Jia, W.; Collins, C.E.; Sun, M. The international food unit: A new measurement aid that can improve portion size estimation. *Int. J. Behav. Nutr. Phys.* **2017**, *14*, 124. [CrossRef] [PubMed]
52. Chandon, P.; Wansink, B. Is obesity caused by calorie underestimation? A psychophysical model of meal size estimation. *J. Mark. Res.* **2007**, *44*, 84–99. [CrossRef]
53. Doherty, A.R.; Hodges, S.E.; King, A.C.; Smeaton, A.F.; Berry, E.; Moulin, C.J.; Lindley, S.; Kelly, P.; Foster, C. Wearable cameras in health: The state of the art and future possibilities. *Am. J. Prev. Med.* **2013**, *44*, 320–323. [CrossRef] [PubMed]

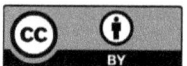

© 2019 by the authors. Licensee MDPI, Basel, Switzerland. This article is an open access article distributed under the terms and conditions of the Creative Commons Attribution (CC BY) license (http://creativecommons.org/licenses/by/4.0/).

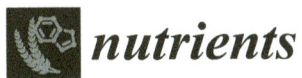 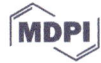

Article

Consumers' Perceptions of Five Front-of-Package Nutrition Labels: An Experimental Study Across 12 Countries

Zenobia Talati [1,*], Manon Egnell [2], Serge Hercberg [2,3], Chantal Julia [2,3,†] and Simone Pettigrew [1,†]

1. School of Psychology, Curtin University, Kent St, Bentley, WA 6102, Australia
2. Nutritional Epidemiology Research Team (EREN), Sorbonne Paris Cité Epidemiology and Statistics Research Center (CRESS), U1153 Inserm, U1125 Inra, Cnam, Paris 13 University, 93000 Bobigny, France
3. Public Health Departmant, Avicenne Hospital, Assistance Publique Hôpitaux de Paris (AP-HP), 93000 Bobigny, France
* Correspondence: zenobia.talati@curtin.edu.au; Tel.: +08-9266-4396
† These authors contributed equally to this work.

Received: 25 July 2019; Accepted: 12 August 2019; Published: 16 August 2019

Abstract: Consumers' perceptions of five front-of-pack nutrition label formats (health star rating (HSR), multiple traffic lights (MTL), Nutri-Score, reference intakes (RI) and warning label) were assessed across 12 countries (Argentina, Australia, Bulgaria, Canada, Denmark, France, Germany, Mexico, Singapore, Spain, the UK and the USA). Perceptions assessed included liking, trust, comprehensibility, salience and desire for the label to be mandatory. A sample of 12,015 respondents completed an online survey in which they rated one of the five (randomly allocated) front-of-pack labels (FoPLs) along the perception dimensions described above. Respondents viewing the MTL provided the most favourable ratings. Perceptions of the other FoPLs were mixed or neutral. No meaningful or consistent patterns were observed in the interactions between country and FoPL type, indicating that culture was not a strong predictor of general perceptions. The overall ranking of the FoPLs differed somewhat from previous research assessing their objective performance in terms of enhancing understanding of product healthiness, in which the Nutri-Score was the clear front-runner. Respondents showed a strong preference for mandatory labelling, regardless of label condition, which is consistent with past research showing that the application of labels across all products leads to healthier choices.

Keywords: front-of-pack nutrition label; traffic light; health star; Nutri-Score; reference intake; warning label

1. Introduction

In response to rising rates of obesity around the world [1], front-of-pack labels (FoPLs) are increasingly being applied to pre-packaged foods to inform consumers about the nutritional value of these foods and help them to make healthier choices [2–4]. A large body of research supports the notion that FoPLs are more effective in achieving these aims compared to the provision of no nutrition information or just a nutrition facts panel (generally found on the back or side of packs) [5–9].

Of the different FoPL formats currently in use around the world, most can be classified as reductive or interpretive [4,10]. Reductive FoPLs provide factual information about a food (such as the amounts of key nutrients within a food) with minimal interpretation (such as the food's contribution to an adult's recommended daily intake). Interpretive FoPLs may contain similar information (i.e., amounts of key nutrients) but also use aids like colour to indicate the healthiness of the food. The reference intakes (RI) and multiple traffic lights (MTL) are prominently studied examples of reductive and interpretive labels respectively [8,9,11,12].

Interpretive FoPLs can further be divided into nutrient-specific or summary indicator formats. Interpretive nutrient-specific formats (such as the MTL) provide information on the individual nutrients within a food, while interpretive summary indicator formats provide an overall evaluation of the nutritional quality of the product. The warning label is an example of another interpretive nutrient-specific format that has recently been mandated in a number of countries [4]. This FoPL typically appears as a black hexagon with the text "High in" followed by saturated fat, salt, sugar, or calories when a predetermined threshold is exceeded. The Nutri-Score is an example of an interpretive summary indicator, assigning foods with a colour-coded rating from A to E. Finally, the health star rating (HSR) similarly features a summary indicator but also displays nutrient-specific information alongside the indicator, making it a hybrid FoPL. Visual depictions of these FoPLs can be found in Figure 1.

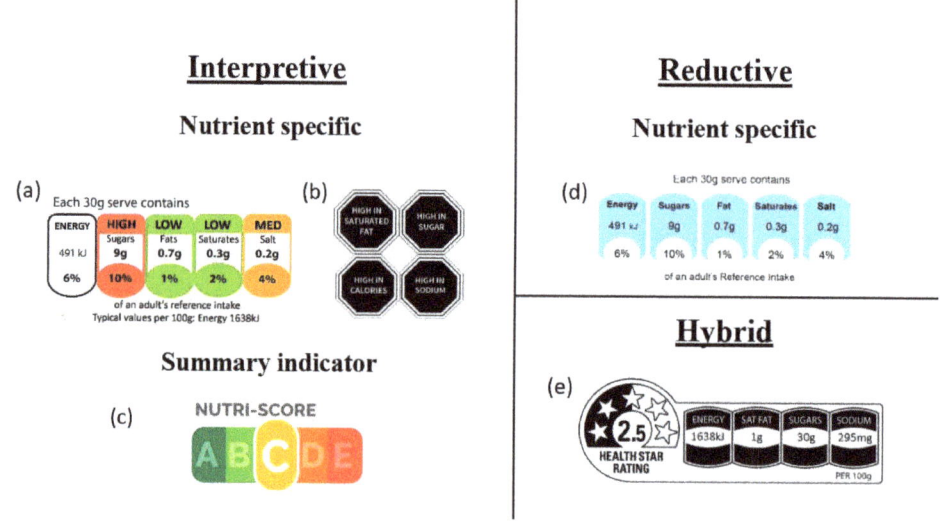

Figure 1. Examples of different front-of-pack label (FoPL) formats and their classifications: (**a**) multiple traffic lights; (**b**) warning labels; (**c**) Nutri-Score; (**d**) reference intakes; and (**e**) health star rating.

Studies have examined how the FoPLs described above influence people's understanding of nutrition information and affect food choices [8,9,11,12]. Given the challenges of conducting research in supermarkets [13], these studies have typically been carried out online or within a laboratory setting [14]. The latter designs allow a high degree of control over the variables being assessed. However, it is possible that respondents are more motivated and less time-pressured to make healthy choices in these contexts. Asking consumers about how they perceive different labels (e.g., whether they like them, trust them, find them easy to use) could provide additional information on how likely shoppers are to actually use a given label. In addition, consumers' attitudes towards FoPLs can affect whether or not governments choose to implement them [12,15]. One example of this comes from France, where consumers petitioned French retailers and food manufacturers to implement the Nutri-Score [15]. This eventually resulted in official recognition from the French government and uptake by some large retailers and manufacturers [15].

Past research on consumers' perceptions of various FoPLs shows that people like simplified labels but want to know how the information underlying the label was derived and do not like to feel they are being coerced [12]. In past studies, consumers have reported positive attitudes towards the MTL [16–25], HSR [26], Nutri-Score [27,28] and RI [20,21,29–31]. However, a direct comparison of perceptions of these FoPLs (and warning labels) has not been performed to date.

FoPL comparison testing has global policy implications. In 2016, the International Association of Consumer Food Organizations proposed that the Codex Committee on Food Labelling develop a new global standard for interpretive FoPLs [32]. A unifying standard was described as having the ability to potentially "protect existing laws from World Trade Organization (WTO) challenge, and encourage and empower other countries to issue nutrition regulations with higher public health impact without fear of WTO disputes" (p. 2, [32]). If a common FoPL standard is to be used across many countries, it is of critical importance to investigate which FoPLs are most effective and well-received across many countries. Testing different FoPL formats provides information that can be considered when determining appropriate elements to include in global FoPL standards.

The FOP-ICE (Front-Of-Pack International Comparative Experiment) project was borne out of efforts to address this issue. Using a randomised experimental design, The FOP-ICE study assessed reactions to five different FoPLs (HSR, MTL, Nutri-Score, RI, warning label) among a large (n = 12,015), diverse sample of consumers from 12 countries (Argentina, Australia, Bulgaria, Canada, Denmark, France, Germany, Mexico, Singapore, Spain, the UK and the USA). Results on the relative effectiveness of the five FoPLs to enhance consumers' understanding of the healthiness of food products showed that the Nutri-Score performed best across all countries, followed by the MTL [33]. The aim of the present study was to further interrogate the FOP-ICE study data by examining how respondents' perceptions of FoPLs vary according to FoPL type and country of residence. Perceptions were assessed in terms of liking, trust, comprehensibility, salience and desire for the label to be compulsory. It was hypothesised that respondents would be most favourable to interpretive labels, as past research has shown that these are most useful in guiding consumers to healthier food choices [8,9,11,12].

2. Materials and Methods

Relevant information on the methodology of the present study is reported below. Further details on the broader FOP-ICE project can be found at http://www.ANZCTR.org.au/ACTRN12618001221246.aspx and elsewhere [33].

2.1. Participants

Respondents (n = 12,015) were recruited from 12 countries (Argentina, Australia, Bulgaria, Canada, Denmark, France, Germany, Mexico, Singapore, Spain, the UK and the USA) to participate in an online survey. All respondents gave their informed consent for inclusion before they participated in the study. The protocol of the present study was approved by the Curtin University Human Research Ethics Committee (approval reference: HRE2017-0760) and the Institutional Review Board of the French Institute for Health and Medical Research (IRB Inserm n_17-404). Recruitment was undertaken by an ISO-accredited international web panel provider (PureProfile). To ensure a diverse sample, quotas were applied so that the sample was evenly split according to gender, age (within the following brackets: 18–30 years, 31–50 years, >50 years) and income level (low, medium and high) within each country. Once a quota had been filled, panel members falling within that demographic group were not eligible to participate. Income brackets for each country were calculated around the median household income (based on various national statistical databases) for that country. A bracket of +/-33% was created around the median income to represent a 'medium' income band. Any incomes that fell below or above those figures were considered low or high, respectively. Key participant demographic data can be found in Table 1.

Table 1. Key respondent demographic information.

n	All Countries		Argentina		Australia		Bulgaria		Canada		Denmark		France		Germany		Mexico		Singapore		Spain		UK		USA	
	11812		992		987		987		984		978		977		985		987		989		984		990		972	
	n	%	n	%	n	%	n	%	n	%	n	%	n	%	n	%	n	%	n	%	n	%	n	%	n	%
Gender																										
Males	5889	50	488	49	492	50	490	50	490	50	492	50	485	50	493	50	495	50	495	50	495	50	493	50	481	49
Females	5923	50	504	51	495	50	497	50	494	50	486	50	492	50	492	50	492	50	494	50	489	50	497	50	491	51
Age, Years																										
18–30	3951	33	329	33	323	33	348	35	332	34	316	32	326	33	334	34	335	34	333	34	332	34	327	33	316	33
31–50	3969	34	330	33	332	34	366	37	323	33	326	33	323	33	326	33	326	33	335	34	325	33	332	34	325	33
>50 years	3892	33	333	34	332	34	273	28	329	33	336	34	328	34	325	33	326	33	321	32	327	33	331	33	331	34
Level of Income																										
Low	3896	33	331	33	321	33	273	28	334	34	329	34	324	33	333	34	333	34	335	34	331	34	323	33	329	34
Medium	3985	34	331	33	332	34	350	35	329	33	336	34	329	34	329	33	325	33	334	34	326	33	334	34	330	34
High	3931	33	330	33	334	34	364	37	321	33	313	32	324	33	323	33	329	33	320	32	327	33	333	34	313	32

2.2. Procedure

The survey began with some background questions (e.g., gender, age, income, grocery buyer status, education level, nutrition knowledge and diet quality). Next, respondents were presented with three sets of three fictional food products with no FoPL on-pack. They were then randomised to one of the five FoPL conditions (HSR, MTL, Nutri-Score, RI, or warning label) and presented with the same food products (this time with a FoPL on-pack). In both the no-FoPL and FoPL scenarios, respondents were asked to (i) rank the three products within each set according to healthiness and (ii) select which product they would be most likely to buy (see [33] for results relating to healthiness rankings). At the conclusion of the study, respondents were presented with 9 items assessing their perception of the FoPL they had just seen. The items, which were assessed on a scale from 1 (strongly disagree) to 9 (strongly agree), were as follows:

- I like this label;
- I trust this label;
- This label is easy to understand;
- This label took too long to understand;
- This label is confusing;
- This label provides me with the information I need;
- This label does not stand out;
- It should be compulsory for this label to be shown on packaged food products;
- Food companies should be able to choose whether they apply this label to their packaged foods.

2.3. Analysis

Data analysis was performed in SPSS (version 25, SPSS Inc., Chicago, IL, USA). Given that some items were positively valanced and others were negatively valanced, respondents who provided the same response across all items (except those who responded with a 5, which was the mid-point of the scale) were removed from analyses ($n = 203$; 2% of the sample). This was a cautionary measure to eliminate potentially invalid responses. A 12 (country) × 5 (FoPL condition) ANCOVA was conducted on each perception item. The interaction between country and FoPL was also included as an independent variable. The p-value cut-off for significance (with a Bonferroni correction for 9 tests) was set to 0.005. Age, gender, income bracket, education, grocery buyer status, nutrition knowledge and diet were included as covariates. Post hoc comparisons among FoPLs and countries were performed with a Sidak correction for multiple comparisons applied to each survey item. The estimated marginal means for the different FoPLs (as well as the aggregated mean) and the FoPL by country interactions were graphed for the perception items where a significant main effect of FoPL or interaction between FoPL and country was observed, along with 99% confidence intervals to facilitate comparisons across all FoPLs.

3. Results

The mean score, standard deviation and intercorrelation for each perception item are shown in Table 2. Liking of and trust in a label were the most highly correlated items ($r = 0.65$). An unexpectedly low correlation ($r = -0.16$) was noted between the items assessing whether the label viewed by the respondent should be compulsory and whether food companies should be able to choose to apply the label. This may have been due to some respondents interpreting the latter item as asking whether food companies should have a choice to include the label vs. no label or interpreting it as asking whether companies should include the label vs. another label format. This item also showed the largest spread (SD = 2.78), indicating that there was less agreement among respondents on this item. Thus, no further analyses are reported on this item. The item assessing whether FoPLs should be compulsory on packs received the highest mean score (M = 7.13), indicating that respondents felt very strongly about this issue. In fact, 36.9% of the sample selected the highest score (9—'strongly agree') on this item.

Table 2. Means, standard deviations and Pearson correlation coefficients between the perception items.

	Mean	Standard Deviation	I Like This Label	I Trust This label	This Label is Easy to Understand	This Label Took Too Long to Understand	This Label is Confusing	This Label Does Not Stand Out	This Label Provides Me with the Information I Need
I like this label+	6.5	2.0							
I trust this label+	6.3	2.0	0.65						
This label is easy to understand+	7.0	2.0	0.58	0.54					
This label took too long to understand−	3.8	2.5	−0.20	−0.15	−0.43				
This label is confusing−	3.7	2.4	−0.29	−0.24	−0.47	0.70			
This label does not stand out−	4.9	2.4	−0.13	−0.06	−0.12	0.39	0.38		
This label provides me with the information I need+	6.6	2.0	0.64	0.64	0.59	−0.22	−0.31	−0.08	
It should be compulsory for this label to be shown on packaged food products+	7.1	2.0	0.52	0.49	0.48	−0.19	−0.26	−0.02[a]	0.55

+ Positively valanced item. − Negatively valanced item [a] $p = 0.04$. All other correlations significant at $p < 0.005$.

FoPL condition and country were significant predictors in the ANCOVAs across all 8 items ($p < 0.0001$). Graphs showing the distribution of means according to the different levels of these variables are presented in Figures 2 and 3.

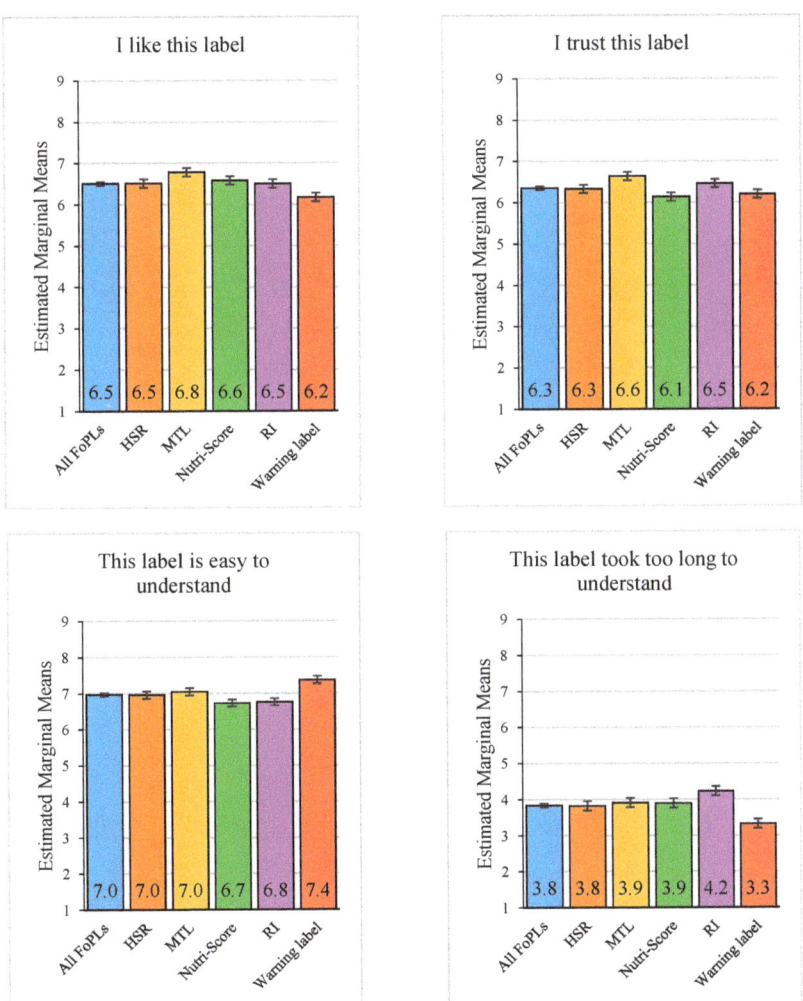

Figure 2. *Cont.*

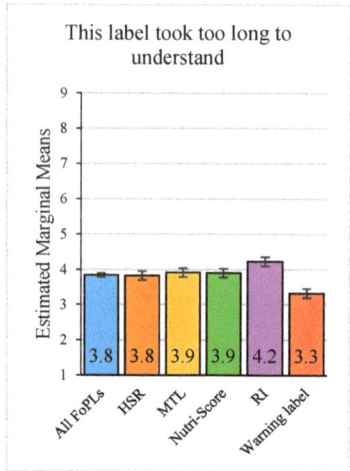
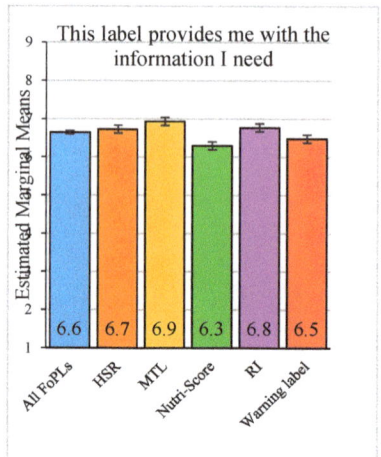
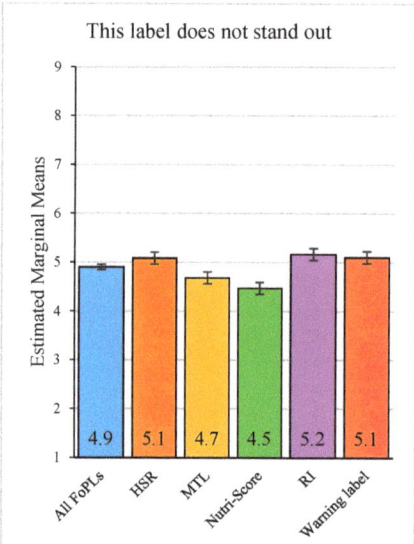
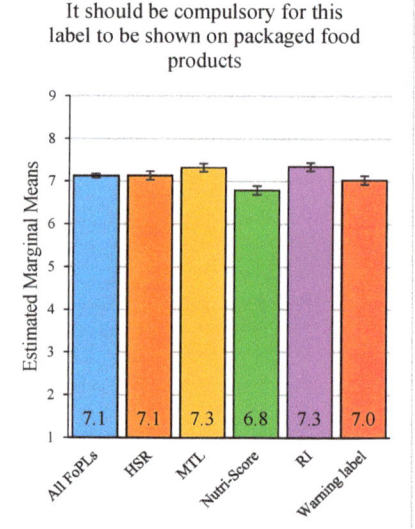

Figure 2. Mean scores across perception items for all FoPLs combined and individually. Note: Graphs show estimated marginal means for FoPL condition adjusted for age, gender, socioeconomic status, grocery buyer status, level of education, diet and nutrition knowledge. Error bars show 99% confidence intervals. HSR = Health Star Rating, MTL = Multiple Traffic Lights, RI = Reference Intakes.

Some notable trends were observed among the FoPLs across the different perception items. Across all the FoPLs included in the present study, the MTL was perceived most favourably. It received the highest scores out of all the FoPLs on four criteria (trust, liking, ease of understanding and providing needed information), the second highest score on the item assessing whether the FoPL should be compulsory and the second lowest score on the item "This label does not stand out". Respondents were ambivalent about the RI and Nutri-Score and neutral about the warning label and HSR. The RI received the highest mean scores for being confusing and not standing out, although it was relatively well trusted and perceived to be appropriate as a compulsory FoPL. The Nutri-Score received the lowest mean scores on trust, being easy to understand, providing enough information and being appropriate as a compulsory label on food packs, but it was relatively well liked and was perceived as standing out more than the other FoPLs. The warning label was the easiest label to interpret (scoring highest on ease of understanding and lowest on being confusing and taking too long to understand) but received the lowest score for liking. Perceptions of the warning label in relation to the other criteria tended to lie somewhere between those of the other FoPLs. The HSR received a relatively high score on the "does not stand out" item and fell somewhere between the other FoPLs for all the other items.

The country x FoPL interaction was significant ($p < 0.005$) for 6 of the 8 perception items: "I trust this label", "This label is easy to understand", "This label took too long to understand", "This label provides me with the information I need", "This label does not stand out" and "It should be compulsory for this label to be shown on packaged food products". Graphs showing the interaction for these items can be seen in Figure 3.

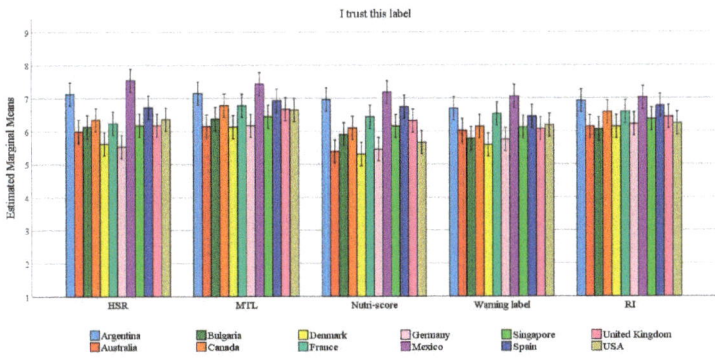

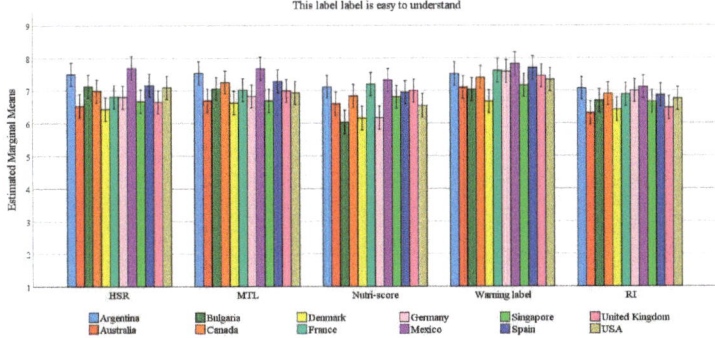

Figure 3. Cont.

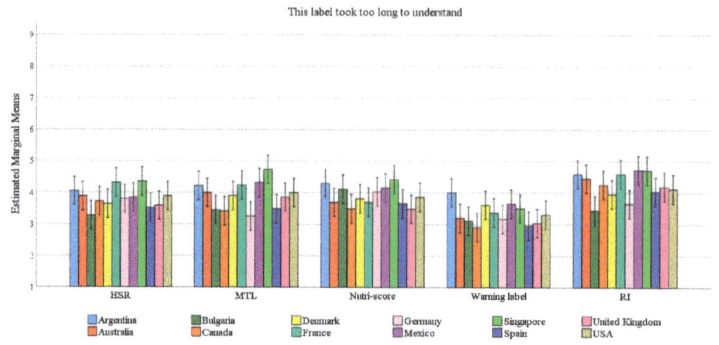
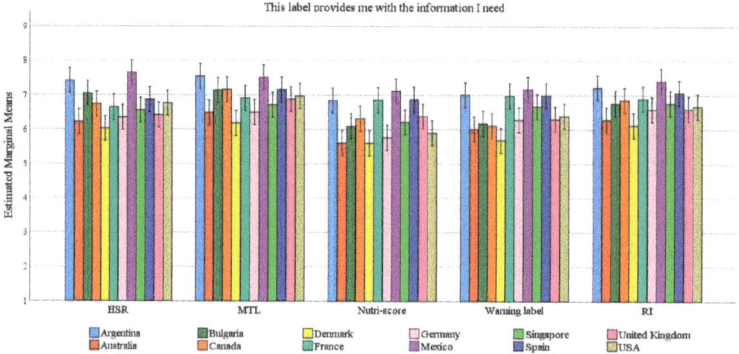
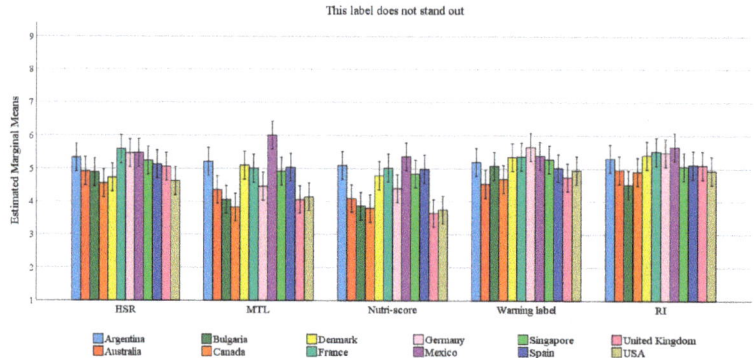

Figure 3. *Cont.*

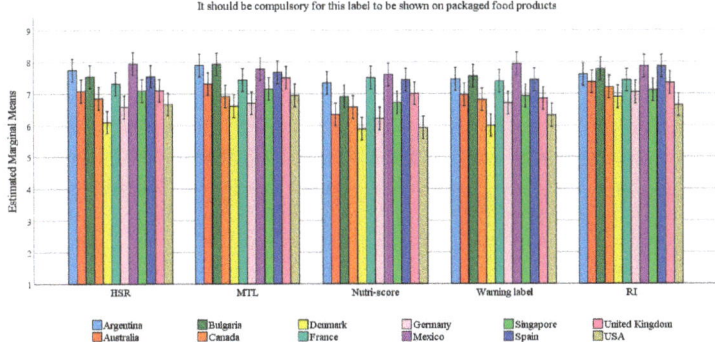

Figure 3. Mean scores across perception items according to country and FoPL type. Note: Graphs show estimated marginal means for countries adjusted for age, gender, SES, grocery buyer status, level of education, diet and nutrition knowledge. Error bars show 99% confidence intervals.

Looking across the interactions, no consistent trends were observed across the items. Patterns of differences between countries were not the same across different FoPL conditions or different perception items.

4. Discussion

This study explored consumers' perceptions of five FoPLs that are currently used around the world. The results show that irrespective of how favourably the different FoPLs were perceived or the country of residence, there was a clear demand for front-of-pack nutrition information to be made available. This was demonstrated in the very high mean score (7 out of 9) and a third of the sample selecting 9 ('strongly agree') for the item assessing whether the FoPL to which they were exposed should be compulsory on packs. Previous research supports the need for mandatory FoPLs, with supermarket studies reporting increased sales of healthier foods when FoPLs are applied to all products within a category rather than just a selection of products [34–37]. Although FoPLs should aid consumers in assessing the healthiness of individual products in isolation, they are most useful when they also allow consumers to compare healthiness across multiple products [38]. Some FoPLs, such as the warning label, only work if they are compulsory given that food manufacturers have no incentive to apply a FoPL across their product range when the aim of the FoPL is to reduce purchases of a product. Furthermore, past experience with the HSR has shown that when FoPLs are not mandatory, they skew towards appearing on healthier products [39], and this can reduce consumer trust in the system as a whole [39,40].

Looking at perceptions of the individual FoPLs studied, it is evident that the MTL was most favourably perceived. Respondents liked and trusted this FoPL the most and felt it provided the information they needed and was the easiest to understand. Perceptions of the RI and Nutri-Score were mixed. Respondents reported that the RI stood out the least and was the most confusing, but they showed relatively high trust in it and felt it should be compulsory on packs. Conversely, the Nutri-Score reportedly stood out the most and was easiest to understand but was the least trusted and least desired as a compulsory FoPL. Although the warning label was considered easiest to interpret, it was least liked. This may be due to the stark negative nature of this label. Finally, the HSR was perceived to stand out the least, which may go some way towards explaining why this FoPL tended to fall somewhere in between the other FoPLs on the other perception dimensions. It is important to note that the absolute differences between the FoPLs tended to be small (i.e., rarely more than 0.5 points difference on the 5-point scale), and thus, in some cases, it is more informative to consider the rating that was averaged across all FoPLs. These findings suggest that, on the whole, respondents were favourable towards FoPLs in general.

Looking at trends among FoPLs that share similar features, it is clear that the coloured FoPLs (MTL and Nutri-Score) stood out the most and were most liked. The more simplified FoPLs (Nutri-Score and warning labels) were seen as not providing enough information and were least trusted and less likely to be desired as compulsory. Other findings from this dataset found the Nutri-Score to be most useful in assisting consumers to accurately identify the healthiest food from a choice set [33]. This is discrepant with the present results showing that this FoPL was perceived to not provide enough information and to be harder to understand. These results suggest that consumers could benefit from education on the credibility of highly interpretive FoPLs such as the Nutri-Score to foster trust in the system, motivate consumers to make use of it and bring perceptions in line with performance.

Respondents were most in favour of the MTL and RI being compulsory on food packs. This is interesting given that other results from this same dataset show that these two FoPLs produce opposite outcomes on objective understanding [33]. Specifically, the MTL led to more positive outcomes (after the Nutri-Score) while the RI performed most poorly. These results are in line with previous studies demonstrating that consumers perceive that more information is better [41]. However, most consumers are not equipped to interpret all this information due to factors such as low levels of nutrition knowledge [42], time pressure [12] and competing priorities [43]. This is evident when results from the perception elements assessed in the present study (which show that consumers desire more information) are compared to the objective understanding results [33] (which show that understanding of food healthiness is not always improved by more information). Fortunately, respondents' perceptions were not always discrepant with objective understanding, as was the case with the MTL, which performed relatively well across both objective understanding and consumer preference. Although some differences were noted between countries, no meaningful or consistent patterns were present in the interactions between country and FoPL type.

It is important to note that certain elements of the study design are likely to have influenced the results. First, the between-subjects design meant that respondents provided ratings for only one FoPL. If respondents had been asked to rank the FoPLs, a clearer hierarchy may have emerged. However, only one FoPL was shown in order to keep the experimental tasks (completed before the perception ratings) to a management time limit. That differences were found among FoPLs using a design that is less sensitive for detecting differences is notable. Second, respondents were asked to provide their opinions directly after using a specific FoPL to make decisions about food healthiness and choice. This means that FoPL perceptions were grounded in the first-hand experience of respondents, which increases the ecological validity of the findings. However, one limitation is that the experimental process did not permit replication of any tactile experiences that would be available to customers in real-world supermarkets.

5. Conclusions

Overall, the results suggest that interpretive aids such as colour are viewed favourably by consumers but oversimplified FoPL formats risk excluding information that is desired by consumers and as a consequence being less trusted. Across the large and diverse sample of respondents, there was strong demand for FoPLs to be compulsory on food packs. This is an important message for policy makers to take away from these findings and is consistent with results from previous studies showing that FoPLs are most effective when applied to all products within a choice set, thus facilitating product comparisons and reducing the cognitive load on shoppers. Perceptions are just one dimension on which consumers' reactions to FoPLs can be assessed. Future work should consider how food choices in the real world are affected across culturally diverse groups.

Author Contributions: Z.T. performed data analyses and interpretation and drafted and revised the paper. C.J. and S.P. conceptualised the project in collaboration with S.H. S.P. supervised the data analyses and interpretation, participated in the writing and critically revised the paper for important intellectual content. C.J. and M.E. interpreted the data and critically revised the paper for important intellectual content. All authors had full access to all of the data in the study and can take responsibility for the integrity of the data and the accuracy of the data analysis. All authors have read and approved the final manuscript.

Funding: The present study received funding from Santé Publique France (French Agency for Public Health) and Curtin University.

Acknowledgments: The authors would like to thank all scientists in charge of the translations: Pilar Galan, Karen Assmann: Valentina Andreeva and Sinne Smed, who contributed to the creation of the different versions of the online survey. We also thank all researchers and doctoral students who tested the online survey.

Conflicts of Interest: The authors declare no conflict of interest.

References

1. NCD Risk Factor Collaboration. Trends in adult body-mass index in 200 countries from 1975 to 2014: A pooled analysis of 1698 population-based measurement studies with 19·2 million participants. *Lancet* **2016**, *387*, 1377–1396. [CrossRef]
2. World Health Organisation. European Food and Nutrition Action Plan 2015–2020. Available online: http://www.euro.who.int/__data/assets/pdf_file/0008/253727/64wd14e_FoodNutAP_140426.pdf (accessed on 18 June 2019).
3. World Health Organisation. Report of the Commission on Ending Childhood Obesity. Available online: Apps.who.int/iris/bitstream/10665/204176/1/9789241510066_eng.pdf (accessed on 31 October 2016).
4. Kanter, R.; Vanderlee, L.; Vandevijvere, S. Front-of-package nutrition labelling policy: Global progress and future directions. *Public Health Nutr.* **2018**, *21*, 1399–1408. [CrossRef] [PubMed]
5. Cowburn, G.; Stockley, L. Consumer understanding and use of nutrition labelling: A systematic review. *Public Health Nutr.* **2005**, *8*, 21–28. [CrossRef] [PubMed]
6. Ni Mhurchu, C.; Gorton, D. Nutrition labels and claims in New Zealand and Australia: A review of use and understanding. *Aust. N. Z. J. Public Health* **2007**, *31*, 105–112. [CrossRef]
7. Nelson, D.; Graham, D.; Harnack, L. An Objective Measure of Nutrition Facts Panel Usage and Nutrient Quality of Food Choice. *J. Nutr. Educ. Behav.* **2014**, *46*, 589–594. [CrossRef] [PubMed]
8. Hersey, J.C.; Wohlgenant, K.C.; Arsenault, J.E.; Kosa, K.M.; Muth, M.K. Effects of front-of-package and shelf nutrition labeling systems on consumers. *Nutr. Rev.* **2013**, *71*, 1–14. [CrossRef]
9. Hawley, K.L.; Roberto, C.A.; Bragg, M.A.; Liu, P.J.; Schwartz, M.B.; Brownell, K.D. The science on front-of-package food labels. *Public Health Nutr.* **2013**, *16*, 430–439. [CrossRef]
10. Kelly, B.; Jewell, J. *What Is the Evidence on the Policy Specifications, Development Processes and Effectiveness of Existing Front-Of-Pack Food Labelling Policies in the WHO European Region*; WHO Regional Office for Europe: Copenhagen, Denmark, 2018.
11. Cecchini, M.; Warin, L. Impact of food labelling systems on food choices and eating behaviours: A systematic review and meta-analysis of randomized studies. *Obes. Rev.* **2016**, *17*, 201–210. [CrossRef]
12. Grunert, K.G.; Wills, J.M. A review of European research on consumer response to nutrition information on food labels. *J. Public Health* **2007**, *15*, 385–399. [CrossRef]
13. Vyth, E.L.; Steenhuis, I.H.; Brandt, H.E.; Roodenburg, A.J.; Brug, J.; Seidell, J.C. Methodological quality of front-of-pack labeling studies: A review plus identification of research challenges. *Nutr. Rev.* **2012**, *70*, 709–720. [CrossRef]
14. Hieke, S.; Taylor, C.R. A Critical Review of the Literature on Nutritional Labeling. *J. Consum. Aff.* **2012**, *46*, 120–156. [CrossRef]
15. Julia, C.; Hercberg, S. Development of a new front-of-pack nutrition label in France: The five-colour Nutri-Score. *Public Health Panor.* **2017**, *3*, 712–725.
16. Maubach, N.; Hoek, J.; Mather, D. Interpretive front-of-pack nutrition labels. Comparing competing recommendations. *Appetite* **2014**, *82*, 67–77. [CrossRef] [PubMed]
17. Méjean, C.; Macouillard, P.; Péneau, S.; Hercberg, S.; Castetbon, K. Perception of front-of-pack labels according to social characteristics, nutritional knowledge and food purchasing habits. *Public Health Nutr.* **2013**, *16*, 392–402. [CrossRef]
18. Méjean, C.; Macouillard, P.; Péneau, S.; Lassale, C.; Hercberg, S.; Castetbon, K. Association of Perception of Front-of-Pack Labels with Dietary, Lifestyle and Health Characteristics. *PLoS ONE* **2014**, *9*, e90971. [CrossRef] [PubMed]
19. Savoie, N.; Barlow, K.; Harvey, K.L.; Binnie, M.A.; Pasut, L. Consumer Perceptions of Front-of-package Labelling Systems and Healthiness of Foods. *Can. J. Public Health* **2013**, *104*, e359–e363. [CrossRef] [PubMed]

20. Emrich, T.E.; Mendoza, J.E.; L'Abbé, M.R. Effectiveness of Front-of-pack nutrition symbols: A pilot study with consumers. *Can. J. Diet. Pract. Res.* **2012**, *73*, 200–203. [CrossRef]
21. Möser, A.; Hoefkens, C.; Van Camp, J.; Verbeke, W. Simplified nutrient labelling: consumers' perceptions in Germany and Belgium. *J. Consum. Prot. Food Saf.* **2010**, *5*, 169–180. [CrossRef]
22. Méjean, C.; Macouillard, P.; Péneau, S.; Hercberg, S.; Castetbon, K. Consumer acceptability and understanding of front-of-pack nutrition labels. *J. Hum. Nutr. Diet.* **2013**, *26*, 494–503. [CrossRef]
23. Gorton, D.; Ni Mhurchu, C.; Chen, M.; Dixon, R. Nutrition labels: A survey of use, understanding and preferences among ethnically diverse shoppers in New Zealand. *Public Health Nutr.* **2008**, *12*, 1359–1365. [CrossRef]
24. Kelly, B.; Hughes, C.; Chapman, K.; Louie, J.C.-Y.; Dixon, H.; Crawford, J.; King, L.; Daube, M.; Slevin, T. Consumer testing of the acceptability and effectiveness of front-of-pack food labelling systems for the Australian grocery market. *Health Promot. Int.* **2009**, *24*, 120–129. [CrossRef] [PubMed]
25. Murphy, M.; Fallows, S.; Bonwick, G. Parents' use and understanding of front-of-pack food labelling, and the impact of socio-economic status. *Proc. Nutr. Soc.* **2008**, *67*, 413. [CrossRef]
26. Pettigrew, S.; Talati, Z.; Miller, C.; Dixon, H.; Kelly, B.; Ball, K. The types and aspects of front-of-pack food labelling schemes preferred by adults and children. *Appetite* **2017**, *109*, 115–123. [CrossRef] [PubMed]
27. Julia, C.; Péneau, S.; Buscail, C.; Gonzalez, R.; Touvier, M.; Hercberg, S.; Kesse-Guyot, E. Perception of different formats of front-of-pack nutrition labels according to sociodemographic, lifestyle and dietary factors in a French population: Cross-sectional study among the NutriNet-Santé cohort participants. *BMJ Open* **2017**, *7*, e016108. [CrossRef] [PubMed]
28. Ducrot, P.; Méjean, C.; Julia, C.; Kesse-Guyot, E.; Touvier, M.; Fezeu, L.; Hercberg, S.; Péneau, S. Effectiveness of front-of-pack nutrition labels in French adults: Results from the NutriNet-Sante cohort study. *PLoS ONE* **2015**, *10*, e0140898. [CrossRef] [PubMed]
29. Babio, N.; Vicent, P.; López, L.; Benito, A.; Basulto, J.; Salas-Salvadó, J. Adolescents' ability to select healthy food using two different front-of-pack food labels: A cross-over study. *Public Health Nutr.* **2014**, *17*, 1403–1409. [CrossRef] [PubMed]
30. Emrich, T.E.; Qi, Y.; Mendoza, J.E.; Lou, W.; Cohen, J.E.; L'Abbé, M.R. Consumer perceptions of the Nutrition Facts table and front-of-pack nutrition rating systems. *Appl. Physiol. Nutr. Metab.* **2013**, *39*, 417–424. [CrossRef] [PubMed]
31. Lowe, B.; de Souza-Monteiro, D.M.; Fraser, I. Nutritional labelling information: Utilisation of new technologies. *J. Mark. Manag.* **2013**, *29*, 1337–1366. [CrossRef]
32. Codex Alimentarius Commission. Proposal for New Work Concerning a Global Standard for Front of Pack Interpretive Nutrition Labelling. Available online: http://www.fao.org/fao-who-codexalimentarius/sh-proxy/en/?lnk=1&url=https%253A%252F%252Fworkspace.fao.org%252Fsites%252Fcodex%252FMeetings%252FCX-714-43%252FCRD%252Ffl43_CRD17x.pdf (accessed on 6 December 2019).
33. Egnell, M.; Talati, Z.; Hercberg, S.; Pettigrew, S.; Julia, C.; Egnell, M.; Talati, Z.; Hercberg, S.; Pettigrew, S.; Julia, C. Objective Understanding of Front-of-Package Nutrition Labels: An International Comparative Experimental Study across 12 Countries. *Nutrients* **2018**, *10*, 1542. [CrossRef] [PubMed]
34. Sutherland, L.A.; Kaley, L.A.; Fischer, L. Guiding Stars: The effect of a nutrition navigation program on consumer purchases at the supermarket. *Am. J. Clin. Nutr.* **2010**, *91*, 1090S–1094S. [CrossRef] [PubMed]
35. Rahkovsky, I.; Lin, B.-H.; Lin, C.-T.J.; Lee, J.-Y. Effects of the Guiding Stars Program on purchases of ready-to-eat cereals with different nutritional attributes. *Food Policy* **2013**, *43*, 100–107. [CrossRef]
36. Sacks, G.; Rayner, M.; Swinburn, B. Impact of front-of-pack 'traffic-light' nutrition labelling on consumer food purchases in the UK. *Health Promot. Int.* **2009**, *24*, 344–352. [CrossRef] [PubMed]
37. Sacks, G.; Tikellis, K.; Millar, L.; Swinburn, B. Impact of 'traffic-light' nutrition information on online food purchases in Australia. *Aust. N. Z. J. Public Health* **2011**, *35*, 122–126. [CrossRef] [PubMed]
38. Newman, C.; Burton, S.; Craig Andrews, J.; Netemeyer, R.; Kees, J. Marketers' Use of Alternative Front-of-Package Nutrition Symbols: An Examination of Effects on Product Evaluations. *J. Acad. Mark. Sci.* **2017**, *46*, 453–476. [CrossRef]
39. Jones, A.; Shahid, M.; Neal, B.; Jones, A.; Shahid, M.; Neal, B. Uptake of Australia's Health Star Rating System. *Nutrients* **2018**, *10*, 997. [CrossRef] [PubMed]

40. Lawrence, M.; Dickie, S.; Woods, J.; Lawrence, M.A.; Dickie, S.; Woods, J.L. Do Nutrient-Based Front-of-Pack Labelling Schemes Support or Undermine Food-Based Dietary Guideline Recommendations? Lessons from the Australian Health Star Rating System. *Nutrients* **2018**, *10*, 32. [CrossRef]
41. Dana, L.M.; Chapman, K.; Talati, Z.; Kelly, B.; Dixon, H.; Miller, C.; Pettigrew, S. Consumers' Views on the Importance of Specific Front-of-Pack Nutrition Information: A Latent Profile Analysis. *Nutrients* **2019**, *11*, 1158. [CrossRef] [PubMed]
42. Miller, L.M.S.; Cassady, D.L. The effects of nutrition knowledge on food label use. A review of the literature. *Appetite* **2015**, *92*, 207–216. [CrossRef]
43. Sanlier, N.; Karakus, S.S. Evaluation of food purchasing behaviour of consumers from supermarkets. *Br. Food J.* **2010**, *112*, 140–150. [CrossRef]

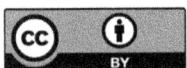

© 2019 by the authors. Licensee MDPI, Basel, Switzerland. This article is an open access article distributed under the terms and conditions of the Creative Commons Attribution (CC BY) license (http://creativecommons.org/licenses/by/4.0/).

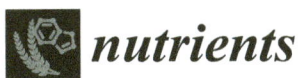 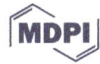

Article

Consumers' Responses to Front-of-Pack Nutrition Labelling: Results from a Sample from The Netherlands

Manon Egnell [1,*], Zenobia Talati [2], Marion Gombaud [1], Pilar Galan [1], Serge Hercberg [1,3], Simone Pettigrew [4,†], and Chantal Julia [1,3,†]

1. Nutritional Epidemiology Research Team (EREN), Sorbonne Paris Cité Epidemiology and Statistics Research Center (CRESS), U1153 Inserm, U1125 Inra, Cnam, Paris 13 University, 93000 Bobigny, France
2. School of Psychology, Curtin University, Kent St, Bentley, WA 6102, Australia
3. Public Health Department, Avicenne Hospital, AP-HP, 93000 Bobigny, France
4. The George Institute for Global Health, Sydney, NSW 2042, Australia
* Correspondence: m.egnell@eren.smbh.univ-paris13.fr
† These authors contributed equally to this work.

Received: 16 July 2019; Accepted: 2 August 2019; Published: 6 August 2019

Abstract: Front-of-pack labels (FoPLs) are efficient tools for helping consumers identify healthier food products. Although discussions on nutritional labelling are currently ongoing in Europe, few studies have compared the effectiveness of FoPLs in European countries, including the Netherlands. This study aimed to compare five FoPLs among Dutch participants (the Health Star Rating (HSR) system, Multiple Traffic Lights (MTL), Nutri-Score, Reference Intakes (RIs), and Warning symbols) in terms of perception and understanding of the labels and food choices. In 2019, 1032 Dutch consumers were recruited and asked to select one product from among a set of three foods with different nutritional profiles, and then rank the products within the sets according to their nutritional quality. These tasks were performed with no label and then with one of the five FoPLs on the package, depending on the randomization arm. Finally, participants were questioned on their perceptions regarding the label to which they were exposed. Regarding perceptions, all FoPLs were favorably perceived but with only marginal differences between FoPLs. While no significant difference across labels was observed for food choices, the Nutri-Score demonstrated the highest overall performance in helping consumers rank the products according to their nutritional quality.

Keywords: nutritional labelling; food choices; comprehension; perception; Dutch consumers; food policies

---

1. Introduction

Front-of-pack labels (FoPLs) have been identified as a promising strategy to help consumers make healthier food choices at the point of purchase [1–3] and encourage manufacturers to improve the nutritional composition of their products [4,5]. Notably, the implementation of FoPLs has been recommended by the World Health Organization as a 'best-buy' measure to help prevent non-communicable diseases [6]. Given their potential to change consumer food choice architecture, by providing readily interpreted nutritional information, the provision of FoPLs has been identified as an effective nudging strategy [7]. However, the multiplicity of existing schemes, potentially in the same market, may increase confusion among consumers [8]. More specifically in the European Union (EU), according to the regulation, FoPLs may only be voluntary, meaning multiple schemes may coexist [9]. In this context, a request for harmonization at the EU level has prompted new discussions by the EU commission since 2018 to modify the existing regulation [10]. Similar political discussions pertaining to the objectives and principles of FoPLs have been included within a Codex Alimentarius e-working group, highlighting government interest in this area [11]. Some European countries have already implemented FoPLs as part of national nutrition prevention programs. Examples of these FoPLs include the Green Keyhole in the Nordic countries since the 1980s [12], the Multiple Traffic Lights (MTL) in the United Kingdom since 2004 [13], the Reference Intakes label (RIs) implemented in 2006 following a voluntary initiative from manufacturers [14], and more recently, the Nutri-Score in France since 2017, and then in Belgium and Spain in 2018 [15]. Other FoPLs have been proposed in recent years, including the Evolved Nutrition Label by a consortium of manufacturers [16], the nutritional circles label proposed by the leading association of the German food sector BLL (*Bund für Lebensmittelrecht und Lebensmittelkunde*), or the battery system proposed by the Italian government. These latter schemes have not been validated by scientific evidence.

Discussions are still on-going in several European countries as to the most efficient FoPL for their population. In the Netherlands, the 'Choices' system was in place between 2006 and 2016. Initially developed by food manufacturers, and then endorsed by the government, this scheme was abandoned following a request from consumers, as it led to confusion as to the ranking of some foods [17]. Recently, the Dutch government announced the possible introduction of a new FoPL in the Netherlands, and noted that further research should be conducted to identify which labels would perform the best for Dutch consumers [18].

Studies investigating consumer responses to different types of FoPLs have explored various dimensions of intrinsic qualities, such as perceptions, understanding, and/or choice. In this context, Grunert et al. proposed a theoretical framework defining the different steps of FoPL use from perception to use in purchasing situations [19]. Although examining each of these elements provides a clearer picture of consumer reactions to different types of FoPLs, the relative contribution of each of these dimensions to help select an effective scheme varies and requires further investigation. Studies investigating perceptions suggest that FoPLs are generally favorably perceived in the population. However, while positive attitudes for a given system are likely to be required for a scheme to be efficient, there may be a discrepancy between consumer preferences and actual performance of the scheme. Indeed, consumers, and especially those with a higher educational level, tend to prefer schemes providing a larger amount of information, although they may not be able to process this information in purchasing situations where decisions are made in very short time frame [20–23]. Objective understanding, defined as the capacity of consumers to understand the information provided by the label in the way that is intended by its designers [19], is usually tested through ranking tasks, in which consumers are exposed to products displaying a FoPL on the pack and are required to rank their relative healthiness compared to a condition with no label. Studies tend to suggest that this type of measure may show a more contrasted performance across FoPLs, thereby providing a better discrimination across different schemes. Studies investigating consumer choices following exposure to FoPLs have shown contrasting results, depending in particular on the type of method that was used (choice task, virtual/experimental supermarket, or in-store study) [24–36]. Globally, the results of these studies suggest that the effect of FoPLs on consumer choices may be of low magnitude, as consumer purchases are guided by a host of influences, of which nutrition may only be one of several drivers, including price and promotion in particular. However, at the population level, such effects would lead to a substantial impact in terms of public health, contributing to the reduction of the nutrition-related disease burden [37].

The aim of the present study was to assess consumer responses to different FoPLs currently implemented in different countries in the world, in a Dutch sample using the methodology of the FOP-ICE study; an international experimental study comparing the effectiveness of various FoPLs in 12 countries [38]. The effectiveness of five front-of-pack nutrition labels corresponding to different types of FoPL formats—Health Star Rating system, Multiple Traffic Lights, Nutri-Score, Reference Intakes, and Warning symbols—was investigated through the three following dimensions: perception, objective understanding, and food choices.

2. Materials and Methods

2.1. Population Study and Individual Characteristics

Participants were recruited in the Netherlands by a web panel provider (Pureprofile), applying quotas for sex (50% women), age (one third in each of the following categories: 18–30 years, 31–50 years, over 51 years), and yearly household income (one third in each of the following categories: low (<13,962 €), medium (13,962 €–28,135 €), and high (>28,135 €)). In the online questionnaire, individuals were first asked to provide information on socio-demographic, lifestyle, and nutrition-related characteristics, including sex, age, monthly household income, educational level, involvement in grocery shopping, self-estimated diet quality, and self-estimated level of knowledge in nutrition. Individuals were also asked to declare the frequency purchasing the tested food categories (pizzas, cakes, and breakfast cereals, with response options as "always", "often", "sometimes", and "never"). Those who responded "never" to at least two of the three food categories were ineligible to participate.

The protocol of the study (similar to the FOP-ICE study) was approved by the Institutional Review Board of the French Institute for Health and Medical Research (IRB Inserm n°17-404 and 17-404 bis) and the Curtin University Human Research Ethics Committee (approval reference: HRE2017-0760). At the beginning of the survey, participants were invited to give their electronic consent.

2.2. Stimuli and Front-of-Pack Nutrition Labels

Three food categories (pizzas, cakes, and breakfast cereals) were selected according to two criteria [38]: (1) commonly available in Dutch supermarkets, and (2) contain products with wide variability in nutritional quality. In each food category, a set of three products with distinct nutrient profiles (higher, medium, and lower nutritional quality) was created, allowing a ranking of products according to their nutritional quality. In order to avoid potential bias on product evaluation (e.g., familiarity, habit), mock packages representing a fictional brand ("Stofer") were developed.

Five FoPLs were tested in the present study (Figure 1), including both nutrient-specific and summary schemes. The nutrient-specific labels were: (1) the Multiple Traffic Lights (implemented in the United Kingdom in 2004), indicating the amounts of energy, fat, saturated fat, sugar, and salt, with a color (green, amber, red) depending on the amount; (2) the Reference Intakes, a monochromatic label displaying the amounts of the same nutrients; and (3) the Warning symbol (implemented in Chile in 2016), advising when the level of a given nutrient exceeds what is considered a healthy amount. Summary FoPLs included: (1) the Nutri-Score, a graded scale of five colors from dark green (associated with the letter A) to dark orange (associated with the letter E), characterizing the overall nutritional quality of the food or beverage and (2) the Health Star Rating system (implemented in Australia and New Zealand in 2014), using a graded scale of stars combined with information on nutrient amounts.

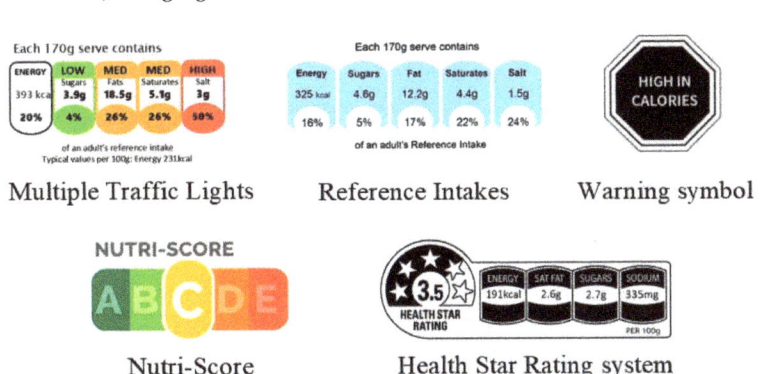

Figure 1. Front-of-pack nutrition labels tested in the present study.

2.3. Procedure

Participants were invited to respond to the online questionnaire that was presented in Dutch. Following the sociodemographic, lifestyle, and nutrition-related questions, participants were asked to complete the choice and understanding tasks, and then answer questions about their perceptions of the FoPL to which they had been assigned.

Given that the first steps of the theoretical framework of FoPL use (perception and understanding) may influence the following step (food choices), the order of the dimensions was reversed in the experiment, starting with choice, followed by understanding and finally perception. First, for each food category, participants were asked to select the product they would be most likely to purchase without any FoPL shown on the mock packages. An "I wouldn't buy any of these products" option was also available. After the choice task, participants were invited to rank the set of three products according to their nutritional quality (1—highest nutritional quality, 2—medium nutritional quality, and 3—lowest nutritional quality), with an "I don't know" option also available and no FoPL on packages. Choice and ranking tasks were completed sequentially for the three food categories. Participants were then randomized to one of the five FoPLs and then invited to fulfill the same tasks, but this time with the assigned FoPL affixed to the mock packages. An example of the choice and ranking tasks for the pizza category is presented in Figure 2.

Participants were then invited to respond to questions about their perceptions on the FoPLs. Various dimensions were assessed including liking (e.g., "I like this label"), awareness (e.g., "this label stands out"), and perceived cognitive workload (e.g., "this label is easy to understand"). For each question, participants provided their responses on a 9-point Likert scale ranging from "strongly disagree" to "strongly agree".

2.4. Statistical Analyses

2.4.1. Food Choice

For the choice analyses, +1 point was attributed when the lowest nutritional quality product was selected by the participant, +2 points for the medium nutritional quality product and +3 points for the highest nutritional quality product, first for the no labelling condition and then for the FoPL condition. Hence, for each food category, a score was computed using the difference of points between the two conditions, resulting in a discrete continuous score ranging from −2 to +2 points. A global score was finally calculated by summing the score of each category, resulting in a final score between −6 and +6 points. The percentage of participants who deteriorated or improved in their food choices between the no label and FoPL conditions was calculated for each FoPL group by food category. An ordinal logistic regression model was conducted to measure the association between the choice score and FoPL type. Only participants selecting a product in both the no label and FoPL conditions were included in the analyses.

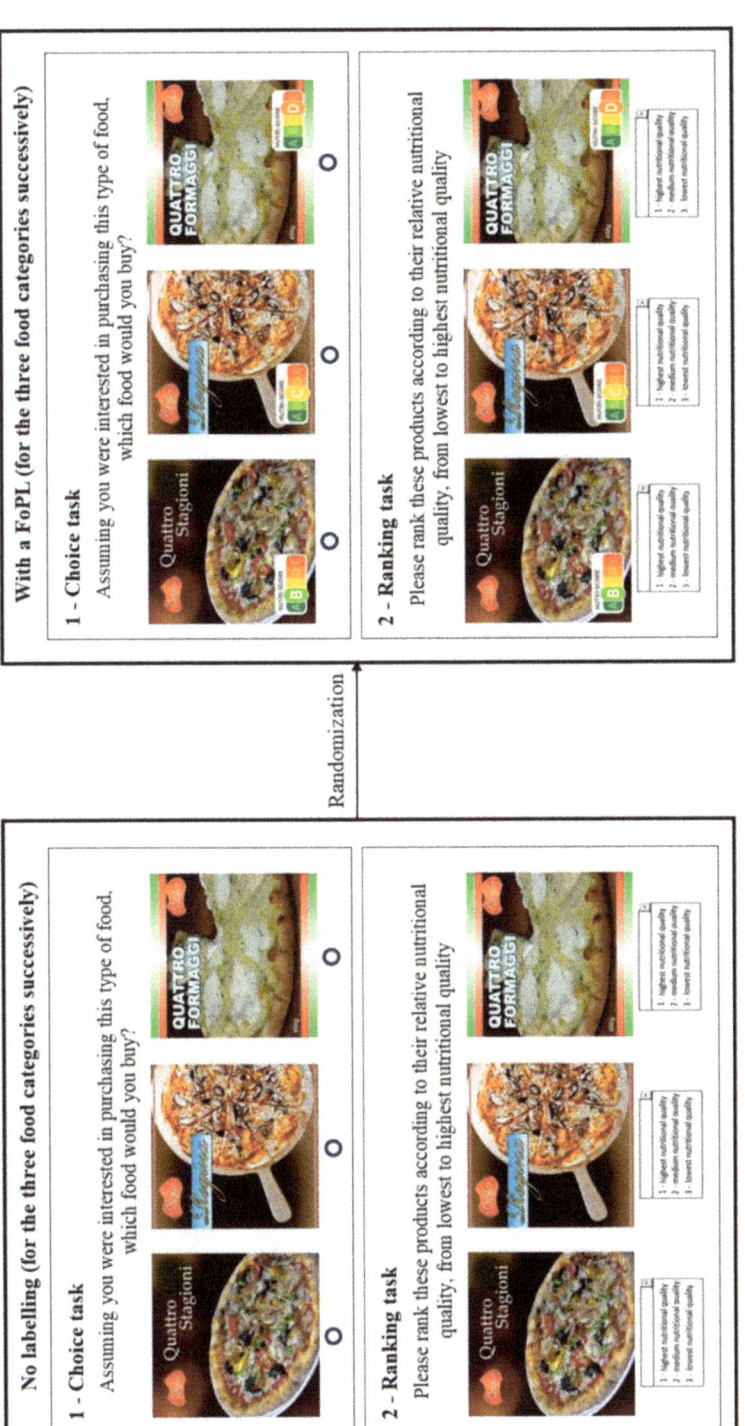

Figure 2. Procedure of the choice and ranking tasks for the pizza category.

2.4.2. Objective Understanding

Objective understanding of the FoPLs by consumers was assessed by the ability of participants to correctly rank the sets of products according to nutritional quality. A response was considered correct when the three products in the set were correctly ranked, leading to a +1 point score for the category. One error (or more) in the ranking task resulted in a −1 point score, while 0 points were attributed when participants selected the "I don't know" answer. Thus, for each food category, a score for ranking ability was calculated using the difference in the number of points between the no label and FoPL conditions, ranging from −2 to +2 points, and leading to a global score of between −6 and +6 points for the three food categories combined. The percentage of correct answers in the no labelling and FoPL conditions was calculated by FoPL type and food category. An ordinal logistic regression model was performed to measure the association between the understanding score and FoPL type.

For the choice and understanding analyses, models were adjusted for individual characteristics including sex, age, level of household monthly income, educational level, involvement in grocery shopping, self-estimated diet quality, and nutrition knowledge, and finally on the response to the question "did you see this label during the survey?". The reference of the models for the FoPL categorical variable was the Reference Intakes label. Interactions between FoPLs and individual characteristics were tested, and stratified analyses were performed when the p-value of the interaction term was ≤0.10.

2.4.3. Perception

The responses for the assessed perception aspects were characterized for each label by using means and standard deviations. To investigate the contribution of the different questions to the overall perception of FoPLs, principal component analysis was performed. Active variables were "this label is confusing", "I like this label", "this label does not stand out", "this label is easy to understand", "this label takes too long to understand", "this label provides me the information I need", and "I trust this label". Dimensions, corresponding to a linear combination of active variables, have an eigenvalue reflecting the total variance explained by the dimension. The number of retained dimensions was chosen to obtain a cumulative percentage of acceptable variance. In the present study, only the first two dimensions were selected, simplifying the presentation. The contribution and coordinates of each active variable on each axis were computed, indicating how variables contribute to dimensions, and to what extent. The label was considered as a qualitative supplementary variable (not used to compute the dimensions, but mapped on the existing axes). Due to the combination of positive and negative framing of the perception questions, participants who provided the same answers to all perception questions were excluded from the analyses, except those consistently giving a score of five, which indicates a neutral perception.

All analyses in the present study were conducted on SAS statistical software (PROC LOGISTIC, PROC PRINCOMP). Statistical tests were two-sided and a p-value ≤ 0.05 was considered statistically significant.

3. Results

3.1. Description of the Sample

Individual characteristics of the study sample are described in Table 1. The present study included 1032 Dutch participants, with 50% women, 33% over 51 years, 32% with a primary or secondary educational level, and 34% with a low household monthly income. Among all participants, 72% were responsible for grocery shopping, 11% had a very or mostly unhealthy diet quality, and 16% had no or little knowledge about nutrition.

Table 1. Individual characteristics of the study sample from Netherlands (N = 1032).

	N	%
Sex		
Men	517	50.1
Women	515	49.9
Age, years		
18–30	345	33.43
31–50	343	33.24
≥ 51	344	33.33
Educational level		
Primary education	13	1.26
Secondary education	314	30.43
Trade certificate	277	26.84
University, undergraduate degree	329	31.88
University postgraduate degree	99	9.59
Level of household monthly income		
High	342	33.14
Medium	343	33.24
Low	347	33.62
Responsible for grocery shopping		
Yes	746	72.29
No	55	5.33
Share job equally	231	22.38
Self-estimated diet quality		
I eat a very unhealthy diet	8	0.78
I eat a mostly unhealthy diet	102	9.88
I eat a mostly healthy diet	865	83.82
I eat a very healthy diet	57	5.52
Nutrition knowledge		
I do not know anything about nutrition	7	0.68
I am not very knowledgeable about nutrition	157	15.21
I am somewhat knowledgeable about nutrition	744	72.09
I am very knowledgeable about nutrition	124	12.02
Did you see the FOP label during the survey?		
No	293	28.39
Unsure	133	12.89
Yes	606	58.72
Participants who recalled seeing the FoPL they were exposed to		
HSR	111	53.62
MTL	135	65.53
Nutri-Score	147	71.36
RIs label	136	53.88
Warning symbol	77	37.20

HSR: Health Star Rating system; MTL: Multiple Traffic Lights; RIs: Reference Intakes.

3.2. Food Choices

The percentage of participants who modified their food choices between the no label and FoPL conditions is described in Figure S1. While within each food category and for all five FoPLs, a large number of participants did not change their choice between the two conditions (between 50% to 63% depending on the food category and the FoPL), or did not select any product (between 22% to 41% depending on the food category and the FoPL), significant modifications in choices occurred in the pizza and cake categories (overall p-value for the Bowker disagreement test = 0.0008 and 0.0001, respectively). Among participants who modified their food choices, a higher percentage demonstrated an improvement in the nutritional quality of their choices (between 2.9% and 10.7% depending on the label and the food category) compared to those demonstrating deterioration (between 2.9% and 5.8% depending on the label and the food category), with similar results found for the five individual labels.

Results of the associations between FoPLs and food choices are displayed in Table 2. Compared to the RIs, no significant association was found between FoPLs and the change in nutritional quality of food choices, overall and by food category, except for the Warning symbol. Exposure to the Warning symbol encouraged participants to select a healthier breakfast cereal.

Table 2. Associations between front-of-pack label type and change in nutritional quality of food choices by food category (N = 1032).

Food Category	N	HSR		MTL		Nutri-Score		Warning Symbol	
		OR (95% CI)	p	OR (95% CI)	p	OR (95% CI)	p	OR (95% CI)	p
All categories	898	1.21 [0.76–1.94]	0.4	0.94 [0.59–1.51]	0.8	1.10 [0.69–1.75]	0.7	1.32 [0.82–2.13]	0.3
Pizzas	692	1.11 [0.58–2.10]	0.8	0.85 [0.45–1.64]	0.6	0.76 [0.40–1.44]	0.4	0.88 [0.45–1.73]	0.7
Cakes	744	0.81 [0.44–1.49]	0.5	0.90 [0.50–1.63]	0.7	1.10 [0.61–1.98]	0.7	0.93 [0.50–1.71]	0.8
Breakfast cereals	643	1.72 [0.84–3.50]	0.1	0.93 [0.46–1.88]	0.8	1.77 [0.87–3.60]	0.1	2.99 [1.45–6.21]	0.003

The reference of the multivariate ordinal logistic regression for the categorical variable 'label' was the Reference Intakes. The multivariate model was adjusted for sex, age, educational level, level of income, responsibility for grocery shopping, self-estimated diet quality, self-estimated nutrition knowledge level, and "did you see this label during the online survey?" HSR: Health Star Rating system; MTL: Multiple Traffic Lights; OR: Odds Ratio; CI: Confidence Interval. Bold values correspond to significant results (p-value ≤ 0.05).

3.3. Objective Understanding

The percentage of correct answers in the nutritional quality ranking task and the improvement between the no label and FoPL conditions are presented (according to FoPL type and food category) in Figure S2. Across all three food categories, the Nutri-Score produced the largest improvement in the percentage of correct answers compared to no label, followed by the MTL. For the other FoPLs, results differed depending on the food category. The associations between FoPL type and the ability to correctly rank products are presented in Table 3, with the RIs label as reference in the models. Overall, the Nutri-Score was the only FoPL to significantly improve participants' ability to correctly rank products according to their nutritional quality compared to the RIs (odds ratio (OR) = 3.60 [2.48–5.24] (p-value < 0.0001)), while the other FoPLs did not show any significant results. Similar results were found for the three food categories, except for cakes where the Warning symbol (OR = 2.10 [1.32–3.34], p-value = 0.002) and MTL (OR = 1.66 [1.05–2.62], p-value = 0.03) also significantly improved the ranking ability of participants compared to the RIs, but Nutri-Score remained the label with the highest performance for cakes as well (OR = 4.52 [2.89–7.06], p-value < 0.0001).

Table 3. Associations between FoPLs and the ability to correctly rank products according to nutritional quality by food category (N = 1032).

Food Category	N	HSR		MTL		Nutri-Score		Warning Symbol	
		OR (95% CI)	p	OR (95% CI)	p	OR (95% CI)	p	OR (95% CI)	p
All categories	1032	1.20 [0.82–1.75]	0.3	1.31 [0.90–1.90]	0.2	3.60 [2.48–5.24]	<0.0001	1.23 [0.84–1.81]	0.3
Pizzas	972	1.37 [0.85–2.21]	0.2	1.17 [0.73–1.88]	0.5	2.12 [1.34–3.37]	0.001	1.00 [0.62–1.62]	1.0
Cakes	1019	1.42 [0.89–2.24]	0.1	1.66 [1.05–2.62]	0.03	4.52 [2.89–7.06]	<0.0001	2.10 [1.32–3.34]	0.002
Breakfast cereals	931	0.90 [0.56–1.47]	0.7	1.00 [0.62–1.62]	1.0	2.66 [1.68–4.21]	<0.0001	0.85 [0.52–1.39]	0.5

The reference of the multivariate ordinal logistic regression for the categorical variable 'label' was the Reference Intakes. The multivariate model was adjusted for sex, age, educational level, level of income, responsibility for grocery shopping, self-estimated diet quality, self-estimated nutrition knowledge level, and "did you see this label during the online survey?" HSR: Health Star Rating system; MTL: Multiple Traffic Lights; OR: Odds Ratio; CI: Confidence Interval. Bold values correspond to significant results (p-value ≤ 0.05).

In sensitivity analyses where respondents who answered "I don't know" were not included, similar trends were observed, though with even higher magnitudes of the effect of FoPLs (Table S1).

No significant interaction with individual characteristics was found, except with sex. However, the interaction was quantitative.

3.4. Perception

The average scores for all perception questions are displayed in Figure S3. Overall, homogeneous results were observed between FoPLs on the various items that were investigated. From principal component analysis, two main dimensions were identified, explaining 44.8% and 21.1% of the total variance, respectively. The contribution values and coordinates of active variables on these two dimensions are displayed in Table 4. The first dimension (horizontal axis) was a linear combination of the responses to the following items: "this label is easy to understand" and "this label provides me the information I need" (which were positively associated with the first dimension), and "this label is confusing" and "this label takes too long to understand" (which were negatively associated with this dimension). The second dimension (vertical axis) was a linear combination of the responses to the following items: "this label takes too long to understand", "this label does not stand out", and "I like this label", which were positively associated with this dimension.

Table 4. Contributions and coordinates of active variables on the two dimensions from the principal component analysis.

Questions	Contributions		Coordinates	
	Dimension 1	Dimension 2	Dimension 1	Dimension 2
This label is confusing	19.59	12.88	−1.65	0.92
I like this label	10.40	18.14	1.20	1.09
This label does not stand out	7.09	20.36	−0.99	1.15
This label is easy to understand	18.51	2.03	1.61	0.36
This label takes too long to understand	15.06	22.64	−1.45	1.22
This label provides me the information I need	16.58	13.28	1.52	0.93
I trust this label	12.76	10.66	1.33	0.84
HSR	-	-	−0.22	0.16
MTL	-	-	0.38	0.44
Nutri-Score	-	-	0.04	−0.43
RIs label	-	-	−0.05	0.32
Warning symbol	-	-	−0.15	−0.49

Labels do not have contribution values given that they were considered as qualitative supplementary variables and were thus not used to compute the dimensions.

When the label was mapped on the two axes as an illustrative variable, the graphic in Figure 3 was obtained. Differences between the FoPLs on the two dimensions appeared to be of very low magnitude (the position on the dimensions was between −0.5 and +0.5), although the MTL appeared opposed to the Nutri-Score and the Warning symbol on the second dimension. The MTL therefore appeared to somewhat be the preferred label, but compared to the Nutri-Score and Warning symbol, the MTL took too long to understand and did not stand out.

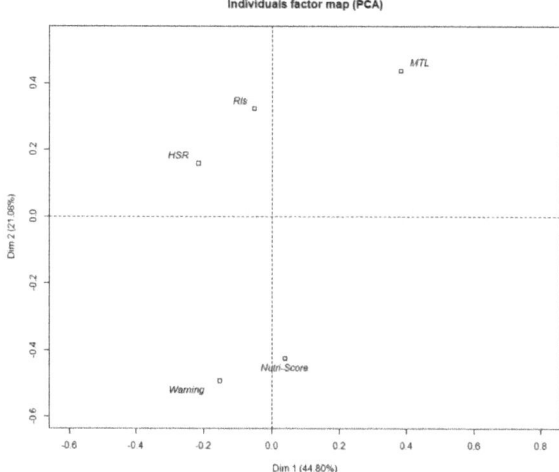

Figure 3. Principal component analysis map showing projection of the labels on the two axes.

4. Discussion

While no significant discrimination across FOPLs was observed in terms of perceptions and effect on food choices, the analyses of objective understanding of the labels showed significant differences across schemes. The Nutri-Score demonstrated the highest performance compared to the Reference Intakes in helping Dutch consumers identify and rank the nutritional quality of foods. The other FoPLs did not show any significant effects compared to the RIs except the MTL and Warning symbol for cake products, but to lesser extents. These results, specific to Dutch consumers, are consistent with the findings of the FOP-ICE study, where stronger overall performance of the Nutri-Score was observed for participants' ability to correctly rank the nutritional quality of products in all countries, including the following European countries: Bulgaria, Denmark, France, Germany, Spain, and the United Kingdom [38–40].

The analyses exploring consumers' perceptions of the FoPLs showed that all five FoPLs were favorably perceived. While variations across participants were substantial on the two dimensions of the principal component analysis, the differences by FoPL type were much smaller in magnitude. Moreover, familiarity appeared to influence perceptions, as RIs—that have been implemented as front-of-pack labels on the majority of food products worldwide since 2006—appeared to be appreciated by consumers compared to other labels. Finally, labels providing more accurate information (nutrient-based approaches with numerical information) appeared to be considered somewhat more trustworthy, especially among individuals with higher educational level or substantial knowledge, according to the literature, although they were less salient and entailed a higher cognitive workload [21–23,41]. The limited ability of studying perception to discriminate across labels might be related to the inter-subject approach used in this study (each participant was exposed to one FoPL only), while an intra-subject approach may have yielded more contrasted results (all participants exposed to all FoPLs).

Most previous studies investigating the effects of FoPLs on food choices have focused on the MTL or the RIs and their variants, and have yielded somewhat mixed results. The findings of these studies have typically shown that the RIs have no or limited effect on food choices [35,42–44], whereas the more interpretive MTL can help guide consumers towards healthier foods [26,28,33,35,45,46]. Few studies have investigated more recent schemes, including the Warning symbol, the HSR, and the Nutri-Score, and even fewer in a comparative design, though the results to date in studies using choice sets or experimental design in supermarkets have suggested that these interpretive labels can have a positive effect on the nutritional quality of food choices [30,32,35,42,44,47–49]. A recent study observed a significant improvement in the nutritional quality of food choices associated with the use of a warning label, while no results were observed for the other tested labels (MTL, HSR, and Nutri-Score); nevertheless larger sets (20 products) were used compared to our study, allowing capture of the differences for some labels [50]. Results of studies using choice sets, as in our study, appear to be influenced by the categories of products selected [49], as well as the size and types of products within the choice set [24]. When the effects of FoPLs were investigated in studies assessing purchasing outcomes, the Nutri-Score appeared to have a significant impact [30,32,47,48], while results were contrasted for other labels [27,34,47,51–57]. The non-significant effects observed on food choice in the present study could be related first to the use of mock packages featuring a fictional brand differing from a real world setting, and second to the type of methodology that was used. Indeed, even if the experimental design allowed control over potential confounding factors and other purchasing determinants, the choice tasks focused on three products from three food categories only, which limits the magnitude of the effects that could be observed compared to studies measuring the overall shopping cart. However, in our case the number of sets and products within the sets had to remain limited given that three dimensions were investigated in the same survey and the questionnaire could not be too long for participants to complete. In addition, choice and ranking tasks were performed on the same sets and included three products only. Indeed, the ranking of products according to nutritional quality had to be similar regardless of the FoPL used, and the higher the number of products within the set, the harder it is to achieve. The balance between the number of products for each task and overall simplicity for participants was carefully considered. Finally, the results could have been impacted by familiarity with and purchasing habits for the food categories used in the study. However, this bias was minimized first by the use of fictional products and a fictional brand, and second by the fact that participants who declared having never purchased one of the food categories were excluded from the analyses on that specific food category.

Our results on consumer understanding confirmed that interpretive systems, and in particular color-coded FoPLs, have greater potential than purely informative systems to improve the capacity of Dutch consumers to correctly rank the nutritional quality of foods. In our study, compared to the RIs, the Nutri-Score outperformed the other FoPLs in improving consumers' ability to correctly rank products according to nutritional quality. These findings are consistent with the results of studies conducted in Uruguay [42,58], Australia [59], and other European countries [38–40,60]. Summary indicators have been demonstrated to be easier to understand by consumers [43,60,61], whereas nutrient-specific labels require greater cognitive workload. Color-coding, using in particular the green/red scale, provides an easy-to-interpret signal, associated with 'stop' and 'go' signals [62], and has been shown to increase attentional capture [58,63]. Moreover, from a biological perspective, red and green are immediately discerned and discriminated by the human eye [64]. Thus, a FoPL combining both summary and color-coded features, such as the Nutri-Score, is associated with a better objective understanding by consumers [38,60,65].

Another interesting issue raised by our results is the relative contribution of the different dimensions (and studies thereof) developed to characterize FoPLs and to compare the efficiency of different models. Overall, this study provides useful information on the relative contribution of each type of dimension to policy-makers in the selection of a FoPL. Consumers' perceptions of FoPLs suggest that all types of labels are considered acceptable by consumers, with a limited discrimination across schemes, especially when using an inter-subject approach. Of greater concern is the finding of discrepancies between label preferences and performance, with the Nutri-Score displaying significantly higher performance on objective understanding compared to the other labels, while at the same time being perceived as less reliable by Dutch participants. By contrast, FoPLs considered more trustworthy and useful (RIs in particular), did not significantly improve the ability of participants to correctly rank the nutritional quality of products. This finding suggests that performance studies relying on the testing of consumer understanding may be one of the most important study types, allowing discrimination across label types, and therefore helping policy-makers in decision-making. Finally, results on choice suggest that FoPLs may yield limited effects on consumer choices, but that the results are highly dependent on the type of study that is performed, and in particular on the choice set and task consumers are asked to perform. Studies involving experimental conditions mimicking real-life purchases with a high number of choices and high variability in the nutritional quality of the foods offered may provide more contrasted results across labels and would be also one of the most important potential effects of FoPLs to investigate.

Strengths of our study include the participation of a large number of Dutch consumers from various sociodemographic groups, the investigation of multiple dimensions of FoPL effectiveness, and the comparison across multiple types of FoPL schemes using a randomized approach. A potential learning effect was also avoided by using a randomization of the presentation order within the sets and across food categories. Nevertheless, some limitations need to be acknowledged. First, Dutch participants were recruited online using set quotas, rather than attempting to generate a population representative sample, which requires caution regarding the extrapolation of the results. Moreover, although we were able to take into account several aspects of socio-cultural background, we did not include information on ethnicity, while it may affect consumer responses to FoPLs. Second, as participants were blinded to the hypotheses, no information was provided as to the objective or meaning of the FoPL to which they were exposed. While this reduced priming, it may have led to less favorable perceptions of less familiar FoPLs and to an underestimation of the labels' effects. Moreover, participants did not have access to the nutritional composition of the products used in the study, which differs from real-life situations and might have led to fewer correct responses in the no label condition in the understanding task compared to what would occur in real life settings. However, this limitation applied equally to all FoPLs included in the study. Finally, participants were randomized to one FoPL, which led to an inter-subject comparison of the effects of FoPLs. Combining intra- and inter-subject approaches may yield more contrasted results across FoPLs, as shown in earlier studies [20,22,41,60].

To conclude, it is of major importance to investigate various dimensions of effectiveness before implementing a FoPL in a country; however, all dimensions do not necessarily have the ability to discriminate FoPL performance. It is important to note that even if a FoPL is favorably perceived and liked by consumers, it does not guarantee that it will be well understood and used to inform food choices. Thus, before selecting a FoPL, it appears essential to investigate consumers' ability to understand and use various schemes, as this ability constitutes an essential step for a label to be effective in influencing food purchases and consumption. Among the different label types tested in the study, the Nutri-Score appears to be a valid alternative to help Dutch consumers identify and rank the nutritional quality of food products.

Supplementary Materials: The following are available online at http://www.mdpi.com/2072-6643/11/8/1817/s1, Table S1: Associations between FoPLs and the ability to correctly rank products according to nutritional quality by food category: sensitivity analyses (N = 1032); Figure S1: Percentage of participants that deteriorated or improved their food choices between the two labelling situations, by food category and FoPL; Figure S2: Percentage of correct answers for the ranking tasks, by food category and FoPL; Figure S3: Average scores with standard deviation of perception questions by FoPL.

Author Contributions: M.E. performed data analyses and interpretation, drafted and revised the paper. C.J. and S.P. conceptualized the project in collaboration with S.H. and Z.T., supervised the data analyses and interpretation, participated in the writing, and critically revised the paper for important intellectual content. C.J. is the guarantor. S.H., Z.T., P.G. and M.G. interpreted the data and critically revised the paper for important intellectual content. All authors had full access to all of the data in the study and can take responsibility for the integrity of the data and the accuracy of the data analysis. All authors have read and approved the final manuscript.

Acknowledgments: The authors would like to thank Mark Orange for creating the mock packages, and all researchers and doctoral students who tested the online survey. We also would like to thank Stefanie Vandevijvere for the Dutch translation of the online survey. The present study received funding from Santé Publique France (French Agency for Public Health).

Conflicts of Interest: The authors declare no conflict of interest.

References

1. World Health Organization. *Global Strategy on Diet, Physical Activity and Health*; WHO: Geneva, Switzerland, 2004; pp. 2–8.
2. Organisation for Economic Co-operation and Development. *Promoting Sustainable Consumption—Good Practices in OECD Countries*; Organisation for Economic Co-operation and Development: Paris, France, 2008.
3. Kleef, E.V.; Dagevos, H. The growing role of front-of-pack nutrition profile labeling: A consumer perspective on key issues and controversies. *Crit. Rev. Food Sci. Nutr.* **2015**, *55*, 291–303. [CrossRef] [PubMed]
4. Vyth, E.L.; Steenhuis, I.H.; Roodenburg, A.J.; Brug, J.; Seidell, J.C. Front-of-pack nutrition label stimulates healthier product development: A quantitative analysis. *Int. J. Behav. Nutr. Phys. Act.* **2010**, *7*, 65. [CrossRef] [PubMed]
5. Ni Mhurchu, C.; Eyles, H.; Choi, Y.-H. Effects of a Voluntary Front-of-Pack Nutrition Labelling System on Packaged Food Reformulation: The Health Star Rating System in New Zealand. *Nutrients* **2017**, *9*, 918. [CrossRef] [PubMed]
6. World Health Organization. *NCDs Tackling NCDs*; World Health Organization: Geneva, Switzerland, 2017; Available online: http://www.who.int/ncds/management/best-buys/en/ (accessed on 9 July 2019).
7. Scrinis, G.; Parker, C. Front-of-Pack Food Labeling and the Politics of Nutritional Nudges. *Law Policy* **2016**, *38*, 234–249. [CrossRef]
8. Draper, A.K.; Adamson, A.J.; Clegg, S.; Malam, S.; Rigg, M.; Duncan, S. Front-of-pack nutrition labelling: Are multiple formats a problem for consumers? *Eur. J. Public Health* **2013**, *23*, 517–521. [CrossRef] [PubMed]
9. Europa Summary of EU legislation. *Labeling of Foodstuffs. Regulation (EU) No. 1169/2011*; European Union: Brussels, Belgium, 2012.
10. Goiana-da-Silva, F.; Cruz-E-Silva, D.; Miraldo, M.; Calhau, C.; Bento, A.; Cruz, D.; Almeida, F.; Darzi, A.; Araújo, F. Front-of-pack labelling policies and the need for guidance. *Lancet Public Health* **2019**, *4*, e15. [CrossRef]
11. Thow, A.M.; Jones, A.; Schneider, C.H.; Labonté, R. Global Governance of Front-of-Pack Nutrition Labelling: A Qualitative Analysis. *Nutrients* **2019**, *11*, 268. [CrossRef]
12. Asp, N.-G. Bryngelsson Susanne Health claims in the labelling and marketing of food products: The Swedish food sector's Code of Practice in a European perspective. *Scand. J. Food Nutr.* **2007**, *15*, 107–126. [CrossRef]
13. Food Standard Agency. *Front-of-Pack Traffic Light Signpost Labelling Technical Guidance*; Food Standard Agency: Kingsway, UK, 2007; pp. 2–12.
14. Food and Drink Federation. *Reference Intakes (Previously Guideline Daily Amounts)*; Food and Drink Federation: London, UK, 2017.
15. Arrêté du 31 Octobre 2017 Fixant la Forme de Présentation Complémentaire à la Déclaration Nutritionnelle Recommandée par l'Etat en Application des Articles L. 3232-8 et R. 3232-7 du Code de la Santé Publique|Legifrance. Available online: https://www.legifrance.gouv.fr/eli/arrete/2017/10/31/SSAP1730474A/jo/texte (accessed on 6 June 2018).
16. ENL Taskforce. Promoting Healthier Diets Through Evolved Nutrition Labelling. ENL Taskforce, 2018. Available online: https://ec.europa.eu/health/sites/health/files/nutrition_physical_activity/docs/ev_20171130_co03_en.pdf (accessed on 5 August 2019).
17. Choices International Foundation Dutch Choices Logo Gets One Year Extra. Available online: https://www.choicesprogramme.org/news-updates/news/dutch-choices-logo-gets-one-year-extra (accessed on 9 July 2019).
18. Niamh Michail Dutch Government Mulls Nutrition Logo. Available online: https://www.foodnavigator.com/Article/2018/04/18/Dutch-government-mulls-nutrition-logo (accessed on 9 July 2019).
19. Grunert, K.G.; Wills, J.M. A review of European research on consumer response to nutrition information on food labels. *J. Public Health* **2007**, *15*, 385–399. [CrossRef]
20. Mejean, C.; Macouillard, P.; Peneau, S.; Hercberg, S.; Castetbon, K. Consumer acceptability and understanding of front-of-pack nutrition labels. *J. Hum. Nutr. Diet.* **2013**, *26*, 494–503. [CrossRef]
21. Julia, C.; Peneau, S.; Buscail, C.; Gonzalez, R.; Touvier, M.; Hercberg, S.; Kesse-Guyot, E. Perception of different formats of front-of-pack nutrition labels according to sociodemographic, lifestyle and dietary factors in a French population: Cross-sectional study among the NutriNet-Sante cohort participants. *BMJ Open* **2017**, *7*, e016108. [CrossRef] [PubMed]

22. Ducrot, P.; Mejean, C.; Julia, C.; Kesse-Guyot, E.; Touvier, M.; Fezeu, L.; Hercberg, S.; Peneau, S. Effectiveness of Front-Of-Pack Nutrition Labels in French Adults: Results from the NutriNet-Sante Cohort Study. *PLoS ONE* **2015**, *10*, e0140898. [CrossRef] [PubMed]
23. Talati, Z.; Pettigrew, S.; Kelly, B.; Ball, K.; Dixon, H.; Shilton, T. Consumers' responses to front-of-pack labels that vary by interpretive content. *Appetite* **2016**, *101*, 205–213. [CrossRef] [PubMed]
24. Aschemann-Witzel, J.; Grunert, K.G.; van Trijp, H.C.; Bialkova, S.; Raats, M.M.; Hodgkins, C.; Wasowicz-Kirylo, G.; Koenigstorfer, J. Effects of nutrition label format and product assortment on the healthfulness of food choice. *Appetite* **2013**, *71*, 63–74. [CrossRef] [PubMed]
25. Balcombe, K.; Fraser, I.; Falco, S.D. Traffic lights and food choice: A choice experiment examining the relationship between nutritional food labels and price. *Food Policy* **2010**, *35*, 211–220. [CrossRef]
26. Borgmeier, I.; Westenhoefer, J. Impact of different food label formats on healthiness evaluation and food choice of consumers: A randomized-controlled study. *BMC Public Health* **2009**, *9*, 184. [CrossRef] [PubMed]
27. Carrad, A.M.; Louie, J.C.-Y.; Milosavljevic, M.; Kelly, B.; Flood, V.M. Consumer support for healthy food and drink vending machines in public places. *Aust. N. Z. J. Public Health* **2015**, *39*, 355–357. [CrossRef] [PubMed]
28. Cecchini, M.; Warin, L. Impact of food labelling systems on food choices and eating behaviours: A systematic review and meta-analysis of randomized studies. *Obes. Rev.* **2016**, *17*, 201–210. [CrossRef] [PubMed]
29. Christoph, M.J.; Ellison, B. A Cross-Sectional Study of the Relationship between Nutrition Label Use and Food Selection, Servings, and Consumption in a University Dining Setting. *J. Acad. Nutr. Diet.* **2017**, *117*, 1528–1537. [CrossRef]
30. Ducrot, P.; Julia, C.; Mejean, C.; Kesse-Guyot, E.; Touvier, M.; Fezeu, L.K.; Hercberg, S.; Peneau, S. Impact of Different Front-of-Pack Nutrition Labels on Consumer Purchasing Intentions: A Randomized Controlled Trial. *Am. J. Prev. Med.* **2016**, *50*, 627–636. [CrossRef]
31. Gorski Findling, M.T.; Werth, P.M.; Musicus, A.A.; Bragg, M.A.; Graham, D.J.; Elbel, B.; Roberto, C.A. Comparing five front-of-pack nutrition labels' influence on consumers' perceptions and purchase intentions. *Prev. Med.* **2018**, *106*, 114–121. [CrossRef] [PubMed]
32. Julia, C.; Blanchet, O.; Mejean, C.; Peneau, S.; Ducrot, P.; Alles, B.; Fezeu, L.K.; Touvier, M.; Kesse-Guyot, E.; Singler, E.; et al. Impact of the front-of-pack 5-colour nutrition label (5-CNL) on the nutritional quality of purchases: An experimental study. *Int. J. Behav. Nutr. Phys. Act.* **2016**, *13*, 101. [CrossRef] [PubMed]
33. Maubach, N.; Hoek, J.; Mather, D. Interpretive front-of-pack nutrition labels. Comparing competing recommendations. *Appetite* **2014**, *82*, 67–77. [CrossRef] [PubMed]
34. Ni Mhurchu, C.; Volkova, E.; Jiang, Y.; Eyles, H.; Michie, J.; Neal, B.; Blakely, T.; Swinburn, B.; Rayner, M. Effects of interpretive nutrition labels on consumer food purchases: The Starlight randomized controlled trial. *Am. J. Clin. Nutr.* **2017**, *105*, 695–704. [CrossRef] [PubMed]
35. Talati, Z.; Norman, R.; Pettigrew, S.; Neal, B.; Kelly, B.; Dixon, H.; Ball, K.; Miller, C.; Shilton, T. The impact of interpretive and reductive front-of-pack labels on food choice and willingness to pay. *Int. J. Behav. Nutr. Phys. Act.* **2017**, *14*, 171. [CrossRef] [PubMed]
36. Waterlander, W.E.; Steenhuis, I.H.M.; de Boer, M.R.; Schuit, A.J.; Seidell, J.C. Effects of different discount levels on healthy products coupled with a healthy choice label, special offer label or both: Results from a web-based supermarket experiment. *Int. J. Behav. Nutr. Phys. Act.* **2013**, *10*, 59. [CrossRef]
37. Egnell, M.; Crosetto, P.; D'Almeida, T.; Kesse-Guyot, E.; Touvier, M.; Ruffieux, B.; Hercberg, S.; Muller, L.; Julia, C. Modelling the impact of different front-of-package nutrition labels on mortality from non-communicable chronic disease. *Int. J. Behav. Nutr. Phys. Act.* **2019**, *16*. [CrossRef]
38. Egnell, M.; Talati, Z.; Hercberg, S.; Pettigrew, S.; Julia, C. Objective Understanding of Front-of-Package Nutrition Labels: An International Comparative Experimental Study across 12 Countries. *Nutrients* **2018**, *10*, 1542. [CrossRef]
39. Egnell, M.; Talati, Z.; Pettigrew, S.; Galan, P.; Hercberg, S.; Julia, C. Comparison of front-of-pack labels to help German consumers understand the nutritional quality of food products. *Ernährungs Umsch.* **2019**, *66*, 76–84.
40. Galan, P.; Egnell, M.; Salas-Salvadó, J.; Babio, N.; Pettigrew, S.; Hercberg, S.; Julia, C. Understanding of different front-of-package labels by the Spanish population: Results of a comparative study. *Endocrinol. Diabetes Nutr.* **2019**. [CrossRef]
41. Mejean, C.; Macouillard, P.; Peneau, S.; Hercberg, S.; Castetbon, K. Perception of front-of-pack labels according to social characteristics, nutritional knowledge and food purchasing habits. *Public Health Nutr.* **2013**, *16*, 392–402. [CrossRef] [PubMed]

42. Arrúa, A.; Machín, L.; Curutchet, M.R.; Martínez, J.; Antúnez, L.; Alcaire, F.; Giménez, A.; Ares, G. Warnings as a directive front-of-pack nutrition labelling scheme: Comparison with the Guideline Daily Amount and traffic-light systems. *Public Health Nutr.* **2017**, *20*, 2308–2317. [CrossRef] [PubMed]
43. Feunekes, G.I.; Gortemaker, I.A.; Willems, A.A.; Lion, R.; van den Kommer, M. Front-of-pack nutrition labelling: Testing effectiveness of different nutrition labelling formats front-of-pack in four European countries. *Appetite* **2008**, *50*, 57–70. [CrossRef] [PubMed]
44. Talati, Z.; Pettigrew, S.; Ball, K.; Hughes, C.; Kelly, B.; Neal, B.; Dixon, H. The relative ability of different front-of-pack labels to assist consumers discriminate between healthy, moderately healthy, and unhealthy foods. *Food Qual. Prefer.* **2017**, *59*, 109–113. [CrossRef]
45. Kelly, B.; Hughes, C.; Chapman, K.; Louie, J.C.; Dixon, H.; Crawford, J.; King, L.; Daube, M.; Slevin, T. Consumer testing of the acceptability and effectiveness of front-of-pack food labelling systems for the Australian grocery market. *Health Promot. Int.* **2009**, *24*, 120–129. [CrossRef] [PubMed]
46. Van Herpen, E.; Hieke, S.; van Trijp, H.C.M. Inferring Product Healthfulness from Nutrition Labelling: The Influence of Reference Points. *Appetite* **2013**, *72*, 138–149. [CrossRef]
47. Crosetto, P.; Muller, L.; Ruffieux, B. Réponses des consommateurs à trois systèmes d'étiquetage nutritionnels en face avant. *Cah. Nutr. Diététique* **2016**, *59*, 124–131. [CrossRef]
48. Crosetto, P.; Lacroix, A.; Muller, L.; Ruffieux, B. Modification des achats alimentaires en réponse à cinq logos nutritionnels. *Cah. Nutr. Diététique* **2017**, *52*, 129–133. [CrossRef]
49. Tórtora, G.; Machín, L.; Ares, G. Influence of nutritional warnings and other label features on consumers' choice: Results from an eye-tracking study. *Food Res. Int.* **2019**, *119*, 605–611. [CrossRef]
50. Acton, R.B.; Jones, A.C.; Kirkpatrick, S.I.; Roberto, C.A.; Hammond, D. Taxes and front-of-package labels improve the healthiness of beverage and snack purchases: A randomized experimental marketplace. *Int. J. Behav. Nutr. Phys. Act.* **2019**, *16*, 46. [CrossRef]
51. Dodds, P.; Wolfenden, L.; Chapman, K.; Wellard, L.; Hughes, C.; Wiggers, J. The effect of energy and traffic light labelling on parent and child fast food selection: A randomised controlled trial. *Appetite* **2014**, *73*, 23–30. [CrossRef] [PubMed]
52. Hamlin, R.; McNeill, L. Does the Australasian "Health Star Rating" Front of Pack Nutritional Label System Work? *Nutrients* **2016**, *8*, 237. [CrossRef] [PubMed]
53. Sacks, G.; Rayner, M.; Swinburn, B. Impact of front-of-pack "traffic-light" nutrition labelling on consumer food purchases in the UK. *Health Promot. Int.* **2009**, *24*, 344–352. [CrossRef] [PubMed]
54. Sacks, G.; Tikellis, K.; Millar, L.; Swinburn, B. Impact of "traffic-light" nutrition information on online food purchases in Australia. *Aust. N. Z. J. Public Health* **2011**, *35*, 122–126. [CrossRef] [PubMed]
55. Seward, M.W.; Block, J.P.; Chatterjee, A. A Traffic-Light Label Intervention and Dietary Choices in College Cafeterias. *Am. J. Public Health* **2016**, *106*, 1808–1814. [CrossRef] [PubMed]
56. Hamlin, R.P.; McNeill, L.S.; Moore, V. The impact of front-of-pack nutrition labels on consumer product evaluation and choice: An experimental study. *Public Health Nutr.* **2015**, *18*, 2126–2134. [CrossRef]
57. Thorndike, A.N.; Riis, J.; Sonnenberg, L.M.; Levy, D.E. Traffic-light labels and choice architecture: Promoting healthy food choices. *Am. J. Prev. Med.* **2014**, *46*, 143–149. [CrossRef]
58. Antúnez, L.; Giménez, A.; Maiche, A.; Ares, G. Influence of Interpretation Aids on Attentional Capture, Visual Processing, and Understanding of Front-of-Package Nutrition Labels. *J. Nutr. Educ. Behav.* **2015**, *47*, 292–299.e1.
59. Carter, O.; Mills, B.; Phan, T. An independent assessment of the Australian food industry's Daily Intake Guide "Energy Alone" label. *Health Promot. J. Aust.* **2011**, *22*, 63–67. [CrossRef]
60. Ducrot, P.; Mejean, C.; Julia, C.; Kesse-Guyot, E.; Touvier, M.; Fezeu, L.K.; Hercberg, S.; Peneau, S. Objective Understanding of Front-of-Package Nutrition Labels among Nutritionally At-Risk Individuals. *Nutrients* **2015**, *7*, 7106–7125. [CrossRef]
61. Hersey, J.C.; Wohlgenant, K.C.; Arsenault, J.E.; Kosa, K.M.; Muth, M.K. Effects of front-of-package and shelf nutrition labeling systems on consumers. *Nutr. Rev.* **2013**, *71*, 1–14. [CrossRef] [PubMed]
62. Vasiljevic, M.; Pechey, R.; Marteau, T.M. Making food labels social: The impact of colour of nutritional labels and injunctive norms on perceptions and choice of snack foods. *Appetite* **2015**, *91*, 56–63. [CrossRef] [PubMed]

63. Bialkova, S.; Grunert, K.G.; Juhl, H.J.; Wasowicz-Kirylo, G.; Stysko-Kunkowska, M.; van Trijp, H.C.M. Attention mediates the effect of nutrition label information on consumers' choice. Evidence from a choice experiment involving eye-tracking. *Appetite* **2014**, *76*, 66–75. [CrossRef] [PubMed]
64. Nagle, M.G.; Osorio, D. The tuning of human photopigments may minimize red-green chromatic signals in natural conditions. *Proc. Biol. Sci.* **1993**, *252*, 209–213. [PubMed]
65. Egnell, M.; Ducrot, P.; Touvier, M.; Allès, B.; Hercberg, S.; Kesse-Guyot, E.; Julia, C. Objective understanding of Nutri-Score Front-Of-Package nutrition label according to individual characteristics of subjects: Comparisons with other format labels. *PLoS ONE* **2018**, *13*, e0202095. [CrossRef]

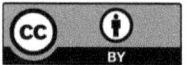

© 2019 by the authors. Licensee MDPI, Basel, Switzerland. This article is an open access article distributed under the terms and conditions of the Creative Commons Attribution (CC BY) license (http://creativecommons.org/licenses/by/4.0/).

MDPI
St. Alban-Anlage 66
4052 Basel
Switzerland
Tel. +41 61 683 77 34
Fax +41 61 302 89 18
www.mdpi.com

Nutrients Editorial Office
E-mail: nutrients@mdpi.com
www.mdpi.com/journal/nutrients

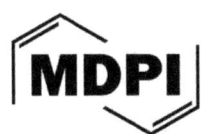